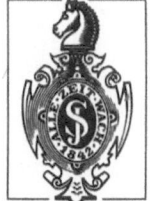

T. Yamamuro (Ed.)

New Developments for Limb Salvage in Musculoskeletal Tumors

Kyocera Orthopaedic Symposium

With 277 Figures

Springer-Verlag
Tokyo Berlin Heidelberg New York London Paris

TAKAO YAMAMURO, M.D., D.M.Sc.
Professor and Chairman
Department of Orthopaedic Surgery
Faculty of Medicine
Kyoto University
Kyoto, 606 Japan

ISBN-13: 978-4-431-68074-1   e-ISBN-13: 978-4-431-68072-7
DOI: 10.1007/978-4-431-68072-7

Library of Congress Cataloging-in-Publication Data
New developments for limb salvage in musculoskeletal tumors. Papers presented at a
symposium held in Kyoto in Oct. 1987. Includes bibliographies and indexes. 1. Limb
salvage — Congresses. 2. Musculoskeletal system — Tumors — Treatment — Congresses.
I. Yamamuro, T. (Takao), 1931-   . [DNLM: 1. Bone Neoplasms — therapy — congresses. 2. Extremities — surgery — congresses. 3. Prosthesis — congresses. 4. Soft
Tissue Neoplasms — therapy — congresses. WE 258 N532 1987]   RD674.N49
1989   616.99'471059   89-5894

The use of registered names, trademarks, etc. in this publication does not
imply, even in the absence of a specific statement, that such names are exempt
from the relevant protective laws and regulations and therefore free for general use.

Product liability: The publisher can give no guarantee for information about
drug dosage and application thereof contained in this book. In every individual
case the respective user must check its accuracy by consulting other pharmaceutical literature.

Typesetting: Asco Trade Typesetting, Hong Kong and Export Aid, Tokyo

Preface

Introduction of new diagnostic methods including various imaging techniques in the field of orthopaedic surgery has enabled us to make early and precise diagnoses of musculoskeletal tumors. In addition, recent progress in the chemotherapy and radiotherapy of malignant tumors has raised the five-year survival rate remarkably, although complete recovery from these treatments alone cannot be expected as yet. These medical advances naturally stimulate the search for ways of limb salvage even in malignant musculoskeletal oncology. To this purpose, not only oncologists, but orthopaedic surgeons, radiologists, engineers, and biomaterials scientists should work together to design suitable surgical procedures and prostheses using autograft, allograft and biomaterials.

The First International Workshop on the Design and Application of Tumor Prostheses for Bone and Joint Reconstruction was held in 1981 in Rochester, Minnesota. Participants were of an interdisciplinary nature in order to establish a basis for cooperative efforts, which have subsequently spread throughout the world. Since then, biennial international symposia have been held successively in Vienna, Florida, and Kyoto. Previous gatherings of this prestigious series were open only to a small number of experts. However, since recent rapid progress in biomaterials, biomechanics, chemotherapy, radiotherapy, oncology, and surgical technique has brought about a substantial increase in the number of researchers involved in limb salvage, the Kyoto Symposium held in October, 1987, accepted some 300 participants with the expectation of young researchers exposed to highly advanced, intensive, and interdisciplinary fields being able to exchange opinions with experts on limb salvage. As a result, nearly 100 papers covering ten different topics were presented at the Kyoto Symposium. In addition to the functional evaluation of limb-saving operations performed earlier, many new approaches to limb salvage were discussed intensively.

This book records the new developments made after the Florida Symposium in the search for ways of complete limb salvage in musculoskeletal oncology. It is our hope that it will provide readers with useful ideas in planning surgery for limb salvage and that it will stimulate research on this difficult subject.

I wish to express my thanks to the contributors, who submitted their manuscripts in time. I am also grateful to the following members of the Planning Committee of the 4th International Symposium on Musculoskeletal Oncology for their tremendous help in making the Kyoto Symposium so successful: Dr. M. Campanacci, Dr. E.Y.S. Chao, Dr. R. Kotz, Dr. F. Langlais, Dr. U. Nilsonne, Dr. D.J. Pritchard, Dr. D. Springfield, Dr. S. Toriyama, and Dr. H.G. Willert. Finally, on behalf of the contributing authors, I would like to express our sincere gratitude to Kyocera Corporation, which sponsored this book for publication by Springer-Verlag Tokyo.

Kyoto, January 1989   TAKAO YAMAMURO

Table of Contents

Chapter 2: Influence of Limb Salvage on the Rate of Long Term Survival in Malignant Tumors

Chapter 3: Limiting Factors for Limb Salvage Operation

Chapter 4: Rationales of Adjuvant Therapies for Limb Salvage

Chapter 5: Biomaterial and Biomechanical Evaluation of Tumor Prostheses

Chapter 6: The Use of Ceramic Prostheses for Replacement of Bone Tumors

Chapter 7: Prosthesis vs. Osteochondral Graft, Alternative Substitute for Bone Tumor

Chapter 8: Reconstruction After Resection of Large Bone Tumors About the Hip and Pelvis

Chapter 9: Functional Results Following Resection of Tumor in the Proximal Humerus and Tibia

Chapter 10: Innovative Techniques

Chapter 1

Functional Evaluation of Reconstruction After Tumor Resection

Kinesiological Measurements in Patients with Various Limb Salvage or Amputation Procedures for Tumor Removal

JAMES C. OTIS[1], JOSEPH M. LANE[1], MICHAEL A. KROLL[2], SHERRY I. BACKUS[2], and JOHN H. HEALEY[1]

Summary. Measurements of energy cost, stride characteristics, and lower extremity strength were obtained for 139 patients who underwent 11 different lower extremity limb salvage or amputation procedures during the past 8 years. These included 70 limb salvage patients, 34 above-the-knee amputations, nine Van Nes procedures, and six patients with only soft tissue resections. Above-the-knee amputees demonstrated the greatest net energy cost of all the groups studied.

Key words: Kinesiology—Limb salvage—Amputation

Introduction

When tumor excision includes en bloc resection or amputation of the lower extremity, some level of ambulatory dysfunction results. It is of great importance for clinicians and for patients with tumors to understand the functional differences which exist among the treatment alternatives available, for the prosthesis designer to understand the outcome of reconstruction procedures, and for the clincan and therapist to monitor progress and evaluate the role of rehabilitation.

Lower limb function can be measured in a quantitative manner by measuring the motion and strength capabilities about individual joints [1, 2], characteristics of gait [2, 3], and energy cost during gait [4, 5]. The capacity of a muscle to generate torque, i.e., a rotational effort, about a joint is measured. These measurements reflect the relation between the salvaged muscles and the kinematics of the implant.

In studying our tumor patients, we have measured stride characteristics derived from foot-floor contact measurements. The quantification of stride parameters during gait provides a measure of the symmetry and stability during gait. Individuals with major alterations of the musculoskeletal system of the lower extremity, however, differ greatly in their methods of gait compensation, making it difficult, if not impossible, to compare their gait performances based on

Memorial Sloan Kettering Cancer Center[1] and Rehabilitation Services[2], Hospital for Special Surgery, New York Hospital–Cornell University Medical College, New York, NY, USA

stride characteristics or even more sophisticated kinematics and kinematic measurements. For example, one individual may compensate primarily by altering motion of the knee joint, whereas another will alter motion of the hip joint, with the result that it is possible to conclude only that their gait patterns are different but not that one is superior to the other.

Oxygen-consumption measurements during gait provide an overall measure of gait performance by determining energy cost per unit of distance traveled and, therefore, overcome the present limitation of interpretation of stride characteristics by permitting the comparison of vastly different compensatory gait patterns. In addition, by correlating heart rate with the rate of oxygen consumption, the percentage maximum aerobic capacity that is required may be estimated [6]. This is particularly important since individuals can sustain prolonged physical activity if they are functioning at less that 50% of their maximum aerobic capacity. For normal individuals, energy cost testing is usually conducted on motorized treadmills. Due to space limitations and the unacceptable features of a motorized treadmill, we designed a walking task, suitable for our patients that would fit in the available space [4]. The walking task required the subject to traverse continuously a 17.4-m rectangular walkway with rounded corners, which was instrumented with a series of pacing lights to control walking velocity.

Materials and Methods

Measurements of torque production about individual joints were obtained using a model 2110H-5K Lebow torque sensor (Lebow Associates, Troy, MI, USA) attached to a Cybex II isokinetic dynamometer (Lmex, Ronkonkoma, NY, USA). Measurements were obtained for knee extensor torque, knee flexor torque, ankle plantar flexor torque, and ankle dorsiflexor torque.

Measurements of stride characteristics including velocity, cadence, stride length, gait cycle time, and right and left single limb support times were obtained using the VA-Rancho Footswitch Stride Analyzer. This instrumentation consists of footswitches, automatic stop/start controller, waistpack recorder, microprocessor, and printer. Testing was conducted at free speed and at slower and faster speeds.

Oxygen consumption was determined by measuring the volume, carbon dioxide content, and oxygen content of expired air while the subject walked on the previously described rectangular walkway. Energy cost was determined using the Douglas bag protocol previously described [4]. Individuals walked around a rounded rectangular track at their preferred rates and at a 20% faster rate as expired air was collected and heart rate monitored. Net cost (ml oxygen/m traveled/kg body mass) was calculated for each walking speed.

A total of 139 patients receiving 11 different lower extremity limb salvage or amputation procedures have been evaluated during the past 8 years. Seventy limb salvage patients required either en bloc resection of proximal (pelvis, proximal femur), middle (knee, distal femur/proximal tibia), or distal (fibula, foot) segments of the lower extremity. Thirty-four amputations were above the knee, 12 were below the knee, and nine were Van Nes procedures. Six patients received only soft tissue resections. Kinesiological studies included measurement of energy cost, stride characteristics, and torque production.

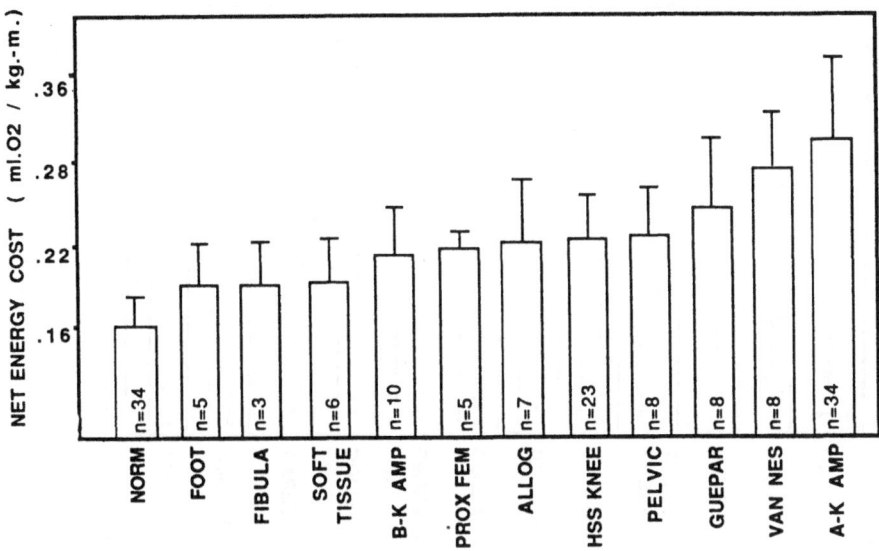

Fig. 1. The net energy cost (mean and 1 SD) for the normal control group and the 11 patient groups

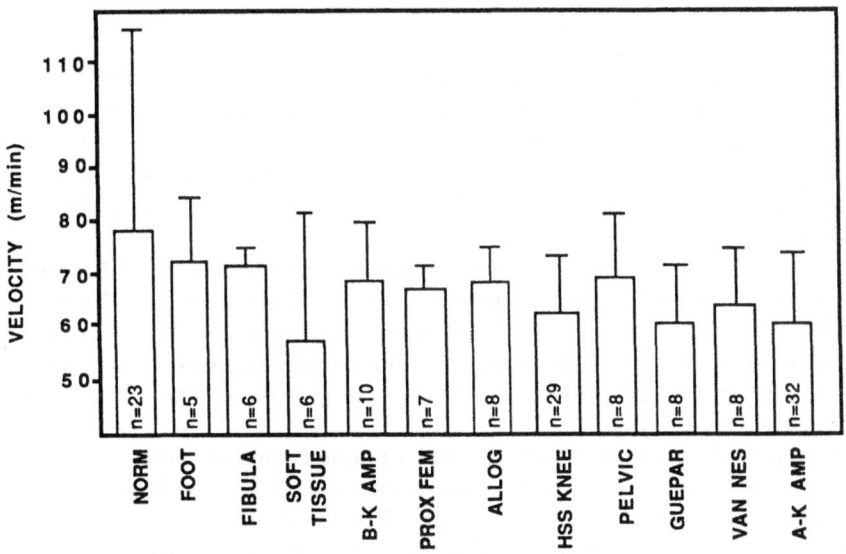

Fig. 2. The preferred walking speed (mean and 1 SD) during energy-cost testing for the normal control group and the 11 patient groups

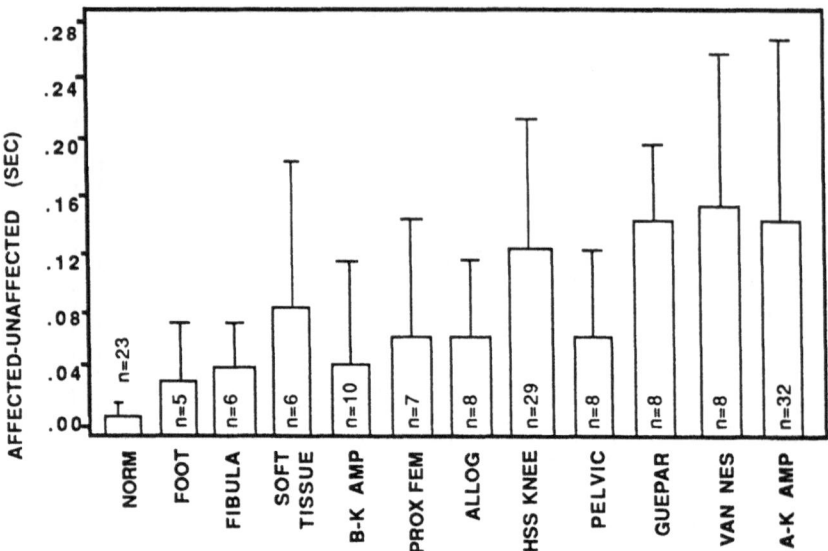

Fig. 3. The difference between affected and unaffected side single-limb stance time for the 11 patient groups studied. The difference for the normal group is between right and left sides

Results

The results for net cost of ambulation, preferred walking velocity, and affected/unaffected single stance time difference are reported in Figs. 1–3. The group means in Fig. 1 are shown in rank order form lowest to highest net cost. In general, dital resections have a lower net cost than proximal and middle resections. The proximal and middle resections have similar net costs, and above-knee amputees have the highest net cost.

The results for velocity (Fig. 2) and single-limb support time difference (Fig. 3) show that above-the-knee amputees walk the slowest and are the most asymmetrical. Patients with a custom-designed endoprosthetic knee replacement are also asymmetrical. In general, the more distal the resection (and/or amputation), the faster the preferred walking rate and more symmetrical the single stance time.

Measurements of residual muscle torque obtained on the same day that measurements of net cost were obtained demonstrated that knee flexor torque was inversely related to net cost. The range of residual knee extensor torque measurements was not great enough to correlate with net cost measurements.

Quantification of function through kinesiological measurements is an important adjunct to the surgical management and postoperative recovery of patients undergoing limb salvage after tumor resection. These measurements provide the information necessary to help patients achieve their maximum level of functions.

Acknowledgment. The authors gratefully acknowledge the support of the Clark Foundation.

References

1. Markhede G, Stener B (1981) Function after removal of various hip and thigh muscles for extirpation of tumor. Acta Orthop Scand 52: 373–395
2. Murray MP, Jacobs PA, Gore, DR, Gardner GM, Mollinger LA (1985) Functional performance after tibial rotationplasty. J Bone Joint Surg 67A: 392–399
3. Otis JC, Fabian DF, Burstein AH, Insall JN (1982) Evaluation of total knee arthroplasty patients using the VA rancho gait analyzer. In: Biomechanics VIII, University Park Press
4. Otis JC, Lane JM, Kroll MA (1985) Energy cost during gait after resection and knee replacement and after above-knee amputation in osteosarcoma patients. J Bone Joint Surg 67A: 606–611
5. Waters RL, Perry J, Antonelli D, Hislop H (1976) Energy cost of walking of amputees: The influence of level of amputation. J Bone Joint Surg 58A: 42–46
6. McArdle WD, Katch FI, Katch VL (1981) Exercise physiology—Energy nutrition and human performance. Lea and Febiger, Philadelphia

Gait Analysis in Patients with Osteosarcoma Treated by Limb Salvage Procedures

Compared with Those Treated by Amputation

RYOHEI SUZUKI, TORU HIRANO, MASAAKI FUJITA, and NOBUOU MATSUSAKA[1]

Summary. Gait analysis by ground reaction force measurement was performed on 17 cases of primary osteosarcoma around the knee treated by limb salvage procedure (eight cases) and by ablative surgery (nine cases). From the patterns of the ground reaction force, it was difficult to distinguish functionally which operative method was better. The only significant difference between them showed the locus of the center of pressure calculated by the vertical component of the ground reaction force. It was was revealed that the limb salvage procedure group had better function than the ablative surgery group, provided that the normal function of the foot could be preserved in the former group. On the other hand, measurement of the ground reaction force was useful in evaluating the recovery process of walking in the same patient.

Key words: Osteosarcoma—Limb salvage procedure—Gait analysis

Introduction

Limb salvage procedures for osteosarcoma have been frequently performed in recent years because of the progress in preoperative adjuvant chemotherapy and radiotherapy as well as in the technique of endoprosthetic replacement. It has been widely discussed how better function may be provided by means of limb salvage operation.

Enneking's method is widely accepted in the field of functional evaluation of the operation, and the modified method is also being commonly used.

The development of artificial limbs for amputees has also progressed. However, comparative functional studies on limb salvage vis-à-vis amputation are rarely undertaken.

In order to reveal the efficiency of the limb salvage procedure, we performed a functional evaluation using a modified version of Enneking's method and gait analysis on the cases with osteosarcoma around the knee treated by the above prodedure and on those patients who received above-knee amputation as well as disarticulation of the hip.

---

[1]Department of Orthopaedic Surgery, Nagasaki University School of Medicine, Nagasaki, Japan

Patients and Methods

Seventeen cases of primary osteosarcoma in the distal end of the femur and proximal end of the tibia were examined in this study.

Limb salvage procedures have been performed on eight patients since 1978. They were treated preoperatively with radiotherapy and multidrug chemotherapy (CTX, MTX, VCR, ADR, CDDP, etc).

Surgical procedures performed on the eight cases were as follows: In five cases preoperatively treated with radiotherapy (3000–5000 cGy, TDF 49–82), wide resection of the tumor was performed. In four of them, the hingeless knee prostheses made by Kyocera Co. was used, and in the remaining patient, arthrodesis of the knee was done using an allograft. In three cases preoperatively treated with a large dose of radiation (more than 7000 cGy, TDF 115), vascularised and/or free bone grafts were performed after wide resection of the tumor. In one case, the knee joint was fused.

The function of the quadriceps muscle could be maintained in every case except for two, in which arthrodesis was carried out.

In the cases in which ablative surgery was finally performed, seven underwent amputation at the proximal third of the thigh, and three disarticulation at the hip. In every case, a skeletal artificial limb with safety knee mechanism was applied.

For gait analysis of the above patients and ten normal adults, large force plates made by Anima Co. were employed. These were embedded in parallel in the center of the walkway for gait analysis, and we recorded three components of the ground reaction force for two or three steps of both limbs separately. Using a computer, the step length, stride length, step width, cadence, walking speed, and center of pressure (COP) were calculated.

The length of the locus of the COP (Lp) obtained by computing the vertical force, the distance in a straight line of the COP (Ls), and the ratio of Lp and Ls were calculated with a computer.

Results

According to the modified Enneking's method, the rating of functional evaluation of a patients treated by limb salvage procedure was as follows: Good, three cases; fair, three cases; and poor, two cases. The functional activity of was good in five cases and fair in three (Table 1).

In each case, including the amputees, patterns of the ground reaction force were noticeably different from those of the normal adults.

In the normal adults (Fig. 1a), the vertical component was the largest and the lateral component the smallest. The curve of the vertical component had two peaks almost equal in height and greater than body weight, corresponding to the reception phase and the thrust phase. The minimum between the peaks was less than the body weight. The curve of the forward-backward component had two peaks, in opposite direction to one another, representing the breaking and driving forces. These were almost equal in height and approximately 20% of the body weight. The lateral component was smallest of all and differed from step to

Table 1. Results of surgery

Case no.	Age (yrs.)	Sex	Site	Surgery	Follow-up	Rating
1	20	M	Tibia	Arthrodesis	n.p. (9 mos.)	Good
2	64	F	Femur	Endoprosthesis	meta. (10 mos.)	Fair
3	15	M	Femur	Endoprosthesis	n.p. (3 yrs.)	Fair
4	16	F	Femur	Endoprosthesis	n.p. (2 yrs.)	Poor
5	16	F	Femur	Endoprosthesis	meta. (1 yr.)	Good
6	15	M	Femur	Endoprosthesis	meta. (11 mos.)	Fair
7	13	M	Femur	Bone graft	n.p. (5 yrs.)	Poor
8	15	F	Femur	Arthrodesis	n.p. (9 yrs.)	Good

n.p. no particular problems, *meta.* metastasis to the lung

step, i.e., its reproducibility was relatively poor.

The following are the ground reaction forces of representative cases.

Case 6. This was a 15-year-old male (Fig. 1b). Wide resection of the distal end of the femur and prosthetic replacement were carried out. Six months after surgery, two peaks of the vertical component on the operated side were small, and driving force of the operated side and breaking force of the sound side in the forward-backward component were weak.

Case 4. This was a 16-year-old female (Fig. 1c). The same operation was performed on the left side, but the sciatic nerve and popliteal vessels were injured. The patient cannot walk without a cane because of paralysis and ischemic contracture of the foot. From the ground reaction force, every component was small on the operated side and the sound side was markedly influenced by the operated side.

Case 7. This was a 13-year-old male (Fig. 2a). Wide resection of the tumor and vascularised bone grafting were performed. At 5 years postoperation, the rating of Enneking's functional evaluation was poor, but the pattern of the ground reaction force was closest of all to the normal pattern.

Case 1. This was a 20-year-old male (Fig. 2b). Osteosarcoma of the proximal end of the tibia was widely resected and arthrodesis was done using an allograft. The rating of Enneking's evaluation was good. The ground reaction force 8 months after surgery showed flattening of the minimum between two peaks of the vertical component on the operated side and weakened driving force of the forward-backward component. Moreover, three peaks were found in the vertical component on the sound side.

Case 9. This was a 34-year-old male (Fig. 2c). Above-knee amputation was carried out in 1973. On the amputated side, the vertical component had three peaks and the driving force of the forward-backward component was weak. On the sound side, the vertical component was influenced by the other side.

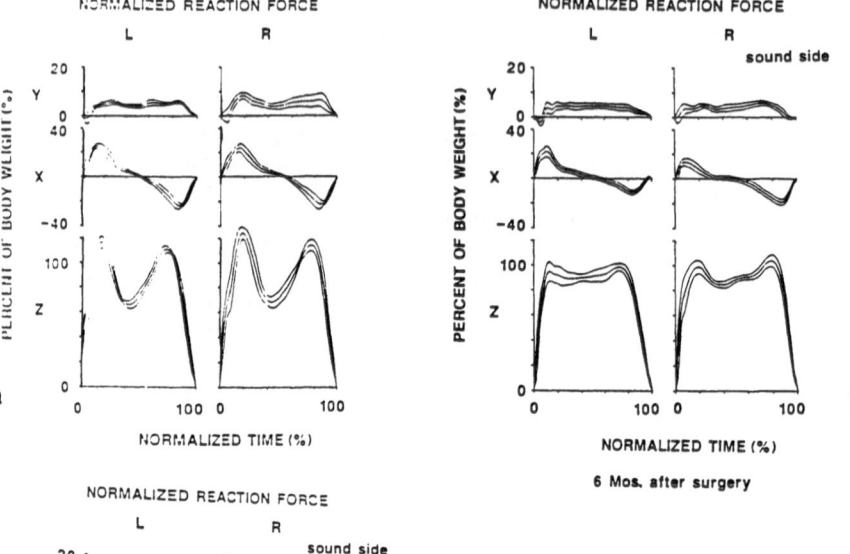

Fig. 1a–c. Ground reaction force **a** in a normal subject (male, 29 years old), **b** endo-prosthesis in case 6 (male, 15 years old; fair), **c** endoprosthesis in case 4 (female, 18 years old; poor)

In the other patients in whom ablative surgery was carried out, the patterns of the ground reaction force were quite different from those in normal subjects. As shown above, it was very difficult to evaluate which operative method was better from the pattern of the ground reaction force (Figs. 1, 2). Furthermore, there was no significant difference between the limb salvage and ablative surgery groups in the step length, stride length, step width, cadence, and walking speed. However, according to the ratio of Lp and Ls, there were significant differences between the normal and ablative surgery groups, as well as between the limb salvage and ablative surgery groups. No significant difference was found between the normal and limb salvage groups (Fig. 3).

The recovery process of gait in a case belonging to the limb salvage group is presented in the following.

Case 5. This was a 16-year-old male (Fig. 4). Wide resection and prosthetic replacement were performed. The rating of Enneking's evaluation 9 months after surgery was good.

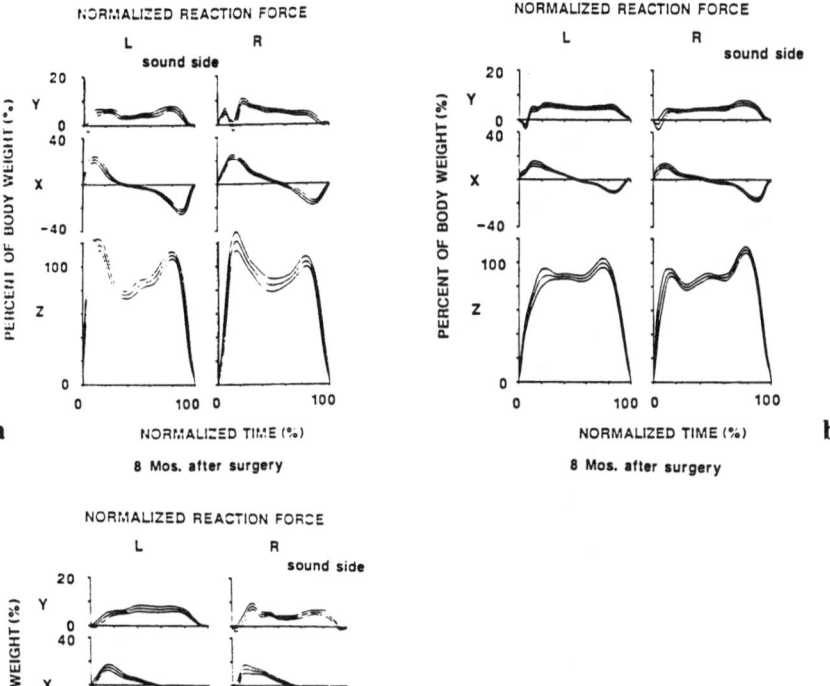

Fig. 2a–c. Ground reaction force in **a** wide resection and bone graft (case 7, poor), **b** arthrodesis (case 1, good), **c** above-knee amputation (case 9)

The ground reaction force examined 4 months after surgery showed that the vertical and forward-backward components were weak, not only on the operated side, but also on the sound side. With time, the pattern of the curves on the sound side gradually normalized, but the breaking force in the forward-backward component was still weak on the operated side; the pattern of the vertical component was also fairly different from the normal pattern even 9 months after surgery.

Repeated examination of gait in case 3 also showed marked recovery in the ground reaction force.

Discussion

The modified Enneking's functional evaluation method widely accepted in limb salvage did not always parallel the results of gait analysis by measurement of the

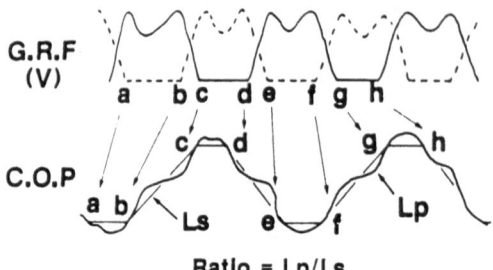

Fig. 3. Ratio of Lp and Ls

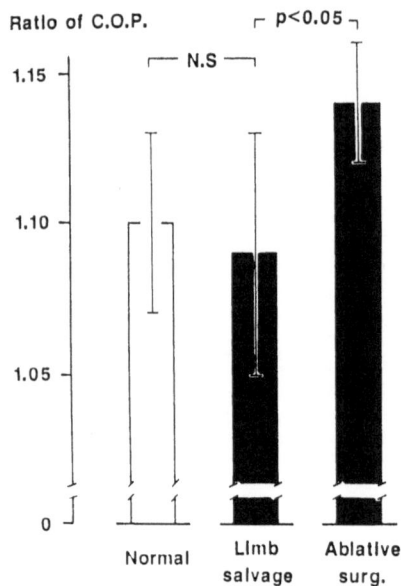

ground reaction force. One purpose of our study was to compare the efficiency of the limb salvage procedure with that of the ablative surgery from the viewpoint of gait analysis. However, from the pattern of the ground reaction force, it was difficult to distinguish which operative method was better. The only significant difference between them was evident in the ratio of Lp and Ls, which is considered to represent the smoothness in shift of the body weight during walking. Using this parameter, it was revealed that the limb salvage prodecure was better than ablative surgery. We believe that this smoothness was obtained by the normal function of the foot.

Conversely, walking was remarkably impaired in the case 4 (Fig. 1c) with a lack of normal function of the foot even thought it belonged to the limb salvage group. This also demonstrates the importance of foot function and suggests that the limb salvage procedure should not be done for patients in whom preservation of normal function of the foot cannot be expected after surgery. On the other hand, measurement of the ground reaction force is very useful for recording and evaluating the recovery process of gait in the same patient. Attention should be paid to the normalization of the ground reaction force pattern in the sound side which has been fairly influenced by the operated side.

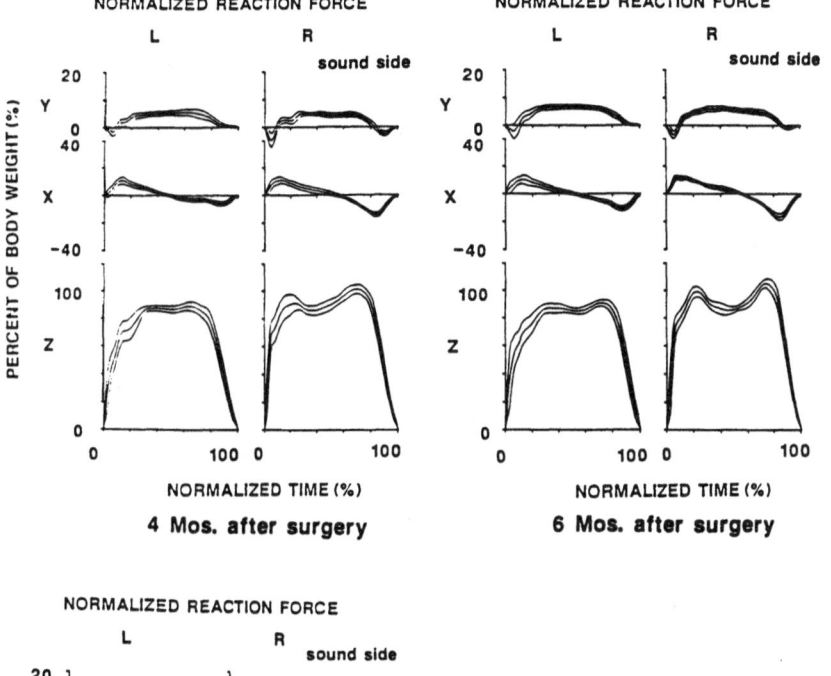

4 Mos. after surgery

6 Mos. after surgery

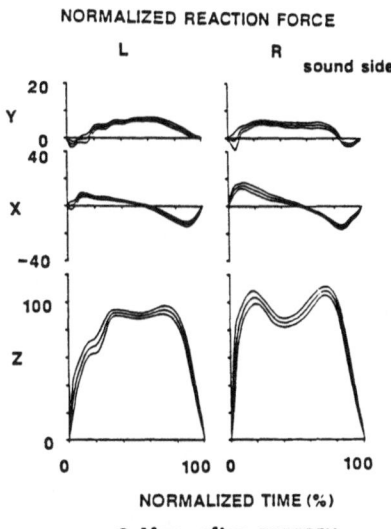

9 Mos. after surgery   **Fig. 4.** Endoprosthesis in case 5 (good)

Conclusion

The limb salvage operation for osteosarcoma around the knee is better than ablative surgery from the viewpoint of gait analysis, provided that the normal function of the foot can be preserved.

The rating of modified Enneking's functional evaluation method for the limb salvage procedure did not always parallel the results of measurement of the ground reaction force.

Limb Salvage in Malignant Pelvic Tumors

A Follow-up Study

MARY I. O'CONNOR[1] and FRANKLIN H. SIM[2]

Summary. Malignant tumors involving the pelvis continue to present a challenging problem. Pelvic limb salvage procedures are becoming more popular and are justified when compared with hemipelvectomy and its resultant disability. These extensive procedures, however, are associated with significant morbidity and a high incidence of complications. The high infection rate (21%) supports the current trend to a delayed reconstruction after an extensive periacetabular resection. Moreover, the risk of recurrence is notably high (26%), particularly so with iliosacral lesions (40%). This suggests the need for more aggressive adjuvant treatment. Also, when preoperative assessment suggests that a satisfactory margin cannot be achieved by resection, amputation should be considered if it is more oncologically sound. The functional results vary with the type of resection performed. The best functional results occur after resection in which pelvic continuity is maintained or restored. A solid arthrodesis was achieved in 55% of the patients with periacetabular reconstruction. This percentage suggests the need for improved internal fixation and reconstructive techniques. However, pseudarthrosis after an unsuccessful arthrodesis still gives a satisfactory result that is superior to having a flail extremity.

Key words: Limb salvage procedure—Limb-saving resection—Malignant pelvic tumor

Introduction

Previous attempts at limb salvage for malignant tumors of the pelvis have resulted in a high incidence of recurrence and poor functional results, necessitating hemipelvectomy with its debilitation and disfiguring sequelae. However, just as advances in orthopedic oncology have stimulated increased interest in limb-saving resections for lesions of the long bones, there has been greater interest in resection for pelvic tumors as well. Improved staging methods such as computed tomography (CT) and magnetic resonance imaging (MRI) provide better assessment of the exact extent of the pelvic tumor, facilitating a decision as to whether resection can be successful. Moreover, successful adjuvant treatment with chemotherapy or radiation therapy and improved reconstructive techniques contribute to the greater current interest in limb-sparing surgery for pelvic tumors.

[1] Department of Orthopedics, Mayo Graduate School of Medicine, Rochester, MN, USA
[2] Department of Orthopedics, Mayo Clinic and Mayo Foundation, Mayo Medical School, Rochester, MN, USA

Table 1. Surgical staging of 51 malignant pelvic tumors

Diagnosis	Stage I (23 pt)		Stage II (27 pt)		Stage III (1 pt)
	A	B	A	B	
Chondrosarcoma	1	19	0	10	0
Osteosarcoma	0	0	0	12	0
Fibrosarcoma	0	1	0	5	0
Other	1	1	0	0	1
Total	2	21	0	27	1

Clinical Series

Between 1970 and 1985, 51 petients with malignant lesions of the pelvis underwent limb-saving resection at the Mayo Clinic. This series included 28 males and 23 females with an age-range of 13–71 years (average 37.5 years). The follow-up ranged from 4 to 197 months, with a mean of 62 months.

Chondrosarcoma was the most frequent tumor, occurring in 30 patients, while 12 patients had osteosaroma and six had fibrosarcoma. In addition, one patient each had malignant fibrous histiocytoma, hemangiopericytoma, and mesenchymal sarcoma. Of the 51 patients, six and recurrent lesions at presentation: Four had chondrosarcomas, one had osteosarcoma, and one had malignant fibrous histiocytoma. Then patients had adjuvant treatment: Four had radiation therapy (two preoperatively and two postoperatively), and six had preoperative or postoperative chemotherapy.

The pathological diagnosis was further subdivided according to the surgical staging system adopted by the Musculoskeletal Tumor Society (Table 1) [1]. The localization of the tumors was classified according to the system proposed by Enneking and Dunham [2]. According to this system, 22 patients had lesions in the iliosacral region (type I), 19 had periacetabular lesions (type II), and ten had lesions in the ischiopubic region (type III). The chondrosarcomas were fairly evenly distributed among the three locations, whereas most of the osteosarcomas and fibrosarcomas occurred in the acetabular or iliosacral region.

Surgical Treatment

Resection

Resection resulted in a wide margin in 29 patients, a contaminated wide margin in eight, a marginal margin in 11, and a lesional margin in three. The resection resulted in disruption of pelvic continuity in 31 of the 51 patients. These included 14 of the 22 patients with iliosacral resections and 17 of the 19 patients with periacetabular resection.

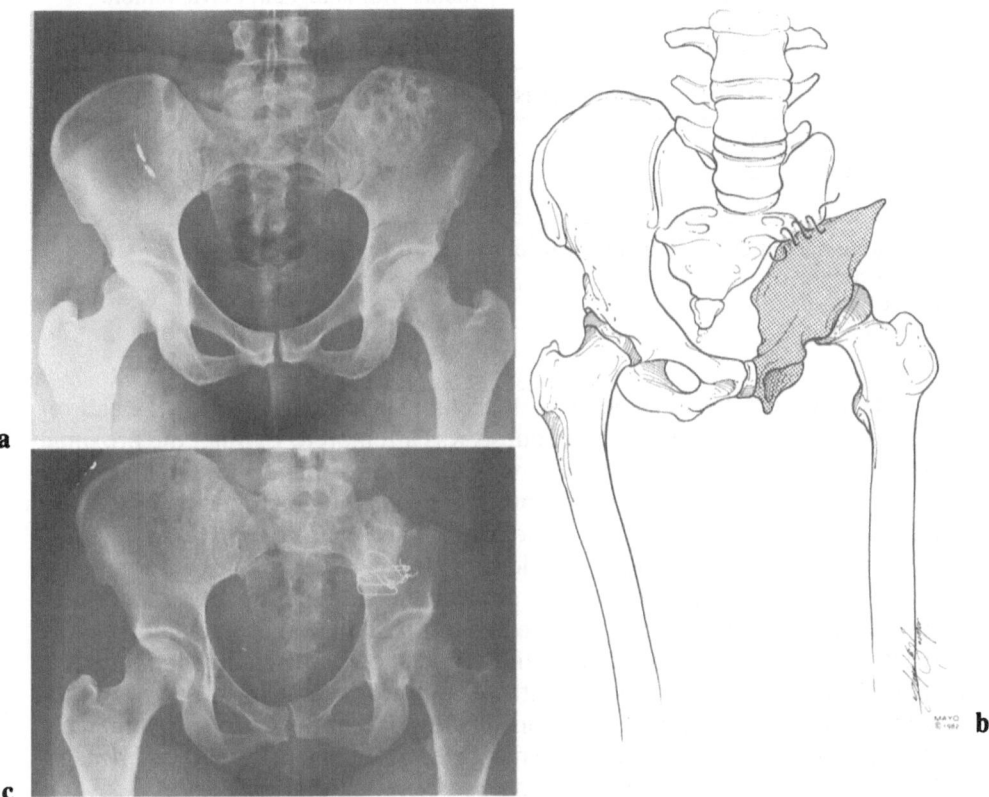

Fig. 1. a Anteroposterior view of pelvis, showing large chondrosarcoma in iliosacral region. **b** Primary closure and wiring. **c** Anteroposterior view of pelvis 36 months after surgery, showing solid iliosacral arthrodesis. **b** Reproduced with permission of Mayo Foundation

Reconstruction

Reconstruction varied according to the anatomical location of the lesion and the extent of the defect.

Ischiopubic. All ten patients with ischiopubic lesions (type III) had maintenance of pelvic continuity and required no reconstruction.

Iliosacral. Of the 14 patients with iliosacral lesions and disruption of pelvic continuity, ten had reconstruction and four were left flail. Of the ten patients who had reconstruction, four had the defect closed and wired (Fig. 1), three had fusion with an intercalary iliac graft, and three had a vascularized graft (two iliac, one fibular). Of the eight patients with sufficient follow-up after attempted iliosacral arthrodesis, six had a successful outcome. This group included all four patients who had primary closure and wiring and two who developed a pseudarthrosis (Table 2).

Table 2. Results of attempted arthrodesis in patients with malignant pelvic tumors

Procedure	No. of patients	Result			
		Arthrodesis	Pseudarthrosis	Flail	Amputation
Iliofemoral	11	5	3	2[b]	1[c]
Ischiofemoral	2	1	0	0	1[d]
Iliosacral	8[a]	6	2	0	0

[a] Two additional patients had insufficient follow-up
[b] For infection
[c] For recurrence
[d] For infection

Periacetabular. Of the 19 patients with acetabular lesions (type II), 14 had reconstruction. In 13 of these, an arthrodesis was attempted. In nine, the proximal femur was anchored to the remaining ilium with a plate, resulting in limb shortening of 2–7 cm (Fig. 2). In two other patients, an intercallary allograft was used to bridge the defect and restore leglength (Fig. 3). In two patients who had removal of the adjacent ilium in addition to the acetabulum, ischiofemoral arthrodesis was attempted: One had a successful result and the other underwent amputation for tumor recurrence. Two patients with partial acetabular resection had intact pelvic continuity. One of these had successful reconstruction of the medial acetabular wall with bone grafts. The other patient, who had no reconstruction, developed medial migration of the femoral head. In four other patients, the soft tissues were closed, leaving a large defect and a flail limb (mega-Girdlestone procedure). Of the patients in whom femoral iliac arthrodesis was attempted, five of the nine (55%) who had a standard arthrodesis with a plate had a successful result (Table 2). However, both patients with intercalary allograft required removal of the graft because of infection, resulting in a flail limb.

Results

Complications and Morbidity

Considerable morbidity may be associated with such extensive limb-sparing procedures, varying with the location of the lesion and the extent of resection. In this series, four patients with extensive iliosacral resections required sacrifice of a nerve root with subsequent neurological dysfunction. Two other patients had reconstructive procedures on the urinary tract, and one patient required a penile implant for organic impotence. One patient with an intact pelvis after an iliosacral resection required a Girdlestone procedure 10 years later because of severe postradiation osteonecrosis. Another patient with a partial acetabular resection developed medial subluxation of the hip. Abdominal peroneal hernias developed in five patients.

In addition to the morbidity associated with the procedure, there may be a high incidence of complications. There were no perioperative deaths in this series. Postoperative wound infection and wound healing problems occurred in

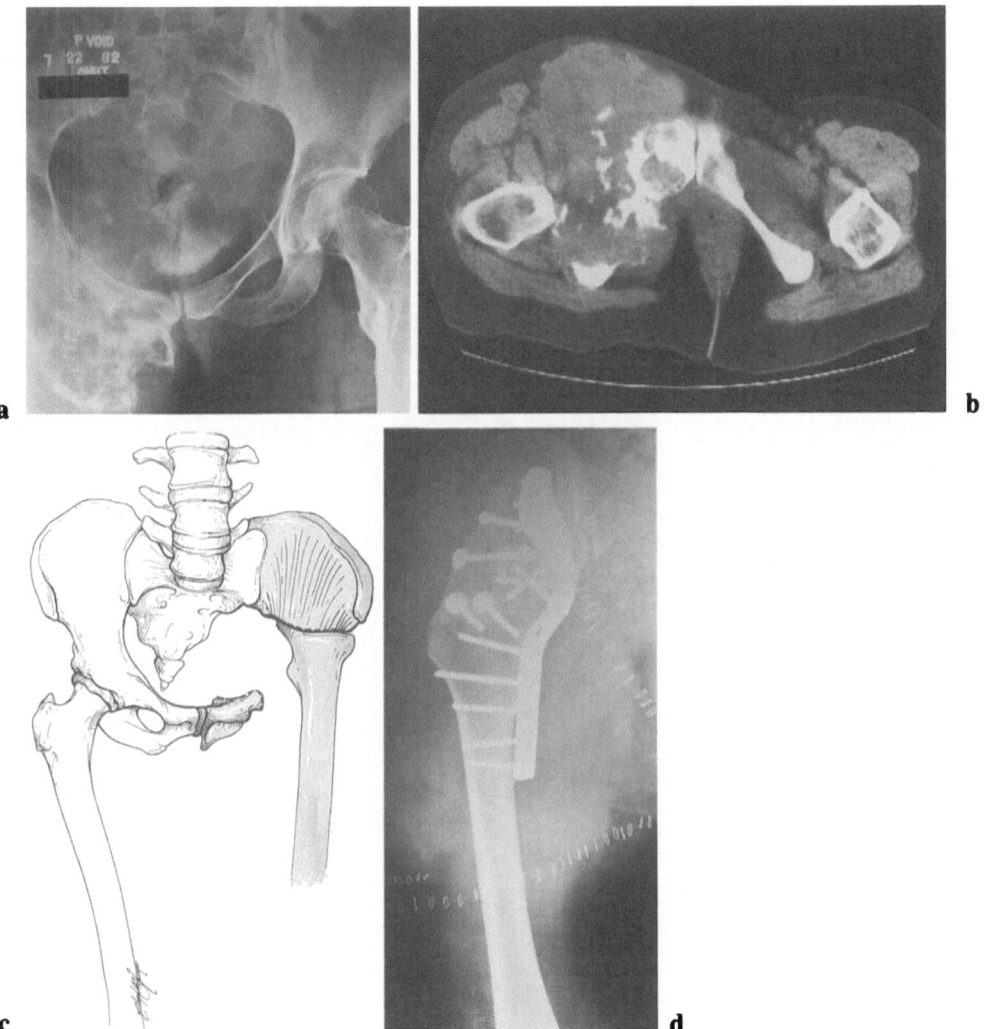

Fig. 2. a Anteroposterior view of pelvis, showing large chondrosarcoma involving anterior pelvis and extending into acetabulum. **b** Computed tomography scan, showing extent of tumor. **c** Femoral iliac fusion. **d** Anteroposterior view of right femur after arthrodesis. **c** Reproduced with Permission of Mayo Foundation

11 of the 51 patients (21%). Five patients in whom arthrodesis was attempted developed a nonunion with a pseudarthrosis. One patient had a decuditus ulcer, and one had a pulmonary embolus.

Survival

At a mean follow-up of 62 months, 32 patients (63%) had no evidence of disease; 25 of the 32 had been continuously disease-free. Thirteen patients died of

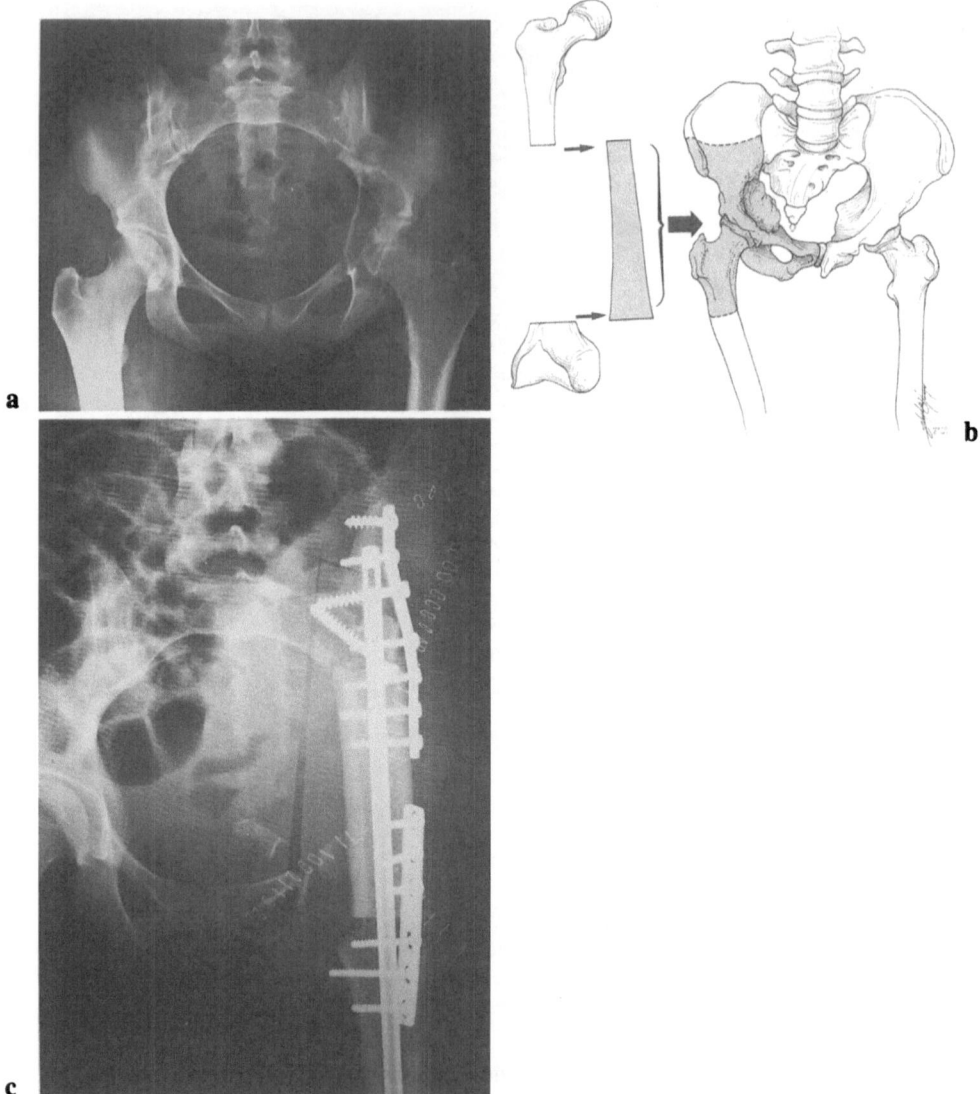

Fig. 3. a Anteroposterior view of pelvis, showing large osteosarcoma involving periace-tabular region of left hip. **b** Intercalary allograft. **c** Anteroposterior view of pelvis and left femur after intercalary allograft to bridge the defect and maintain leg length. **b** Repro-duced with permission of Mayo Foundation

their disease, three were alive with the disease, and three died of other causes. Disease progression was more evident in the patients with iliosacral and acetabu-lar lesions. Of the patients who were either alive with the disease or had died of disease, 41% had iliosacral lesions and 32% had acetabular lesions, compared with 10% who had ischiopubic lesions.

Local Recurrence

In this series, the incidence of local recurrence was analyzed according to the histology, surgical stage, and location of the lesion, as well as the surgical margin achieved with the resection. Of 49 patients in whom en bloc tumor resection was attempted, 13 (26%) had local recurrence, with an average time to recurrence of 19 months. Moreover, an additional two patients had persistence of tumor after debulking procedures despite postoperative radiation treatment. Three of the six patients who presented with local recurrence had a further recurrence after pelvic resection, and two of these developed pulmonary metastasis. Of the 20 patients with chondrosarcomas, seven (23%) had recurrence: Six were surgical stage IB and one was stage IIB. Five of the twelve patients with osteosarcomas (41%) and three of the six with fibrosarcomas (50%), all with stage IIB lesions, developed local recurrence.

Of the 15 patients with local recurrences in this series, nine (40%) were in the group of 22 patients with iliosacral lesions. Of the 19 patients with periacetabular resections, four developed local recurrence (21%), as did two of the ten patients with ischiopubic resection (20%).

The incidence of local recurrence correlated closely with the margin achieved at the time of surgical resection: Recurrences were noted in six of the eleven patients with a marginal margin, two of the three patients with a lesional margin, two of the eight patients with a contaminated wide margin, and 5 of the 29 patients with a wide margin. The influence of the surgical margin was most apparent in patients with iliosacral lesions—patients in whom it is often difficult to obtain a wide margin when the tumor involves the sacrum and extends to the spinal column. Eight of the nine patients with recurrences in this region had lesions that were resected with less than a wide margin.

Functional Evaluation

The functional results were analyzed according to the modified system adopted by the Musculoskeletal Tumor Society [3]. The overall rating was then determined by combining the rating for each of the individual factors, and in addition a numerical score was given. Thirty-seven patients were available for functional assessment 2 years or more after surgery. The other 14 patients had died or required conversion to hemipelvectomy because of recurrence or infection within 2 years after operation.

Among the 37 patients available for evaluation, 17 had excellent results, seven good, seven fair, and six poor. The results varied with the location of the lesion resection, being better in the iliosacral and ischiopubic regions when the acetabulum was preserved. None of the nine patients with ischiopubic lesions required reconstruction. Eight had excellent results and one had a good result. In the iliosacral region, when the continuity of the pelvis remained intact (that is, resection was above the sciatic notch), the results were uniformly excellent (Table 3). When a solid iliosacral fusion was achieved, the results were superior to either pseudarthrosis after attempted fusion or a flail articulation (no reconstruction).

Of the 11 patients with periacetabular lesions who were available for evalua-

Table 3. Results of resection according to site of malignant pelvic tumor and outcome

Lesion and outcome	No. of patients	Excellent	Good	Fair	Poor
Iliosacral (type I)	17 6	9	3	4	1
Intact pelvis	6	6	0	0	0
Arthrodesis	2	3	2	1	0
Pseudarthrosis	3	0	0	2	0
Flail	11	0	1	1	1
Acetabular (type II)	2	0	3	3	5
Intact pelvis	3	0	2	0	0
Arthrodesis	3	0	1	2	0
Pseudarthrosis	3	0	0	1	2
Flail	9	0	0	0	3
Ischiopubic (type III)	9	8	1	0	0
Intact pelvis		8	1	0	0
Total	37	17	7	7	6

tion 2 years or more after surgery, none had an excellent result. Both patients with partial acetabular resection had a good result. Of the three patients with a solid arthrodesis, two had a fair result and one had a good result. Of the three patients who developed a pseudarthrosis, one had a fair results and two had a poor result. All three patients with flail limbs (mega-Girdlestone procedure) had a poor result.

When the numerical score was utilized weighing the functional parameters, 14 of the 17 patients with iliosacral lesions had a satisfactory result. All nine of the patients with ischiopubic lesions had a satisfactory result. Four of the six patients with periacetabular lesions who had either an arthrodesis or a pseudarthrosis had a satisfactory result, with the scores being better when a solid arthrodesis was achieved. All three patients with flail limbs had unsatisfactory results.

In addition to the location of the lesion and type of reconstruction, the functional result varied according to the pelvic stability obtained. When the pelvis was left intact after resection, the numerical score was 33.3, indicating an excellent result. When the reconstruction restored pelvic continuity after resection, as it did in nine patients, the score was 27.3 (a good result). However, in the 11 patients in whom stability could not be restored, the score was 13.2 (a poor rating).

Discussion

Malignant tumors of the pelvis remain a challenge. While overall survival does not seem to be compromised by local resection, significant problems remain in terms of local control after internal hemipelvectomy. In this series, the overall incidence of local recurrence was 29% (including three patients who had debulking procedures and six who presented with local recurrence). The location of the tumor and the surgical margin achieved were the most important factors. This was particularly true in patients with iliosacral lesions in whom only a lesional or marginal resection is often possible, whether amputation or respection is performed. This experience suggests the need of continued search for effective adjuvant treatment of these lesions.

In addition to achieving local control, justification for these procedures is dependent on restoration of a functional status which is better than that achieved by hemipelvectomy. In this series, the results varied with the location of the resection and the maintenance or restoration of pelvic continuity. In ischiopubic or iliac resections above the sciatic notch when pelvic continuity is maintained, the functional results are uniformly excellent. Thus, the functional results in these patients are difficult to compare with those in patients who have a flail extremity after resection of the entire hemipelvis, in whom reconstruction is not possible. Without reconstruction, there is a great deal of instability necesstating heavier walking aids as well as loss of strength and endurance and diminution in functional activities. However, most patients regain reasonable functional capabilities and are satisfied with their status, especially when they consider the option of hemipelvectomy. Moreover, concerning the location of the tumor, a superior result can be expected after either resection of an iliosacral or ischiopubic lesion than after removal of the acetabulum. Moreover, in a patient who undergoes an extensive resection with attempted reconstruction, such as a solid arthrodesis or a successful pseudarthrosis, the result cannot be rated unsatisfactory because of shortening, muscle weakness, or the use of walking aids.

However, to facilitate comparisons of similar procedures among different institutions, the present modified Musculoskeletal Tumor Society Rating System can be used to reflect the different functional expectations in each location by modifying the numerical scoring system. Thus, a weighted numerical score of 25–30 for a periacetabular resection would represent an excellent result, compared with 25–30 for an iliosacral resection and 30–35 for an ischiopubic resection. In this way, various reconstructive options in each location can be evaluated and compared with realistic expectations.

References

1. Enneking WF, Spanier SS, Goodman MA (1980) A system for the surgical staging of musculoskeletal sarcoma. Clin Orthop 153: 106–120
2. Enneking WF, Dunham WK (1978) Resection and reconstruction for primary neoplasms involving the innominate bone. J Bone Joint Surg (Am) 60: 731–746
3. Enneking WF, Menendez LR (1987) Functional evaluation of various reconstructions after periacetabular resection of iliac lesions. In: Enneking WF (ed) Limb salvage in musculoskeletal oncology. Churchill Livingstone, New York, pp 117–135

Functional Evaluation of Limb Salvage Operation for Malignant Bone and Soft Tissue Tumors Using the Evaluation System of the Musculoskeletal Tumor Society

Katsuhisa Amino[1], Noriyoshi Kawaguchi[1], Seiichi Matsumoto[1], Jun Manabe[1], Kohtaro Furuya[2], and Yasushi Isobe[2]

Summary. A total of 158 cases of bone and soft tissue sarcomas treated by limb salvage operations were evaluated using the evaluation system of the Musculoskeletal Tumor Society. They overall rating was 41% excellent, 31% good, 17% fair, and 11% poor. From the viewpoint of the value "satisfactory" for the categories "excellent" and "good," soft tissue sarcomas were found to be better than bone sarcomas, high-malignant tumors were better than low-malignant ones, intracompartmental tumors were better than extracompartmental ones, and smaller soft tissue sarcomas were better than larger ones. To make this functional evaluation system more useful, recurrent cases should be excluded as failures, and more emphasis should be placed on the factor of functional activity. To determine the successfulness of the limb salvage operation itself, a new evaluation system was tried. Under this sytem, 78% of the cases were rated as satisfactory, while 24 (15%) were rated as poor.

Key words: Functional evaluation—Limb salvage operation—Malignant bone and soft tissue tumors

Introduction

The functional evaluation system of the Musculoskeletal Tumor Society (MTS), which was modified for use in the Fourth International Symposium on Limb Salvage in Musculoskeletal Oncology held in Kyoto [1], was applied in a study of our limb salvage operations. To determine how the extent of resection or the type of operation most influences postoperative function, we would like to show the usefulness of the functional evaluation system and raise several points of constructive criticism without engaging in a "rating competition" of patient success rates. We think that if the result of the rating is poor and yet the saved limb is in fact more useful than an amputated limb, then the rating system is not adequate and should be improved.

[1]Department of Orthopedic Surgery, Cancer Institute Hospital, Tokyo, Japan
[2]Department of Orthopedic Surgery, Tokyo Medical and Dental University, Tokyo, Japan

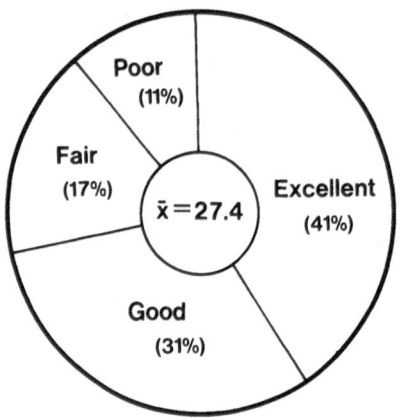

Fig. 1. Overall rating of functional evaluation by the system of the Musculoskeletal Tumor Society ($n = 158$)

Material and Methods

In the 10 years beginning January 1977, at the Department of Orthopedic Surgery of the Cancer Institute Hospital in Tokyo, limb salvage operations were performed for 158 malignant bone and soft tissue tumors of the extremities. These 158 tumors included 51 bone sarcomas and 107 soft tissue sarcomas. The 51 bone sarcomas comprised 27 osteosarcomas, 12 chondrosarcomas, and 12 other sarcomas. The 107 soft tissue sarcomas comprised 36 MFHs, 27 liposarcomas, eight synovial sarcomas, and 36 other sarcomas. According to the Surgical Staging System [2], they were classified as 22 cases of I A, 21 cases of I B, 40 cases of II A, 61 cases of II b, and 14 cases of III. For 45 of the patients, such skeletal reconstruction as total knee replacement, arthrodesis, intercalary grafting was required after tumor resection. Three types of radical surgery were performed for limb salvage. Those were curative wide resection, wide resection, and adjunctive operation after chemo- and/or radiotherapy. We usually use curative wide resections for almost all cases of bone and soft tissue sarcoma. "Curative wide resection" can be classified as extensive wide excision based on biological barrier effects. These barriers include fascia, periosteum, vessel sheath, and joint capsule [3].

Results and Discussion

Results of treatment of all 158 cases were 12% for recurrent cases, 38% for metastasis, and 67% for 5-year survival. Analysis of the functional status of the 158 cases by the rating system used for this symposium showed 41% as excellent, 31% as good, 17% as fair, and 11% as poor (Fig. 1). The average score was 27.4, and the overall values for the cases were determined to be almost 72% satisfactory for the categories of "excellent" and "good." From the viewpoint of the value "satisfactory," soft tissue sarcomas were better than high-grade malignant tumors, and intracompartmental tumors were better than larger soft tissue sarcomas (Fig. 2). However, in the case of soft tissue sarcomas, the histological

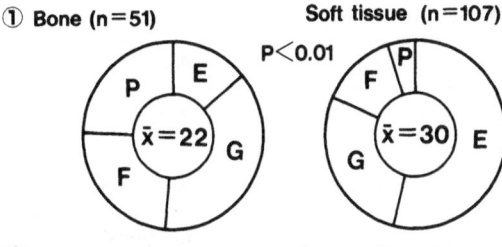

① Bone (n=51)   Soft tissue (n=107)

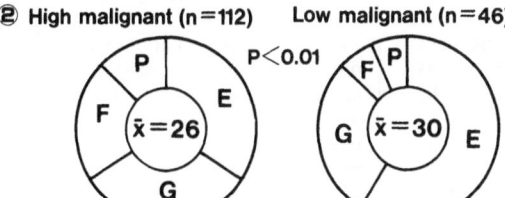

② High malignant (n=112)   Low malignant (n=46)

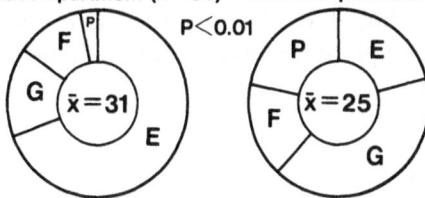

③ Interacompartment (n=66)   Extracompartment (n=92)

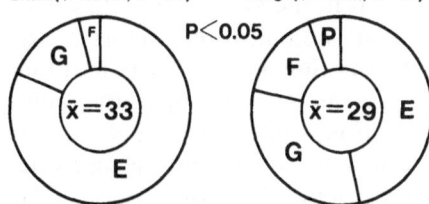

④ Soft Tissue Sarcomas (n=107)
Small($\phi <$5cm, n=26)   Large($\phi \geq$5cm, n=81)

Fig. 2. Comparative study of overall rating of limb salvage operations. *E* excellent, *G* good, *F* fair, *P* poor

grade did not influence postoperative functions so much.

For eight soft tissue sarcomas of the posterior high, resection of the sciatic nerves combined with limb salvage operations was performed. The results for knee function were 75% satisfactory, while the ankle had a 0% satisfactory rate. In this evaluation system, the appropriate anatomical region should be selected, but in some cases evaluation should include the distal regions and, especially, the functional activities of the entire extremity.

There were 17 cases graded as "poor" by this system. We attached most importance to functional activity among the seven factors. The functional activities were six good, six fair, a dn 5 poor, while the mean score for the overall rating "poor" was 13 ± 5. The causes of a poor result were determined to be major infections in four, recurrences in three, shoulder cases in five, and other causes in five. Apart from the infected or recurrent cases, ten patients had useful limbs following treatment. As a rule, overall ratings involving the shoulder region were worse than those of other regions; while there were some useful limbs

Table 1. A new system for evaluating the limb salvage operation

	Excellent	Good	Fair	Poor
Local recurrence or complication requiring ablation	No	No	No	Yes
Emotional acceptance	—	—	Acceptable	Not acceptable even if "fair" in functional ability
Functional activity				
Low extremity	normal	Patient capable of outdoor activity	Patient capable of outdoor activity	Patient requires assistance
Upper extremity	normal	Patient essentially capable of self-care	Limb is somewhat useful, with a few functions preserved	All functions lost

among the poor cases as determined by the evaluation system. To make this functional evaluation system more useful, it is recommended that recurrent cases be excluded as failures and more emphasis be placed on functional activity [4].

New System for Evaluating Limb Salvage Operation

To evaluate the limb salvage operation itself, we are employing a new system [5] because it is felt that the rating system used in the symposium does not always reflect the actual usefulness of limbs. In our system, three factors are used for evaluation: recurrence and complication, emotional acceptance, and functional activity (Table 1). In this system, the poor rating means operative failure, the fair rating is a suspended state of limb function, while excellent and good results are considered to be satisfactory. The results of our 158 limb salvage operations with our rating system were 78% satisfactory and 15% poor (24 cases). The poor cases comprised 19 local recurrences and five major infections requiring ablative operations.

References

1. Enneking WF (1987) Modification of the system for functional evaluation of surgical management of musculoskeletal tumors. In: Enneking WF (ed) Limb salvage in musculoskeletal oncology. Churchill Livingstone, New York, pp 626–639
2. Enneking WF (1986) A system of staging musculoskeletal neoplasms. Clinic Orthop 204: 9–24
3. Kawaguchi N, Amino K, Matsumoto S, Manabe J, Furuya K, Isobe Y (1987) Limb salvage operation of osteosarcoma. Rinsho Seikei Geka 22: 1189–1197
4. Amino K, Kawaguchi N, Matsumoto S, Manab J, Tago M, Takakura Y, Furuya K, Wada S, Isobe Y (1986) Functional evaluation of limb saving operation for malignant soft tissue tumors. Rinsho Seikei Geka 21: 977–984
5. Mankin HJ, Doppelt SH, Sullivan TR, Tomford WW (1982) Osteoarticular and intercalary allograft transplantation in the managment of malignant tumors of bone. Cancer 50: 613–630

Functional Results of Rotationplasty

Analysis and Commentary of the Enneking Evaluation System

K. Knahr, J. Sekera, and M. Salzer[1]

Summary. Rotationplasty is a standard method of surgery for treatment of malignant bone tumors of the distal part of the femur. Compared with the hitherto accepted methods of limb salvage—endoprosthesis, allogruft, and resection arthrodesis—rotationplasty seems to give better oncological and functional results. Thus far, at the Orthopedic Hospital Vienna, we have had experience of 49 cases of rotationplasty with a follow-up of 3–10 years. With respect to the emotional acceptance of this method, the results of this study were particularly revealing.

The functional results according to the evaluation schema of Enneking show in most cases good and excellent results. More than 80% of the patients actively and regularly engage in sporting activities. From these results, it is no longer justifiable to reject rotationplasty in principle as a therapeutic alternative in treating malignant bone tumors of the distal part of the femur.

Key words: Bone tumor—Rotationplasty—Functional evaluation system

It is a well-known fact that the knee joint is the main location of primary malignant bone tumors. For this reason, the local treatment of tumors of this region occupies a central position in therapeutic considerations.

The objectives of surgical treatment are as follows: (a) Improvement of survival, i.e., oncologically sufficient elimination of the primary tumor; (b) optimal functional rehabilitation.

There are four possibilities in the surgical treatment of tumors around the knee joint: above-knee amputation, rotationplasty, endoprosthesis, and resection arthrodesis. Which of these measures should be given preference in an individual case is largely dependent on the primary objective—the survival of the patient. In principle, the method of operation selected should be the one which gives the patient the greatest chance of survival. The question of functional rehabilitation arises when equal or similar chances of survival are offered by several methods.

The choice of the method of operation depends to some extent on the patient, but mainly it depends on the attitude of the treatment center in each case. As a result of their own experience, physicians generally prefer one or other of the

---

[1] Orthopedic Hospital Wien-Gersthof, Vienna, Austria

four possible methods of operation. For this reason, it is very difficult to compare the results, as no one center has equal experience of all four methods of operation.

In 1983, Enneking in Vienna presented a system of classification that was designed to facilitate comparison of the functional results of different surgical approaches [1]. This system represented a first step toward the uniform evaluation of different methods, but it still requires modification.

As mentioned above, four very different methods of operation must be compared for the anatomical region of the knee joint. In view of the fact that our own department has many years of experience with rotationplasty [3–5] (the first operation of this kind we did took place as long ago as 1974), the present paper sets out to analyze the extent to which the system of classification recommended by Enneking can be applied to this method of operation.

Knee Evaluation System (Enneking)

It is virtually impossible to compare the four methods with regard to evaluation of the first criterion, the mobility of the knee joint, as the situation is different in each case. In the case of arthrodesis, there is a complete absence of mobility of the knee joint, and in the case of amputation this mobility depends on the design of the prosthesis. Only rotationplasty and the endoprosthesis are comparable, as both methods offer both passive and active mobility.

The subjective perception of pain is a parameter that can be applied to all four methods.

The evaluation of varus/valgus instability or giving way specified under stability cannot meaningfully be applied to either rotationplasty or above-knee amputation, as these problems are not encountered if a suitable prosthesis is fitted. Evaluation should be confined to the loadability of the extremity. A clearly defined criterion would be the necessity of using supports.

The three criteria listed under deformity—varus/valgus position, flexion contraction, and shortening of the leg—are also not applicable to rotationplasty or amputation. The only sensible common criterion here is the evaluation of gait—based on the degree, constancy, and severity of the limp.

Strength, measured in terms of the ability to overcome gravity in an extended position, is hardly applicable as a common criterion for evaluation either, as only rotationplasty and the endoprosthesis offer an active possibility of extending the lower leg. Such active extension is not possible with arthrodesis or above-knee amputation.

The criteria of functional activity and emotional acceptance are suitable for the evaluation of all four methods of operation and thus represent suitable evaluative parameters.

In view of these circumstances, there is no overall rating incorporating all seven evaluative criteria specified by Enneking that would be suitable for an objective comparison of the results of rotationplasty with the alternatives of amputation, endoprosthesis, and resection arthrodesis. In any evaluation of results, it is, therefore, necessary to apply only criteria that are equally applicable to all four methods.

Knee Evaluation System (Modified)

For the functional evaluation of tumors around the knee joint, we therefore propose a system of classification based on three subjective and three objective criteria (Table 1). The three subjective criteria are pain, functional activity, and emotional acceptance. These three parameters can be adopted unchanged in the form specified by Enneking. They can be applied without restriction to amputation, endoprosthesis, rotationplasty, and arthrodesis. It would seem expedient to subdivide the results into excellent, good, fair, and poor ratings by the number of points awarded: 5, 3, 1 and 0 points.

Three objective criteria should also be included: The use of supports, walking ability, and gait are three criteria that can be evaluated for all four methods of operation. In principle, these three criteria do not represent a departure from the previous system, as mobility, stability, deformity, and strength are reflected in walking ability, gait, and the need for supports. Once again, it would be possible to give a rating of excellent, good, fair, and poor based on the corresponding number of points.

Overall evaluation is carried out on the basis of a combination of the subjective and objective data, 26–30 points being required for a rating of excellent; 21–25 points represents a good result, and 16–20 points a moderate result, while a rating of 15 or fewer points must be regarded as a poor result, and thus as a failure of the method.

Material and Results

This system of evaluation was applied to our own patients with rotationplasty and compared with the system proposed by Enneking. For comparison, we took the group of patients used in the meeting in Orlando in 1985 (Table 2) [2]. A total of 18 patients received rotationplasty in the years 1977–1983. In 13 cases, the primary tumor was an osteosarcoma, in two cases each a periosteal osteosarcoma and Ewing's sarcoma, and in one case a malignant fibrous histiocytoma.

Three patients died within the first 2 years postoperation, and one in the 4th year postoperation. It was, therefore, possible to carry out a comparative investigation of 14 patients.

The analysis based on Enneking's criteria showed that no change in condition occurred between the 2nd and 4th years after operation. This is an indication that the degree of rehabilitation achieved after 2 years subsequently neither improved nor deteriorated.

In ten cases, the patients analyzedusing Enneking's criteria displayed excellent results, in three cases good results, and in one case a bad result (Table 3). Analysis of the same sample of patients according to the modified evaluation system gave the following picture: Judged by the three subjective criteria, ten had excellent results, three good results, and one poor result; judged by the objective data, there were excellent results, one good and one poor result. The overall result was nine excellent and four good ratings, and one poor rating. These approximately similar results are an indication that the modified system does not represent a fundamental change in the evaluation.

Table 1. Modified evaluation system for the anatomical region of the knee

	Subjective data			Objective data		
	Pain	Functional activity	Emotional acceptance	Support	Walking ability	Limp
Excellent (5 points)	None	No restriction	Enthusiastic	None	Unlimited	No
Good (3 points)	Modest	Recreational restriction only	Satisfied	Brace/prosthesis	1 km	Slight, only with fatigue
Fair (1 point)	Moderate	Partial disability	Acceptance	One cane/crutch	Only at home	Moderate
Poor (0 points)	Severe	Total disability	Dislike	Two canes/crutches	Wheelchair	Habitual limp

Table 2. Tumor resection and rotationplasty 1977–1983 ($n = 18$)

	Patient	Follow-up >2 years	Follow-up >4 years
Osteosarcoma	13	11	11
Periosteal osteosarcoma	2	2	2
Ewing's sarcoma	2	1	1
Malignant fibrous histiocytomas	1	1	—
Total	18	15	14

Table 3. Functional evaluation of patients with rotationplasty with a follow-up of more than 4 years ($n = 14$)

	Enneking's system (overall results)	Modified system		
		Subjective data	Objective data	Overall results
Excellent	10	10	11	9
Good	3	3	2	4
Fair	—	—	—	—
Poor	1	1	1	1

Conclusion

In contrast to the original Enneking system, all six criteria of our modified system apply without exception to all four methods of operation in region of the knee. Reducing the number of criteria to six clearly defined and easily measurable parameters also facilitates the recording of results. For this reason, we are of the opinion that the proposed modification of the evaluation system represents a practicable alternative to the previous method of classification.

Acknowledgment. The authors are indebted to the Verein für orthopädische Forschung und Rehabilitation for its support in the preparation of this paper.

References

1. Enneking WF (1983) Functional evaluation of reconstruction after tumor resection. In: Kotz R (ed) Proceedings of 2nd international workshop on the design and application of tumor prostheses for bone and joint reconstruction, Vienna, Sept. 5–8, 1983. Egermann, Vienna, pp 5–10
2. Knahr K, Kotz R, Kristen H, Ramach W, Salzer-Kuntschik M, Salzer M, Sekera J (1987) Clinical evaluation of patients with rotationplasty. In: Enneking WF (ed) Limb salvage in musculoskeletal oncology. Churchill Livingstone, New York, pp 429–434
3. Knahr K, Kristen H, Ritschl P, Sekera J, Salzer M (1987) Prosthetic management and functional evaluation of patients with resection of the distal femur and rotationplasty. Orthopedics 1241–1248
4. Kotz R, Salzer M (1982) Rotationplasty for childhood osteosarcoma of the distal part of the femur. J Bone Joint Surg 65A: 959–969
5. Salzer M, Knahr K, Kotz R, Kristen H (1981) Treatment of osteosarcoma of the distal femur by rotation-plasty. Arch Orthop Trauma Surg 99: 131–136

Modular Kotz Prosthesis

The Rizzoli Experience

Rodolfo Capanna[1], Cesare Leonessa[1], Graziano Bettelli[1],
Battista Borghi[2], Roberto de Cristofaro[1], Cristina Martelli[1],
Pietro Ruggieri[1], and Mario Campanacci[1]

Summary. The functional results of 94 cementless Kotz prostheses are reported according to Enneking's system. Excellent or good results were obtained in 61% of the patients who had a proximal femur resection and in 75% of the patients who had a knee resection. Only 10% of the patients had a complication that altered the functional status, and only 5% required surgical treatment for their complications. No case of loosening was observed at a mean follow-up of 2 years.

Key words: Bone tumors—Modular prostheses—Resections

Material and Methods

Between 1983 and 1987, 100 KMFTR (Kotz modular femur and tibia reconstruction) prostheses were implanted at the Istituto Ortopedico Rizzoli. There were 63 male and 37 female patients ranging from 11 to 71 years. Fifteen patients had a benign tumor (two stage 2, 13 stage 3); 83 had a malignant tumor (four stage IA, nine stage IB, four stage IIA, 64 stage IIB; two stage III) (Fig. 1) [5–7].

The KMFTR prosthesis was inserted to replace the proximal femur in 26 patients, the distal femur in 66 patients, the proximal tibia in seven and the entire knee in one case. The resection was extra-articular in 15 patients (13 distal femur resections and two proximal femur resections) and intra-articular in 85. The resection length ranged from 11 to 28 cm (mean 16.4 cm).

In this study, 94 cases were included (63 distal femur, 23 proximal femur, seven proximal tibia, and one total knee). Six cases were excluded: three cases because the prosthesis was cemented (one Charcot joint, one metastatic tumor, and one stem size inadequate to provide a good press fit in the medullary canal), two cases of postoperative death (pulmonary embolism), and one case of postoperative amputation (ensuing thrombosis in a previous femoropopliteal bypass).

---

[1] Bone Tumor Center and 1st Orthopaedic Clinic Istituto Ortopedico Rizzoli, Bologna, Italy
[2] Anaesthesiology Department, University of Bologna, Bologna, Italy

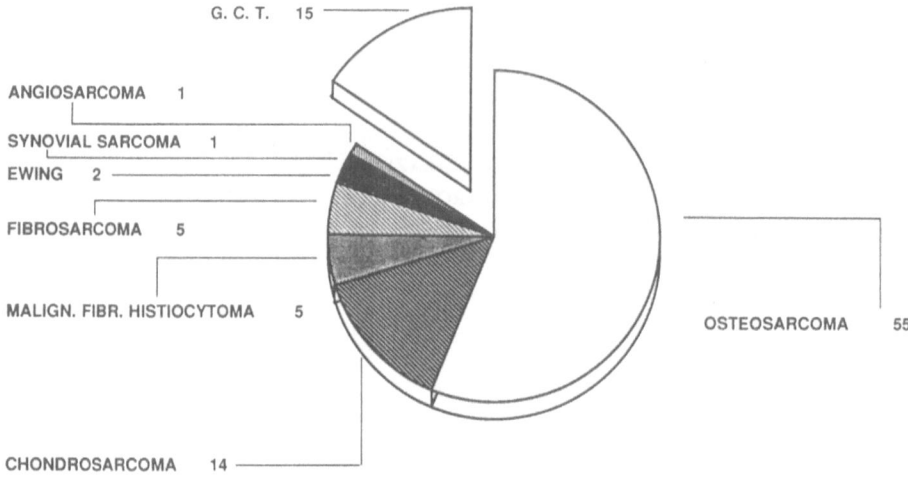

Fig. 1. Histological diagnosis (primary bone tumors)

In proximal femur resection (23 cases), part of the pelvic-trochanteric and quadriceps muscles was also resected. Two patients had an extra-articular resection and reconstruction of the acetabulum with autogenous grafts. A double-cup endoprosthesis was used in 18 patients, and a screwed ring in five. The gluteal muscles were inserted to the prosthesis or the fascia lata.

In the distal femur resections (63 cases), the prosthesis was used as a primary reconstruction in 53 cases. In ten patients, the prosthesis was inserted as a salvage procedure following failure of a previous surgical treatment (five broken and five infected Kuntscher rods and cement).

Nine patients had excision of the vastus intermedius (type A), 11 of the vastus medialis, and 18 of the vastus lateralis (type B). Nine cases had complete excision of the vastus, preserving the rectus (type C); 16 cases had excision of the entire quadriceps or a previous arthrodesis (type D).

Muscles transfers (flexors proextensors) were used in nine patients, ten patients had patellar replacement, and five had myocutaneous flap (gastrocnemius).

In proximal tibia or knee resections (eight cases), the patellar tendon was always anchored to the prosthesis and sutured to the anteposed gastrocnemius.

The prosthesis was press-fitted in the medullary canal and no cement was used.

According to Enneking's classification [5–7], the surgical margins were wide in 75 cases, wide but contaminated in five, marginal in ten, and intralesional in four.

Complications

Minor complications such as delayed wound healing (three patients), local hematoma (six), and transient Sudeck's atrophy (three) were observed in 12 patients.

Table 1. Complications in proximal femur resection

Complication	Number	Percent	Result
Knee motion restriction	3	12	Impaired function
Peroneal nerve palsy	2	8	Transient
Deep infection	1	4	Healed after surgical debridement
Luxation	1	4	Closed reduction

Table 2. Complications in distal femur or proximal tibia resections

Complication	Number	Percent	Result
Patellar subluxation	3	4	Impaired function
Deep infection	4	6	Amputation (1), persistence (1), healed with surgical debridement (2)
Tibial compound fracture	6	9	Healed without consequence
Peroneal nerve palsy	2	3	Transient
Wear of polyethylene bushes	2	3	Varus/valgus instability

Major complications were found in 28% of the proximal femur resections and in 25% of the distal femur or proximal tibia resections (Tables 1, 2). The infection rate was low (5%): In three patients the infection healed after surgical debridement, one patient had persistent infection, and one patient underwent amputation. In this last patient, the prosthesis was implanted as a salvage procedure in a previously infected Kuntscher rod and cement. There were three lateral patellar subluxations with resulting limitation of the knee motion, all in patients who had had patellar replacement. Dislocation of the proximal femoral prosthesis was rarely observed (4%): it was prevented by the extensive use of a double-cup endoprosthesis. Only eight patients (three patellar subluxation, two deep infection, three knee motion limitation) out of 24 major complications had bad functional results.

Oncological Results

At a mean follow-up of 22 months (range 10–48 months), only three cases developed a local recurrence (3%). There were two local recurrences in proximal femur resection (9%) and one local recurrence in distal femur resection (1.5%). All patients had a high-grade extracompartmental tumor (two osteosarcoma, one dedifferentiated chondrosarcoma). The resection was wide in one patient and marginal in two. In all patients, pulmonary metastases followed the local recurrence. No local recurrences were observed in benign or low-grade tumors.

Two patients had pulmonary metastases at the onset. Distant metastases developed in 18 of the 67 high-grade lesions (27%) and in one of the twelve low-grade tumors (8%). At the follow-up, 73 patients (13 benign, 11 low-grade, and 49 high-grade tumors) were alive without evidence of disease.

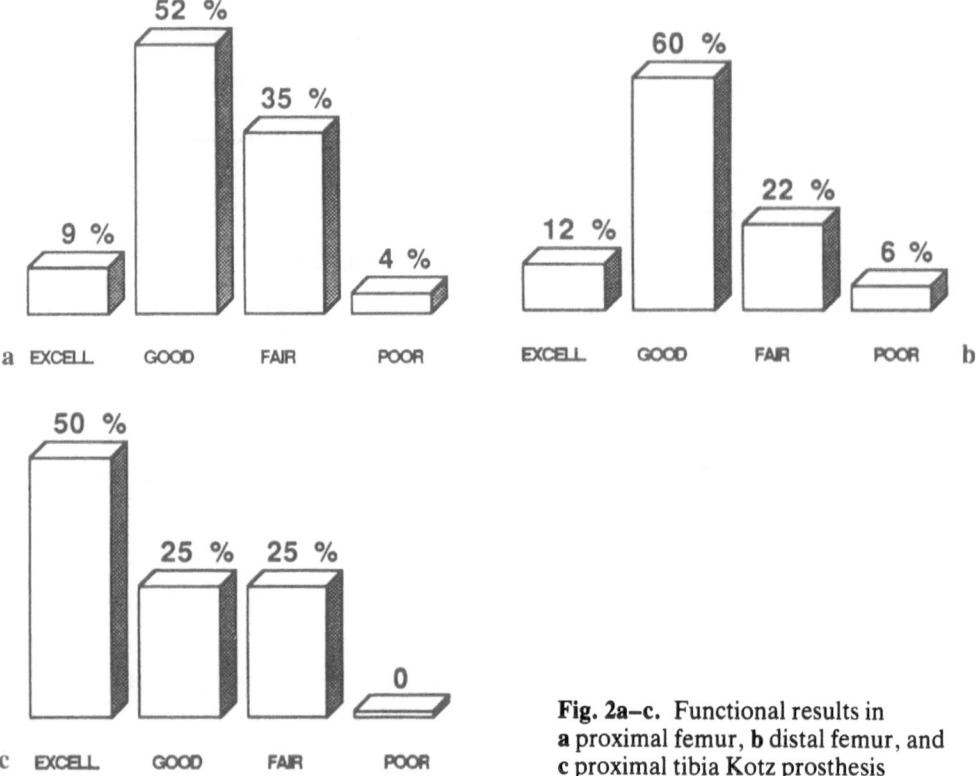

Fig. 2a–c. Functional results in
a proximal femur, **b** distal femur, and
c proximal tibia Kotz prosthesis

Functional Results

The functional results were rated according to the modified Enneking classification. Excellent or good results were obtained in about 75% of the patients having replacement of the distal femur or proximal tibia and in 61% of the patients
having a proximal femur replacement (Fig. 2). The rate of excellent or good
results observed for each parameter (motion, pain, stability, deformity, functional activity, emotional acceptance) is reported separately for replacement of
the proximal femur (Fig. 3), distal femur (Fig. 4), and proximal tibia (Fig. 5).

For distal femur replacement, the detailed functional status of the patients
who had resection of the entire quadriceps and/or a previous arthrodesis (type
D) was recorded separately from that of patients who had a partial resection of
the quadriceps muscle (types A, B, C).

Radiographic Evaluation

In 30% of the cases, a periosteal ossification developed during the first 12
months at the body-stem junction. This phenomenon is similar to that observed
in cemented prostheses.

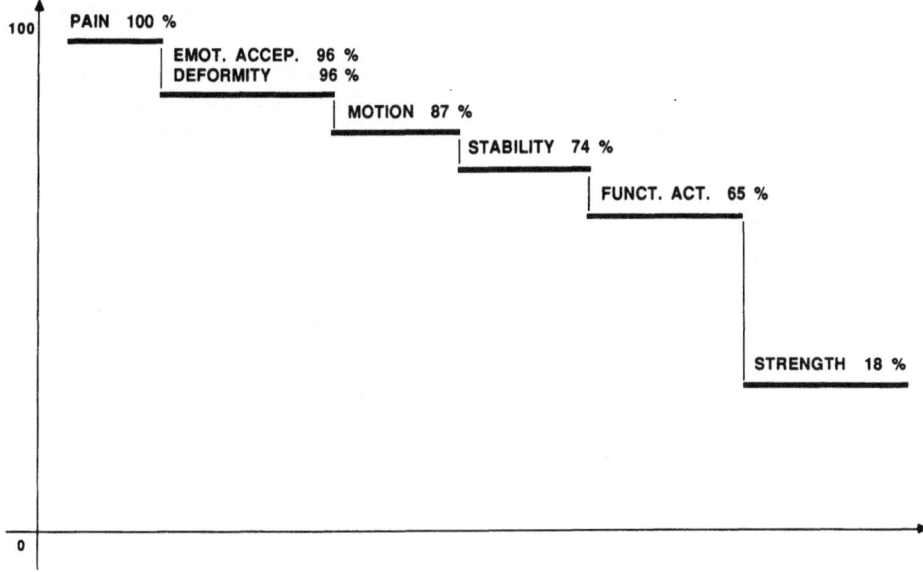

Fig. 3. Detailed functional status in proximal femur Kotz prostheses (% of satisfactory results; i.e., excellent or good)

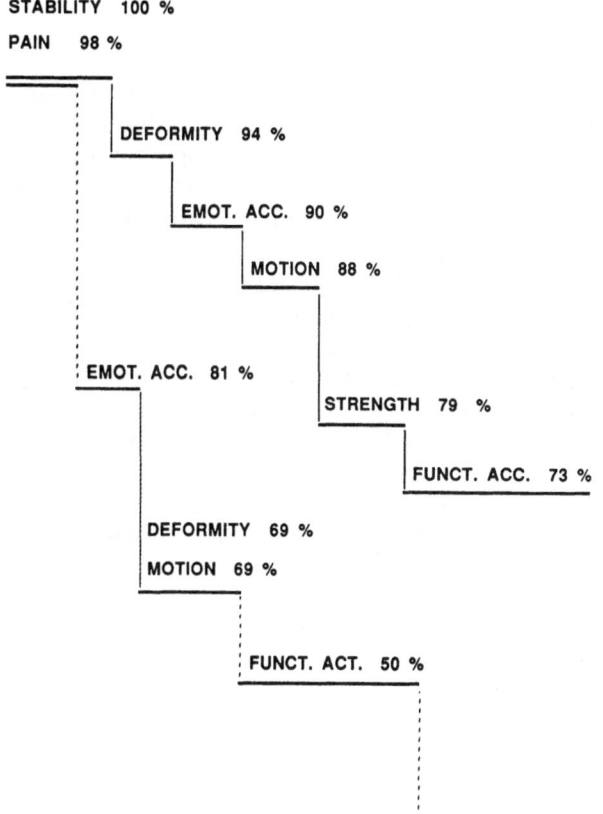

Fig. 4. Detailed functional status in distal femur Kotz prostheses. *Unbroken line* types A–C, *broken line* type D (% of satisfactory results; i.e., excellent or good)

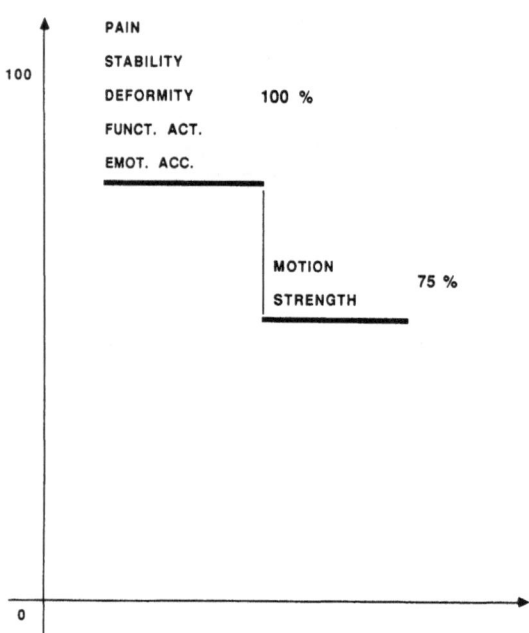

Fig. 5. Detailed functional status in proximal tibia Kotz prostheses (% of satisfactory results; i.e., excellent or good)

Five types of response of the cortex around the stem were observed: no reaction (type 1), hypertrophy (type 2), diffuse osteoporosis (type 3), distal hypertrophy and proximal osteoporosis (type 4), and distal hypertrophy and proximal reabsorption of the cortex (type 5). These radiographic changes in the cortex became evident within 6 months in 56% of the patients, within 12 months in 38%, and within 18 months in 6%. Regressive changes of the cortex were more frequently observed in proximal femur than in distal femur replacement; they were rarely observed in proximal tibia replacement.

Although the two groups of patients have a different mean follow-up (28 months vs. 12 months), type 3, 4, or 5 response was more frequent (43%) in cases with a complete fixation of both plates, while it was rarely observed (6%) in patients who had an incomplete fixation (three screws in the short plate; Fig. 6). A type 2 response was usually observed after breaking of the screws.

No radiographic changes around the tip of the stem were observed in 64% of the patients; trabecular thickening developed in 12%, and a "halo" sign in 24% of patients. All of these changes developed in the first 18 months and showed no modification later.

Even when radiographic signs of bone resorption appeared, no patient had clinical symptoms suggesting mechanical loosening.

Discussion

In our experience, the modularity of the KMFTR prosthesis proved to be adequate in all cases in coping with the length of the resected bone. The functional results in replacement of both the proximal and distal femur were similar with

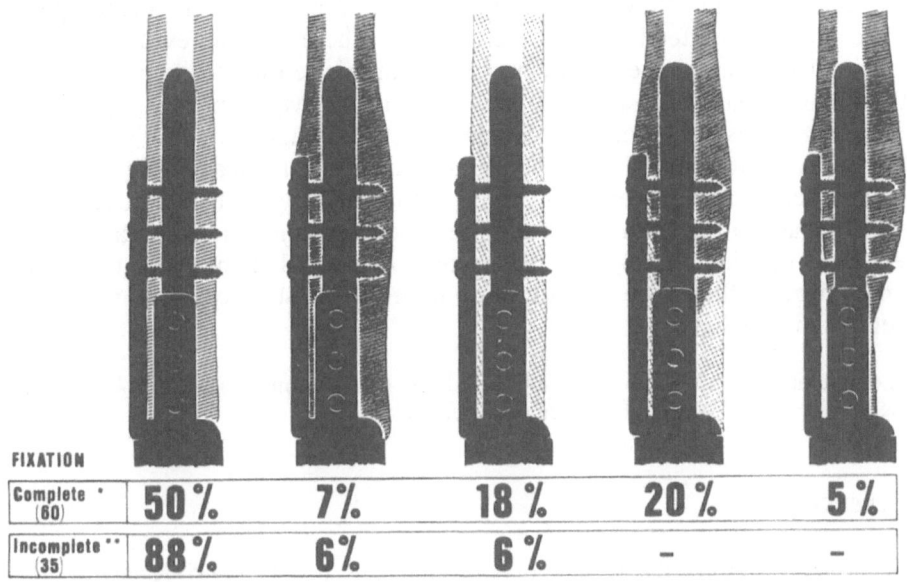

FIXATION					
Complete * (60)	**50%**	**7%**	**18%**	**20%**	**5%**
Incomplete ** (35)	**88%**	**6%**	**6%**	–	–

Fig. 6. Results of fixation. *Follow-up 28 months, **follow-up 12 months

those we previously reported with cemented prostheses [2, 3]. In replacement of the proximal femur, postoperative dislocation is a frequent complication (4%–25% of cases). The extensive use of a double-cup endoprosthesis (which is intrinsically more stable), careful muscle reconstruction around the prosthesis, and the use of a plaster cast for 40 days reduced the incidence of this complication (4%).

The infection rate was lower (5%) than those reported with a Kuntscher rod and cement (13%) or the Putti-Juvara arthrodesis (17%) [1, 4]; this is due to the fact that the prosthesis can be assembled more quickly, reducing the operative time. It is probably also related to the better biocompatibility of vitallium with respect to cement in large quantities [2].

In knee prostheses, we prefer not to replace routinely the patella with a prosthesis [3] for the following reasons: (a) to preserve the valuable effect of the quadriceps; (b) to maintain better stability of the patella; and (c) to enhance resistance to the stresses produced by the hinged prosthesis.

In resections of the distal femur, the posteriorly positioned hinge gives the prosthesis an intrinsic stability that does not depend on the integrity of the quadriceps. This means that these prostheses can be used in patients in whom extensive excision of the quadriceps is required. Initially, we felt doubtful about using these prostheses in patients who were receiving intensive chemotherapy before and after the operation, since we feared that this might adversely affect the osteogenic response of the bone in contact with the madreporic surface. However, the clinical trial seems to show that the anchorage of the prosthesis in these patients was just as good as in patients not receiving chemotherapy and it was achieved in the same time [2].

At the short-term follow-up (mean follow-up 22 months), the anchorage of the prosthesis was effective in all the patients. There is some evidence that a press-fitted stem supplemented by two plates and six screws, while providing an initial optimal stability, may sometimes cause regressive changes in the cortex; the artophy seems to be due to stress-shielding phenomena.

We believe that a curved stem (being more anatomical and avoiding the three-point contact of a linear stem in a curved intramedullary canal), without a madreporic surface in the distal third and the tip of the stem (thus diminishing the stress concentration there), and having only one supplementary plate for immediate fixation should be considered to improve the stem configuration of an uncemented prosthesis.

Acknowledgment. This study was supported by grant number 86.02679.44, Special Project "Oncology," National Council of Research.

References

1. Campanacci M, Cervellati C, Guerra A, Biagini R, Ruggieri P (1985) Knee resection-arthrodesis. In: Proceedings of international symposium on limb salvage in musculo-skeletal oncology, Orlando, Oct. 1985
2. Capanna R, Guerra A, Ruggieri P, Biagini R, Campanacci M (1985) The Kotz modular prosthesis in massive osteo-articular resection for bone tumors: preliminary results in 27 cases. It J Orthop Traum. 9: 271–281
3. Chao EYS, Ivins JC (eds) (1983) Tumor prostheses for bone and joint reconstruction. The design and application. Thieme-Stratton, New York, pp 207–214, 311–314, 321–328, 399–408
4. Enneking WF, Shirley PD (1977) Resection-arthrodesis for malignant and potentially malignant lesions about the knee using an intramedullary rod and local bone grafts. J Bone Joint Surg 59/A; 223–236
5. Enneking WF, Spanier SS, Goodman MA (1980) A system for the surgical staging of musculoskeletal sarcoma. Clin Orthop 153: 106–120
6. Enneking WF (1985) Staging of musculoskeletal neoplasms. Skel Radiol 13: 183–194
7. Enneking WF (1986) A system of staging musculoskeletal neoplasms. Clin Orthop 204: 9–24

Functional Evaluation of Musculoskeletal Sarcomas by Hokkaido Orthopedic Oncology Group

Tomonori Yagi[1], Takeo Matsuno[1], Seiichi Ishii[2], Masamichi Usui[2], Tetsuto Sasaki[2], Shinya Yamawaki[3], and Kazuo Isu[3]

Summary. Functional evaluation of the surgical management of musculoskeletal sarcomas treated by the Hokkaido Orthopedic Oncology Group was performed according to the Enneking's modified system. Sixty malignant or semimalignant musculoskeletal tumors were studied over a period of 5 years. There were 40 bone tumors, including 25 osteosarcomas and 20 soft tissue tumors. There were 30 amputations and 30 limb salvage procedures. The limb salvage group included four bone graft cavities, six arthrodeses, four biological arthroplasties using osteochondral allograft, eight prosthetic arthroplasties, and eight no reconstructions.

The overall results of functional evaluation of these patients showed 35% satisfactory (limb salavage 43%, amputation 27%) and 65% unsatisfactory ratings (57% and 73%, respectively). In 29 osteosarcomas of the knee, half the total knee replacement (TKR) cases were evaluated as good. However, the mean score was lower than in the arthrodesis cases. The evaluation of amputation and arthrodesis in Japan is lower than in the United States because of the difference in life-style. Especially, the primary factor of emotional acceptance generally tends to be evaluated low in Japan because of cultural differences. Therefore, this factor should be evaluated separately.

Key words: Functional evaluation—Musculoskeletal sarcoma—Life-style

Introduction

Limb salvage procedure for musculoskeletal sarcoma of the extremity followed by adjuvant chemotherapy has become more and more common. Within the Hokkaido Orthopedic Oncology Group (HOOG), this procedure, with preoperative and postoperative chemotherapy, has been commonly used in recent years. Functional evaluation of the surgical management of musculoskeletal sarcomas treated by our group was performed according to Enneking's modified system (Enneking, personal communication). The results of the functional evaluation were analyzed and compared with each procedure.

[1] Department of Orthopedic Surgery, Bibai Rousai Hospital, Bibai, Hokkaido, Japan
[2] Department of Orthopedic Surgery, Sapporo Medical College, Sapporo, Japan
[3] Department of Orthopedic Surgery, National Sapporo Hospital, Sapporo, Japan

Material and Methods

Sixty malignant or semimalignant musculoskeletal tumors were studied over a period of 5 years. There were bone tumors, which included 25 osteosarcomas, two chondrosarcomas, two malignant fibrous histiocytomas (MFH), eight giant cell tumors, and three others. There were 20 soft tissue tumors, which included ten MFH, two rhabdomyosarcomas, and six others.

Surgical Procedures

There were 30 amputations and 30 limb salvage procedures. The 30 amputations included 25 bone tumors and five soft tissue tumors. The 30 limb salvage procedures included 15 bone tumors and 15 soft tissue tumors. The amputation group included 24 amputations and six disarticulations. Among the 24 amputations, there were 20 above-knee (AK) one below-knee (BK) amputation, one hemipelvectomy, and two others. There were six disarticulations, which included four hip, one shoulder, and one thoracoscapular disarticulation.

Limb Salvage Group

Reconstruction after tumor resection included four bone graft cavities, six arthrodeses, four biological arthroplasties using an osteochondral allograft, eight prosthetic arthroplasties, and eight no reconstructions.

Evaluation was performed according to Enneking's modified systems based on six anatomical sites and seven primary factors: (a) motion, (b) pain, (c) stability, (d) deformity, (e) strength, (f) functional activity, and (g) emotional acceptance. The criteria for the ratings are essentially the same as in the previous system [1]. In addition, the score is calculated on the basis of: 5 as "excellent," 3 as "good," 1 as "fair," and 0 as "poor" for each primary factor. Furthermore, excellent and good scores were considered satisfactory cases, fair and poor unsatisfactory cases.

Results

In the limb salvage group, there were 13 satisfactory and 17 unsatisfactory cases. In the amputation group, there were 8 satisfactory and 22 unsatisfactory cases.

The amputation and disarticulation group included 20 AK amputations, four hip disarticulations, and six others. Most cases in this group showed unsatisfactory results because of lack of strength, restricted functional activity, and poor emotional acceptance.

The arthrodesis group included three knees, two ankles, and one shoulder arthrodesis. The evaluation of this group showed three good and three fair results. Every case showed a relatively high rating because there was no pain, good stability, little deformity, and good strength. The main causes of fair ratings were absence of motion, restricted functional activity, and fair emotional acceptance.

The prosthetic arthroplasty group which included six TKR cases showed three

Table 1. Functional evaluation for osteosarcomas of the knee joint

Procedure	No. of patients	Evaluation				Average score
		E	G	F	P	
Arthrodesis	3	0	0	3	0	20.7
Total knee replacement	6	0	3	3	0	19.6
Amputation	20	0	5	12	3	17.5

E excellent, *G* good, *F* fair, *P* poor

Table 2. Results of arthrodesis and amputation in Hokkaido Orthopedic Oncology Group and Florida University

Procedure	Institute	No. of patients	Excellent	Good	Fair	Poor
Arthrodesis	HOOG	6	0	3	3	0
	USA	18	2	10	3	3
Amputation	HOOG	30	0	5	21	4
	USA	10	2	5	0	3

HOOG Hokkaido Orthopedic Oncology Group, *USA* Florida University

good and three fair results upon evaluation. Most of the TKR cases scored well on the primary factor of functional activity and emotional acceptance, but there was no consistent score on good motion.

No reconstruction after tumor resection was performed in most of the soft tissue tumors, which were within the compartment [2]. The results showed nine satisfactory and three unsatisfactory evaluations. Biological arthroplasty was indicated for semimalignant bone tumors, such as giant cell tumor and chondroblastoma [3]. All four biological arthroplasties showed excellent or good results. The mean score in this group was high.

There were 29 osteosarcomas of the knee joint (Table 1): three arthrodeses, six TKRs, and 20 amputations. All cases of arthrodesis were evaluated as fair because there was no motion and fair functional activity. However, the patients gained good evaluation in terms of stability, deformity, and strength, and their mean score was more than 20. Half of the TKR cases were evaluated as good and the other half as fair; however, their mean score was less than 20 because of a lower evaluation of stability and strength. The amputation group had a lower evaluation: five cases scored good, 12 fair, and three poor with a mean score of 17.5.

As compared with the United States, amputation and arthrodesis are usually evaluated lower in Japan. In the amputation group, only 5 of 30 cases in our series showed satisfactory functional evaluation, in contrast to seven of ten in the United States. The same tendency can be seen in the arthrodesis group. In most cases, the primary factors of functional activity and emotional acceptance were evaluated lower (Table 2).

Discussion

There are many adverse living conditions that could bring about the lower functional evaluation in Japan. One is having small houses with several steps at the entrance; these become especially problematic in Hokkaido because of the heavy snow in winter. Japanese frequently sit by kneeling on the floor. In addition, it is common for houses to have steep stairs, and small, deep baths. These could be resons why all the-cases with knee arthrodesis and most AK amputation showed fair results. In Japan, functional evaluation has a tendency to be lower than in the United States because of the difference in life-style.

Finally, we suggest that the primary factor of emotional acceptance should be evaluated separately from the other factors because of what we believe to be a cultural difference. It is sometimes said that Japanese show little sympathy to the handicapped. Japanese generally tend not to want to impose upon others, the more so in the case of handicapped people. This characteristic and the fear of becoming handicapped and dependent on others could be valid reasons for our subjects having scored low on the primary factor of emotional acceptance. If emotional acceptance is evaluated, separately, the overall rating on the basis of a four-stage evaluation will have a close correlation with the score.

References

1. Yagi T, Enneking FW (1985) Evaluation of surgical management of musculoskeletal tumors. Orthopedic Surgery 36: 1342–1349
2. Enneking WF, Spanier SS, Goodman MA (1980). A system for the surgical staging of musculoskeletal sarcoma. Clin Orthop 153: 106–120
3. Sasaki T, Yagi T, Aoki M, Tsuge H (1985) Clinical results of osteochondral allograft in the treatment of osteochondral defects. J Jpn Orthop Ass 59: 1073–1088

Functional Evaluation of Reconstructed Extremities in Patients with Osteosarcoma After Limb Salvage Surgery

Norihiko Takada[1]

Summary. We compared both Enneking's functional criteria and the ADL criteria for evaluation of the extremities following surgical treatment. Evaluation according to the ADL criteria involves a subdivision of Enneking's criteria in terms of functional activity. However, some discrepancies between these two criteria were found. In cases of total knee replacement, for instance, the ADL score was high but Enneking's score was low. This might be attributed to limited motion and high deformity. Moreover, in cases of below-knee amputation, although there was a high score with ADL, there appeared to be a markedly low score because of different evaluation points with Enneking's criteria, such as evaluation of the ankle joint of the prosthetic foot. Functional activity, according to Enneking's criteria assesses whole body activity and the criteria are rather narrow. In the evaluation of a function of the affected limbs following surgery satisfactory daily life capability may be taken into consideration even if the recreational capability is low.

Key words: Functional evaluation—Limb salvage—Amputation

Introduction

Recent advances in chemotherapy against malignant tumors of bone and soft tissue have dramatically improved the cure rate and made it possible to introduce salvage operations of the affected limbs. However, there are some problems to be solved in terms of functional status of the preserved limbs and prosthetic limbs.

The purpose of this study is to compare functional aspects of preserved and amputated limbs according to Enneking's criteria and to introduce our activity of daily living (ADL) evaluation criteria for a comparison of preserved and amputated limbs to supplement Enneking's criteria.

[1] Department of Orthopedic Surgery, Chiba Cancer Center Hospital, Chiba, Japan

Table 1. Surgical modalities and sites of disease in 59 patients (1975–1985)

		Lower extremity		Upper extremity	
Limb preservation group (35)	Total knee replacement	15		Prosthetic replacement of shoulder joint	4
	Total hip replacement	3		Tumor resection only	3
	Hemiarthroplasty	3		Arthrodesis (wrist)	4
	Bone graft	1			
	Tumor resection only	2			
	Total	24 (69%)		Total	11 (31%)
Amputation group (24)	Hemipelvectomy	1		Shoulder amputation	2
	Disarticulation of hip	8		Disarticulation	2
	Above-knee amputation	6			
	Below-knee amputation	3			
	Rotationplasty	2			
	Total	20 (84%)		Total	4 (16%)

Materials and Methods

Distribution and Sites of Disease

Fifty-nine patients with malignant bone and soft tissue tumors, who were treated in our hospital from 1975 to 1986, were evaluated for present functional activity. The cases consisted of 43 osteosarcomas, four chondrosarcomas, three malignant fibrous histiocytomas, two malignant giant cell tumors, one Ewing's sarcoma, and six soft tissue sarcomas. Forty-four lesions were located in the lower extremities and 15 in the upper.

Surgical Modalities

The surgical modalities employed are shown in Table 1. In 24 cases of limb preservation for the lower extremity, prosthetic replacement of the limb was carried out in 21 patients (88%), and for the upper humerus in four of seven patients. For the distal radius, arthrodesis was done in all patients. The amputation group was composed of 24 patients.

Functional Evaluation

Initially, all of the 59 patients were functionally evaluated according to Enneking's criteria and were divided into two groups—a limb preservation group and an amputation group. For the purpose of supplementary understanding of the functional profile in addition to Enneking's criteria, we introduced ADL evaluation criteria. This system was based on an evaluation of seven primary daily-life factors. For the upper extremities, these were the ability: (a) to use chopsticks; (b) to button a shirt; (c) to put on and take off a T-shirt; (d) to put on socks; (e) to wash the face; (f) to comb hair; (g) to wring towel. For the lower extremities, these were the ability: (a) to walk fast; (b) to walk a long distance; (c) to go up and down stairs; (d) to stand up from the floor; (e) to put on trousers; (f) to put on socks; (g) to get in and out of the bath. The results of evaluation were excellent, good, fair, and poor, as in Enneking's system.

Table 2. Functional evaluation of the limb according to Enneking's criteria in 59 patients

	Average points in lower extremity (44)		Average points in upper extremity (15)	
	Limb-salvage group (24)	Amputation group (20)	Limb-salvage group (11)	Amputation group (4)
Motion	1.0	4.2	0	0
Pain	4.9	5.0	5.0	5.0
Stability	4.5	5.0	2.6	3.0
Deformity	2.9	5.0	2.0	5.0
Strength	3.7	0	2.5	0
Functional activity	2.2	2.2	2.2	1.0
Emotional acceptance	3.5	1.6	3.6	1.0

Results and Discussion

Results According to Enneking's Functional Evaluation Criteria

The 44 patients with surgically treated lower extremities eligible for evaluation were followed for at least 2 years (Table 2). Motion of the joint in the two groups undergoing lower extremity surgery showed quite different scores. The low score in the limb preservation group was attributed to the removal of a large amount of the muscle group surrounding the tumor and late effects of the radiation given to the tumor area. A marked difference in the score in the deformity category between the preservation and amputation groups was definitely dependent on the delayed growth of the limbs. Evaluation of strength in the amputated group was carried out in an identical manner to test the prosthesis. In 15 patients with surgical treatment of the upper extremity, motion of the joint was poorly maintained according to the score system in both the shoulder and wrist.

Results According to ADL Functional Evaluation Criteria

In 44 patients with a surgically treated lower extremity, the amputation group was superior to the other group in terms of two factors—the ability to walk a long distance and put on socks (Table 3). Limitation in the ability to walk a long distance in the limb preservation group was due to pain in the limb. On the other hand, the limb preservation group was significantly superior to the amputated group in terms of two factors—the ability to put on trousers and to get in and out of the tub. These two required standing capability of the affected limbs. In 15 patients with a surgically treated upper extremity, the limb preservation group was overwhelmingly superior to the amputated group according to the ADL functional evaluation.

Table 3. Functional evaluation of usefulness of the limb on ADL

	Limb-preservation surgery group	Amputation surgery group
Lower extremity		
Walk fast	4.3	3.8
Walk long way	4.5	4.9
Go up and down stairs	3.4	3.1
Stand up from floor	3.9	3.6
Put on trousers	4.6	3.4
Put on socks	4.1	4.4
Get in and out of bath	4.1	2.3
Upper extremity		
Use chopsticks	1.8	—
Button shirt	3.7	—
Put on and take off T-shirt	3.2	3.0
Put on socks	5.0	—
Wash face	2.1	—
Comb hair	1.2	—
Wring towel	3.2	—

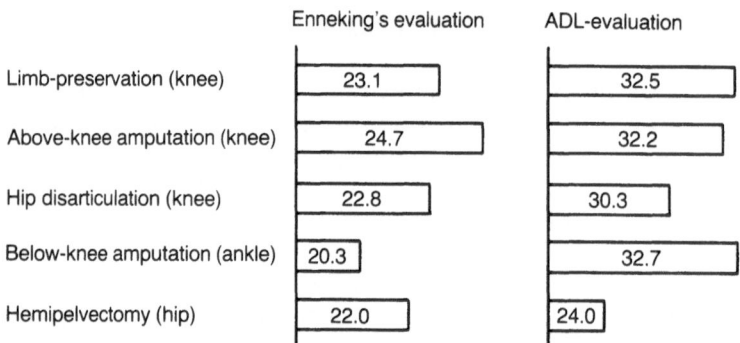

Fig. 1. Functional evaluation of lower extremity

Comparative Evaluation of Function by Both Criteria

Comparative evaluation of the function in the lower extremities was performed according to the criteria of both Enneking and ADL in each surgical modality (Fig. 1). Below-knee amputation received a low score with Enneking's criteria because of the extremely low score points given to a prosthetic ankle. On the other hand, with the ADL criteria, below-knee amputation gained a high score, because of the inherent limited function of the ankle joint. Therefore, the introduction of one aspect of evaluation of the affected joint, namely, optimal but minimal function of the joint concept to estimate the function of the joint is quite reasonable. In functional evaluation of the upper extremities, amputated limbs obtained higher points with Enneking's criteria than with the ADL criteria. Since the prosthesis of the upper extremity is useful only for cosmetic purposes it seems reasonable that the ADL score is lower.

Overall Results and Functional Evaluation of Limb Salvage for Osteosarcoma

Assessment and Proposed Reorganization of Functional Evaluation System

KATSURO TOMITA, YASUO AOTAKE, MAKOTO SUGIHARA, and HIROYUKI TSUCHIYA[1]

Summary. A report is presented of the Intergroup Study of Osteosarcoma by 22 university hospitals and cancer centers in Japan with an assessment and proposal for reorganization of the functional evaluation system. Between 1980 and 1985, 248 patients with osteosarcoma were treated and 105 patients (42.3%) underwent limb salvage surgery. For these cases, functional evaluation was studied in July 1987. The follow-up period was 2–7 years. The cumulative survival rate was 71.0% at 5 years in the limb salvage group, while in the amputation group it was 45.7%. The results of overall functional evaluation of the preserved limbs according to the standard system is that the number of cases rating excellent or good was relatively high in the 2- to 4-year follow-up period; however, this later decreased. Cases rating fair or poor increased after 4 years. Based on our data, we clarified a few problems in the present functional evaluation system and revised it; we separated physical function (factors 1–6) and mental evaluation (factor 7). We also put a higher value on factor 6 to attach importance to the whole preserved limb function. We believe that salvaged limbs are much more objectively evaluated by our new revised system.

Key words: Osteosarcoma—Limb salvage surgery—Functional evaluation

Introduction

Since 1980, when enthusiasm for limb salvage in osteosarcoma increased among Japanese orthopedic oncologists, the Intergroup Study of Osteosarcoma has been carried out by 22 university hospital and cancer centers in Japan. The purposes of this study are as follows: (a) study on the trend of limb salvage surgery in Japan, (b) functional evaluation of salvaged limbs, (c) clarification of the problems of Enneking's evaluation system, and (d) reorganization of functional evaluation system.

Materials

Between January 1980 and April 1985, 248 patients with osteosarcoma were treated, and 105 patients (42.3%) underwent limb salvage surgery [1]. In 1980,

[1] Bone Tumor Group, Department of Orthopaedic Surgery, Kanazawa University School of Medicine, Kanazawa, Japan

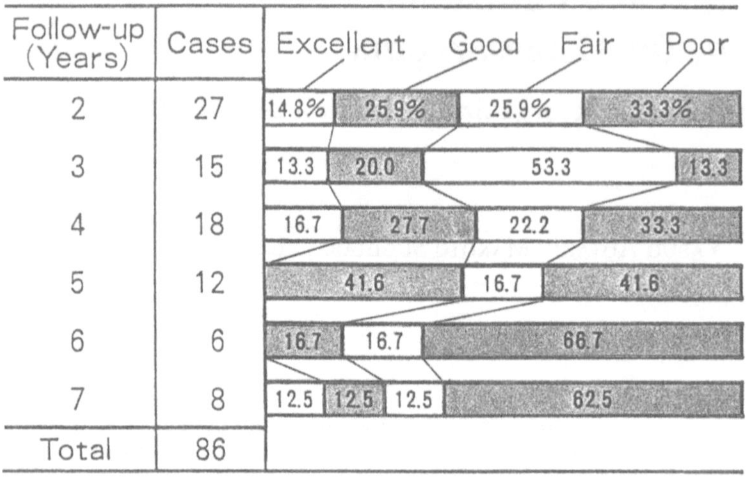

Follow-up (Years)	Cases	Excellent	Good	Fair	Poor
2	27	14.8%	25.9%	25.9%	33.3%
3	15	13.3	20.0	53.3	13.3
4	18	16.7	27.7	22.2	33.3
5	12		41.6	16.7	41.6
6	6	16.7	16.7		66.7
7	8	12.5	12.5	12.5	62.5
Total	86				

Fig. 1. Overall functional evaluation

16.7% of all osteosarcoma patients received limb salvage surgery; this figure had risen to 62% by 1985. Surgery was performed on 54 male and 51 female patients, and the average age was 19.7 years. The anatomical regions concerned were the proximal arm-shoulder-shoulder girdle (22 cases), distal forearm (one), proximal thigh-hip-pelvis (nine), proximal leg-knee-distal thigh (72), and distal leg (one). According to the surgical staging system, 90% of the patients were classified as IIB, and most of them received wide resection. Reconstruction was performed using a metal prosthesis in 43 cases (41.0%), ceramic prosthesis in 17 (16.2%), spacer in 16 (15.2%), bone graft in six (5.7%), and arthrodesis in two (1.9%). These cases were studied for functional evaluation in July 1987. The follow-up period was 2–7 years, the average being 38 months.

Results

The cumulative survival rate (Cutler-Ederer method) excluding stage III cases was 79.0% at 2 years and 71.0% at 5 years in the limb salvage group (101 cases), while in the amputation group (126 cases) it was 65.3% and 45.7%, respectively. The disease-free rate was 59%. Pulmonary metastasis was observed in 41% of cases and local recurrence was seen in 12.4% (13 cases).

The results of overall functional evaluation of the preserved limb by Enneking's system [2] are shown in Fig. 1. The number of cases rating excellent or good was relatively high in the 2-to 4-year follow-up period; however, this later decreased. Fair or poor cases increased after 4 years. These data indicate that the postoperative condition of the preserved limbs was relatively good for about 4 years. However, because of late complications, such as prosthesis destruction, loosening, or deep infection, the number of fair and poor cases subsequently increased, even though most of the limbs were able to be preserved. This figure will improve with the development of better prosthesis and surgical techniques.

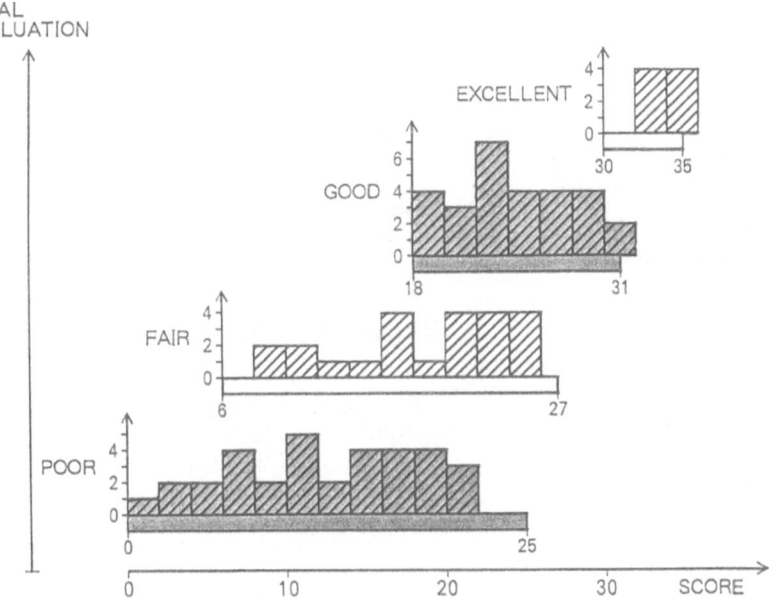

Fig. 2. Distribution of cases

Discussion

The better survival rate in the limb salvaged group is thought to be due to proper selection of cases for limb salvage operation. This was considered to be due to good local control by chemotherapy and radiotherapy, carefully planned surgery, and proper selection of patients in the early stage. On the other hand, the overall results of functional evaluation were not quite satisfactory, especially in long-term follow-up cases. Therefore, we recommend that certain developments be made, such as better material and design of the prosthesis, reduction of the surgical margin by intensive local control, further refinement of the surgical technique, and prevention of complications [3].

As we analyzed our data in detail based on this evaluation system, a few, but nevertheless unacceptable, problems became apparent. The overall evaluation in some cases was far from that which we expected. Firstly, the overall evaluation of "excellent," "good," "fair," or "poor" is not reflected accurately in the score system. "Excellent" can be scored in the range from 35 to 30 points in total, "good" from 31 to 18, "fair" from 27 to 6, and "poor" from 25 or less. Thus, the tolerance for each grade is too wide. In other words, the same score can be evaluated as "good," "fair," or even "poor." Our data shown in Fig. 2 demonstrate this inconsistency. Another question is whether these seven factors are equal in value. We believe that factors 1–6 reflect physical evaluation. Factor 7, emotional acceptance, reflects mental evaluation. Factor 7 can vary significantly according to how much the patient is aware of his disease and limb salvage operative techniques. These two elements, physical and mental, i.e.,

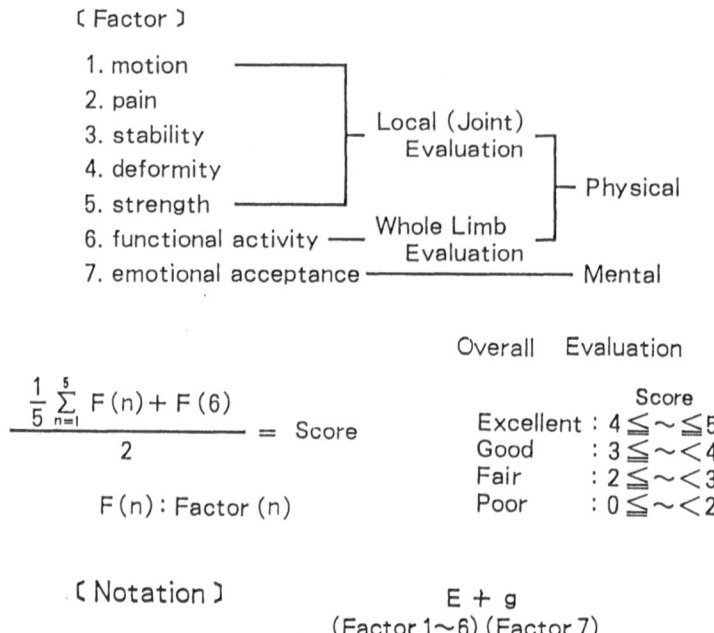

〔 Factor 〕

1. motion
2. pain
3. stability
4. deformity
5. strength   Local (Joint) Evaluation
6. functional activity — Whole Limb Evaluation
7. emotional acceptance ——————— Mental

Physical

Overall   Evaluation

$$\frac{\frac{1}{5}\sum_{n=1}^{5} F(n) + F(6)}{2} = Score$$

F(n) : Factor (n)

	Score
Excellent :	$4 \leqq \sim \leqq 5$
Good	: $3 \leqq \sim < 4$
Fair	: $2 \leqq \sim < 3$
Poor	: $0 \leqq \sim < 2$

〔 Notation 〕

E + g
(Factor 1~6) (Factor 7)

Fig. 3. Revised evaluation system

objective and subjective elements, cannot be evaluated together on the same scale. Furthermore, among the physical factors, 1–5 reflect local joint function, and factor 6 reflects the functional activity of the whole limb, which is the most important factor and of course the goal for limb salvage patients. For example, there are some cases including arthrodesis and the Tikhof-Linberg operation in which factors 1–5 are given lower scores and factor 6 gets a high score, resulting in lower total scores. We believe these cases should be evaluated higher.

For this reason, we propose a revised evaluation system. Scores are given in the same way as the standard system, such as "excellent" = 5, "good" = 3, "fair" = 1, and "poor" = 0, according to the rating in each evaluation factor. Then, the scores of factors 1–5 are calculated and mean values are obtained, which are again calculated with the score of factor 6, then divided by 2 to obtain mean values again; this thus gives more importance to functional activity. The overall rating is set up as shown in Fig. 3. Additionally, factor 7 is rated and noted in lowercase letters—e, g, f, and p. Thus, each case can be reported, e.g., E + g, G + p.

Case Presentation

Case 1. Osteosarcoma of the proximal humerus in a 13-year-old male was replaced by a ceramic prosthesis following wide resection. The overall evaluation by the standard system 3 years later was "poor" (EPFGPEE = P). However, by our new evaluation system it is "GOOD + e" with a score of 3.4 [(1/5(5 + 0 + 1 + 3 + 5) + 5)/2]. In fact, the patient is quite adept in operating a personal computer with his preserved arm and has hopes of becoming a professional computer operator.

Case 2. In the case of a 26-year-old male with an osteosarcoma on the distal tibia, vascularized bone graft with arthrodesis was performed after wide resection. The standard evaluation at the 2 year follow-up "poor" was (PEEEPEE = P), but by our new system, it is "excellent + e," with a score of 4.0 $((1/5(0 + 5 + 5 + 5 + 0) + 5)/2)$. At the 2-year follow-up the patients gait, even though the range of motion of the ankle joint was zero. He has returned to his former job as a blue collar worker and is quite satisfied with the results of the surgery.

In conclusion, with our revised evaluation system, physical function and mental evaluation are clearly separated, thus avoiding confusion. By putting a higher value on factor 6, the functional evaluation of the preserved limb as a whole is more clearly indicated. We hope that this paper will stimulate further advances in functional evaluation.

Acknowledgments. Other main co-workers at university hospitals (UH), cancer centers (CC), and national hospitals (NH) are (from north to south): S. Yamawaki (Sapporo NH), T. Yagi (Hokkaido UH), S. Ishii (Sapporo UH), H. Kakizaki (Hirosaki UH), N. Takada (Chiba CC), F. Endo (Chiba UH), H. Umeda (Kashiwa NH), A. Tateishi, S. Takeyama, H. Miki (Teikyo UH), S. Higaki (Tokyo UH), H. Kawano, S. Osaka (Nippon UH), S. Inoue (Juntendo UH), S. Takeuchi (Gifu UH), K. Shinjo (Nagoya NH), S. Tatezaki (Toyama UH), J. Uchida, H. Hayashi (Osaka UH), O. Inoue (Ryukyu UH), and A. Yokogawa (Kanazawa UH)

References

1. Tomita K et al. (1987) A trend of limb saving surgery for osteosarcoma from 1980 to 1985. Clin Orthop Surg 22: 1147–1153 (in Japanese)
2. Enneking WF (1986) A system of staging musculoskeletal neoplasms. Clin Orthop 204: 9–24
3. Tomita K (1985) Functional and device evaluations of patients with custom-made or modular-system tumor prosthesis in the lower extremity. In: Proceedings of international symposium on limb salvage in musculoskeletal oncology, Orlando, Oct. 1985. pp III-18–19

Chapter 2

Influence of Limb Salvage on the Rate of Long Term Survival in Malignant Tumors

A Multi-Institutional Cooperative Study of Osteosarcoma

Partial Report with Emphasis on Survival After Limb Salvage

JOHN C. IVINS[1], WILLIAM F. TAYLOR[2], and HELEN GOLENZER[2]

Summary. Malignant musculoskeletal tumors, notably osteosarcoma, continue to pose difficult problems in diagnosis and treatment. One medical institution is unlikely to see enough patients with osteosarcoma to provide material for an adequate study, hence, the attraction of cooperative multi-institutional studies.

Few clinical trials have been designed to compare treatments among randomly selected patients with osteosarcoma. The need for adequate controls or comparison groups is acknowledged, but having patients and physicians agree on randomization is extremely difficult, particularly in osteosarcoma. The question arises: How can we learn more about osteosarcoma, its management, and its survival prospects without randomization, utilizing only observational data?

These considerations led to the project "Exploratory Studies of Osteosarcoma Prognosis," in which 13 comprehensive cancer centers in the United States participated. The study cohort consisted of patients with osteosarcoma who were seen and treated during the period July 1977 to December 1982. All of the patients had tumors that fulfilled Dahlin's definition of osteosarcoma. The 13 centers provided 1005 patients, of whom 543 fulfilled all the study requirements.

Choosing variables carefully, we compared the expected outcome with the observed outcome. The observed and expected survival curves after amputation and after limb-salvage resection were essentially identical.

Key words: Osteosarcoma—Patient variables—Prediction of outcome

Introduction

Osteosarcoma has long presented major challenges that so far have been unresolved in spite of the efforts of knowledgeable persons. A retrospective study of osteosarcoma can be divided into the prechemotherapy and postchemotherapy periods and now, in addition, the emerging period of limb salvage.

At the base of the observation period were the early days, as when a destructive swelling was diagnosed as "sarcoma," and amputation was performed. Few of these patients survived more than 2 or 3 years [1]. Survival to 3 years ranged from near 0% to the 20s.

Department of Orthopedic[1] and Department of Health and Science Research[2], Mayo Clinic and Mayo Foundation, Rochester, MI, USA

During the late 1960s and early 1970s, the reports of Cortes et al. [2] and Jaffe [3] describing the use of doxorubicin and methotrexate, first for metastatic disease and later as ingredients of adjuvant treatment programs, maked a turning point for the better. Much has been accomplished since then, but many questions about the effectiveness of treatment remain unanswered.

Two decades have passed, during which a great many reports have been published, detailing a wide variety of studies of osteosarcoma, many of which are of fundamental importance. Key items in this new knowledge include the following:

a) The recognition of a dozen or more different types of osteosarcoma, each having its own peculiar biological behavior [4]

b) The design and general acceptance of logical staging schemes and the effort at developing a reliable uniform record system to assure the validity of comparisons among studies [5]

c) The increasing availability and reliability of sophisticated imaging techniques

d) The development of medical and surgical oncology training programs

e) The formation of organizations, such as the Musculoskeletal Tumor Society, which foster free interchange of experience and ideas

f) The proliferation of cooperative multiinstitutional studies

Saving life has always been the principal goal. An increasing effort to save the affected limb also has evolved whenever there is reasonable promise that such "limb salvage" will not decrease the chances of saving life. In recent years, treatment directed at limb salvage has become popular at cancer centers all over the world, and evidence is emerging concerning its efficacy in saving life and limb [6, 7].

We studied a group of patients with osteosarcoma in an attempt to determine if survival after surgical resection for limb salvage was different from survival after amputation. The study did not evaluate morbidity or functional results.

Any study has a number of inherent problems, among which are: a comparison of treatment requires sizeable samples, direct comparison of two groups treated differently may be fallacious, patients selected for one treatment may be different from those selected for another, and observed differences in treatment response may merely reflect patient differences [8].

Material and Methods

We present our data and the patient characteristics found to be associated with recurrence and death from osteosarcoma. We applied a method for comparing groups of patients who may differ with respect to their characteristics and their prognosis for survival from osteosarcoma.

A group of 13 comprehensive cancer centers pooled their data (Table 1). All centers were members of the Centralized Cancer Patient Date System (CCPDS) and had a uniform cancer data system based on cooperation and quality control. The records of all patients with osteosarcoma treated at these institutions from 1 July 1977 to 31 December 1982 were collected. These records were complete

Table 1. Comprehensive cancer centers participating (cooperating institutions)

Institution	Location
University of Alabama in Birmingham Comprehensive Cancer Center	Birmingham, AL
Columbia University Comprehensive Cancer Center	New York, NY
Comprehensive Cancer Center of Metropolitan Detroit	Detroit, MI
Duke Comprehensive Cancer Center, Duke University Medical Center	Durham, NC
Fred Hutchinson Cancer Research Center	Seattle, WA
Fox Chase/University of Pennsylvania Comprehensive Cancer Center	Philadelphia, PA
Illinois Cancer Council Comprehensive Cancer Center	Chicago, IL
Johns Hopkins Oncology Center	Baltimore, MD
NCI Designated Mayo Comprehensive Cancer Center	Rochester, MN
Roswell Park Memorial Institute	Buffalo, NY
Wisconsin Clinical Cancer Center	Madison, WI
UCLA Jonsson Comprehensive Cancer Center	Los Angeles, CA
Yale Comprehensive Cancer Center	New Haven, CT

because of the care taken in maintaining the data system; they do not reflect favorite subgroup of cases.

Of the patients, 91% were followed up for a minimum of 3 years; 9% were lost to follow-up. All cases were confirmed by microscopic study of the lesion, and all patients received at least part of the first definitive course of treatment at the cooperating institution. Morphological classification and anatomical site were those of the International Classification of Diseases Oncology (ICDO). A manual was developed, and data collection forms were constructed. As a further attempt to ensure uniformity, all the abstracting was done by professionals who received special training for this project. They repeatedly visited the cooperating institutions, examining case records and recording their findings on the data collection forms developed for this study. All the data were then edited and entered into a computer.

In an effort to achieve further uniformity, radiographs and representative pathology slides of the primary lesion were submitted to a "pathology center," where they were examined by a surgical pathologist and an oncological radiologist, both with much experience in evaluating osteosarcoma.

As another check on the accuracy of tissue interpretation, a panel of pathologists (Table 2) not primarily involved in the study visited the pathology center on two occasions and independently assessed the morphology and grade of randomly selected lesions.

To be certain that all cases of osteosarcoma were included in the study, there was a deliberate oversampling by including all cases of chondrosarcoma and fibrosarcoma. The total number of cases processed was 1005. Of these, 543 were confirmed by Dahlin's definition as osteosarcoma, i.e., the proliferating malignant cells were producing osteoid substance [4].

Table 2. Consulting pathologists participating in pathology confirmation study

Pathologist	Institute
Ayala, Alberto G.	MD Anderson Hospital and Tumor Institute, Texas Medical Center, Houston, TX
Dahlin, David C.	Section of Surgical Pathology, Mayo Clinic and Mayo Foundation, Rochester, MN
Dorfman, Howard D.	Albert Einstein College of Medicine, Bronx, New York, NY
Fechner, Robert E.	Department of Pathology, University of Virginia Medical Center, Charlottesville, VA
Huvos, Andrew	Department of Pathology, Memorial Center for Cancer, New York, NY
Mirra, Joseph M.	Division of Surgical Pathology, UCLA School of Medicine, Los Angeles, CA
Spjut, Harlan J.	Baylor College of Medicine, Texas Medical Center, Houston, TX
Unni, K. Krishnan	Section of Surgical Pathology, Mayo Clinic and Mayo Foundation, Rochester, MN

Results and Discussion

Comparison of Amputation and Resection

Because attempts at limb salvage nearly always involve tumors of the humerus, femur, or proximal tibia or fibula, the study concentrated on these sites.

The 3-year survival rate was 52% for the 227 patients with osteosarcoma who underwent resection and 41% for the 119 patients with osteosarcoma who underwent amputations (Fig. 1); the difference for survival to 3 years was statistically significant ($P = 0.02$). The question is: Could the difference be due to differences in the patients and not in the treatment?

A principal goal of this study was to determine, if possible, whether or not certain patient characteristics (or variables) were predictive of length of survival. A study of survival curves of several subgroups of patients revealed that nearly all differences in survival were found only during the first 3 years after surgery. Therefore, we chose the death rate R (or the progression rate) for the first 3 years as an index of risk of death from osteosarcoma (or progression of osteosarcoma) and used it in the evaluation of possible prognostic variables. Because the usual index is in terms of survival, we also considered the expected 3-year survival percentage P_3 obtained from the death rate R by the expression $P(3) = e^{-3R}$. (This is a reliable approximation for the first 3 years and reflects the assumption of "exponential" survival.)

From an extensive list that was entered into the record system, the prognostically useful variables were chosen. These variables were chosen on the basis of our general knowledge of osteosarcoma and its biological behavior, as well as of some variables that we thought were important on the basis of our experience. Some, such as patient age and sex, anatomical site of tumor, diameter of tumor, morphology of tumor, duration of symptoms, stage of disease, and treatment modality, were chosen on the basis of earlier findings.

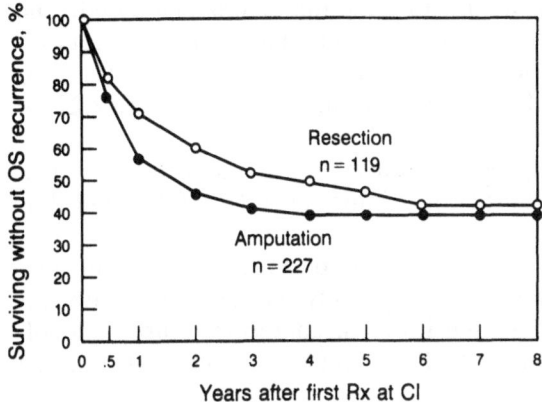

Fig. 1. Observed survival to first recurrence of osteosarcoma (*OS*) for 227 patients with amputation and 119 with resection (limb salvage). At 3 years, survival rates were 41% and 52%, respectively ($P = 0.02$; log-rank test based on first 3 years only)

The study began with approximately 40 variables excluding treatment. After each variable was studied separately, about half were deleted because either they did not indicate a significant association or there were too few patients with each variable to study. The Cox stepwise regression method was applied to the remaining variables to determine their significance [9, 10].

The first analysis revealed a set of variables and their regression coefficients that were significantly predictive of death from osteosarcoma. The second analysis revealed a set of variables that wer significantly predictive of disease progression. As expected, these sets overlapped considerably.

The score that was predictive of death from osteosarcoma is defined as follows:

Death score = +1.30, if morphology class was Paget's disease
-1.49, if morphology class was juxtacortical
$+1.95$, if distant metastasis was present at admission
$+0.77$, if regional spread of disease was present at admission (no metastasis)
$+0.50$, if tumor site was head (not jaws), body, humerus, or proximal femur
$+0.77$, if tumor size was more than 20 cm or surgery was not done
$+0.47$, if patient age was more than 50 years
$+0.47$, if weight loss was 10 lb (4.5 kg) or more
$+1.03$, if duration of symptoms was less than 12 months
$+0.71$, if time from diagnosis to treatment was less than 1 month
$+0.41$, if number of symptoms was more than four
$+2.27$, if there was no erythema at primary site

Illustrative example. A 17-year-old boy had an osteoblastic osteosarcoma of the distal femur. The tumor involved both bone and soft tissue and was 15 cm in maximal diameter. The patient had not lost weight and had symptoms for 5 months. Treatment was started on the day that the tumor was diagnosed. The patient had three symptoms and no erythema. Tabulation of these factors resulted in the patient having a score of 4.07 for death from osteosarcoma (0.77 for regional spread, 1.03 for duration of symptoms less than 12 months, and 2.27 for no erythema).

The absence of tumor grade as a prognostic variable was unexpected; we had found tumor grade to be only of "borderline" importance ($P = 0.06$) and thus excluded it.

Erythema at the primary site was of borderline importance for death in spite of being recorded for only 21 patients, of whom only one died. We have not seen this reported before and suggest that it be considered in future data collections from patients with osteosarcoma. The immunity implications may be of importance.

The score significantly related to progression of disease is defined as:
Progression score = +1.05, if morphology class was Paget's disease
$\qquad$ −1.68, if morphology class was juxtacortical
$\qquad$ +0.77, if distant metastasis was present
$\qquad$ +0.53, if regional spread of disease was present at admission (no metastasis)
$\qquad$ +0.35, if tumor site was head (not jaws), body, humerus, or proximal femur
$\qquad$ +0.57, if tumor size was more than 20 cm or surgery was not done
$\qquad$ +1.04, if tumor was of high or unknown grade
$\qquad$ +0.45, if weight loss was 10 lb (4.5 kg) or more
$\qquad$ +0.76, if duration of symptoms was less than 12 months
$\qquad$ +0.45, if time from diagnosis to treatment was less than 1 month

In this score, high grade appears as a strongly deleterious variable, but patient age, presence of erythema, and number of symptoms were not significant and were deleted.

Interpretation of Scores: Relation to Death Rate

The scores for all 543 patients in the study ranged from 0.78 to 9.00, with a median of 4.78 (Fig. 2). Most scores were between 3.00 and 7.00.

When the range of scores was divided into intervals and then for each interval, and the 3-year death rate was computed and plotted (logarithmic scale), the significance of the score became clear. The death rate was closely related to score, and the expected death rate is represented by the straight line in Fig. 3. If a patient had a score of 4.07, as in the example above, the expected death rate, shown on the scale on the left in Fig. 3, was 5.9/100 person-years. The expected 3-year survival was 84%, as seen on the scale on the right in Fig. 3. The expected group death rate and the expected group 3-year survival percentage or the expected survival curve can be obtained for both the group with amputation and the group with resection (Fig. 4).

The expected 3-year survival was worse for the group with amputation (35%) than for the group with resection (52%). This difference reflects the fact that

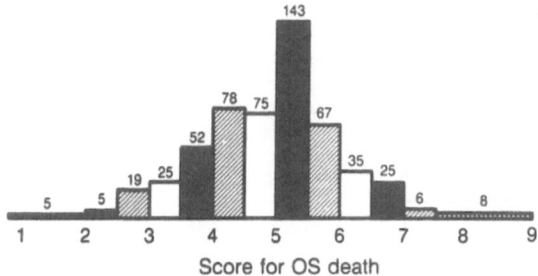

Fig. 2. Distribution of scores for death from osteosarcoma (*OS*) for all 543 patients in the study. The patients presented here are subgroups, and the scores apply to them as well as to this total

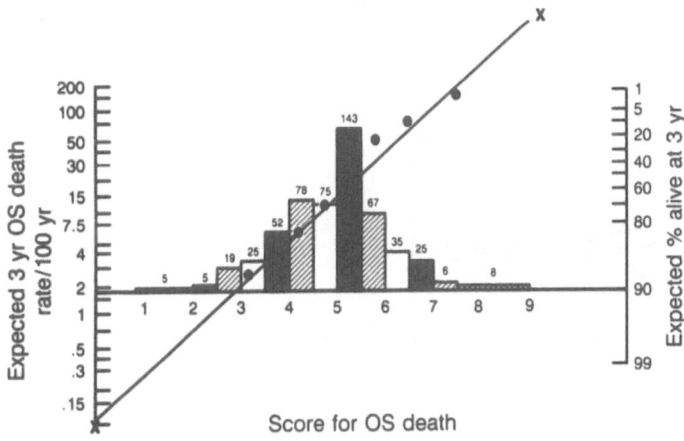

Fig. 3. Distribution of scores for death from osteosarcoma (*OS*) for all 543 patients in the study. The scores were grouped (<4, 4–4.5, 4.5–5, 5.5–6, 6–7, 7–9), and for each group the 3-year death rate and the mean score were computed. Each *dot* represents the logarithm of a group rate plotted at the corresponding mean score for the group. The *straight line* shows the relation ^{l}n rate $= {^{l}n}\lambda_0 +$ score. On the *right* is the *scale* that translated the death rate R to the expected 3-year survival. $P(3) = e^{-3R}$

patients with amputation have a higher score (mean 5.8) than patients with resection (mean, 5.4). Thus, the difference in score alone leads to a sizeable difference in survival. The observed difference in survival at 3 years, which was considered significant, now can be explained as a difference in the patients themselves, as revealed through their scores. Thus, we cannot justify a treatment effect. We argue that if an observed treatment effect is explainable by patient differences, then a treatment effect was not demonstrated and the effect would seem to be inconsequential.

We examined the same patients, using death from osteosarcoma instead of osteosarcoma progression. There was no significant difference in either the

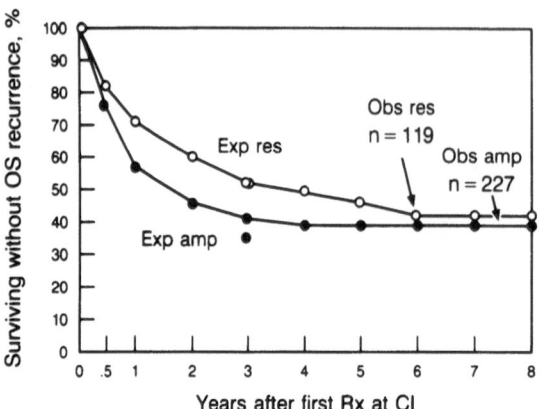

Fig. 4. Observed survival to first recurrence of osteosarcoma (*OS*) for 227 patients with amputation and 119 with resection (limb salvage). Three-year expected survival rates are also shown

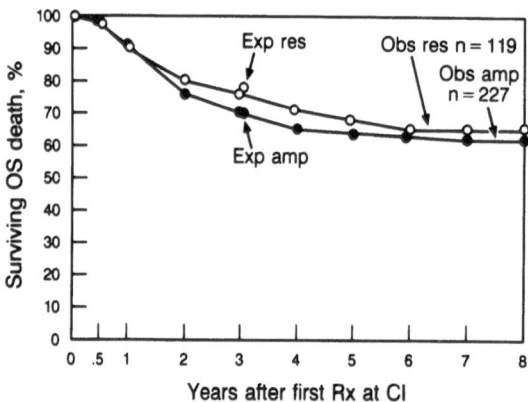

Fig. 5. Observed survival to death from osteosarcoma (*OS*) for 227 patients with amputation and 119 with resection. Three-year expected survival rates are also shown

observed 3-year survival rates or the expected 3-year survival rates (Fig. 5).

Because many data on "classic high-grade osteosarcoma" are available, we examined this subgroup of 237 cases, 52 of resection and 185 of amputation. A comparison of these subgroups revealed no appreciable differences either for osteosarcoma recurrence or death from osteosarcoma.

Conclusions

This study indicated that survival after resection for limb salvage was similar to that after amputation when the patient's scores were taken into account. A continuing examination into patient variables and characteristics is indicated. This should be done as a multi-institutional effort, with carefully structured data collection and recording and analysis methods. In addition to the usual variables already examined, a new study should include immunological profiling, viral studies, and perhaps others. As this is an early report of work in progress, the definitive papers on this study are still in preparation. Information can be obtained about them by writing to the authors.

References

1. Marcove RC, Mike V, Hajek JV, Levin AG, Hutter RV (1971) Osteogenic sarcoma in childhood. NY State J Med 71: 855–859
2. Cortes EP, Holland JF, Wang JJ, Sinks LF (1972) Doxorubicin in disseminated osteosarcoma. JAMA 221: 1132–1138
3. Jaffe N (1972) Recent advances in the chemotherapy of metastatic osteogenic sarcoma. Cancer 30: 1627–1631
4. Dahlin DC, Unni KK (1986) Bone tumors: general aspects and data on 8,542 cases, 4th edn. Thomas, Springfield, p 286
5. Enneking WF, Spanier SS, Goodman MA (1980) Current concepts review. The surgical staging of musculoskeletal sarcoma. J Bone Joint Surg (Am) 62: 1027–1030
6. Consensus Conference (1985) Limb-sparing treatment of adult soft-tissue sarcomas and osteosarcomas. JAMA 254: 1791–1794
7. Simon MA, Aschliman MA, Thomas N, Mankin HJ (1986) Limb-salvage treatment versus amputation for osteosarcoma of the distal end of the femur. J Bone Joint Surg (Am) 68: 1331–1337
8. Taylor WF, Ivins JC, Pritchard DJ, Dahlin DC, Gilchrist GS, Edmonson JH (1985) Trends and variability in survival among patients with osteosarcoma: a 7-year update. Mayo Clin Proc 60: 91–104
9. Cox DR (1972) Regression models and life-tables. JR Stat Soc (B) 34: 187–202
10. Kaplan EL, Meier P (1958) Nonparametric estimation from incomplete observations. J Am Stat Assoc 53: 457–481

Limb Salvage for Osteosarcoma

Michael A. Simon[1]

Summary. Though limb salvage increases the local recurrence rate to 10%, it does not appear to affect disease-free and long-term survival rates adversely. When perfomed by experienced surgeons using wide surgical margins with adjuvant or neoadjuvant chemotherapy, there is no risk of increased mortality. Unless there are significant factors preventing wide surgical margins, most patients should be considered candidates for this procedure.

Key words: Limb Salvage—Local recurrence—Long-term survival rate

Five issues need to be addressed when considering limb salvage instead of amputation for osteosarcoma of the extremities. Is there any decrease in survival with limb salvage when compared with amputation? What are the differences in the immediate morbidity between the two surgical procedures? What is the durability of the reconstructions and the delayed morbidity of each type of limb salvage surgical procedure? How does the salvaged limb function when compared with amputation at the homologous anatomical site? Lastly, are there any psychosocial benefits for patients who have limb salvage instead of amputation? I will only address the impact of limb salvage on the incidence and consequences of local recurrence, the length of the disease-free interval, and the rate of long-term survival for patients who have osteosarcoma of the extremities.

Recent single institutional studies have found that limb salvage while possibly increasing the local recurrence rate to 10% (almost exclusively in femur tumors) does not seem to have an adverse impact on disease-free and long-term survival rates. These studies have the distinct disadvantage of observer bias, small patient accrual, variable anatomical sites and patient ages included in the study, and significant patient selection. However, each institution had fairly consistent adjuvant or neoadjuvant chemotherapy regimens, pathological support, and surgical strategy for limb salvage and thoracotomy.

One multi-institutional study also confirms data that limb salvage will also have about a 10% local recurrence rate for distal femur osteosarcomas. But, again, there is little, if any, compromise of disease-free or long-term survival

---

[1]University of Chicago Medical Center, Chicago, IL, USA

rates compared with amputation. Again, although the study was nonrandomized, observer bias and patient selection were diluted by the inclusion of many
institutions. In addition, when compared with single-institutional studies, this
study had the advantage of investigating over a short period of time a large
number of patients who were under the age of 30 years and who had tumors at
only one anatomical site. The disadvantage of the study was the variability of the
chemotherapy regimens administered, the lack of a central pathological review,
and the potential variability in the surgical technique and strategy for limb
salvage and thoracotomy.

In spite of the potential drawbacks to the above studies, it appears that limb
salvage when performed by experienced surgeons with wide surgical margins in
an adjuvant or neoadjuvant chemotherapy setting does not cause a significantly
increased rate of death. Therefore, unless there are significant factors which
preclude the achievement of wide surgical margins, such as an extensive tumor,
anatomical locations that have significant technical problems (i.e., distal tibia),
or markedly displaced pathological fractures, most patients are candidates for
limb salvage if they and their families understand the ambiguities of the other
four issues.

Limb Salvage Versus Amputation for Malignant Tumors Other Than Osteogenic Sarcoma

Jeffrey J. Eckardt[1,2], Frederick R. Eilber[2,3], Gerald Rosen[4], Michael H. Kody[1], Joseph M. Mirra[5], and F.J. Dorey[1]

Summary. Seventy-seven patients with malignant tumors other than osteosarcoma were treated at UCLA between 1973 and 1987. Chondrosarcoma (39 cases), Ewing's sarcoma (19 cases), and a third group composed primarily of fibrosarcoma and MFH were identified. Amputation was used as the surgical means of local control in only 6% (5/77) of the patients. Limb sparing surgery was performed in 94% (72/77), generally in conjunction with adjuvant protocols. Of the limb salvage patients, 32% experienced some sort of complication, of whom only 15 required additional surgery. Only one limb salvage patient went on to have an amputation and no deaths were associated with the limb salvage procedures. Local recurrence was observed in 4.2% (3/72) of patients undergoing limb salvage and 20% (1/5) of those undergoing primary amputation. The Musculoskeletal Tumor Society's functional analysis revealed a 50% good to excellent rating in the limb salvage group, with the best results seen in intercalary and partial resection-reconstructions. Endoprosthetic reconstructions generally resulted in improved function when compared with their amputation counterparts who receive an obligatory "poor" by this schema. Kaplan-Meier survivor analysis for the 72 limb salvage patients revealed a 1- and 2-year survival for Ewing's patients of 78% and 32%, respectively; for chondrosarcoma, it was 97% at 1 year and 69% at 5 years, and for the FS/MFH group it was 70% at 1 year and 40% at 5 years. Chemotherapy as applied in this present chondrosarcoma group did not give any survival advantage and has been deleted from present chondrosarcoma protocols. Careful longitudinal follow-up of both the oncological outcome and reconstruction techniques will be important to determine where each limb salvage technique should be utilized.

Key words: Endoprosthesis—Limb salvage—Malignant bone tumor

Introduction

The traditional approach to skeletal tumors other than osteosarcoma has, like osteosarcoma, been amputation. Seventy-seven patients with malignant bone tumors other than osteosarcoma who have been treated at the UCLA Center for Health Sciences since 1973 were reviewed. Chondrosarcoma, Ewing's sarcoma,

Division of Orthopaedic Surgery[1], Jonsson Comprehensive Cancer Center[2], Division of Surgical Oncology[3], Department of Pediatrics[4], and Department of Surgical Pathology[5], UCLA Center for the Health Sciences, Los Angeles, CA, USA

fibrosarcoma, and malignant fibrohistiocytoma comprised the most common histological types and these groups were analyzed separately in terms of the means of primary surgical control, survival, and function. Of the 77 patients, 72 (94%) underwent primary limb salvage procedures for control of the primary lesion, whereas only five patients (6%) underwent primary amputation. As anticipated, survival, function, and adjuvant treatments varied considerably between the histological groups. Functional analyses were made on available patients utilizing the Musculoskeletal Tumor Society functional analysis [1].

Methods and Materials

A retrospective analysis was made of 77 patients with malignant bone tumors, other than osteosarcoma, treated at the UCLA Center for the Health Sciences between March 1973 and March 1987. Three histological groupings were identified: chondrosarcoma ($n = 39$), Ewing's sarcoma ($n = 19$), and a third group of 19 patients made up of 11 patients with fibrosarcoma, four with malignant fibrocystiocytoma (MFH), three with leiomyosarcoma, and a single patient with an undifferentiated bone sarcoma (hereafter referred to as the FS/MFH group). The 39 patients with chondrosarcoma consisted of 15 females and 24 males who ranged in age from 17 to 80 years and had a mean age of 52 years. The 19 patients with Ewing's sarcoma consisted of ten females and nine males, ranging in age from 6 to 38 years with a mean age of 21 years. The FS/MFH group with 19 patients had nine females and ten males, ranging in age from 25 to 72 years with a mean of 53 years. Location of the primary tumor at presentation was the ilium in 25 patients, femur in 23, scapula in ten, humerus in six, tibia in five, pubis in three, ischium in two, and in single instances the sacrum, radius, and metacarpal. The Musculo-skeletal Tumor Society stage and grade at presentation is presented in Table 1. Nineteen patients had low-grade lesions (IA five patients, IB 14), and 58 patients had high-grade lesions (IIA two patients, IIB 46, III ten). Seven of the 67 patients with localized disease actually presented with local recurrences, having been treated elsewhere prior to presenting at UCLA; they did not have metastases at presentation.

Adjuvant radiation and chemotherapy varied both within and between the histological groups. Of the 39 patients with chondrosarcoma, 16 received preoperative intra-arterial doxorubicin (90 mg) over 3 days followed by 17.5 Gy in five fractions [2, 3]. Only one patient with chondrosarcoma received immediate postoperative adjuvant chemotherapy, and this was because of positive surgical margins. Since 1984, patients with chondrosarcoma have not received pre- or postoperative adjuvant therapy except for two patients who received neutron radiation preoperatively.

All 19 patients with Ewing's sarcoma received preoperative adjuvant chemotherapy and 18 received 30–66 Gy preoperatively. Of the 19 Ewing's patients, 18 received post-operative chemotherapy (one patient refused). Since 1984, patients with Ewing's sarcoma have received a standardized adjuvant protocol. Four cycles of chemotherapy are combined with a reduced dose of radiation introduced after the first phase of the first cycle. Phase 1 of the first cycle consists of cyclo-phsophamide (1200 mg/m^2) on day 1, doxorubicin (30 mg/m^2) on

Table 1. Stage and grade at presentation according to Enneking and Musculoskeletal Tumor Society

Stage	Chondrosarcoma ($n = 39$)	Ewing's ($n = 19$)	FS/MFH ($n = 19$)	Total ($n = 77$)
IA	5	0	1	5
IB	13	0	1	14
IIA	0	0	2	2
IIB	20	14	12	46
III	1	5	4	10

days 1 and 2, and methotrexate (18 mg/m^2) on days 1 and 2. This is followed after 3 weeks by phase 2: cyclophosphamide (1200 mg/m^2) on 2 consecutive days. After 3 weeks phase 3 (the same combination chemotherapy as phase 1) is given to complete cycle 1. After the initial phase of cycle 1, radiation therapy is begun at 180–200 cGy/day. This is administered five times a week until a total whole bone dose of 40–45 Gy is reached. An additional three cycles of chemotherapy are administered for a total of four cycles or 12 treatments. There is generally a 3- to 4-week rest between the cycles. Surgery is generally introduced between the first and second or the second and third cycles, depending on the size of the primary tumor, its location, and the intended means of reconstruction. When excision with soft tissue reconstruction alone is to be the surgical procedure, it is generally done between the first and the second cycles. When an endoprosthesis is to be used for reconstruction, surgery is then done between the second and third of the four cycles.

Of the 19 patients in the FS/MFH group, 16 had preoperative chemo- and radiation therapy (90 mg intra-arterial doxorubicin over 3 days and radiation—17.5 Gy in eight patients, 22.8 Gy in four patients, 35 Gy in three patients, and 50 Gy in one patient). Only six received immediate postoperative chemotherapy—doxorubicin, doxorubicin and methotrexate, doxorubicin and BCD (bleomycin, cyclophosphamide, and dactinomycin), Rosen T-10 protocol, CYVADIC (cyclophosphamide, vincristine, adriamycin, and dacarbazine), and methotrexate with doxorubicin and cis-platinum. Since 1984, patients with fibrosarcoma or MFH primary of bone have been treated with our osteosarcoma protocols. Preoperatively, they receive methotrexate, 8–10 gm/m^2 for adults and 12 gm/m^2 for children followed after 2 weeks by a course of bleomycin (20 mg/m^2/day) for 2 days, cyclophosphamide (600 mg/m^2/day) for 2 days, and dactinomycin (0.6 mg/m^2/day) for 2 days. This is followed after 2 weeks by another course of methotrexate with two additional methotrexate courses at weekly intervals prior to surgery. If histological review of the surgical specimen reveals a complete response (100% tumor necrosis), the patients receive an abbreviated postoperative course of a single cycle of BCD followed after 2 weeks by two courses of methotrexate with a 1-week interval. Incomplete responders, those with less than 100% tumor necrosis, receive six cycles of doxorubicin and cis-platinum. Each cycle consists of doxorubicin (60 mg/m^2) over 48 h and cis-platinum (120 mg/m^2) with a manitol diuresis. This cycle is repeated every 3 weeks for six cycles.

Patients generally received additional radiation, chemotherapy, and slected surgery when progression of disesase was observed.

Limb salvage procedures were performed via a longitudinal incision, ellipsing previous biopsy sites. The neurovascular bundles were dissected free in the sub-adventitial plane and the resections that were routinely intracompartmental and intra-articular were carried out in a manner aimed at achieving wide margins at all times. All the pathological study was reviewed by one of us (JM) at the Department of Surgical Pathology at UCLA and survival analyses were based on the Kaplan-Meier survivorship plots [4].

Results

Of the 77 patients, 72 (94%) underwent primary limb salvage procedures. Following resection, 34 underwent endoprosthetic reconstruction, two underwent allograft reconstruction, and in one a knee arthrodesis was performed. Nineteen patients had excision alone of the involved part and 16 underwent total internal hemipelvectomy, including the hip joint, for primary pelvic lesions. Of the 34 endoprosthetic reconstructions, there were eight proximal femoral replacements, six distal femoral replacements, six scapula-total shoulder replacements, five proximal humeral replacements, three total femur replacements, and there were single instances of a total humerus replacement, proximal tibia replacement, an intercalary endoprosthesis, expandable total femur, expandable proximal femoral replacement, and expandable total humerus replacement; the latter three were in skeletally immature Ewing's patients. Allograft reconstruction and resection arthrodesis have not been performed at UCLA since 1979 for patients with malignant bone tumors.

Of the 72 limb salvage patients, 72 (68%) were without any complications; 23 of the 72 (32%) had a total of 28 complications. Wound dehiscence was the most requent and seen in 11 patients. Local recurrence was seen in three (4.2%), positive margins in two, deep endoprosthetic infection in two, and there were single instances of extremity edema, hip fracture, total femur replacement dislocation at the hip, perforated diverticulum, temporary peroneal palsy, nonfatal pulmonary embolism, femoral nerve entrapment following internal hemipelvectomy, dural leak, proximal femoral osteomyelitis in a distal femoral replacement, and a nonunion of a knee arthrodesis. Only the patient with a nonunion of a knee arthrodesis went on to amputation. The patient with the proximal femoral osteomyelitis was converted to a total femur replacement. Of the 28 complications, 15 were treated with surgical measures and the remainder were managed with medical treatment, radiation, and/or chemotherapy or observation. Forty-three of the limb salvage patients had adequate data for evaluation. Excellent results were seen in eight, good in 13, fair in 13, and poor in nine (Table 2).

Amputation was utilized as the primary surgical means of local control in only five patients (6%) in this series. A total of three hemipelvectomies and two above-the-knee amputations were carried out, all for stage IIB lesions. The histology was chondrosarcoma in four and MFH in one. Three lesions were located in the ilium and two in the proximal tibia. Three patients had received pre- and postoperative adjuvant chemotherapy. Three died of progressive disease at 17, 31, and 41 months and two remain continuously disease-free at 11 and 29

Table 2. Musculoskeletal Tumor Society functional rating for the 43 limb salvage procedures for nonosteosarcoma primary bone malignancies according to location and type of reconstruction

	Excellent	Good	Fair	Poor
Knee				
Distal Femoral endo.	2	1	2	0
Excision	1	0	0	0
Proximal tibial endo.	0	1	0	0
Arthrodesis	0	0	0	1
Shoulder				
Total/proximal humeral endo.	0	0	3	2
Scapula-total shoulder endo.	0	4	2	0
Scapulectomy	0	0	0	2
Partial scapulectomy	1	0	0	0
Tikhor-Linberg	0	0	0	1
Hip				
Partial pelvic resection	2	1	2	1
Internal hemipelvectomy	0	0	2	1
Proximal femoral endo.	1	6	2	0
Total femoral endo.	0	0	0	1
Intercalary femoral endo.	1	0	0	0
Total	8	13	13	9

endo. endoprosthesis

months. One hemipelvectomy patient with an iliac wing primary had a local recurrence that was treated with palliative chemotherapy. The only other complication in the amputation group was a dural leak, which was treated surgically. All five of the amputees received a poor rating on the Musculoskeletal Tumors Society rating system.

Follow-up for the 77 patients ranged from 1 to 133 months. At the last follow-up, 25 had died of disease progression: chondrosarcoma in 12, Ewing's in five, FS/MFH in eight Three patients remain alive with disease, one from each histological group. Two patients are alive without disease postthoracotomy. Forty-seven patients (61%) remain continuously disease-free: chondrosarcoma in 25, Ewing's in 13, and FS/MFH in nine. The median follow-up for the continuously disease-free patients was 36 months for those with chondrosarcoma, 8 months for those with Ewing's, and 37 months for the FS/MFH group.

Survival for the 72 patients undergoing limb sparing surgery was estimated by Kaplan-Meier survival curves (Fig. 1). For the 19 patients with Ewing's sarcoma, the survival was 78% at 1 year and 32% at 2 years. For the 35 patients with chondrosarcoma who underwent primary limb sparing surgery, the survival was 97% at 1 year, 74% at 2 years, and 69% at 5 years. For the 18 limb salvage patients with FS/MFH, the survival was 70% at 1 year, 54% at 3 years, and 40% at 5 years. Pre- and postoperative adjuvant treatments added no statistical survival advantage for patients with chondrosarcoma.

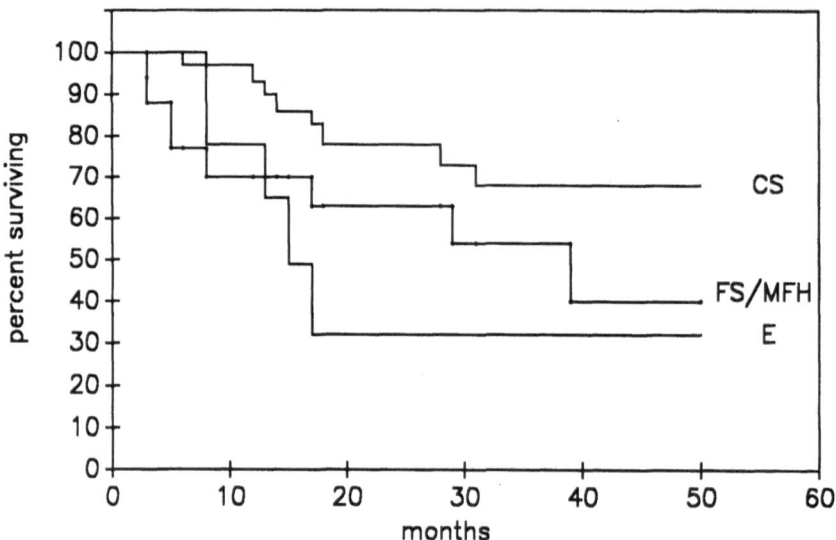

Fig. 1. Kaplan-Meier survival curves for limb salvage patients according to histological type. *CS* chondrosarcoma ($n = 35$), *FS* fibrosarcoma/MFH ($n = 18$), *E* Ewing's sarcoma ($n = 18$)

Discussion

Only 5 of the 77 patients in this retrospective analysis had amputation as the primary treatment for the malignant bone tumor. The two complications in this group consisted of a single instance of local recurrence and a single instance of a dural leak, both after a hemipelvectomy. All these patients whether the utilized a prosthesis or not received a poor rating on the Musculoskeletal Tumor Society (MSTS) rating because amputees receive a poor evaluation in the deformity and strength categories. In general, patients who undergo amputation surgery adapt to their disability, though they generally would have preferred limb sparing surgery should the result be uncomplicated.

The small numbers within the histological group precluded survival analysis with regard to adjuvant therapy except for those patients with chondrosarcoma where no survival advantage was seen for those receiving adjuvant therapy, leaving wide surgical resection as the only therapeutic regimen effective for this histological group.

The role of surgery in the management of Ewing's sarcoma patients had recently evolved to the point where it is now felt that removal of the involved bone is desirable whenever possible [5]. This is based on reports of persistent disease at the primary site in spite of the best adjuvant chemotherapy and high-dose radiation, concern of secondary malignancies in long-term Ewing's survivors, problems with the management of late Ewing's pathological fractures, and because of evidence of improved survival in patients undergoing surgical excision of the primary tumor [6–8]. Until recently, the only surgical option for management of these skeletally immature patients was amputation. Now, however, rotationplasty or reconstruction with an expandable endoprosthesis gives the

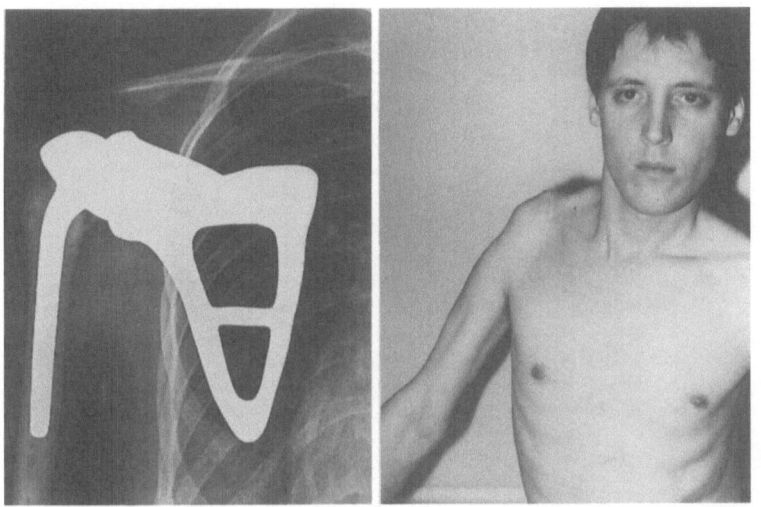

a   b

Fig. 2. a Postoperative radiographic and **b** clinical photograph demonstrating active abduction 1 year following total scapula-total shoulder implantation for a IIA fibrosarcoma of the scapula

treating surgeons other surgical options for the skeletally immature child [9, 10].

A wide variety of limb salvage procedures were performed on these 72 patients. Resection arthrodesis and allograft reconstruction have not been used at this institution since 1979 because of our unsatisfactory results with these techniques [2, 3]. The only patient in this limb salvage series undergoing amputation was the resection arthrodesis of the knee, which was done for nonunion. Intercalary reconstructions, whether it be an endoprosthesis or an allograft, routinely result in excellent functional results because the joints proximal and distal tend not to be involved. Total femur and total humeral functional results are hampered by the necessity of rehabilitating two joints in the series with one generally turning out fair to poor and the other joint good to fair. In spite of the fact that the hand and elbow are retained, the Tikhor-Linberg reconstruction leaves a significant cosmetic deformity and the instability of the shoulder girdle coupled with poor motion and poor strength results in an overall poor functional evaluation. Proximal humeral replacements generally rate only a fair result because of the tendency for subluxation, limited active motion, and limited power. Total scapular replacement in conjunction with total shoulder resurfacing gave good results in four and fair results in two, an improvement over the Tikhor-Linberg resection because of the enhanced stability of the shoulder girdle (Fig. 2). Partial scapulectomy as well as partial pelvic resection tend to result in good to excellent result. Total internal hemipelvectomies as well as major pelvic resections that retain the hip joint achieve only a fair rating at best on the MSTS evaluation score because of shortening and lack of strength. Yet they remain an improvement over amputation not only because of the psychological advantage of the retained extremity but because of improved function, in so far as younger patients can eventually become free of ambulatory aids. Routinely good results are

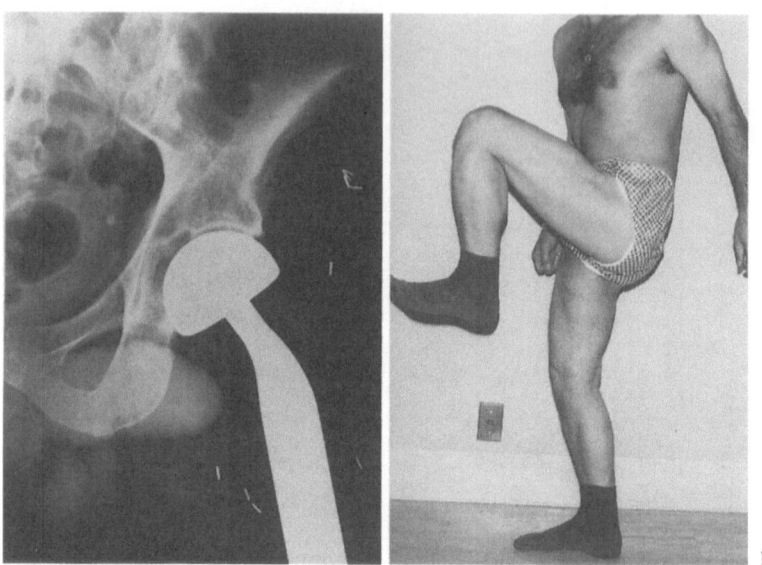

a   b

Fig. 3. a Postoperative radiograph and **b** clinical photograph demonstrating 130° of active hip flexion with good (+) strength 1 year after replacement of the proximal 32 cm of the femur with a proximal femoral endoprosthesis for IIA fibrosarcoma

seen with proximal femoral replacements where the majority of patients eventually learn to abduct with fair strength and ambulate without ambulatory aids (Fig. 3). The poor results in this series were most often associated with local complications, advanced age, deteriorating health associated with progression of disease, or a lack of effort on the patient's part. Typically, a total internal hemipelvectomy in a young, otherwise healthy patient can result in an individual who has no pain, requires only a shoe lift, and who ambulates without ambulatory aids. The same total internal hemipelvectomy in an elderly patient with associated medical problems, generalized weakness, or problems associated with progression of disease may in fact have no significant advantage over a classic hip disarticulation or hemipelvectomy, where the patient can learn at least to transfer early in the postoperative period and eventually ambulate with a walker. The functional results of limb salvage surgery seen in this study are multifactorial with patient selection a critical component. The tumor size and grade, the types of adjuvant therapies, the extent of the resection, reconstructive technique, prosthetic design, materials, fixation techniques, along with rehabilitation effort, not to mention the patient's weight, activity level, motivation, and cooperation all affect the ultimate functional result.

References

1. Enneking WF (1987) Modification of the system for functional evaluation of surgical management of musculoskeletal tumors. In: Enneking WF (ed) Limb salvage in musculoskeletal oncology. Churchill Livingstone, New York, p 626

2. Eckardt JJ, Eilber FR, Grant TT, Mirra JM, Weisenberger TH, Dorey FJ (1985) The UCLA experience in the management of stage IIB osteogenic sarcoma. Cancer Treatment Symposia 3: 117
3. Eckardt JJ, Eilber FR, Dorey FJ, Mirra JM (1985) The UCLA experience in limb salvage surgery for malignant tumors. Orthopedics 8: 612
4. Kaplan EL, Meier P (1958) Nonparametric estimation from incomplete observations. J Am Stat Ass 53: 457
5. Rosen G (1976) Multidisciplinary management of Ewing's sarcoma. In: Donaldson MH, Gunter-Seydel H (eds) Trends in childhood cancer. Wiley, New York, pp 89–106
6. Telles NC, Rabson AS, Pomeroy TC (1978) Ewing's sarcoma: An autopsy study. Cancer 41: 2321–2329
7. Wilkins RM, Pritchard DJ, Burgert EO, Unni KK (1986) Ewing's sarcoma of bone: Experience with 140 patients. Cancer 48: 2551–2555
8. Strong LC, Herson J, Osborn BM, Sutow WW (1979) Risk of radiation-related subsequent malignant tumor in survivors of Ewing's sarcoma. J Nat Cancer Inst 62: 1401–1406
9. Kotz R, Salzer M (1982) Rotation-plasty for childhood osteosarcoma of the distal part of the femur. J Bone Joint Surg 64A: 959
10. Lewis MM (1986) The use of an expandable and adjustable prosthesis in the treatment of childhood malignant bone tumors of the extremity. Cancer 57: 499

Surgical Margins Influencing Oncological Results in Osteosarcoma

RAINER KOTZ[1], KURT WINKLER[2], MECHTHILD SALZER-KUNTSCHIK[3],
FLORIAN GOTTSAUNER-WOLF[1], WOLFGANG KICKINGER[1], CHRISTIAN SCHILLER[1],
PETER RITSCHL[1], ULRICH HEISE[4], and SILVA TORGGLER[2]

Summary. A total of 118 patients with osteosarcoma underwent operation at the Orthopaedic University Clinic from 1976 until 1986. There were 57 female and 61 male patients with an age of 20.2 ± 11.9 years in the female and 19.5 ± 9.7 in the male group. In 25 cases, amputation was performed, of which 13 were above the knee. Resectional therapy was carried out in 93 cases, 49 of them with tumors in the distal femur, 14 in the proximal tibia, and 13 in the proximal humerus; there were 17 at other locations.

Twenty-six cases underwent resection and reconstruction as rotationplasty; in 49 cases a tumor endoprosthesis was implanted. Nine cases had a bone graft reconstruction; no reconstruction was necessary in nine. The distribution of endoprostheses was: 23 in the femur, 15 in the humerus, and 11 in the tibia. The radicality of surgery was investigated and it was seen to be wide and radical in 104 cases (88.2%). In 14 cases, marginal or intralesional surgery was done (11.8%), and this influenced the end result. Amputation and rotationplasty as the more aggressive therapy was compared with resection with or without an endoprosthesis but preserving the full length of the extremity.

The 3-year survival in 68 cases with a minimum follow-up of 3 years showed 72% in the group with amputation and rotationplasty (32 cases) and 75% in the group with resection and resection with an endoprosthesis (36 cases). Therefore, no influence on the long-term survival was seen in limb-preserving surgery versus amputation and rotationplasty.

Key words: Osteosarcoma—Surgical margins—Limb salvage—Survival rates

The success of chemotherapy improving the prognosis of patients with osteosarcoma has changed the surgical treatment from amputation to limb salvaging procedures. Extremity tumors constitute up to 90% of osteosarcomas where rotationplasty, endoprostheses, and reconstruction with extensive bone grafting are used. A total of 117 patients with osteosarcoma were investigated. Amputation and resection are compared with regard to clinical results in local recurrence, systemic metastases, and radicality of surgery.

---

[1] Department of Orthopedics, University of Vienna, Vienna, Austria
[2] Pediatric University Clinic, Hamburg, Federal Republic of Germany
[3] Vienna Bone Tumor Registry, Institute of Pathological Anatomy, University of Vienna, Vienna, Austria
[4] Orthopedic University Clinic, Hamburg, Federal Republic of Germany

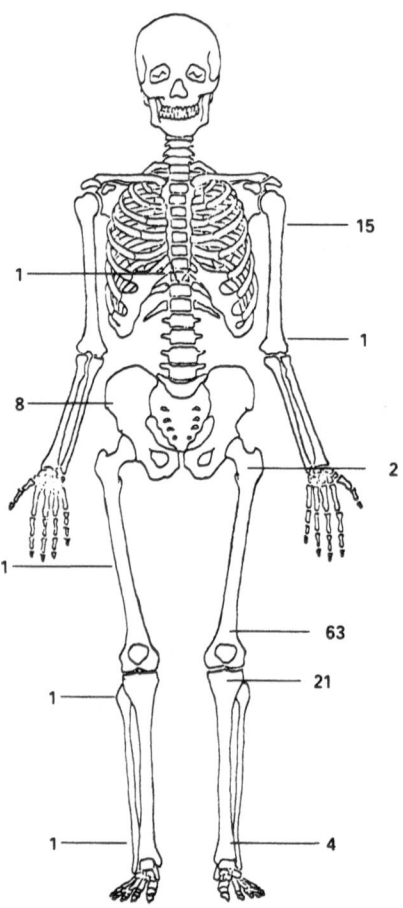

Fig. 1. Location of osteosarcoma
(1976–1986; $n = 118$, 117 patients)

Methods and Material

From 1976 to 1986, 117 patients with osteosarcoma were treated at the Department of Orthopedics of the University of Vienna. One patient suffered from two primary osteosarcomas. We report, therefore, on 118 tumors. Sex distribution was found to be well balanced (male 60, female 57) with a mean age of 20 years (male 19.5 range 6–55 years). More than two-thirds of the tumors were located in the knee region (distal femur 63, proximal tibia 21), followed by the proximal humerus (15), the pelvic region (eight), and rare locations like the thoracic spine (one), distal tibia (four), proximal femur (three), fibula (two), and distal humerus (one; Fig. 1).

In 25 patients, amputation was performed, whereas 93 had a resection or rotationplasty. Based on macroscopic and histological evaluation, they were divided into wide and radical or marginal and intralesional resections, according to Enneking et al. [1] with regard to their location (Tables 1, 2). The methods of reconstruction were rotationplasty in 26 cases, en bloc resection with endoprostheses in 49, bone transplantation in nine, and resection without recon-

Table 1. Results of amputation ($n = 25$)

Location	Wide, radical	Marginal, intralesional
Above knee	14	—
Knee exarticulation	3	1
Below knee	3	—
Hip exarticulation	3	—
Hemipelvectomy	1	—
Total	24	1

Table 2. Results of resection ($n = 93$)

Location	Wide, radical	Marginal, intralesional
Distal femur	49	2
Proximal tibia	14	—
Proximal humerus	14	1
Others	9	4
Total	86	7

Table 3. Reconstructional methods in resectional surgery

		Local[a] failure	Total[b] failure
Rotationplasty	26	—	8
Endoprosthesis	49	2	9
Bone graft	9	1	3
Without reconstruction	9	2	6
Total	93	5	26

[a] Local recurrence alone, without distant recurrence after surgical treatment
[b] Distant recurrence with and without local recurrence

struction in another nine. Autologous or homologous bone was transplanted to fill up bony defects in resection arthrodesis. In two cases, a pediculated transplantation of the fibula for bridging of large defects of the femur was performed; a resection in the pelvic region and thoracic spine did not necessarily involve reconstruction in every case. Tumor endoprostheses were used altogether in 49 cases, replacing the distal femur (23 cases), proximal humerus (15), and the proximal tibia (11).

Clinical results are determined by local recurrence (local failure) or postoperatively appearing systemic metastases with or without local recurrence (total failure). A total failure is not equivalent to the death of the patient (Table 3).

Chemotherapy

Chemotherapy has developed fast in the past 10 years and protocols change every 2–3 years. In 1976, HD-MTX (7.5 g/m² BS) was used at the Orthopedic University Clinic in Vienna. The protocol from 1976–1977 also included Adriamycin (2 × 45 mg/m² BS) and cyclophosphamide (1200 mg/m² BS) in 2-week intervals, lasting for 1 year [2]. In 1977–1980, a modified type of COSS 77 (Cooperative Osteosarcoma Study) with a combination of bleomycin, cyclo-phosphamide, and Actinomycin-D—BCD [3] instead of cyclophosphamide alone was used [4].

From 1980–1986, protocols COSS 80, COSS 82, COSS 85, and COSS 86 were used as described by Winkler et al. [5–7] (Winkler, unpublished data). Since 1979, preoperative chemotherapy has been used routinely. Tumor regression is defined by morphological evaluation of the tumor necrosis according to the staging of Salzer-Kuntschik et al. [8].

Wide and Radical Surgery

In 110 patients (93.2%), a wide or radical margin was achieved (Table 4). There were 24 amputations (total 25) and 86 resections (total 93). Indication for resection was based on careful exploration of the local tumor extension, clinically, and by routine investigations (computed tomography, angiography, bone scan, and in some cases nuclear magnetic resonance). The radicality was verified in-traoperatively by macroscopic and microscopic examination (frozen sections) and postoperatively by histopathological evaluation.

Marginal and Intralesional Surgery

In spite of careful preoperative investigations, marginal and intralesional surgery was carried out in eight patients (Table 5). The reasons for this are outlined in the following selected case reports.

Case 1 (S.F., aged 13, male; osteosarcoma right femoral diaphysis). Preoperative chemotherapy was performed according to study COSS-80. An intralesional resection was made through an undetected skip lesion, which was not connected to the main tumor mass, at distal femoral osteotomy. Intraoperative frozen section showed completely unviable tumor cells as a result of chemotherapy (total tumor regression according to Salzer-Kuntschik grade 1) in this skip lesion. After resection of the skip lesion, reconstruction with pediculated fibular transplantation. The patient died by chemotherapy complication without local recurrence.

Case 2 (S.J., aged 21, male; osteosarcoma right distal femur). Pulmonary metastases were detected at presentation and preoperative chemotherapy was carried out. Intraoperative examination indicated radical resection, and pediculated fibular transplantation was done. Definite histological examination revealed marginal resection with 2 mm of soft tissue to a periosteal protuberance of a viable tumor area, rising 1.5 cm above the intraosseous tumor. Overall tumor

Table 4. Radicality of surgery wide and radical ($n = 110$; 93.2%)

	Amputation	Resection
Number	24	86
Local failure	1 (4.2%)	4 (4.7%)
Total failure	4 (16.7%)	22 (25.5%)

Table 5. Radicality of surgery—marginal and intralesional ($n = 8$; 6.8%)

	Amputation	Tumor[a] regression	Resection	Tumor[a] regression
Number	1		7	
Local failure	—	—	1 (14.3%)	5, V
Total Failure	1 (100%)	5, V[b]	4 (57.2%)	6, V
				5, V
				5, V
				1, D[c]

[a] Tumor regression after preoperative chemotherapy, according to Salzer-Kuntschik staging
[b] Marginal or intralesional surgery through vital tumor areas
[c] Died by chemotherapy complication
V vital, *D* devital

regression was staged at 5 (50%–80% viable tumor tissue). Local recurrence occurred 15 months later and was treated by with above-knee amputation. The patient died from systemic metastases 2 months later.

Case 3 (P.G., aged 13, female; osteosarcoma right proximal tibia). Preoperative chemotherapy was undertaken with methotrexate (MTX). Following MTX intoxication, knee exarticulation was performed. At the dorsal joint capsule, an extraosseous viable tumor mass was entered accidentally and verified by frozen sections intraoperatively. Tumor regression was staged at 5. Wide resection of infiltrated area was followed with chemotherapy. No local recurrence has thus far occurred, though one solitary pulmonary metastasis was resected.

Results

In 110 patients with osteosarcoma, a wide or radical margin was achieved and in eight cases only could marginal or intralesional surgery be performed. After wide and radical surgery, a slight increase in total failures (systemic metastases with or without local recurrence) was found in resected as compared with amputated patients (25.5% vs. 16.7%; Table 4).

The incidence of recurrences increased significantly for resections in the pelvic region. Marginal or intralesional resections mainly occurred at this location. The incidence of systemic failure was observed to be highly increased in (marginal or intralesional) resected patients (4/8). However, only one local recurrence was

Table 6. Details of survival (1976–1983)

	Number	3-year survival
Amputation and rotationplasty	32	23 (71.9%)
Resection	36	27 (75.0%)

Minimum follow-up was 3 years

observed in these cases; the tumor regression in this patient after preoperative chemotherapy was only 5 (50%–80% viable tumor tissue) according to Salzer-Kuntschik and the marginal resection was performed in an area of mostly viable tumor cells. Two patients with a poor chemotherapy response (grades 5 and 6) died of systemic metastases (Table 5). Two patients survived without local recurrence or metastases; in one case, intralesional resection occurred through a totally devitalized tumor area (regression 2), and in the other with an osteosarcoma of the fifth thoracic vertebrae body no preoperative but postoperative chemotherapy and local radiation were performed. Both patients have been disease-free for 3 years.

The best results were achieved in tumors of the knee region, which is the most frequent location. The overall survival rate after a follow-up of at least 3 years is not different after resection (75%) as compared with amputation and rotationplasty (71.9%; Table 6).

Discussion

Resectional tumor surgery in osteogenic sarcoma has to be considered with respect to the curability of the majority of patients after wide or radical surgery and adjuvant chemotherapy [9–11]. The primary task of surgery is the cure of the patient. Limb salvage is secondary and its risk and benefits have to be throughly considered. Careful preoperative investigation (computed tomography, nuclear magnetic resonance, scintigram, angiogram) is indispensable for preoperative definition of the margins for radical or wide resection. In addition, limb salvage procedures should be left to surgeons qualified in this field [12].

The small number of local recurrences we observed may be due to the early death of some patients prior to clinical manifestation of a local recurrence. Review of the COSS studies [6, 7, 9, Winkler; unpublished data] shows that the relation of amputation and rotationplasty versus resection has changed since 1977 (Fig. 2). In the COSS-80 study, patients after ablative surgery showed a higher metastasis-free surival rate than after resection (Fig. 3). This led to a decreasing number of resections in the subsequent COSS-82 study (Fig. 2). In the COSS-82 study, however, the results were slightly better in the resection group (Fig. 4). The frequency of resections has clearly increased since 1985 (Fig. 2). We would attribute these results prior to 1982 to inexperience in surgery, which in the euphoria following the successes reported in the early literature was performed either inadequately or in unsuitable tumors [10]. Amputation nowadays is also clearly indicated if the size and location of the tumor endanger

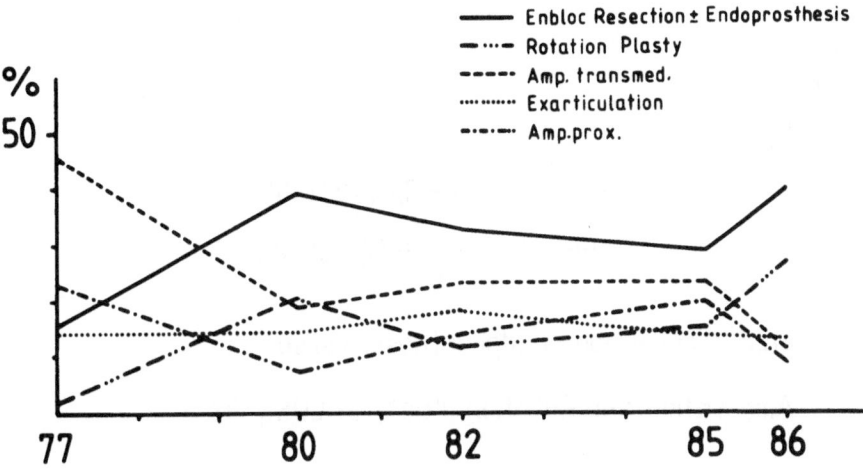

Fig. 2. Operations performed in the Cooperative Osteosarcoma Study ($n = 603$)

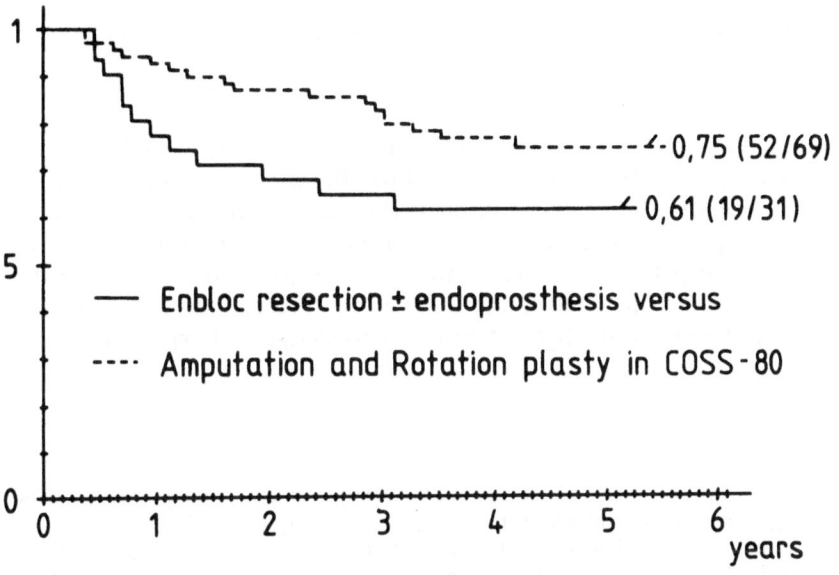

Fig. 3. Resection and amputation in COSS 80. Life table analysis (Kaplan/Meier)

radical resection and if it seems preferable in all tumors unresponsive to primary chemotherapy [13]. Highly complicated reconstruction, such as pediculated fibular transplant, also implicates the risk for nonradical surgery since the resection procedure may be compromised by the needs and difficulty of adequate reconstruction. In addition, if continuation of chemotherapy as scheduled is hampered by unexpected toxicity or major wound healing problems, amputation as an alternative has to be seriously considered. Nonradical resections considerably increase the risk for the patient.

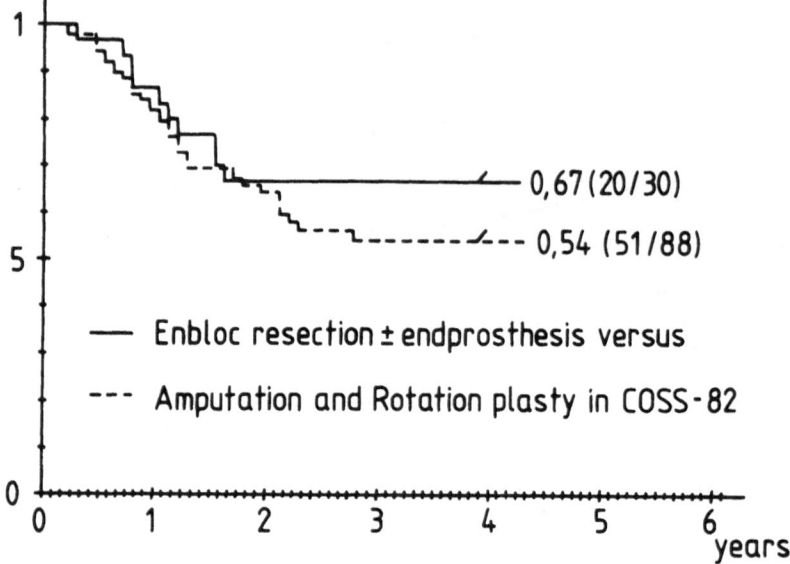

Fig. 4. Resection and amputation in COSS 82. Life table analysis (Kaplan/Meier)

Though we have a small number of cases, our results indicate a similar chance for disease-free survival after amputation and rotationplasty as with en bloc resection, with successful limb salvage in properly selected cases. Slightly worse results in the group of rotationplasty (Table 3) may be due to a higher risk of metastases for these patients by greater tumor extension. Considering all the above-mentioned guide lines and limitations, en bloc resections with limb salvage seem to be justified in the light of current knowledge and experience.

References

1. Enneking WF, Spanier MA, Godmann MA (1980) Current concept review. The surgical staging of musculoskeletal sarcoma. J Bone Jt Surg 62: 1027–1030
2. Kotz R, Leber H, Ramach W, Arbes H, Wolf A (1977) Erfahrungen mit der Durchführung der hochdosierten Methotrexatbehandlung beim Osteosarkom. Wien Klin Wschr 89 (14) 474
3. Mosende C, Guiterrez M, Caparros B, Rosen G (1977) Combination chemotherapy with bleomycin, cyclophosphamide and Dactinomycin for the treatment of osteogenic sarcoma. Cancer 37: 2779
4. Kotz R, Salzer-Kuntschik M, Lechner G, Immenkamp M, Kogelnik HD, Salzer M (1984) Orthopädie in Praxis und Klinik. In: Witt AN, Rettig H, Schlegel KF, Hackenbroch M, Hupfauer W (eds) Tumoren und tumorähnliche Erkrankungen, vol. 3, part 2. Thieme, Stuttgart
5. Winkler K, Beron G, Schellong G, Stollmann B, Prindull G, Lasson U, Brandeis W, Henze G, Ritter J, Russe W, Stengel-Rutkowski L, Treuner J, Landbeck G (1982) Kooperative Osteosarkomstudie COSS 77: Ergebnisse nach über 4 Jahren. Klin Pädiatr 194: 251–256
6. Winkler K, Beron G, Kotz R, Salzer-Kuntschik M, Beck J, Beck W, Brandeis W,

Ebell W, Erttmann R, Göbel U, Havers W, Henze G, Hinderfeld L, Höcker P, Jobke A, Jürgens H, Kabisch H, Preusser P, Prindull G, Ramach W, Ritter J, Sekera J, Treuner J, Wüst G, Landbeck G (1984) Neoadjuvant chemotherapy of osteogenic sarcoma: Results of a cooperative German/Austrian study (COSS 80). J Clin Oncolog 2: 617–624

7. Winkler K, Beron G, Delling G, Heise U, Kabisch H, Purfürst C, Berger J, Ritter J, Jürgens H, Gerein V, Graf N, Russe W, Qruenmayer ER, Ertelt W, Kotz R, Preusser P, Prindull G, Brandeis W, Landbeck G (1988) Neoadjuvant chemotherapy of osteosarcoma: Results of a randomized cooperative trial (COSS-82) with salvage chemotherapy based on histological tumor response. J Clin Oncol 6: 329–337

8. Salzer-Kuntschik M, Delling G, Beron G, Sigmund R (1983) Morphological grade of regression in osteosarcoma after polychemotherapy—Study COSS 80. J Cancer Res Clin Oncol 106: (Suppl)/21

9. Kotz R, Salzer M (1982) Rotationplasty for childhood osteosarcoma of the distal part of the femur. J Bone Jt Surg 64-A: 959–969

10. Rosen G, Tan CH, Sanmanechai A, Beattie EJ Jr, Marcove RC, Murphy ML (1975) The rationale for mutliple drug chemotherapy in the treatment of osteogenic sarcoma. Cancer (Philad) 35: 936–945

11. Salzer M, Knahr K (1976) Resection treatment of malignant bone tumors. Recent Res Cancer Res 54: 239

12. Wilson PD, Lance EM (1965) Surgical reconstruction of the skeleton following segmental resection for bone tumors. J Bone Jt Surg 47-A: 1629–1656

13. Winkler K, Beron G, Kotz R, Salzer-Kuntschik M, Beck J, Beck W, Brandeis W, Ebell W, Erttmann R, Göbel U, Havers W, Henze G, Hinderfeld L, Höcker P, Jobke A, Jürgens H, Kabisch H, Preusser P, Prindull G, Ramach W, Ritter J, Sekera J, Treuner J, Wüst G, Landbeck G (1986) Einfluß des lokalchirurgischen Vorgehens auf die Inzidenz von Metastasen nach neoadjuvanter Chemotherapie des Osteosarkoms Zschr Orthopad Grenzgebiete. 124: 22–29

A Cooperative Study on Limb Salvage Treatment for Osteosarcoma

Kiyoo Furuse[1], Sachio Masuda[2], Shinya Yamawaki[3], Akio Tateishi[4],
Yasuo Beppu[5], and Noriyoshi Kawaguchi[6]

Summary. Between 1973 and 1986, 225 patients with nonmetastatic primary osteosarcoma (OS) of the limbs were registered and treated. The cumulative survival rate was analyzed in several aspects. When classified into the limb salvaged group (72 patients), amputated or disarticulated group (153 patients), and total group (total patients), the 5-year (10-year) cumulative survival rate was 54.6% (49.3%), 51.3% (46.4%), and 62.1% (55.6%), respectively. When classified by the regimen of adjuvant chemotherapy to groups administered adriamycin alone (ADR) for 21 patients, ADR and high-dose methotrexate (MTX) for 108 patients, carcinostatics combined with cisplatin (+CDDP) for 62 patients, and 34 unclassifiable patients, the 5-year (8-year) cumulative survival rate was 15.1% (10.1%) for the ADR group, 62.4% (57.5%) for the ADR + MTX group, and 57.3% (57.3%) for the +CDDP group. The 10-year rate was 10.1% for the ADR group and 57.5% for the ADR + MTX group. The level was significantly lower in the ADR group than in other two groups ($P < 0.001$). Of 72 limb salvaged patients, 38 were involved with some complications. Of the 38 patients, secondary ablation was performed in 14 patients due to local recurrence (eight patients), infection (four patients), and circulatory disturbance (two patients). The serum alkaline phosphatase level, lactate dehydrogenase level, and pulmonary metastasis were studied as the prognostic factors.

Key words: Osteosarcoma—Limb salvage treatment—Cooperative statistical analysis

This paper reports a cooperative study on limb salvage treatment for osteosarcoma (OS) by six Japanese institutions.

Subjects and Methods

Between 1973 and 1986, 225 patients with primary OS of the limbs, non-metastatic at diagnosis, were treated with systemic chemotherapy and surgery in

---

[1] Department of Orthopedic Surgery, Tottori University, School of Medicine, Yonago, Japan
[2] Department of Orthopedic Surgery, Faculty of Medicine, Kyushu University, Fukuoka, Japan
[3] Department of Orthopedic Surgery, National Sapporo Hospital, Sapporo, Japan
[4] Department of Orthopedic Surgery, Teikyo University, School of Medicine, Tokyo, Japan
[5] Department of Orthopedic Surgery, National Cancer Center Hospital, Tokyo, Japan
[6] Department of Orthopedic Surgery, Cancer Institute Hospital, Tokyo, Japan

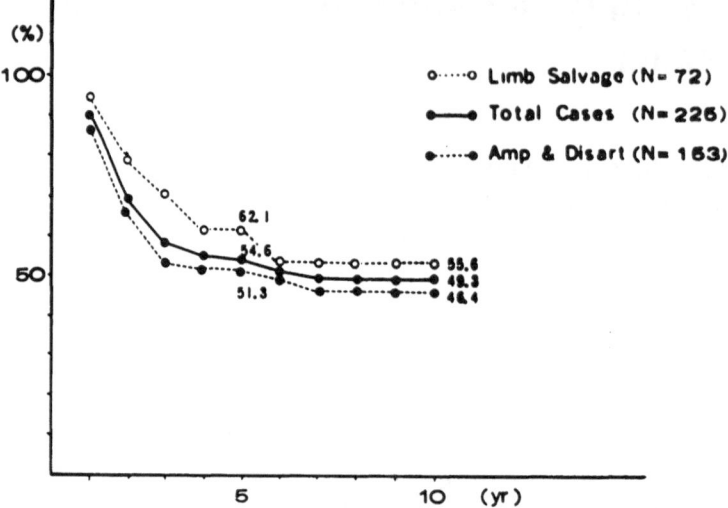

Fig. 1. Cumulative survival rate in osteosarcoma. Cumulative 10-year survival rates presented by dividing subjects into three groups of limb salvaged patients, limb-amputated or -disarticulated (*Amp & Disart*) patients, and total patients. There is no significant difference in level between salvaged and Amp & Disart groups

the six institutions. The limb salvage treatment was first applied in 1975, and to date 72 patients (32%) have undergone limb salvage treatment. During the last 5 years, except 1984, the rate of limb salvaged patients has constituted 47.8%–81.3% of the yearly total.

As of December 1986, we carried out a retrospective, nonrandomized statistical analysis of the 225 patients, dividing them into three groups of the total, 153 limb amputated or disarticulated, and 72 limb-salvaged patients (total, amp/disart, and salvaged groups) and studied the items detailed in the following section.

Results

Survival Rate

The 5-year (10-year) cumulative survival rate was 54.6% (49.3%), 51.3% (46.3%), and 62.1% (55.6%) in the total, amp/disart, and salvaged groups, respectively. Comparisons among the three groups showed on intergroup significant differences (Fig. 1).

Effects of Chemotherapy on Survival Rate

According to the regimens of adjuvant chemotherapy, patients were divided into three groups except for 34 unclassifiable patients: 21 patients were given adriamycin (ADR) alone, 108 were given ADR and high-dose methotrexate

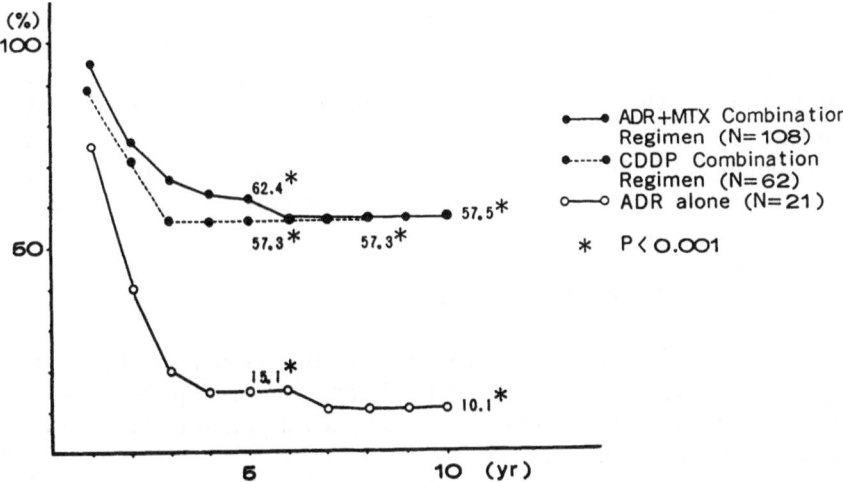

Fig. 2. Comparison of cumulative survival rate among three regimens of adjuvant chemotherapy. Cumulative 10-year survival rates for the adriamycin alone (*ADR*) and ADR and methotrexate (*ADR + MTX*) groups and 8-year survival rates for the carcinostatics combined with cis-platin (*CDDP*) group. The level decrease in the ADR group is much more significant than in the other two

(MTX), and 62 were given carcinostatics combined with cisplatin (+CDDP group).

The 5-year (8-year) cumulative survival rate was 15.1% (10.1%), 62.4% (57.5%), and 57.3% (57.3%) in the ADR, ADR + MTX, and +CDDP groups, respectively. The 10-year cumulative survival rate was 10.1% in the ADR group and 57.5% in the ADR + MTX group. The ADR group showed a significant decrease ($P < 0.001$) to both the ADR + MTX and +CDDP groups (Fig. 2).

Effects of Prognostic Factors on Survival Rate

The serum alkaline phosphatase (ALP) level measured at diagnosis was normal in 40 patients (24.0%; ALP-normal group), increased in 127 (76.0%; ALP-abnormal group), and not described in 58. The 5-year (10-year) cumulative survival rate was 65.3% (56.9%) in the ALP-normal group and 47.0% (43.5%) in the ALP-abnormal group, showing a significant intergroup difference ($P < 0.05$) in 5-year but not 10-year level.

Serum lactate dehydrogenase (LDH) measured at diagnosis was normal in 99 patients (60.0%; LDH-normal group), increased in 66 (40.0%; LDH-abnormal group), and not described in 60. The 5-year (10-year) cumulative survival rate was 64.7% (57.3%) in the LDH-normal group and 26.8% (26.8%) in the LDH-abnormal group. Both rates differed significantly between the groups ($P < 0.001$). In 62 patients showing abnormal ALP and LDH levels, 5- and 10-year cumulative survival rates were 26.2% each. In 102 patients showing normal levels of either ALP or LDH, the 5- and 10-year cumulative rates were 64.5% and 57.3%, respectively. The survival rate was significantly higher ($P < 0.001$) for the latter group.

Distant metastases appeared in 112 patients (49.5%) of the 225 during the course of treatment. Thoracotomy was performed in 61 (54.5%) of the 112 (thoracotomy group), and 51 (45.5%) were treated palliatively (nonthoracotomy group). The 5-year (7-year) cumulative survival rate—33.5% (25.5%) in the thoracotomy group and 7.6% (4.6%) in the nonthoracotomy group—was significantly higher for the former group ($P < 0.01$ for the 5-year level and $P < 0.005$ for the 7-year level). The 10-year cumulative survival rate for the thoracotomy group was 25.5%.

Complications with Limb Salvage Treatment

Of the 72 limb salvaged patients, 38 (52.8%) were involved with complication. Secondary ablative surgery was needed in 14 (36.8%) of the 38 patients due to local recurrence (eight patients), infection (four patients), and circulatory disturbances (two patients; Table 1).

The incidence of complications classified by the site of primary OS was 75.0% (3/4) for the fibula, 53.3% (8/15) for the humerus, 51.4% (18/35) for the femur, and 50.0% (9/18) for the tibia.

The ratio of secondary ablation to the whole complications after limb salvage treatment was classified by the site of primary tumor. The levels were 33.3% (1/3) for the fibula, 37.5% (3/8) for the humerus, 27.8% (5/18) for the femur, and 55.6% (5/9) for the tibia.

Local recurrence was observed in nine patients (12.5%). Six of them died of the tumor, and the remaining three have survived including one suffering from the disease. The ratio of local recurrence to the whole causes of secondary ablation, analyzed by the site of primary tumor, was 100.0% for the fibula (1/1) and humerus (3/3), 60.0% (3/5) for the femur, and 20.0% (1/5) for the tibia.

Discussion

The 5-year cumulative survival rate for the 225 collected patients with OS was 54.6%, consistent with the mean Japanese level [1]. The level did not differ significantly between amp/disart and salvaged patients, as in other reports [2, 3].

Adjuvant chemotherapy is commonly lasted for 1 year or $1\frac{1}{2}$ years in Japan. As reported previously [4], the ADR + MTX group was superior in cumulative survival rate to the ADR group, but the +CDDP group was similar in level to the ADR + MTX group in this study. The results obtained but not described here proved no effects of preoperative adjuvant chemotherapy on the cumulative survival rate, as reported by the COSS Study Group [5].

The prognosis of OS is evaluated in Japan mainly by the size of lesion, ALP level, and distant metastasis [6]. The size of lesion was not measured in this study. However, an individual strategy is needed for each patient according to the data of ALP and LDH levels at diagnosis, and distant metastasis (including the size of lesion) at diagnosis and during treatment.

Limb salvage treatment was performed in 32.0% of the registered patients. It is unclear, however, whether the level is valid or not, since reports published thus far have not offered definite opinions with regard to the rate of limb salvage

Table 1. Limb salvage treatment and complications (as of December 1986)

	No. of cases	Percent
Limb salvage treatment	72	
Complications	38	52.8
Secondary ablative surgery	14	37.0
Local recurrence	8	57.0
Infection	4	29.0
Circulatory disturbance	2	14.0

treatment in all types of surgery for OS because of a paucity of accumulated data for the treatment and of the peculiar surgical procedure for OS [3, 7].

The incidence of complications with limb salvage treatment may differ with the selection of the case for limb salvage surgery and the method of replacement after resection [2, 7, 8]. In this study, prosthetic material was used most frequently (48 patients, 66.7%), and the incidence of secondary ablation was higher than previously reported [8, 9]. The rate of local recurrence was similar to that reported [8, 9].

The incidence of such complications as local recurrence or other causes needing secondary ablation has rapidly reduced over the past 3 years. Advances in surgical manipulation may have contributed to this improvement, as well as the strict choice of limb salvage treatment based on an understanding of biological behavior in local extension of OS. Study of the functional evaluation of the salvaged limb is ongoing by the cooperative group.

Acknowledgment. This work was supported in part by a Grant-in-Aid for Cancer Research (60-14) from the Ministry of Health and Welfare, Japan.

References

1. Furuse K (1987) Bone and soft tissue tumors. In: Ota K (ed) Handbook of clinical pharmacology and therapeutics. Tumor, Jyoho Kaihatsu Kenkyusho, Tokyo, pp 284–297 (in Japanese)
2. Eckhardt JJ. Eilber FR, Grant TT, Mirra JM, Weisenberger TH, Dorey FJ (1985) Management of stage IIB osteogenic sarcoma: Experience at the University of California, Loss Angeles. Cancer Treat Symp 3: 117–130
3. Sim FH, Ivins, JC, Taylor WF, Chao EY-S (1985) Limb-sparing surgery for osteosarcoma: Mayo Clinic experience. Cancer Treat Symp 3: 139–154
4. Furuse K, Maeyama I, Yamawaki S, Abe M, Tateishi A, Furuya K, Takeyama S, Fukuma H, Akaboshi Y, Shinohara N, Sakoh T, Nomura S (1986) Adjuvant chemotherapy for osteosarcoma with adriamycin alone versus adriamycin-vincristine and high-dose methotrexate with citrovorum factor rescue. In: Kimura K, Wang Y-M (eds) Methotrexate in cancer therapy. Raven, New York, pp 249–255
5. Winkler K, Beron G, Kotz R, Saltzer-Kuntschik M (1986) Adjuvant and neoadjuvant chemotherapy of osteosarcoma: Experience of the German-Austrian Cooperative Osteosarcoma Studies (COSS). In: van Oosterom At, van Unnik JAM (eds) Management of soft tissue and bone sarcomas. Monograph series of the European organization for research on treatment of cancer, vol. 16. Raven, New York, pp 275–288

6. Fukuma K, Beppu Y, Shiba K, Nishikawa K (1982) TNM classification of bone tumors. Nippon Seikeigeka Gakkai Zasshi 56: 1475–1476 (in Japanese)
7. Eilber FR, Grant TT, Eckhardt J, Morton DL (1983) Prosthetic replacement after segmental bone and joint resection for malignant bone tumors. Experience at UCLA. In: Chao EY-S, Ivins JC (eds) Tumor prostheses for bone and joint reconstruction—the design and application. Thieme-Stratton, New York, pp 321–327
8. Mankin HJ, Doppelt SH, Sullivan TR, Tomford WW (1982) Osteoarticular and intercalary allograft transplantation in the management of malignant tumors of bone. Cancer 50: 613–630
9. Eilber FR, Eckhardt J, Morton DL (1984) Advances in the treatment of sarcomas of the extremity. Cancer 54: 2695–2701

Long-Term Results of Limb Salvage and Amputation in Extremity Osteosarcoma

DFCI/TCH Results in Patients Receiving Postoperative Weekly High-Dose Methotrexate and Doxorubicin

Mark C. Gebhardt, Allen M. Goorin, Jeffrey Traina, Antonio Perez-Atayde, Janet W. Anderson, H.G. Watts, and Norman Jaffe[1]

Summary. Between July 1976 and December 1981, 46 patients seen at the Dana Farber Cancer Institute and the Children's Hospital (DFCI/TCH) who met the criteria of being less than 30 years of age, without evidence of metastatic disease by plain chest radiograph, bone scan, and whole lung or computed tomography, were entered into this study. Detailed discussions relative to the merits and safety of limb salvage (LS) surgery were carried out in each case felt by the surgeon (HGW) to be a candidate for LS. Criteria for LS were: proximal humeral primaries if the brachial artery was univolved, midfemur lesions if the distal growth plate could be safely spared, distal femur or proximal fibular lesions if sufficient linear growth had been achieved, and lesions in an expendable bone (e.g., fibula). In all cases, a minimum of a wide margin was attempted. The chemotherapy regimen included vincristine (2 mg/m^2), methotrexate (7.5 gm/m^2) with leucovorin rescue, and doxorubicin (75 mg/m^2) to a total of 450 mg/m^2. All operative reports and staging studies were reviewed and the operative procedures classified as marginal, wide, or radical. Survival median curves were estimated by the method of Kaplan and Meier. Sixty-one patients who met the eligibility requirements for this study and were treated at the DFCI/TCH between 1948 and 1972 served as historical controls.

The 46 patients were 3–28 years old (median 14 years), and 31 (67%) were males. Twenty-seven patients remain continuously disease-free with a follow-up of 5.8–8.6 years. Life-table analysis revealed the 6-year disease-free survival (DFS) to be 59%, and the overall survival rate to be 73%, which was significantly improved compared with historical controls ($P < 0.0001$).

Of 46 patients, 20 (43%) had LS resections, while 26 patients had wide or radical amputations. The age and sex of the two groups were similar, as were the tumor sizes. The LS group contained more humeral, while the amputation group had more tibial lesions. There were 6 MSTS stage IIA patients in each group; the remainder were stage IIB. The surgical margins were radical (one patient), wide (16), and marginal (three) in the LS group and radical (15) and wide (ten) in the amputation group (one patient information unavailable).

The DFS at 6 years of patients undergoing LS procedures was 55% (11/20 remain disease-free), and for the amputation group it was 62% (16/26 disease-free; $P = 0.52$). Similarly, survival in the LS group was 67% (12/20 alive) versus 78% (20/26 alive) in the amputation group ($P = 0.24$). One local recurrence occured in the LS group. Six patients initially underwent LS but subsequently required amputation for local recurrence (one patient) and infection (five).

This study suggests that limb salvage surgery does not adversely affect DFS or survival in patients with nonmetastatic extremity osteosarcoma receiving postoperative adjuvant

---

[1] Dana Farber Cancer Institute and Children's Hospital, Boston, MA, USA

chemotherapy, but the results must be viewed with caution. With the small number of patients, this study only had a 32% power to detect a 20% difference between outcome based upon initial surgical procedure. There was a slight DFS advantage to those patients who had radical margins versus wide/marginal margins, but the difference was not significant ($P = 0.19$, univariate analysis). Although limb sparing resections are now commonly performed in many centers, both the safety and function of these procedures require further evaluation.

Key words: Osteosarcoma—Chemotherapy—Long-term results—Limb salvage surgery—Adjuvant chemotherapy—Bone sarcomas—High dose methotrexate—Doxorubicin

The prognosis for patients with osteosarcoma has improved dramatically in the last 15 years [1]. Recently, in a randomized multi-institutional trial, the historical experience of patients treated before the 1970s was confirmed and the benefit of adjuvant chemotherapy in increasing the chances of relapse-free survival in patients was demonstrated [2].

Nonrandomized adjuvant chemetherapy trials for presumed nonmetastatic osteosarcoma were initiated in the early 1970s at the Dana-Farber Cancer Institute/The Children's Hospital (DFCI/TCH) [3]. As only ten new patients per year with the diagnosis of osteosarcoma presented at DFCI/TCH, randomized studies were not feasible.

This is a report of an adjuvant combination chemotherapy trial of high-dose methotrexate (HDMTX) with doxorubicin used at DFCI/TCH denoted as study III. The objectives of this postoperative chemotherapy trial were: (a) to investigate the efficacy of segmental limb resection, and (b) to determine if intensification of chemotherapy by increasing the frequency of administration of HDMTX compared with the previous study II [4] would improve the replase-free survival (RFS). This report presents results with a minimum of 4.7 year follow-up for patients treated on study III. The complete details of this report have recently been published elsewhere [5].

Materials and Methods

Patient Eligibility

Eligibility required that patients be under 30 years of age, without evidence of metastatic disease at presentation as diagnosed by plain chest X-ray, bone scan, and whole-body lung tomography or computed tomography (CT) scan of the lungs. Additional eligibility requirements included no history of other malignant disease, no previous chemotherapy, and primary tumors that were completely resected by amputation or segmental limb resection surgery, i.e., intralesional excisions were prospectively excluded. Detailed discussions relative to the safety and functional outcome of limb salvage operations were carried out in each case, emphasizing that amputation was probably the safest and certainly the standard form of treatment of extremity osteosarcoma.

Patients with tumors in the following locations were candidates for limb resec-

Intensive HDMTX and Dox

HDMTX	HDMTX-Dox	HDMTX	HDMTX	HDMTX
qwk x 4	q3wk x 6	qwk x 4	q3wk x 6	qwk x 4

(Treatment Period of 12 Months)

Drug Doses:

HDMTX-   Vincristine 2.0 mg/m^2 (2.0 mg maximum)
           Methotrexate 7.5 gm/m^2
           Calcium Leucovorin 15 mg/dose

Dox-   Doxorubicin 75 mg/m^2 (450 mg/m^2 total dose)

Fig. 1. Chemotherapy regimen for patients treated on study III. Adjuvant chemotherapy began 1–3 weeks following definitive surgical procedure

tion rather than amputation: (a) all patients with proximal humerus lesions when possible, i.e., the axillary/brachial artery and brachial plexus were univolved with tumor; (b) midfemur lesions if the distal growth plate could be safely spared; (c) distal femur or proximal tibia lesions if >90% of linear growth was achieved; and (d) disease was in an expendable bone, e.g., fibula. Preoperative staging studies were reviewed to assess the site of the soft tissue mass and its relation to the major peripheral nerves and vascular structures. For patients to be considered for limb sparing resection, a tumor-free plane of tissue between these structures and the tumor mass had to be evident at the time of operation. In all cases, a minimum of a wide resection margin was attempted.

Chemotherapy Regimen

The chemotherapy regimen (Fig. 1) included vincristine 2 mg/m^2 followed after 30 min by HDMTX (7.5 g/m^2). Leucovorin (15 mg) rescue was administered after the completion of HDMTX and was continued intravenously (IV) every 3 h for a total of eight doses. Oral leucovorin was continued at the same dose every 6 h for eight doses. Doxorubicin (75 mg/m^2) was administered on days 6–8 after HDMTX to a total of 450 mg/m^2.

Follow-up procedures included monthly chest X-rays for 2 years, and thereafter at increasing time intervals. CT of the chest (plain tomography before April 1979) was performed initially and every 6 months for 2 years. Radionuclide bone scans were performed initially and every 6 months for 2 years. Primary site plain X-rays were also performed initially and every 6 months for 2 years.

The study III program was approved by the institutional review boards at DFCI/TCH. Patients were registered with the protocol office at DFCI after they gave informed consent to participate in this study.

Pathology Review

The pathological status of all 46 cases was reviewed independently by one of the investigators (APA) without knowledge of the patients' clinical outcome. Histological sections included at least one entire cut surface of each tumor. All cases were classified as high-grade osteosarcoma based on the degree of anaplasia, pleomorphism, necrosis, and a number of mitoses.

Surgery Review

Review of all operative reports and X-rays from 45 of 46 patients on this study by investigators MG, APA, RW, and AG was performed to define the site and extent of primary tumor and category of the operative procedure. Operative procedures (limb resections or amputations) were retrospectively defined according to the Musculoskeletal Tumor Society (MSTS) system as described by Enneking et al. [6]: marginal excision if the tumor pseudocapsule formed the periphery of resection (no evidence of gross residual disease, but there was a suspicion of microscopic satellite disease); wide excision if a cuff of noraml tissue of variable amount formed the periphery of the specimen; and radical excision if all noraml tissues of the involved compartments were resected with the tumor. Intralesional excision was defined as a tumor forming the periphery of part or all of the specimen leaving probable gross, and definite microscopic residual disease. Such patients with surgically suspected or pathologically confirmed intralesional excisions were prospectively exclused from entry to study III.

Statistical Methods

Relapse was defined as recurrence of tumor at any site. RFS was calculated from the data of biopsy to the date of relapse or date of last follow-up.

Continuous and graded on-study characteristics were coded to be dichotomous. Where there was no a priori split point for a continuous variable, the sample was dichotomized at the median. The univariate association between dichotomous variables and the experience of RFS ≥ 3 years was evaluated with Fisher's exact test. Difference in the distributions of RFS and overall survival was compared between groups using a log rank test [7]. Survival medians and curves were estimated by the method of Kaplan and Meier [8]. The 95% confidence intervals (CI) around estimated RFS and survival percentages at 5 years were calculated using Greenwood's formula [9] and exact binomial 95% CIs were calculated around observed (no censoring before 3 years) RFS and survival at 3 years. Multivariate logistic regression [10], performed in generalized linear interactive modeling (GLIM), was used to identify variables jointly associated with RFS ≥ 3 years. P values were generated by maximum likelihood procedures in GLIM due to the singularity of the design matrix and are approximate.

Historical Controls

Sixty-one patients seen at DFCI/TCH between 1948 and 1972 constitute the historical control patients. These 61 patients meet the eligibility criteria of study III. Patient characteristics and treatment received by these historical control patients were previously described.

Results

Between July 1976 and December 1981, 90 patients with osteosarcoma were seen at DFCI/TCH and 46 were eligible for treatment on adjuvant study III. Reasons for ineligibility of 44 patients included: metastases at diagnosis in 22; prior chemotherapy in three; prior history of cancer in two; age >30 years in two; nonextremity primaries in two; suspected intralesional excision of primary tumor in four (all four patients had surgery performed before being seen at DFCI/TCH); treatment on other chemotherapy regimens in six; and the wrong diagnosis in three.

Patient Characteristics

The 46 eligible patients were 3–28 years old (median, 14 years). Thirty-one (67%) were males. Twenty-two patients (48%) had femur lesions; 15 (32%) had tibial lesions; five (11%) had humerus lesions; three (7%) had fibula lesions; and one patient had a primary tumor in the os cales. The primary tumor of 12 patients had no associated soft tissue mass.

Relapse-Free Survival

Twenty-seven patients remain relapse-free with a follow-up of 4.8–8.6 years. Life-table analysis reveals the 5-year RFS to be 59% (95% CI, 43%, 74%). This RFS represents a significant improvement when compared with a nonconcurrent historical group of patients from the same institution ($P < 0.0001$; Fig. 2). Of the 19 patients who relapsed, the initial site of relapse was the lung in 16 and bone in three (one local).

Overall Survival

The life-table analysis of overall survival is shown in Fig 3. Thirty-four patients remain alive and the 5-year survival is 78% (95% CI, 65%, 91%), which is significantly improved when compared with historical controls ($P < 0.0001$). Following thoracotomies, with or without further chemotherapy and/or radiation therapy, 7 of the 34 survivors who relapsed are currently free of disease.

Surgery of Primary Tumor

Of 46 patients, 20 (43%) had limb-sparing resections, while 26 patients (57%) had wide or radical amputations. The median age of the patients having resections was 15 years compared with 13 for those having amputations. The male to female ratio was 14:6 for the patients having resections and 17:9 for those having amputations. The median largest dimension of the primary tumor was 9.0 cm for both groups of patients. Location of the primary tumors and type of surgery

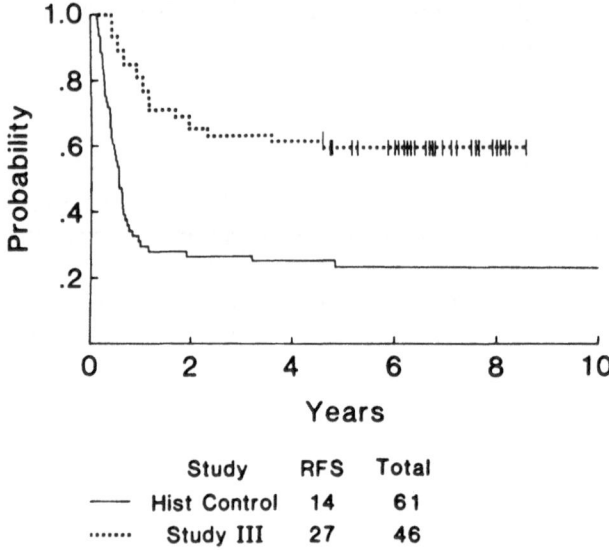

Fig. 2. Life-table analysis of relapse-free survival for patients treated on study III compared with DFCI historical control patients

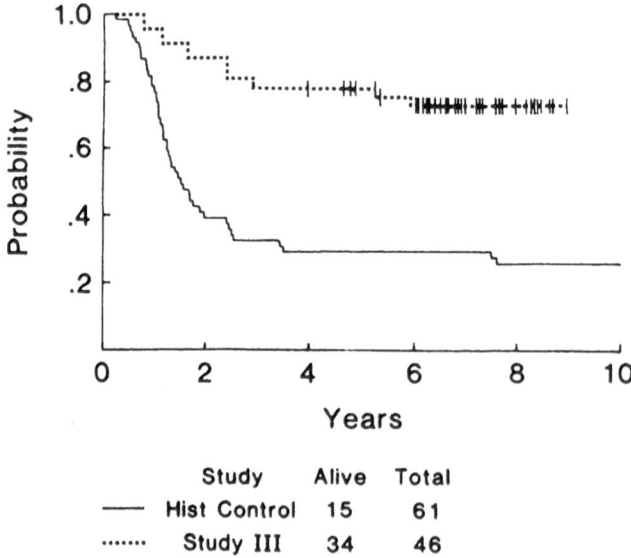

Fig. 3. Life-table analysis of overall survival for patients treated on study III compared with DFCI historical control patients

Table 1. Tumor location and surgical procedure performed on 46 patients

Location	Resection (n = 20)		Amputation (n = 26)	
	No.	Percent	No.	Percent
Humerus	4	80	1	20
Femur	11	50	11	50
Tibia	2	13	13	87
Fibula	3	100	—	—
Calcaneus	—	—	1	100

Table 2. Percentage of patients relapse-free at ≥ 3 years by surgical procedure, staging, resection margins, and growth plate involvement

	Resection			Amputation		
	No. RFS	Total		No. RFS	Total	
		No.	Percent		No.	Percent
Staging[a]						
2A	4	6	67	4	6	67
2B	8	14	57	12	19	63
Resection margins						
Radical	1	1	100	11	15	73
Wide	10	16	62	5	10	50
Marginal	1	3	33	—	—	—
Growth plate						
Open	5	10	50	9	13	69
Closed	7	10	70	7	12	58

One patient, currently relapse-free but with no available X-ray, is excluded from this table

[a] Musculoskeletal Tumor Society staging system (see text) [6]

for the 46 patients are given in Table 1. Six patients initially underwent limb sparing surgery but subsequently needed to have amputations for local recurrence (one case) and for infection (five cases).

Using the MSTS surgical staging system [4], six patients had stage IIA lesions treated with resection and six patients had stage IIA lesions treated with amputation (Table 2). Only 1 of 20 patients who had a limb resection procedure underwent a radical operative procedure, compared with 15 of 25 who had initial amputations. Three of twenty patients had marginal excisions with limb resections, compared with none undergoing amputation. Eleven of twenty-three patients had tumor crossing open epiphyses.

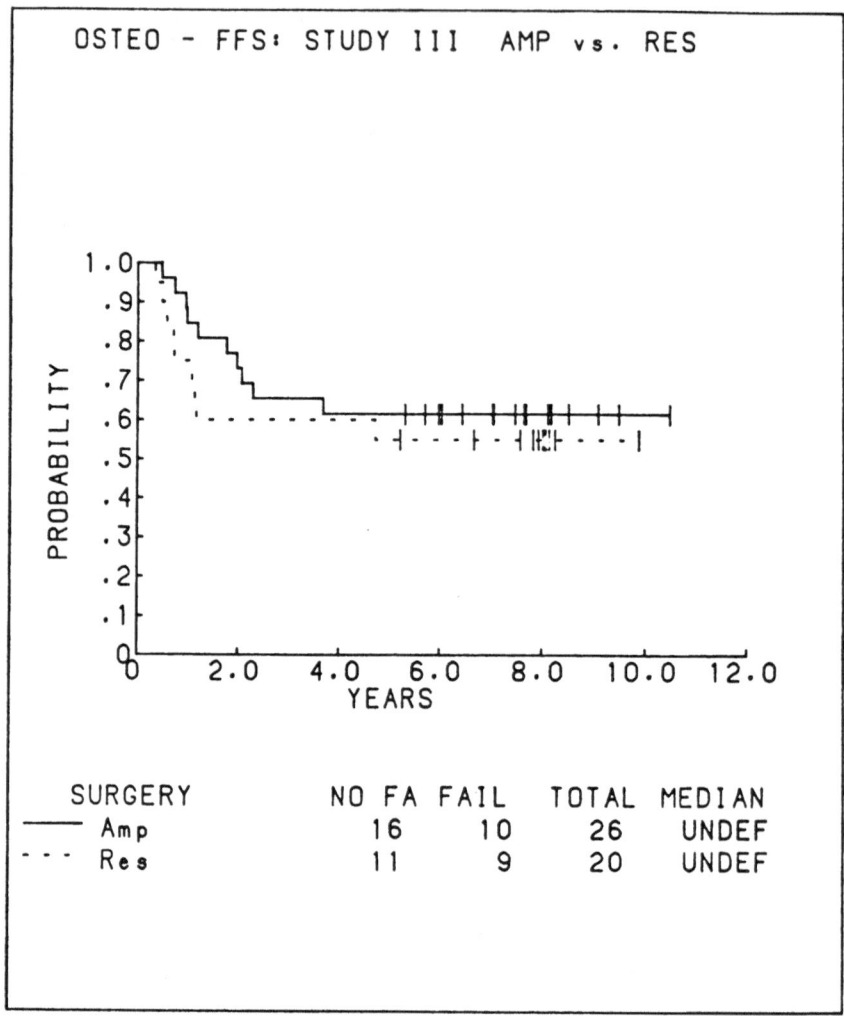

Fig. 4. Life-table analysis of relapse-free survival for patients treated on study III by type of surgical procedure

RFS by Type of Surgery

Life-table analysis of RFS of patients undergoing segmental resection surgery of the primary tumor versus amputation is shown in Fig 4. Eleven of the twenty patients who had limb resections remain relapse-free with a follow-up of 5.3–8.6 years. The 5-year RFS for patients who initially were treated with a limb resection procedure is 55% (95% CI, 32%, 77%). Of 26 patients who had initial amputations, 16 remain relapse-free with a follow-up of 4.7–8.6 years. The 5-year RFS is 62% (95% CI, 43%, 81%). The RFS of patients who underwent limb resection surgery is not significantly different from those who had amputations ($P = 0.52$).

Table 3. Toxicity of Chemotherapy regimen

	Percentage of total patients receiving chemotherapy[a]	
	Moderate-severe	Life-threatening
Fever and neutropenia	7	22
Muscositis	41	4
Renal	15	2
Hepatic	26	2
Neurological	9	4
Cardiac	0	7
Wound healing	9	4
Diarrhea	37	0

[a] National Cancer Institute recommendations for grading toxic effects (October 1985)

Analysis of overall survival by surgical treatment of the primary tumor shows 13 of 20 patients having limb resections and 21 of 26 patients having an initial amputation survive. The predicted 5-year overall survival is 70% (95% CI, 46%, 88%) for patients who had limb resections, compared with 85% (95% CI, 68%, 99%) for patients who had amputations. This survival difference is not significantly different ($P = 0.24$)

Toxicity of Chemotherapy

Of the 46 patients on study III, chemotherapy was stopped in two at 2 and 4 months, and chemotherapy was discontinued in one additional patient at 7 months because of CNS toxicity. All 46 patients are included in the statistical analysis. There were no deaths among these 46 patients as a result of drug toxicity. Toxicities from the chemotherapy regimens were as previously described (Table 3) [4]. The most serious complications included CNS changes attributable to HDMTX, and congestive heart failure (CHF) attributable to doxorubicin. Six patients (13%) had CNS changes that occurred within 2 weeks of receiving HDTMX. Two of six had seizures, while the other four had migrain-type headaches. One of the two patients with seizures had severe hypertension as well. All six patients had complete clinical resolution of the CNS changes. Three patients (7%) developed CHF following completion of 450 mg/m² doxorubicin. Of these three patients, two are clinically well, and one died of progressive osteosarcoma. Less serious complications such as fever, neutropenia, mucositis, elevated liver function studies, and diarrhea occurred. Wound healing was a problem in four patients after limb resection procedures.

Prognostic Variable

Using multivariate analyses, only the presence of moderate or marked lymphocytic infiltration of the primary tumor was a significant predictor of RFS ⩾3 years ($P < 0.002$); only the primary site in the proximal humerus ($P < 0.005$) or predominance of an osteoblastic pattern ($P < 0.03$) were significant predictors of RFS >3 years.

Discussion

One of the objectives of study III was to evaluate the feasibility of performing immediate limb resection surgery for patients with nonmetastatic osteosarcoma of an extremity without giving preoperative chemotherapy (all patients received adjuvant chemotherapy). Forty-three percent (20 of 46) of patients on this study were selected to undergo limb sparing operations. Only one of twenty patients with limb resection surgery had a local recurrence, and this compares favorably with reports of 5% local recurrence after cross bone amputation [11]. RFS and overall survival based on the type of initial operative procedure are not statistically different in our study, even though proximal humerus lesions (poor prognostic group) are weighted in the segmental resection group. However, with this number of patients, this study had only a 32% power to detect a 20% difference between the outcome based on the initial operative procedure.

Of 16 patients who had a radical surgical procedure, 15 had amputations as their initial surgery (Table 2). When radical operation vs. wide/marginal excision are compared as a predictor of RFS ≥ 3 years, the P value is ≤ 0.2. Although this is not statistically significant and is associated with multiple variables, the extent of the operative procedure in determining RFS may be important. One group study [12] recently reported an RFS advantage for patients treated with amputation or turnabout plasty of the primary tumor vs. local limb resection.

By multivariate analyses, the only prognostic variables found statistically to be predictive in this study included location of the primary in the proximal humerus, moderate to marked lymphocytic infiltration of the primary tumor, and predominance of an osteoblastic pattern. In all, 24 variables were independently analyzed to determine prognostic importance in this study. With such a small number of patients (46), only variables of major importance would be expected to be identified as prognostically significant.

A conceptually ineresting and, until now, undescribed histopathological indication of a favorable outcome in patients with osteosarcoma was moderate to marked lymphocytic infiltration of the primary tumor. None of the ten patients with this finding have relapsed $(P < 0.002)$. With various types of tumors, Rosenberg et al. [13] demonstrated that tumor-infiltrating lymphocytes are 50–100 times more effective in their therapeutic potency than are lymphokine-activated killer cells (LAK). This tumor-infiltrating lymphocyte cell population was recently identified in tumor-bearing patients and constitutes a subpopulation of lymphocytes that infiltrate into growing cancers and can be expanded with interleukin-2.

In conclusion, almost 60% of patients with nonmetastatic osteosarcoma are relapse-free and almost 80% are surviving without evidence of disease beyond 5 years from diagnosis following surgery plus adjuvant HDMTX and doxorubicin. Moreover, limb-sparing surgery was an option for 43% of patients entered on this study without the administration of preoperative chemotherapy. There are few data concerning functional results of limb resection surgery. In our study, 20% of patients who initially underwent limb resection surgery subsequently required amputation as late as 4 years after surgery because of infection. Although limb sparing segmental resection surgery is commonly performed in many centers [12, 14, 15], both the safety and function of these procedures require further evaluation.

References

1. Goorin AM, Abelson HT, Frei E III (1985) Osteosarcoma: Fifteen years later. N Engl J Med 313: 1637–1643
2. Link MP, Goorin AM, Miser AW, et al. (1986) The effect of adjuvant chemotherapy on relapse-free survival in patients with osteosarcoma of the extremity. N Eng J Med 314: 1600–1606
3. Jaffe N, Frei E III, Traggis D et al. (1974) Adjuvant methotrexate citovorumfactor treatment of osteogenic sarcoma. N Engl J Med 291: 994–997
4. Cortes EP, Holland JF, Wang JJ et al. (1974) Amputation and adriamycin primary osteosarcoma. N Engl J Med 291: 998–1000
4. Goorin AM, Delorey M, Gelber R et al. (1985) The Dana-Farber Cancer Institute/The Children's Hospital adjuvant chemotherapy trials of osteosarcoma: Three sequential studies. Cancer Treat Symp 3: 155
5. Goorin AM, Atayde-Perez A, Gebhardt MC et al. (1987) Weekly high-dose methotrexate and doxorubicin of osteosarcoma: The Dana-Farber Cancer Institute/The Children's Hospital-study III. J Clin Oncol 5: 1178–1184
6. Enneking WF, Spanier SS, Goodman MA (1980) The surgical staging of musculoskeletal sarcoma. J Bone Joint Surg 62A: 1027–1030
7. Peto R, Peto J (1972) Asymtomatically efficient rank invariant test procedures. JR Stat Soc (A) 135: 185–198
8. Kaplan EL, Meier R (1958) Nonparametric estimation from incomplete observation. J Am Stat Assoc 53: 457–481
9. Cox DR, Oakes D (1984) Analysis of survival data. Chapman and Hall, London
10. Cox DR (1970) Analysis of binary data. Chapman and Hall, London
11. Campanacci M, Laus M (1980) Local recurrence after amputation for osteosarcoma. J Bone Joint Surg 62: 201–207
12. Winkler K, Beron G, Kotz R et al. (1984) Neoadjuvant chemotherapy of osteogenic sarcoma: Results of a cooperative German/Austrian study. Clin Oncol 2: 617–624
13. Rosenberg SA, Spiess P, Lafreniere R (1986) A new approach to the immunotherapy of cancer with tumor-infiltrating lymphocytes. Sci 233: 1318–1321
14. Eilber FR, Moron DL, Echardt J et al. (1984) Limb salvage for skeletal and soft tissue sarcomas: Multidisciplinary preoperative therapy. Cancer 53: 2579–2584
15. Jaffe N, Knapp J, Chuang YP et al. (1983) Osteosarcoma: Intraarterial treatment of the primary tumor with cis-diamminedichloroplatinum (CDP): Angiographic, pathologic, and pharmacologic studies. Cancer 51: 402–407
15. Rosen G, Murphy ML, Huvos AG et al. (1976) Chemotherapy, en bloc resection, and prosthetic bone replacement in the treatment of osteogenic sarcoma. Cancer 37: 1–11
16. Johnston JO, Harries TJ, Alexander CE et al. (1983) Limb salvage procedure for neoplasms about the knee by spherocentric total knee arthroplasty and autogenous autoclaved bone grafting. Clin Orthop 181: 137–145

Surgical Management of Osteosarcoma in Extremities

Survival Between Limb Salvage and Amputation

Takafumi Ueda[1], Atsumasa Uchida[1], Hideki Yoshikawa[1], Hideki Hamada[2], Hideki Hayashi[3], Yasuaki Aoki[3], and Keiro Ono[1]

Summary. Forty-four patients with stage IIB osteosarcoma in the first to third decades of life with the primary tumors located in the femur, tibia, or humerus were investigated to evaluate the utility of limb salvage procedures as treatment for osteosarcoma. They were treated by wide resection (26 patients) or amputation (18 patients), combined with pre- and/or postoperative adjuvant chemotherapy. Radiation therapy was not performed in any case. The actuarial 5-year survival rates of the limb salvage and amputation groups were 51.1% and 51.9%, respectively. There was no significant difference between these two groups. The 5-year disease-free survival rate (65.8%) of the limb salvage group was significantly better than that (33.3%) of the amputation group ($P < 0.05$). However, the limb salvage group included more good responders for adjuvant chemotherapy (63.2%) than the amputation group (37.5%), suggesting the important role of adjuvant chemo-therapy for the improvement of disease-free survival. Local recurrence associated with systemic relapse was detected in only 1 (3.8%) of 26 patients treated by wide resection. The present results showed that when adjuvant chemotherapy was effectively done, limb salvage procedures can replace amputation for the surgical treatment of patients with osteosarcoma in the extremities.

Key words: Osteosarcoma—Limb-salvage procedure—Adjuvant chemotherapy

Introduction

Osteosarcoma is the most common malignant bone tumor in childhood and adolescence and frequently affects major long bones, especially around the knee. Until the early 1970s, patients with osteosarcoma of the extremities have exclusively been treated by radical amputation or disarticulation. However, their prognosis was poor with the 5-year survival rate ranging from 10% to 20% [1, 2]. Recent advances in the mode of therapy, such as adjuvant chemotherapy, wide resection, and aggressive thoracotomy for pulmonary metastasis, have improved the survival of patients [3, 4] and subsequently led to the proposal of limb salvage procedures as possible surgical treatment for osteosarcoma [5]. In this study, we examined whether limb salvage procedures can replace amputation for

---

[1]Department of Orthopaedic Surgery, Osaka University Medical School, Osaka, Japan
[2]Department of Orthopaedic Surgery, Osaka Prefectural Hospital, Osaka, Japan
[3]Department of Orthopaedic Surgery, Center for Adult Diseases, Osaka, Japan

the treatment of osteosarcoma in the extremities by comparing the prognosis of patients treated with limb-salvage procedures and amputation.

Materials and Methods

Among 72 consecutive patients with osteosarcoma admitted to our hospitals during the period 1976–1986, 44 patients, in the first to third decades of life with the primary tumors located in the femur, tibia, or humerus were selected for the current study. The remaining 28 patients were excluded for the following reasons: (a) age over 30 years (five cases); (b) primary tumor location other than the femur, tibia, and humerus (five cases); (c) inadequate surgical margin (two cases); (d) definitive therapy elsewhere (two cases); (e) pulmonary metastases at first admission (13 cases); and (f) periosteal osteosarcoma (one case). Primary tumors were located in the proximal femur in three patients, femoral diaphysis in one, distal femur in 21, proximal tibia in 15, distal tibia in one, and proximal humerus in three. The age of patients ranged from 4 to 24 years (median 14 years). The male to female ratio was 2.1:1. The stage of all patients was stage IIB according to the surgical staging system by Enneking et al. [6]

The patients were treated with both radical surgery and pre- and/or post-operative adjuvant chemotherapy. Radiation therapy was not performed in any case. Four patients received postoperative adjuvant chemotherapy alone. The remaining 40 patients received preoperative regional (intra-arterial) chemotherapy combined with or without systemic chemotherapy and postoperative adjuvant chemotherapy with single or multiple chemotherapeutic agents, consisting of adriamycin (ADR), high-dose methotrexate with citrovorum factor (HD-MTX-CF), cis-platinum (CDDP), and bleomycin plus cyclophosphamide plus actinomycin-D (BCD). Of 44 patients, 18 were treated by either amputation or disarticulation. The remaining 26 patients were treated by wide resection followed by reconstructive surgery with endoprosthesis (limb salvage procedure). Normal bone of 5–10 cm proximal to the tumor margin was removed without exposing the pseudocapsule of the tumor. In the case of tumor involvement into the surrounding soft tissue, wide resection was indicated only when a good response to chemotherapy was confirmed and, thus, a curable surgical margin was securely obtained.

The specimens were carefully evaluated postoperatively for the effect of preoperative chemotherapy in 35 of 44 patients. Based on the rate of tumor necrosis, the histological response was categorized as "good" or "poor." A good response was defined as more than 90% of tumor necrosis in multiple sections, and a poor response as less than 90%. Actuarial survival curves of 26 limb salvaged patients by wide resection and 18 patients treated by amputation were calculated by the method of Kaplan and Meier [7], and differences were estimated by the log rank rank test [8] to analyze the influence of limb salvage procedure for survival. These two groups were almost comparable with each other in the distribution of their age, sex, and location of the primary tumors (Table 1). The follow-up period calculated from the date of first treatment ranged from 4 to 116 months (median 37 months).

Table 1. Distribution of age, sex, and location of primary tumors in 44 patients with osteosarcoma

Surgical procedure	Number of patients	Age (yrs)		Sex		Location		
		Range	Median	Male	Female	Femur	Tibia	Humerus
Limb salvage	26	11–24	14.0	18	8	15[a]	8[b]	3[c]
Amputation	18	4–21	13.5	12	6	10[d]	8[e]	0
Total	44	4–24	14.0	30	14	25	16	3

[a] Proximal 1, distal 14 [b] Proximal 8 [c] Proximal 3 [d] Proximal 2, diaphysis 1, distal 7
[e] Proximal 7, distal 1

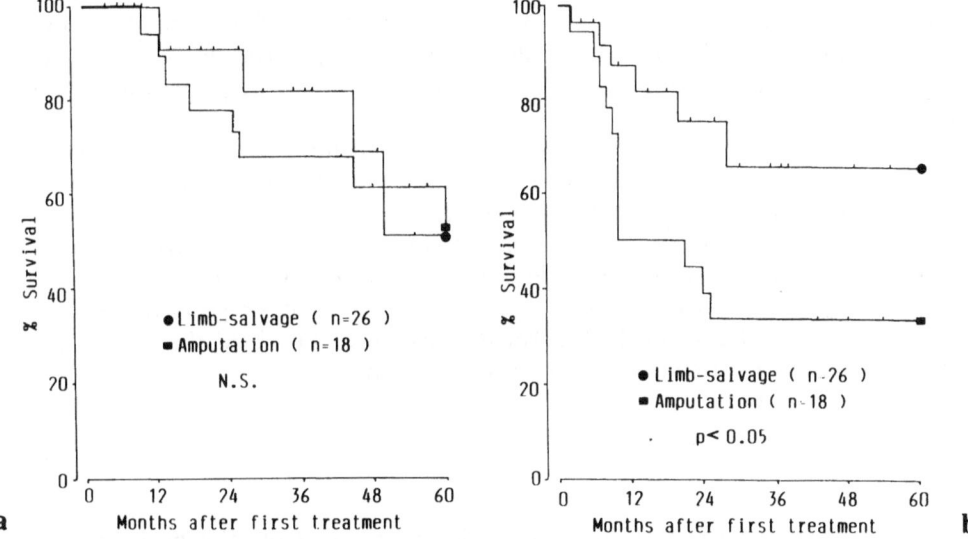

Fig. 1. a Actuarial overall survival and **b** continuous disease-free survival in patients treated with limb salvage procedures and amputation

Results and Discussion

The actuarial 5-year overall survival rates of the patients treated by limb salvage procedures and amputation were 51.1% and 51.9%, respectively (Fig. 1a). There was no significant difference between these two groups, indicating that the limb salvage procedure never reduced survival. In relation to the location of primary tumors, there was also no significant difference between them, neither with the femur (42.3% vs. 45.0%) nor tibia (53.3% vs. 60.0%). All three patients with a tumor in the humerus were treated by wide resection, and all of them were alive with no evidence of disease for 7–20 months (median 18 months). The 5-year continuous disease-free survival rate (65.8%) of the limb salvage group was significantly better than that (33.3%) of the amputation group

($P < 0.05$; Fig. 1b). On histological evaluation of the response for preoperative chemotherapy, however, the limb salvage group included 12 (63.2%) patients with a good response, whereas only six (37.5%) patients showed a good response in the amputation group. These results might be attributed to the difference in chemotherapeutic regimen between the limb salvage and amputation group.

Local recurrence was detected in only 1 (3.8%) of 26 patients treated by wide resection. This patient belonged to a poor response group for preoperative chemotherapy and had systemic relapse simultaneously with local recurrence. Pulmonary metastases developed in 12 (66.7%) of 18 patients treated by amputation, and 6 (23.1%) of 26 patients by wide resection at 2–28 months after first treatment (median 10 months). Thoracotomies were performed in 15 (83.3%) patients, and among them five (33.3%) patients were alive with no evidence of disease for 27–71 months (median 35 months) after initial thoracotomy. Complications, such as skin necrosis or superficial infection, were observed in six (23.1%) patients treated by limb salvage procedures, especially in the proximal tibial lesions, though none of these patients required revision of the prosthesis or amputation.

The present results show that when adjuvant chemotherapy was effectively done, amputation did not show any significant favorable effect on survival compared with limb salvage procedures. Therefore, limb salvage procedures based on reliable reconstructive methods are recommended for the treatment of osteosarcoma in the extremities under effective per- and postoperative adjuvant chemotherapy. Moreover, the presence of pulmonary metastasis at the time of diagnosis does not exclude limb salvage procedures, provided the pulmonary lesion is resectable or controllable by chemotherapy.

References

1. Dahlin DC, Coventry MB (1967) Osteogenic sarcoma: A study of six hundred cases. J Bone Joint Surg 49-A: 101–110
2. Friedman MA, Carter SK (1972) The therapy of osteogenic sarcoma: Current status and thoughts for the future. J Surg Oncol 4: 482–510
3. Rosen G, Marcove RC, Caparros B, Nirenberg A, Kosloff C, Huvos AG (1979) Primary osteogenic sarcoma: The rationale for preoperative chemotherapy and delayed surgery. Cancer 43: 2163–2177
4. Putnam JB Jr, Roth JA, Wesley MN, Johnston MR, Rosenberg SA (1983) Survival following aggressive resection of pulmonary metastases from osteogenic sarcoma: Analysis of prognostic factors. Ann Thorac Surg 36: 516–523
5. Eilber FR, Mirra JJ, Grant TT, Weisenburger T, Morton DL (1980) Is amputation necessary for sarcomas?: A seven-year experience with limb salvage. Ann Surg 192: 431–438
6. Enneking WF, Spanier SS, Goodman MA (1980) Current concepts review: The surgical staging of musculoskeletal sarcoma. J Bone Joint Surg 62-A: 1027–1030
7. Kaplan EL, Meier P (1958) Nonparametric estimation from incomplete observations. J Am Stat Assoc 53: 457–481
8. Peto R, Peto J (1972) Asymptotically efficient rank invariant test procedures. JR Stat Soc [A] 135: 185–198

A Comparative Study of Amputation and Limb Salvage for Musculoskeletal Sarcoma

The EUSM Experience Before and After the Adoption of the Surgical Staging System

Taihoh Shibata, Masatoshi Sasaki, Hideo Kushibe, Kiyoshi Komi, and Motoo Nojima[1]

Summary. Fifty-three rimary musculoskeletal sarcomata (36 with bone and 17 with soft tissue lesions) were operated on over a period of 11 years. Before July 1981, the Surgical Staging System (SSS) introduced by Enneking had not yet been adopted by our institute (pre-SSS), 16 sarcomas had undergone operation. After adoption of SSS, 34 patients with musculoskeletal sarcoma were treated. The cumulative survival rate (CSR) of the pre-SSS group was as follows: 1 year, 81.2%; 3 years, 37.5%; and 5 years, 36.8%. On the other hand, the CSR of the post-SSS group was as follows: 1 year, 84.1%; 3 years, 76.1%; and 5 years, 67.7% retrospectively. A statistically significant difference was evident. With respect to stage II lesions, 5-year-CSR of the pre-SSS is calculated as 30.7%, while that of the post-SSS is 61.7%. There was high incidence of advanced and high-grade malignancies in the pre-SSS group. Surgical procedures performed in the pre-SSS group were mainly wide or radical amputation. However in the post-SSS group, limb saving procedure ($n = 23$) and amputation ($n = 8$) were initially carried out. Five-year-CSR of limb salvage is calculated as 78.5%, while that of amputation is 62.5%. Local recurrence was seen in 5 of 16 cases in the pre-SSS. Surgical margin of these recurrent cases was estimated as marginal or intralesional. We conclude that a limb salvage procedure does not increase the frequency of local recurrences and that both limb salvage and amputation offer a similarly good prognosis if the surgical stagig system is strictly adapted.

Key words: Musculoskeletal sarcoma—Surgical staging—Cumulative survival rate

In our institute, established and started in 1976, 53 primary musculoskeletal sarcomas were operated over a period of 11 years. On the treatment of these lesions, there was a major development with the introduction of Enneking's Surgical Staging System [1, 2], which was first proposed in 1979. We started to utilize the surgical staging system in July 1981. We then divided our cases into two groups for the purpose of this study: before, presurgical staging system period (pre-SSS), and after, postsurgical staging system period (post-SSS), the adoption of the system [3].

The aims of this study are to clarify the following three concerns: that the

---

[1]Department of Orthopedic Surgery, Ehime University School of Medicine, Ehime, Japan

incidence of local recurrence is more frequent in the limb saving group, that the survival rate is less in the limb saving than the amputation group, and that an improvement can been achieved after the adoption of Enneking's surgical staging system.

Materials

Seventeen musculoskeletal sarcomas were operated on in the pre-SSS period; however, one patient died from a postoperative complication, so the patient was excluded from this study. In the post-SSS period, 36 sarcoma patients were operated on, but we lost two patients due to cardiac arrest, which occurred close to the time of preoperative chemotherapy in one young patient and relatively close to the time of ampuation in another older patient. So, 34 patients were eligible for analysis.

The mean age of the pre-SSS patients was 44.9 years and that of the post-SSS was 39. There were 12 males and four females in the pre-SSS group, and 15 males and 19 females in the post-SSS group. Twelve sarcomas were primary bone tumors and four were soft tissue tumors in the pre-SSS group, while in the post-SSS group 20 sarcomas originated in bone and 14 in soft tissue.

The pathohistological diagnoses in the pre-SSS group were eight osteosarcomas, two chondrosarcomas, two malignant giant cell tumors, and one each of malignant fibrous histiocytoma, leiomyosarcoma, and liposarcoma. While in the post-SSS group, the histological diagnoses were ten MFHs (malignant fibrous histiocytomas) (seven from bone and three from soft tissue), seven osteosarcomas, four chondrosarcomas, three rhabdomyosarcomas, three liposarcomas, two synovial sarcomas, and one each of malignant hemangiopericytoma, chordoma, Ewing's sarcoma, extranodal malignant lymphoma, and malignant Schwannoma.

The surgical stages of Enneking were done retrospectively in the pre-SSS group and the patients were classified as: IA, nil; IB, one; IIA, nil; IIB, 13; and III, two. The surgical stages in the post-SSS group were classified as: IA, four; IB, seven; IIA, four; IIB, 16; and III, three. Two types of surgical procedure for local control—amputation and limb salvage—were performed in both the pre- and post-SSS groups, though the criteria of the indications were different. In the pre-SSS period, the treatment of choice of a musculoskeletal sarcoma was amputation, and limb saving procedures were chosen in only four cases under criteria which were summarized retrospectively as follows: (a) the histological malignancy was low; (b) the location of the tumors was in a proximal part of the extremities; (c) the reconstruction was fairly easy, as in the Tikoff-Leinberg procedure; and (d) the will of the family of the patient coincided with the surgeon's opinion. On the other hand, limb saving procedures (including those in which a local resection for a lesion that could not be amputed because of the anatomical situation, such as a spine lesion, was involved), were increased in the post-SSS period.

The criteria for limb salvage in the post-SSS period were settled upon as follows: (a) there had to be wide surgical margins in all surgical planes of dissection, as well as a consiserable barrier between a tumor and a neurovascular bundle; (b) the location of the tumor had to be in the proximal or middle part of the extremity; (c) an intracompartmental sarcoma was more suitable for local resection than an extracompartmental one; (d) a soft tissue sarcoma was more suitable than a skeletal sarcoma due to the possibility of saving the supportive structure; and (e) patients had to be in a skeletally matured state.

With regard to the surgical stage of the amputation patients, 9 of 12 in the pre-SSS period and five of eight cases in the post-SSS period were IIB lesions. While in limb salvage cases, four IIB lesions received the procedure in the pre-SSS period, but in the post-SSS group three IA, seven IB, four IIA, eight IIB lesions, and one III lesion received limb saving operations under the criteria described above. Three patients (one each of chondrosarcoma of the thoracic vertebra, osteosarcoma of the lumbar vertebra, and Ewing's sarcoma of the sacrum) were excluded from this part of analysis. The reason was that they had lesions that were only partially excisable.

Several—rather arbitrary—regimens of chemotherapy were administered to 24 patients. All of the osteosarcoma patients and half of the MFH ones who were under 40 years of age received chemotherapy, while chondrosarcoma and older patients of this series were routinely not candidates for chemotherapy. Osteosarcoma patients received adriamycin systemically in the pre-SSS period, while in the post-SSS period, high-density methotrexate and cis-platinum were chosen. With respect to compliance with postoperative chemotherapy, approximately half of the selected patients dropped out because of complications and/ or social conditions such as school activities. Conclusively, 11 cases received and completed the postoperative adjuvant chemotherapy regimens, however 13 were estimated as incomplete patients. So, the effect of the chemotherapy could not be analyzed statistically.

Results

There was a local recurrence of tumor in one of the 12 patients who underwent amputation and in all of the limb saving patients in the pre-SSS group, while in the post-SSS group, there was a local recurrence in one of the eight patients who had undergone an amputation, and in 5 of the 23 patients who had had a limb saving procedure. The local recurrence rate of the limb saving patients in the post-SSS group is statistically lower than that of the pre-SSS group.

Metastasis was detected in eight of ten amputation patients (80%) in the pre-SSS group and in four of eight amputees (50%) in the post-SSS group. The rate of metastasis in the limb salvage patients was 75% and 22% in the pre- and post-SSS groups, respectively. The metastatic rates are significantly lower in the post-SSS group than in the pre-SSS. The cumulative survival rates (CSR) of the pre-SSS group were: 1 year, 81.2%; 3 years, 37.5%; and 5 years, 36.8%. On the other hand, the CSRs of the post-SSS group were: 1 year, 84.1%; 3 years, 76.1%; and 5 years, 67.7%. A statistically significant difference was evident in this study.

The Kaplan-Meier estimates of the proportion of the surviving patients in the post-SSS group are shown in Fig. 1. The survival rate for the limb saving procedure was better than for amputation. The 5-year cumulative survival rate of the

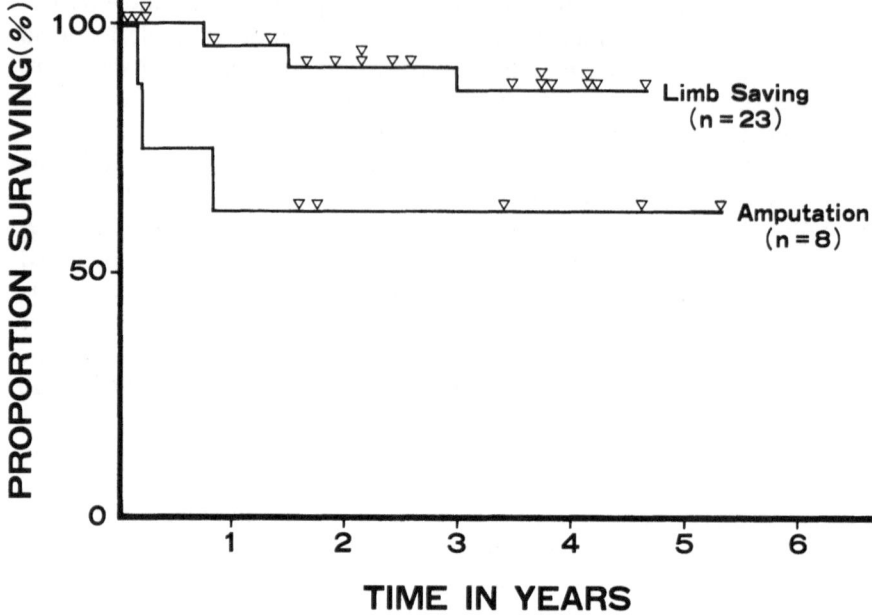

Fig. 1. Comparison of the survival function between limb saving and amputation (post-SSS)

limb salvage group was calculated as 78.5%, while that of the amputation group was 62.5%.

The survival rates of the patients in Enneking's surgical stages I, II, and III in the post-SSS group are shown in Fig. 2. The 5-year cumulative survival rate in stage I was 100% in the post-SSS period. Concerning stage II lesions, the 5-year CSR of the post-SSS group was calculated as 61.7%, while that of the pre-SSS period was 30.7%.

A comparison of the CSRs of every surgical margin evaluated in 43 patients, regardless of pre- or post-SSS group status, is shown in Fig. 3. The 5-year CSRs were 100% in the wide margin group, 56% in the radical amputation group, 28% in the wide amputation group, and 0% in the marginal excision group. This discrepancy occurred chiefly because of the difference in the metastatic rates of each group in this series.

Discussion and Conclusion

Recently, there has been increasing interest in limb saving surgery for musculo-skeletal sarcomas. When limb salvage procedures were compared with amputation in our institute, the following three questions had to be answered: (a) in the case of limb saving, did the number of local recurrences increase? (b) after the adoption of Enneking's surgical staging system, did the number of local recurrences decrease? and (c) when using Enneking's surgical staging system, could the same prognosis be promised for limb saving procedures and amputations?

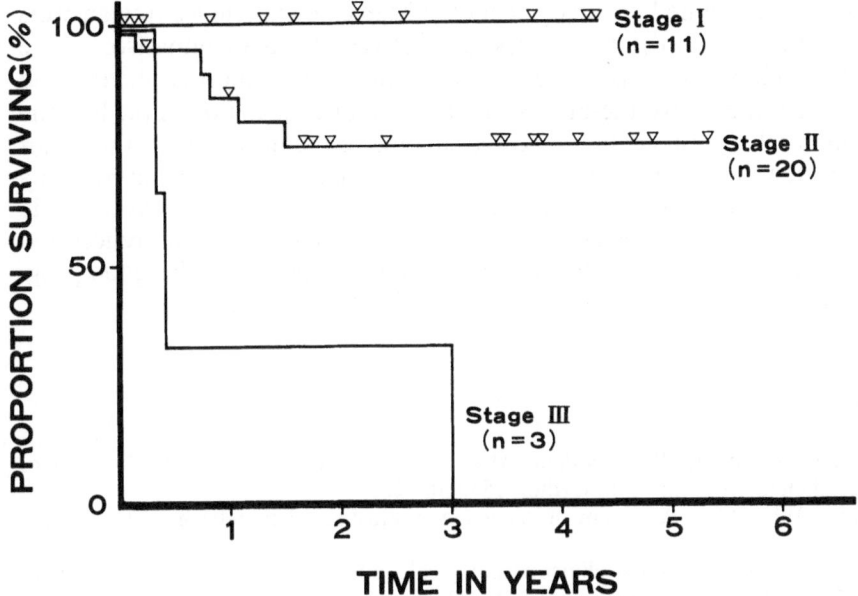

Fig. 2. Comparison of survival rate and surgical stages (life-table method)

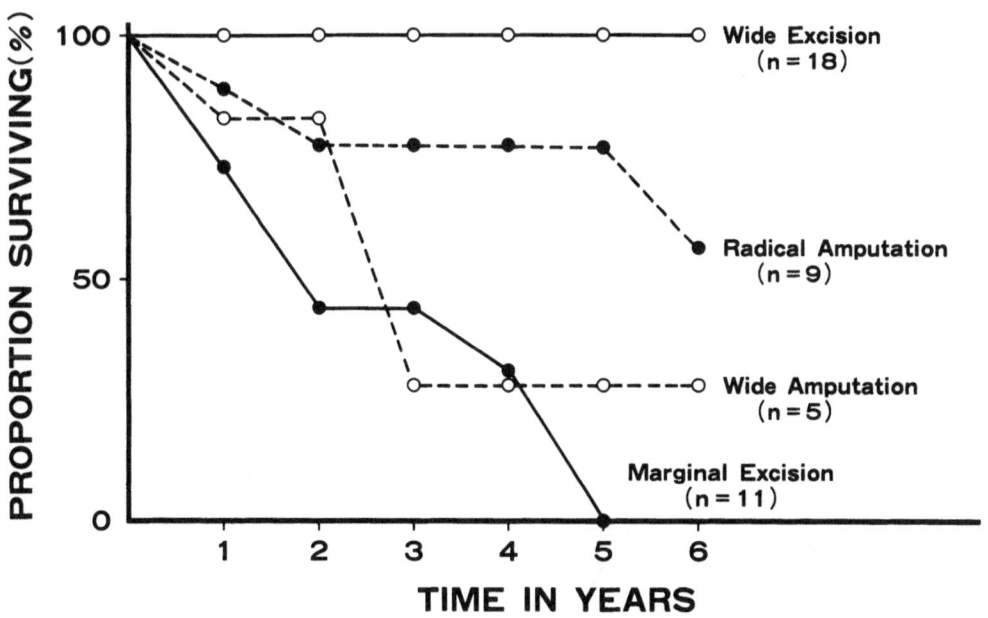

Fig. 3. Comparison of the cumulative survival rate of surgical margin

According to the Ehime University School of Medicine experience, the answers for the questions were: (a) no, (b) yes, and (c) yes. As to a comparison of the results of the limb salvage procedures and amputations, Simon et al. reported that compared with above-the-knee amputation or disarticulation of the hip, the use of a limb salvage procedure for osteosarcoma of the distal end of the femur did not shorten the disease-free interval or compromise long-term survival in a retrospective multi-institutional study of 227 patients [4]. So now, we conclude that limb salvage procedures do not increase incidence of local recurrences and that both limb salvage procedures and amputations promise similar good prognoses if the appropriate surgical staging system is strictly utilized.

References

1. Enneking WF, Spanier SS, Goodman MA (1980) A system for the surgical staging of musculoskeletal sarcoma. Clin Orthop 153: 106–120
2. Enneking WF (1986) A system of staging musculoskeletal neoplasms. Clin Orthop 204: 9–24
3. Shibata T, Komi K (1986) A clinicopathological study on local extension in musculoskeletal sarcoma. Arch Jpn Chir 55: 224–241
4. Simon MA, Aschliman MA, Thomas N, Mankin HJ (1986) Limb-salvage treatment versus amputation for the distal end of the femur. J Bone Joint Surg 68-A: 1331–1337

European Osteosarcoma Intergroup

An Interim Analysis of Surgical Data

JAN W. VAN DER EIJKEN[1]

Summary. A preliminary analysis is made of 307 patients who were entered into a randomized study comparing the tolerability and efficacy of two chemotherapies is done. Special attention is given to the surgical part of this study. Amputation was done in 31.6% of cases and conservative surgery in 58%. Local recurrences appeared in 17 cases after a period of 10 months. There were postoperative complications in 34 patients. There was no significant difference in the recurrences in the two chemotherapy. The recurrences were as frequent in the ampuation group as in the group which receiving conservative treatment.

Key words: Osteosarcoma—Recurrences

Materials and Methods

The entry of the first patient in this protocol was in July 1983. This report is based on an analysis carried out in September 1987. A total of 307 patients were entered into a randomized study comparing the tolerability and efficacy of two chemotherapy regimens. In one of the regimens, adriamycin and *cis*-platinum was used, and in the other adriamycin, cis-platinum, and high-dose methotrexate (HDMTX; Fig. 1).

The eligibility criteria were as follows: under 40 years of age; a biopsy-proven osteosarcoma; start of chemotherapy within 4 weeks after biopsy or surgery; normal hepatic, renal, cardiac, and hematological function. The following were excluded: parosteal and periosteal Pagetoid sarcomas; post XRT sarcomas; prior chemotherapy; other malignancies. A preliminary analysis was done of 307 patients. Of these patients, 46 had metastases at entry, 24 were inoperable at entry, and 30 had already undergone operation before chemotherapy.

In the characteristics of the registered patients, we noted an almost equal sex and age distribution. The on-study form was missing for 25 patients for whom we do not know the tumor side, sex, and exact age. The median age for 122 males was 16.9 years and for 92 females 14.5 years. The follow-up in March 1987 was after 18 months. A total of 127 patients were followed up for more than 1 year; 51 patients were followed up for more than 2 years.

---

[1] OLVG/Werkgroep Kindertumoren EKZ/AVL, Amsterdam, The Netherlands

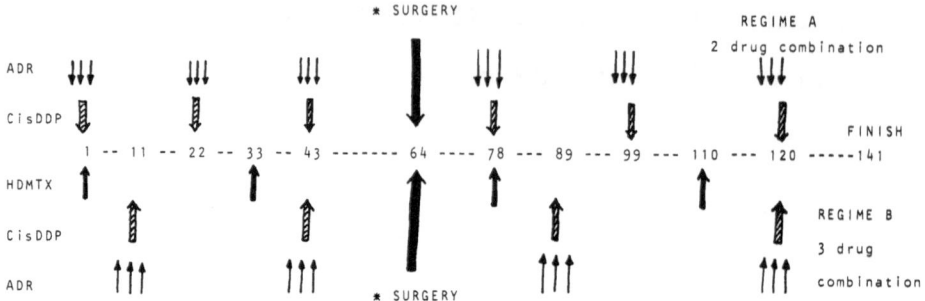

Fig. 1. Treatment regime. *ADR* adriamycin 25 mg/m² IV daily × 3, *CisDDP* Cisplatinium 100 mg/m² 24 h IV infusion, *HDMTX* High-dose methotrexate 8 g/m² 6 h IV infusion, folinic acid rescue 12 mg/m² IV or 15 mg/m² oral, commencing 24 h from start of infusion × 10 doses

Table 1. Patient characteristics at entry

	No.	ADM-DDP 1	ADM-DDP MTX 2	Total
Neoadjuvant	1	111	117	228
		72.5	76.0	74.3
Adjuvant-postop	2	11	12	23
		7.2	7.8	7.5
Recurrent	3	1	1	2
		0.7	0.6	0.7
Axial tumor	5	5	3	8
		3.3	1.9	2.6
Metastatic	6	25	21	46
		16.3	13.6	15.0
Total		153	154	307
		49.8	50.2	100.0

ADM-DDP adriamycin cisplatinum, *ADM-DDP MTX* adriamycin cisplatinum methotrexate

The patients were stratified into six categories. Group 1 consisted of all non-metastatic patients with limb tumors registered before surgery for neoadjuvant chemotherapy. Group 2 was all nonmetastatic patients with limb tumors operated before chemotherapy without recurrence. Group 3 included all nonmetastatic patients with limb tumors already operated and recurrent. Group 5 was all nonmetastatic patients with axial (nonlimb, including ribs) tumors independently of the declared operability status. Group 6 was made up of all metastatic patients independently of the stage of the primary tumor (Table 1).

Results

The tumor localization in both regimens arms showed no difference. Of 307 patients, 227 tumors were localized around the knee (Table 2).

Table 2. Tumor localization at entry

	No.	ADM-DDP 1	ADM-DDP MTX 2	Total
		13	12	25
		8.5	7.8	8.1
	1	70	68	138
Femur		45.8	44.2	45.0
	2	39	36	75
Tibia		25.5	23.4	24.4
	3	6	8	14
Fibula		3.9	5.2	4.6
	4	18	25	43
Humerus		11.8	16.2	14.0
	7	2	1	3
Ribs		1.3	0.6	1.0
	8	1	1	2
Other limb		0.7	0.6	0.7
	9	4	3	7
Other axial		2.6	1.9	2.3
Total		153	154	307
		49.8	50.2	100.0

Of the 237 patients who stopped chemotherapy, 106 (71%) completed the schedule, 69 (29%) terminated chemotherapy early. Twenty-four (9%) progressed during chemotherapy and 22 stopped because of excessive toxicity, seven because of protocol violation, 12 because of refusal, and four for miscellaneous reasons. Hematological and GI toxicity were slightly greater in the regimen without methotrexate.

The overall survival curve, which has to be considered a preliminary screening of the data is shown in Fig. 2. Of the 220 evaluable patients 80 had a relapse, of whom 17 had a local recurrence.

The surgical procedures were documented for 209 nonmetastatic operable patients. Of these patients, amputation was performed in 66 cases (31.6%). In 123 cases, different forms of conservative surgery were performed (58.8%; Table 3). The kind of operation was divided equally between the two treatment regimens.

Surgery was performed about 4 weeks after the end of the last chemotherapeutic cycle, while it was possible to start chemotherapy about 21 days after surgery. There was no significant difference between the two treatment regimens.

The type of surgery actually performed, extracted from the surgery form as a function of the type of surgery planned at registration, was studied. The patient declared inoperable at registration was probably due to a misunderstanding on the telephone. A planned amputation was changed in conservative surgery in 18 cases, while planned prosthetic surgery was changed for amputation in 27 cases.

Postoperative complications were seen in 34 cases (18%) with a slight prefer-

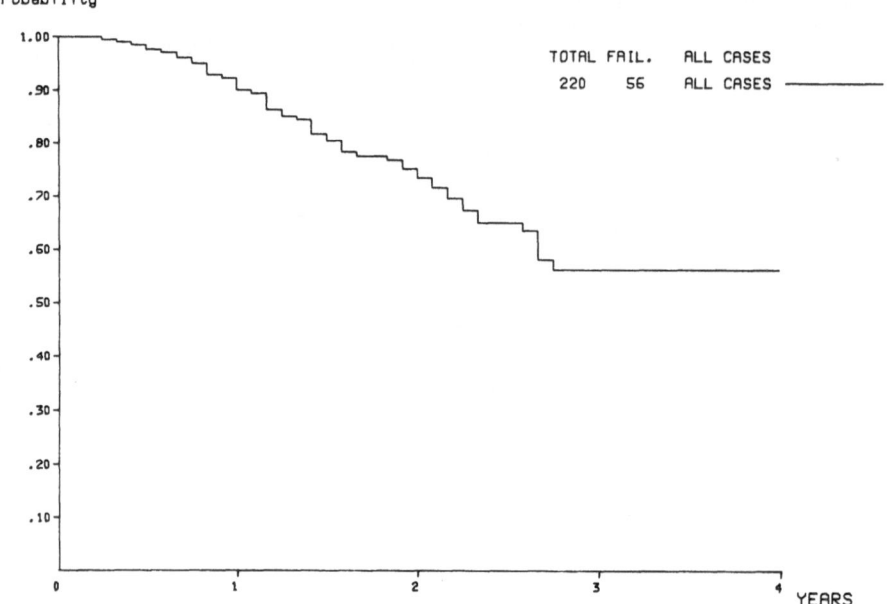

Fig. 2. Survival curve

Table 3. Surgical operation

	No.	Amputation 2	Prosthetic 3	Inoperable 4	Total
		5	15	0	20
					9.6
Amputation	1	39	27	0	66
					31.6
Cons + bone graft	2	3	8	0	11
					5.3
Cons + prostheses	3	9	83	1	93
					44.5
Rotationplasty	4	3	10	0	13
					6.2
Cons-no reconstruction	5	3	2	0	5
					2.4
Other	8	0	1	0	1
					5
				1	
Total		62	146	0.5	209
		29.7	69.9		100.0

Table 4. Local tumor status

	−0	Femur	Tibia	Fibula	Humerus	Other limb	Total
Remission	7	105	56	9	24	2	203
Recurrences	1	6	4	1	5	—	17
Total							220

ence for the regimen with adriamycin, cis-platinum and methotrexate. There were nine superficial infections and two deep infections.

From the surgical point of view, local recurrences can be a measure of the quality of a radical or wide excision. There were local recurrences in 17 cases. Most recurrences were in tumors localized in the humerus and femur (Table 4).

It is notable that just as many or even more local recurrences were observed in patients who underwent amputation. There does seem not to be any significant difference in survival in the different kinds of surgery. The recurrence appeared after a median time of 9.5 months. Nine patients died after a median time of 12.5 months. The patients with a local recurrence are analyzed separately.

Even from X-rays and the operation sheet, it is very difficult to judge the possibility of performing a wide resection. It appeared to be difficult to obtain the necessary data. Also, there is the possibility that a recurrence is not the result of inadequate resection, but the result of a skip metastasis.

Analysis of seven patients with a local recurrence shows that further study is absolutely necessary. In studying the figures of the 80831 osteosarcoma trial, one should always bear in mind that this is only a preliminary report. Final data will be given later.

Acknowledgments. The European Osteosarcoma Intergroup is composed of members representing the following groups:

Medical Research Council (MRC)
United Kingdom Children Cancer Study Group (UKCCSG)
European Organisation for Research into Treatment of Cancer (EORTC)
International Paediatric Oncology Society (SIOP)
Canadien Sarcoma Group
National Institute of Canada Clinical Trials
New Zealand Bone Sarcoma Group
 Martine van Glabbeke, statistician (EORTC)
 Dirk Crabeels, data manager (EORTC)
 Laurence Friedman, statistician (MRC)
 Bethan Smith, data manager (MRC)
The surgical subcommittee of the EOI consists of:
 G. Delepine, Hopital Paul Brousse, Villejuif, France
 J.W. van der Eijken, Onze Lieve Vrouwe Gasthuis Emma Kinder Ziekenhuis, Antoni van Leeuwenhoek Huis, Amsterdam, Holland
 J. Genin, Hopital Paul Brousse, Villejuif, France
 M. Rock, University Hospital, London, Canada
 R. Sneath, Royal Orthopaedic Hospital, Birmingham, England
 A. Taminiau, Academisch Ziekenhuis, Leiden, Holland
 A. Triffaud, Institute J. Paoli Calmettes, Marseille, France

Extremity Soft Tissue Sarcomas Treated with Limb Salvage Surgery and Amputation

A Comparison of Survival

Örjan Berlin[1], Bertil Stener[1], Lennart Angervall[2], Lars-Gunnar Kindblom[2], Anders Odén[3], and Björn Gunterberg[1]

Summary. A total of 137 consecutive patients treated surgically for an extremity soft tissue sarcoma during a 20-year period were followed up for at least 10 years. Prognostic factors were subjected to a multivariate statistical analysis. Independent significant factors related to poor survival were older age, high malignancy grade, and surgical treatment by amputation with radical or wide margins. The 10-year survival was 50% (38/76) after limb salvage surgery with radical or wide margins and 37% (13/35) after amputation with such margins; the difference was significant ($P < 0.05$). The difference in outcome may at least partly be related to an uneven distribution of diagnostic procedures. The diagnosis was obtained by a surgical intervention much more often before amputation than before limb salvage surgery (83% versus 29%).

Key words: Soft tissue tumors—Amputation—Prognosis

Introduction

Each case of soft tissue sarcoma of the extremities poses a challenge to the responsible surgeon in his aim to preserve as much function as possible, yet to remove the tumor safely, with a minimal risk of local recurrence. In attempts to increase these possibilities, adjuvant radiation and chemotherapy have been used in many centers [1–3]. This report gives the results of surgical treatment alone with special reference to the difference in survival after limb salvage surgery versus amputation.

Material and Methods

A total of 137 consecutive patients treated surgically for an extremity soft tissue sarcoma during a 20-year period (1956–1976) were reviewed. They all had received their definite treatment at our institution and were followed up for a

Departments of Orthopaedics[1] and Pathology[2], Sahlgren Hospital, Gothenburg University, Gothenburg, Sweden
Department of Mathematics and Statistics[3], Chalmers University of Technology, Gothenburg, Sweden

minimum of 10 years. No patient was lost to follow-up. The referral pattern and 16 factors related to host, tumor, diagnostic procedures, and surgery were registered and evaluated using a nonparametric multivariate statistical analysis. When feasible, the following surgical principle (suggested by one of the senior authors, B.S.) was applied: Biopsy can be omitted when the history, a careful physical examination, and various radiographic studies all agree on the diagnosis of malignancy and the location of the tumor allows its complete removal without significant loss of function; this enables good function to be preserved while still obtaining an adequate surgical margin.

A prerequisite for the application of this principle is that the patient is referred with the primary tumor intact.

Results

The male/female distribution was 78/59. The median age was 58 years (range 13–90). Eighty-nine patients were primarily referred with a virgin tumor (potentially suitable for the use of the previously mentioned surgical principle). Forty-eight patients were secondarily referred, after incisional or excisional biopsy, or with a local recurrence after previous surgery. Of the primarily referred patients, 15% underwent amputation versus 48% in the secondarily referred group. The most common tumors were malignant fibrous histiocytoma and liposarcoma.

Tumor-Related Death

Independent unfavorable prognostic factors were increasing age, increasing histological grade of malignancy, and ablative versus local surgery (radical and wide margins). The factor site in the Surgical Staging System [4], in contrast to grade, did not have any significant influence on tumor-related death. Deep tumor location and large tumor size had an unfavorable influence, but the depth and size factors were not independent. The multivariate analysis revealed a reciprocal dependence.

Of the 137 patients, 101 had limb salvage surgery (76 with a radical or wide margin and 25 with a marginal margin); 36 patients underwent amputation (35 with a radical or wide margin and one with a marginal margin). For the patients operated on with radical or wide margins, a comparison was made between the limb salvage group and the amputated group in terms of prognostic factors: Age—the limb salvage patients were significantly older; grade—there was no significant difference (approximately 90% high-grade tumors in both groups); site—in the amputated group, extracompartmental tumor site (stages IB and IIB) was found nearly three times more often than in the limb salvage group; death—the amputated patients had a significantly larger proportion of deeply located tumors; size—the proportion of tumors exceeding 5 cm did not differ significantly between the two groups.

A notable difference was related to the *diagnostic procedures*. The diagnosis was based on noninvasive methods in 50% in the limb salvage group versus 3% in the amputated group. Fine-needle aspiration cytology was used in 21% in the limb salvage group versus 14% in the amputated group. The diagnosis was

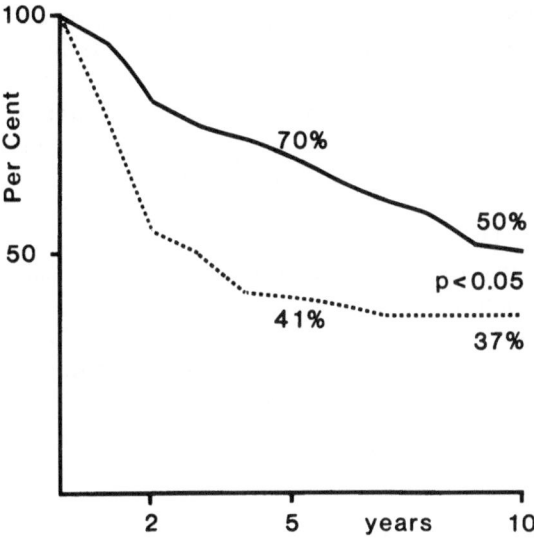

Fig. 1. Survival after limb salvage surgery (*upper curve*) and amputation (*lower curve*, radical and wide margins) with a minimum follow-up of 10 years

obtained by a surgical intervention in 29% in the limb salvage group versus 83% in the amputated group.

Survival After Limb Salvage Surgery Versus Amputation

With radical or wide margins, the 10-year survival was 50% in the limb salvage group versus 37% in the amputated group, which is a significant difference ($P < 0.05$; Fig. 1). If patients with marginal margins were included, the 10-year survival was 48% versus 35%, which is not a significant difference ($P = 0.084$). The observed overall 5- and 10-year survival (137 patients) was 56% and 44%, respectively.

Discussion

Independent significant factors related to poor survival were older age, high malignancy grade, and surgical treatment by amputation with radical or wide margins. Other tumor factors with an adverse effect on survival were deep location and large size in combination. These factors were mutually dependent as shown by multivariate analysis.

The malignancy grade did not differ between the amputated patients and the limb salvage patients. The amputated patients had a larger proportion of extra-compartmental tumors, but then it should be remembered that site had no significant influence on survival. The amputated patients had a larger proportion of deeply located tumors, but the limb salvage patients also had an unfavorable factor: they were older. One, at least contributing reason for the higher risk of tumor-related death after amputation seems to be that the diagnosis was ascertained by cutting into tumor tissue, with the ensuing risk of distant spread, three times as often before amputation as before limb salvage surgery.

Collin and co-workers [5] have reported a similar poor prognosis for amputated patients in comparison with limb salvage patients. In their study, the amputated group had many more risk factors than the limb salvage group. They concluded that the poorer survival for the amputated patients could hardly be attributed to the operation itself. However, it remains that amputation, as an isolated factor, entails a higher risk of tumor-related death than limb salvage surgery. Thus, it should be emphasized that limb salvage can be achieved more frequently (85%) if the patient is referred with a virgin tumor than if he is referred after surgical biopsy or local recurrence, when limb salvage, without adjuvant treatment, is possible only in approximately 50%.

References

1. Eilber FR, Mirra JJ, Grant TT, Weisenburger T, Morton DL (1980) Is amputation necessary for sarcoma? A seven-year experience with limb-salvage. Ann Surg 192: 431–438
2. Suit HD, Proppe KH, Mankin HJ, Wood WC (1981) Preoperative radiation therapy for sarcoma of soft tissue. Cancer 47: 2269–2274
3. Shiu MH, Turnbull AD, Nori D, Hajdu S, Hilaris B (1984) Control of locally advanced extremity soft tissue sarcomas by function-saving resection and brachytherapy. Cancer 53: 1385–1392
4. Enneking WF (1985) Staging of musculoskeletal neoplasms. Skel Radiol 13: 183–194
5. Collin CF, Godbold J, Hajdu S, Brennan M (1987) Localized extremity soft tissue sarcoma: An analysis of factors affecting survival. J Clin Oncol 5: 601–612

Chapter 3

Limiting Factors for Limb Salvage Operation

The Impact of MRI on Staging Malignant Musculoskeletal Tumors

A Prospective Study of 65 Patients

A.H.M. TAMINIAU[1] and J.L. BLOEM[2]

Summary. In 65 patients with primary malignant musculoskeletal tumors, a prospective correlative study including MRI, magnetic resonance imaging (MRI), computed tomography (CT) scan, ^{99m}Tc methylene diphosphate (MDP) scintigraphy, and angiography was performed to establish the role of MRI for diagnosis and treatment planning. The results of the imaging studies were correlated with the surgical and pathological finding.

MRI is significantly better than CT in staging intraosseous and extraosseous tumor extension and cortical involvement. MRI, CT scan, and angiography are equally accurate in demonstrating involvement of the vascular bundle when precise staging is required in musculoskeletal tumors.

Key words: MRI—CT scan—Musculoskeletal tumors

Introduction

Reduction of the magnitude of surgery has become the modern approach to treatment in patients with primary malignant musculoskeletal tumors. Successful management of these patients depends to a large extent on meticulous local tumor staging, because the anatomical setting is the key factor in selecting how a tumor-free margin should be accomplished.

Accurate imaging studies in determining the stage of the disease are extermely important for diagnosis and treatment planning. Limb salvage and reconstructive surgical procedures can only be performed after accurate preoperative correlative study, including MRI, CT scan, ^{99m}Tc MDP scintigraphy, and angiography.

Material and Methods

All patients with suspected primary malignant musculoskeletal tumors who were analyzed between February 1984 and February 1987 were candidates for the study. Sixty-five patients with primary malignant musculoskeletal tumors who

---

Departments of Orthopaedic Surgery[1] and Radiology[2], State University Leiden, Leiden, The Netherlands

were surgically treated were entered into the study; these included nine soft tissue and 56 skeletal tumors. Preoperative MRI was performed in all 65 patients, CT in 62, ^{99m}Tc MDP scintigraphy in 35, and angiography in 31 patients.

The results of the diagnostic studies were correlated in all cases with surgical and pathological findings. The tumor were staged for: (a) marrow involvement; (b) cortical destruction; (c) involvement of all muscle compartments in three different regions—the knee, pelvis, and shoulder; (d) involvement of the neuro-vascular bundle; and (e) involvement of joints.

Results

The sensitivity of MRI for pathological tissue is very high (90%–100%) on TL-weighted images for intraosseous tumor extension and T2-weighted images for soft tissue extension. MRI cannot reliably differentiate benign from malignant tumors. In approximately 50% of patients, MRI provides more clinical important information than a combination of CT scan, ^{99m}Tc MDP scintigraphy, and angiography. In the other 50% of patients, MRI provides as much information as this combination of conventional radiological studies.

The tumor volume in bone marrow and soft tissue is significantly better determined by MRI and CT than by ^{99m}TC MDP scintigraphy.

MRI is more accurate than CT in determining the extent of bone marrow involvement. Although Tc bone scan also displays bone marrow involvement in a longitudinal plane, it is less accurate than MRI because Tc scan detects marrow disease indirectly, it has a poor spatial resolution, and it shows increased uptake in areas of tumor-related hyperemia.

The correlation factor of MRI by pathological examination for bone marrow involvement was 0.99, the CT correlation factor was 0.93, the ^{99m}Tc correlation factor was 79%.

Soft tissue and muscle involvement are significantly better predicted by MRI than by CT.

The results of MRI were not influenced by the anatomical location (knee, pelvis, shoulder.)

The sensitivity of MRI for muscle involvement was 96%, the sensitivity for CT was 70%. MRI is significantly better than CT in identifying cortical involvement. The sensitivity of MRI for cortical involvement was 98%. MRI, CT, and angiography are equally accurate in demonstrating involvement of the neuro-vascular bundle (sensitivity 89%.) MRI is not significantly better than CT in identifying joint involvement (sensitivity 92%.)

Conclusions

MRI is highly accurate in staging primary malignant musculoskeletal tumors at 0.5 T when short and long SE sequences are used in at least two different planes. MRI is significantly better than CT in staging intramedullary extension when TL-weighted images are used. For intraosseous extension, extraosseous extension, involvement of major vessels and nerves, as well as visualization of extension in special localizsations (pelvis, vertebral colum), MRI was in many cases the most accurate imaging study. Hyperemic osteoporosis can only be differentiated from intramedullary tumor extension by MRI and not by CT or Tc bone scan.

MRI is significantly better than CT, ^{99m}Tc MDP scintigraphy, and angiography and should, therefore, be the primary imaging modality when accurate staging is required.

In patients with malignant bone tumors, MRI is indispensable, especially when limb salvage surgery is considered because exact delineation of intraosseous and extraosseous tumor extension is required.

Superior soft tissue demarcation, flexible image planes, and vascular imaging in relation to pathology are responsible for the increased value of MRI in the field of staging malignant musculoskeletal tumors.

References

1. Bloem JL, Falke THM, Taminiau AHM, van Oosterom AT, Steiner RM, Overbosch EH (1985) Ziedses des plantes Jr.B. MRI of primary malignant bone tumors. Radiographics 5 (6): 853–886
2. Bloem JL, Bluemm RG, Taminiau AHM, van Oosterom AT, Stolk J, Doornbos J (1987) MRI of primary malignant bone tumors. Radiographics 7 (3): 425–445

Limiting Factors of Limb Salvage Operation for Musculoskeletal Sarcoma

Noriyoshi Kawaguchi[1], Katsuhisa Amino[1], Seiichi Matsumoto[1], Jun Manabe[1], Kohtaro Furuya[2], and Yasushi Isobe[2]

Summary. Based on the therapeutic results of 158 musculoskeletal sarcomas treated by limb salvage operation, the limiting factors were analyzed. As a result, we concluded that the Surgical Staging System advocated by Enneking is not satisfactory as an indicator of surgical procedures in the treatment of musculoskeletal sarcoma. Also, the Functional Evaluation System does not adequately determine the appropriateness of the limb salvage operation. Therefore, in this analysis, a different standard was applied.

According to these criteria, two groups of limiting factors relating to postoperatively acquired functional deficit were determined. The first group included: (a) patients of younger age in bone sarcoma of lower extremities; (b) involvement of bone and vessel; and (c) extensive involvement exceeding three compartments. The second group of limiting factors, considered to be more important, involved local recurrence relating to inadequate surgical margin which comprised: (a) multicentric sarcoma; (b) skip metastasis; (c) venous invasion; (d) lymph node metastasis; (e) dissemination caused by pathological fracture or multiple inadequate surgery; and (f) the infiltrative character of the tumor. However, some of these limiting factors should be resolved by recent advances in surgical techniques.

Key words: Limiting factors—Limb salvage operation—Bone and soft tissue sarcoma

Introduction

Recently, limb salvage operations have become more commonly accepted procedures in the treatment of musculoskeletal malignancy of extremities. But there continues much spirited debate over when limb salvage operations should be performed. Therefore, in this paper, we attempted to analyze the limiting factors of limb salvage operations based on our clinical experience.

Material and Methods

In the 10 years beginning January 1977, we performed limb salvage operations for 158 musculoskeletal sarcomas of extremities. These 158 sarcomas included

[1] Department of Orthopaedic Surgery, Cancer Institute Hospital, Tokyo, Japan
[2] Department of Orthopaedic Surgery, Tokyo Medical and Dental University, Tokyo, Japan

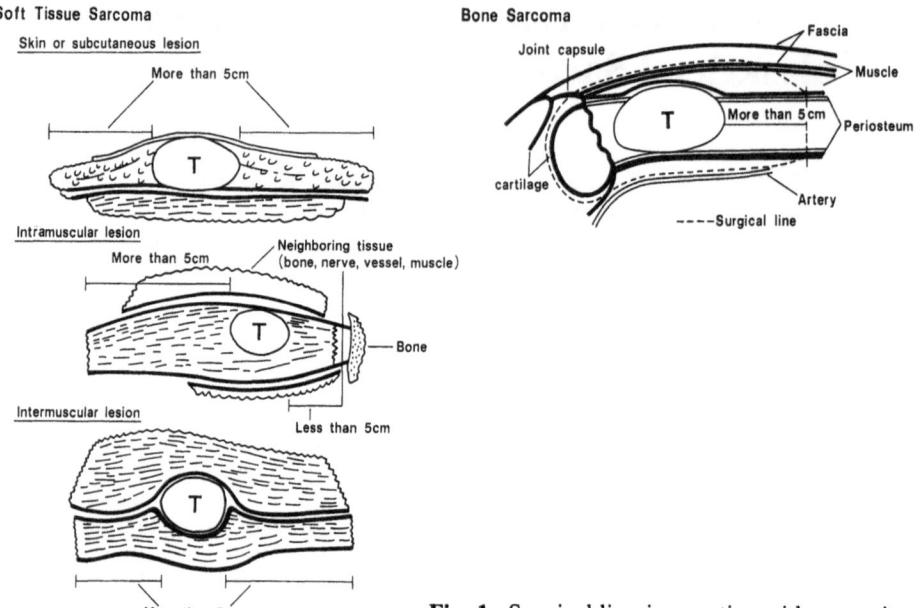

Fig. 1. Surgical line in curative wide resection

51 bone sarcomas and 107 soft tissue sarcomas. The 51 bone sarcomas comprised 27 osteosarcomas, 12 chondrosarcomas, and 12 other sarcomas. The 107 soft tissue sarcomas comprised 36 malignant fibrous histiosarcomas, 27 liposarcomas, eight synovial sarcomas, and 36 other sarcomas. According to the Surgical Staging System advocated by Enneking [1], the 158 cases fell into the following categories: 22 cases of IA, 21 cases of IB, 40 cases of IIA, 61 cases of IIB, and 14 cases of III. We principally performed curative wide resection, wide or marginal excision with preoperative adjunctive therapy, and ablation as radical surgical procedures for musculoskeletal malignancy.

Curative wide resection [2–4], which might be classified according to Enneking's surgical classification as "extensive wide excision," is indicated for almost all soft tissue sarcoma patients. In the remaining cases of soft tissue sarcoma (those in an advanced stage), ablation or excision with preoperative chemo-radiotherapy is chosen. In the treatment of bone sarcoma, we principally perform a combination therapy with preoperative chemotherapy and curative wide resection for high-malignant lesions. However, for high-malignant sarcoma patients who respond effectively to preoperative chemotherapy and for low-malignant sarcoma, we usually carry out less extensive wide excision. Curative wide resection is based on biological barrier effects. These barriers include fascia, cartilage, periosteum, vessel sheath, epineurium, and joint capsule. In the operation, the tumor is removed en bloc on being enclosed with the barrier in transverse section. In longitudinal section, in which no barrier is formed, the surgical line is increased to at least 5 cm beyond the tumor boundary. To carry out the principle of curative wide resection, different procedures are required for lesions in superficial, intramuscular, intermuscular, and osseous locations. (Fig. 1)

Table 1. Surgical staging and therapeutic result

Stage	No. of cases	Recurrence (%)	Metastasis (%)	5-y survival (%)
IA	22	5	9	100
IB	21	14	14	87
IIA	40	8	28	77
IIB	61	16	52	49
III	14	14	86	10
Total	158	12	38	67

Results and Discussion

The results of the 158 limb salvage operations were as follows: 12% local recurrence, 38% metastasis, and 67% cumulative 5-year survival (Table 1). Also, as seen in the result in Table 1, we could find an obvious relation between survival rate and staging but no relation between surgical stage and the efficacy of limb salvage operation. Therefore, the surgical staging system advocated by Enneking is not so helpful as an indicator of surgical procedures in the treatment of musculoskeletal sarcoma. However, to establish an adequate surgical margin and obtain local curability for soft tissue sarcoma, we performed limb salvage operations combined with special procedures. These comprised bone resection (20 cases), vascular surgery (ten cases), nerve resection (24 cases), and musculocutaneous (MC) flap (six cases). Generally, in the treatment of soft tissue sarcoma, resection of nerve, main vessel, or bone does not necessitate ablative operation. The reason is that bone and vessel can be reconstructed and loss of nerve function does not always result in definite disability of the affected limb. Moreover, as concerns predictive functional deficit by other anatomical defect, a defect in one set of compartmental muscles (for instance, the loss of entire extensors of flexors) does not sufficiently justify ablative surgery.

On the other hand, in the treatment of bone sarcoma, removal of the tumor more commonly requires various reconstructive procedures. Reconstructive procedures included the following: bone graft and arthrodesis performed for seven cases (commonly for lesion of shoulder joint), replacement of endoprosthesis for 36 lesions of knee or hip joints, combined with MC flap (two cases), and vascular surgery (one cases). No reconstruction was done for the lesions of the scapula and fibula (eight cases).

With regard to predictive functional defects in these procedures for bone sarcomas, the result does not sufficiently justify ablative surgery, too. For example, a patient with a functional defect of the quadriceps requiring replacement by a hinge-type knee endoprosthesis after removal of a femoral osteosarcoma can walk easily without crutches as if he were wearing a prosthetic device after an above-knee (A–K) amputation. The same result could be produced after replacement using a hinge-type prosthesis for a tibial lesion. Moreover, even if three compartments of the thigh (quadriceps, hamstring, bone and vessel) were resected in the treatment for osteosarcoma of the distal femur, the patient could walk easily without crutches. In this case, the knee was reconstructed by a hinge-type knee endoprosthesis and the femoral artery was reconstructed by autograft. However, it would usually not be appropriate to apply those procedures to bone lesions of lower extremities in younger children because of late discrepancy of limb length. Also, in the treatment for musculoskeletal lesion of the upper extremities, the limb salvage operation may especially be acceptable whenever at least some function can be preserved. The reason is that the functional results after ablation of an upper extremity were poor without exception even if prosthetic devices were used.

Adjunctive preoperative therapy occasionally plays an effective role in limb preservation. If preoperative therapy is effective, local control could be achieved with less extensive wide resection (done in conjunction with chemotherapy) or a marginal margin (done in conjunction with radiotherapy). The effectiveness of those therapies can be evaluated by medical imaging.

The effectiveness of preoperative therapy on bone sarcoma was ascertained as follows. In 27 osteosarcoma cases, chemotherapy was effective in four cases (but not in 13 cases), while chemoradiotherapy was effective in ten cases. All four cases of Ewing's sarcoma responded effectively to chemotherapy but one case of malignant fibrous histiocytoma (MFH) did not respond to chemotherapy at all. In the treatment of soft tissue sarcomas, we performed combination therapy of preoperative therapy and limb salvage operation for 27 cases of locally or systemically advanced lesions. In those cases, three showed no evidence of effectiveness on medical imaging and were followed by ablation.

Moreover, we felt that the Functional Evaluation System [5] advocated by Enneking does not adequately reflect the requirements of normal living. Therefore, in this analysis of the limiting factors, a different standard (as shown in Table 1, Page 30) was applied to assess the appropriateness of limb salvage operations. In this system, the minimum appropriateness of operation is considered to be the preservation of fair functional activity, fair emotional acceptance by the patient, and no local recurrence.

Based on these criteria, 85% of the patients seemed to accept the postoperatively acquired functional deficit, while those deemed "poor" in the appropriateness of limb salvage operation were 15% (Fig. 2). Consequently, the limiting factors on the appropriateness of the limb salvage operation were mainly whether or not there was local recurrence of the tumor, infectious complication requiring ablative operation, and extensive removal of normal structures causing the limb to be useless.

To prevent infectious complications, it seems to be important that the radiation dose and field be decreased and skin coverage be carefully done in the treatment of osteosarcoma. However, infectious complications are excluded here as a limiting factor because the problem of infection is a separate issue and not within the focus of this paper. To control local recurrence, an adequate surgical margin should be established. But, for limited conditions, it is difficult to obtain an adequate surgical margin by common curative wide resection. These conditions are as follows: (a) multicentric sarcoma (cutaneous angiosarcoma, lymphosarcoma); (b) skip metastasis (osteosarcoma, alveolar soft part sarcoma); (c) venous invasion; (d) lymph node metastasis; (e) dissemination caused by pathological fracture or multiple inadequate surgery; and (f) the infiltrative character of the tumor (MFH of soft parts). In conditions a–d, ablative pro-

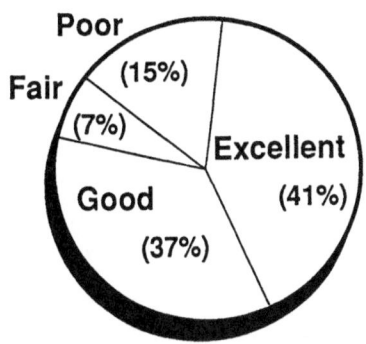

Fig. 2. Evaluation of limb salvage operations ($n = 158$). Poor cases ($n = 24$). Local recurrence: bone sarcoma, 7 cases; soft tissue sarcoma, 12 cases. Infection: bone sarcoma, 5 cases. Useless Limb: soft tissue sarcoma, 1 case

cedures are recommended rather than limb salvage procedures. Therefore, to detect when they exist, more meticulous examination by medical imaging is essential.

Still, the incidence of these particular conditions in the study was only about 15%. The remainder may be controlled using curative wide resection (with or without preoperative therapy) by paying special attention to the extent of surgery. For example, the postoperative local recurrence rate of relapsed soft tissue sarcoma cases (44%, or 7 of 16 cases) was higher than the rate of primary operation (6%, or 4 of 7 cases) or additionally operated cases after inadequate operation (8%, or one twelve cases), and the results of the later two groups were almost the same.

Consequently, if the first operation is not adequate, additional surgery should be done as soon as possible. Moreover, for recurrent cases, more extensive surgery may be required, i.e., both the tumor and the area of hemorrhage indicated by the operation scar should be removed extracompartmentally.

References

1. Enneking WF (1986) A system of staging musculoskeletal neoplasm. Clinic Orthop 204: 9–24
2. Kawaguchi N, Amino K, Matsumoto S, Manabe J, Furuya K, Isobe Y (1982) Radical (curative) wide resection for malignant soft tissue sarcoma. Rinsho Seikei Geka 17: 1192–1206
3. Kawaguchi N, Amino K, Matsumoto S, Manabe J, Furuya K, Isobe Y (1987) Limb salvage operation of osteosarcoma. Rinsho Seikei Geka 22: 1189–1197
4. Kawaguchi N, Amino K, Matsumoto S, Manabe J, Furuya K, Isobe Y (1987) The limb salvage operation of bone and soft tissue sarcomas Orthop Traum Surg 30: 1339–1351
5. Enneking WF (1987) Modification of the system for functional evaluation of surgical management of musculoskeletal tumors. In: Enneking WF (ed) Limb salvage in musculoskeletal oncology. Churchill Livingstone, New York, pp 628–630

Results of Multidisciplinary Limb Salvage in 272 Consecutive Sarcomas

Is Amputation Still Indicated in 1987?

Gerard Delepine[1, 2], Nicole Delepine[2, 3], Claude Jasmin[3], Leon Schwarzenberg[3], Georgei Mathe[3], and Mario Ricci[4]

Summary. From 1979 to 1986, 272 bone and soft tissue sarcomas were treated by a multidisciplinary limb salvage protocol, which included adjuvant radiotherapy in most cases. These patients represented 96% of patients with limb sarcoma treated during this period. The 5-year disease free survival rate was 65%. Local recurrence was observed in 17 cases (6%), mostly in patients referred after biopsy or where disease reccured after radiotherapy.

The functional results were encouraging (79% excellent or good results) and constitute the best argument for limb salvage. These promising results show that most patients can benefit from limb salvage irrespective of the age, location or size of tumor, and fractures without too high a risk of local recurrence if the surgical team has sufficient experience (at least two new patients a month). Amputation is better in infected cases if there is local recurrence following radiotherapy, if there is a lack of experience on the part of the surgical team, or if refined imaging techniques or adopting a multidisciplinary approach are not possible.

Key words: Bone sarcoma—Soft tissue sarcoma—Limb salvage surgery

Introduction

The results of limb salvage surgery are often evaluated through multicentric studies where surgical procedures, adjuvant therapies, and follow-up are not homogenous enough to permit definitive conclusions. The present study, based on 272 consecutive limb sarcomas treated by the same team, tries to answer the main questions about limb salvage: (a) Is it usually feasible? (b) is it worthwhile? (c) is it not too dangerous?

Material

From 1979 to 1987, 272 soft tissue and bone sarcomas of the limbs were treated by a multidisciplinary limb salvage protocol. The average age of the patients was

---

[1] Orthopeadic Oncologic Unit, Pré-Gentil, Rosny, Paris, France
[2] Pédiatric Oncologic Unit, H. Herold, Paris, France
[3] Services des maladies tumorales, H. Paul Brousse, Villejuif, France
[4] Casa di Cura, Siracusa, Italy

33.5 years (range, 3 months to 91 years). The average size of the tumor was 12.5 cm (range, 3–43 cm). Histological study revealed 80 osteosarcomas, 42 chondrosarcomas, 37 liposarcomas, 25 tenosynovial sarcomas, 23 fibrosarcomas, 17 malignant histiocytofibromas, 22 Ewing's sarcomas, 13 rhabdomyosarcomas, and two others. The tumoral locations were the femur or thigh in 128 patients, pelvis or hip in 45, leg in 40, arm or humerus in 27, scapula area in 16, and forearm hand or foot in 16. Tumoral staging was grade IA in 25 patients, grade IB in 39, grade IIA in 25, grade IIB in 141, grade IIIA in 26, and grade IIIB in 16. Ninety-nine patients were seen before biopsy, 74 were referred after biopsy, 37 after local recurrence (without radiotherapy or metastasis), 20 after post-radiotherapy recurrence, and 42 were already metastatic.

Methods

En bloc resection was performed by the same surgeon. Histological examination of the margins showed that the resection was large in 141 patients, marginal in 121, and intrafocal in ten. Adjuvant therapies where adapted to the age of the patient, histological finding, and location of tumor. Postoperative radiotherapy was performed on adult soft tissue sarcomas (65 Gy) and on osteosarcomas and Ewing's sarcomas whose histological response to neoadjuvant chemotherapy was bad (35–50 Gy). High-grade sarcomas received chemotherapy, either neoadjuvant (osteosarcomas and Ewing's sarcomas) or postoperative (soft tissue sarcoma).

After en bloc resection reconstructive, the following procedures were performed: plastic surgery in 15 cases, vascular procedures in ten, and major orthopedic reconstruction in 152 cases (six total femur, 19 upper femoral, 51 distal femoral, 24 iliac, 22 tibial, and 27 upper humeral reconstruction).

All patients were followed up by the same physician with clinical examination, lung and local computed tomography, and bone scan every 3 months for 2 years, then every 6 months for 3 years, and then every year.

Results

Overall Survival

To date, 162 patients are alive without evolutive disease, 22 are still receiving treatment, and 88 have died. Of the deaths, 83 were due to illness, three to complications, and two to intercurrent disease. The actuarial disease-free survival (DFS) rate of patients seen with localized disease was 73% at 3 years and 65% at 5 years.

Local Control

Seventeen local recurrences occurred, most of them in patients who were referred after biopsy or ineffective radiotherapy at other centers.

Functional Result

The functional result was excellent in 134 patients (49%), good in 81 (30%), fair in 35 (12%), and poor in 22 (8%). It depended mainly on the tumors's size and location and could be altered by radiotherapy or complications.

Statistical Analysis

This confirmed the *worst prognosis of visible metastasis* (2-year DFS was only 10% in group III), *proximal location* (3-year DFS was 30% in proximal location adn 80% for distal sites), and large tumor sizes (3-year DFS was 32% for tumors greater than 15 cm compared with 90% for tumors less than 5 cm).

Statistical analysis pointed out the major prognostic value of the following therapeutic factors.

In osteosarcoma, prognosis depended on the effectiveness of chemotherapy: The 5-year DFS rate was 65% in the S04 78 protocol of GETO (postoperative adjuvant chemotherapy of two alternating cycles for 1 year and early lung radiotherapy), under 35% in the European 04 protocol (preoperative and post-operative adriamycin and platinum), and 90% with Rosen T 10 with short preoperative high-dose weekly methotrexate administration adjusted to individual pharmacokinetic findings.

In Ewing's sarcoma, prognosis improved with en bloc resection of the primary: 85% (19/22) of patients who underwent en bloc resection remained disease free compared with 45% of patients treated by radiotherapy.

In low grade chondrosarcoma and soft tissue sarcoma, immediate local control seems to be the major predictive factor of DFS: 85% of patients with local control remained disease free, whereas this was only 60% of those who experienced local recurrence).

The local recurrence rate did not depend on size of the tumor, age of the patient, or type of resection (marginal and large resection have the same local recurrence rate), but only on the experience of surgeon and on the circumstances under which the patients were seen.

The local recurrence rate was 2% in patients seen before biopsy, 5% in patients referred after biopsy or local recurrence after surgery, and 35% for patients seen after local recurrence following radiotherapy.

Comments and Conclusions

This analysis of our results permits some answers to be given to the following problems.

Is Conservative Surgery Dangerous?

Local recurrence is the main fear after limb salvage for high-grade sarcoma because it often appears with metastasis. In this study (with adjuvant local radiotherapy), the local recurrence risk and the DFS are quite similar to those

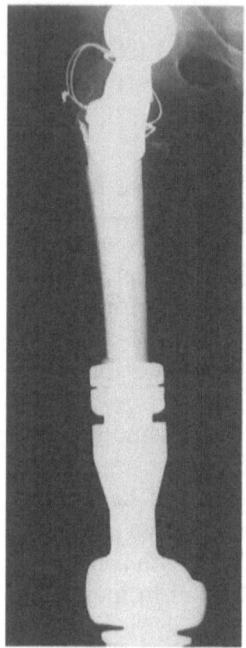
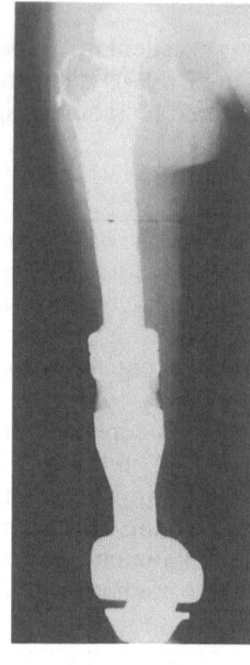

Fig. 1   Fig. 2

Fig. 1. Total femur resection in a 8-year-old girl with very large osteosarcoma

Fig. 2. Total femur replacement including growing distal prosthesis. Two years after 4 cm lengthening

observed after amputation, except for patients referred after local recurrence and after radiotherapy. With a highly trained team (treating at least two sarcomas/month), conservative surgery does not appear to be dangerous.

Is It Worth While?

The functional result is the best argument for limb salvage: 95% of our patients enjoy a much better life than if they had undergone amputation. This functional advantage is greater for small tumors and after surgery which is "not too extensive," guided by refined computed imaging, and completed by adjuvant regional radiotherapy. Moreover, it is necessary to underline the social and professional implications of limb salvage. Most of our patients are adolescents or young adults whose illness appears when they are planning organizing their future life. If functional results are good, the patient can go ahead and fulfill his plans. Conversely, amputation often entails problems with work, friends, partner. Even with large tumors, the functional result is important.

Is Limb Salvage Usually Feasible?

The indication for limb salvage depends on the experience of the surgeon and ability of the team.

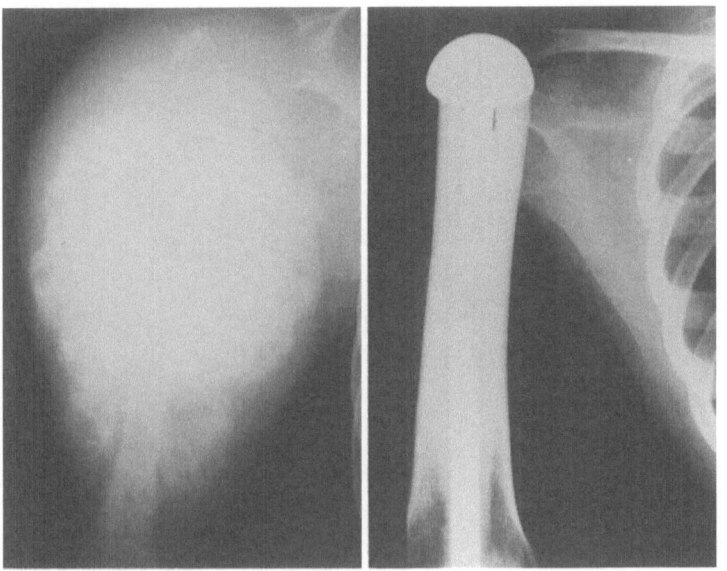

a   b

Fig. 3. a Huge osteosarcoma developed in a 5-year-old boy. **b** Total humerus resection and prosthetic replacent

To illustrate the findings given in this chapter, we will present here the classical indications for amputation and our opinion.

Young age of the patient is not a logical indication for amputation if the treatment involves limb egalization. Our young patients with Ewing's sarcoma or osteosarcoma of the lower limb benefitted from a growing prosthesis that permitted egalization without operation on the safe limb (Figs. 1, 2).

A tumor size of over 15 cm gave the worst functional results and DFS but did not seen to give greater local recurrence. As we choose limb salvage since the functional result is better than with amputation (Fig. 3).

Fracture can be treated by limb salvage after 2 or 3 weeks of orthopedic treatment if hematomas can be resected "en bloc" with the tumor.

multifocal or metastasized osteosarcoma should not be amputated if it is possible to resect every tumor as a primary. If lung metastases are seen, thoracotomy is easier to accept by patients who have not undergone amputation.

The only indications for amputation seems us: appear to us to be: (a) Infected tumors if infection compels discontinuing chemotherapy; (b) local recurrence after radiotherapy.

Role of Vascular Resection and Reconstruction in Rotationplasty

A.H.M. Taminiau[1], J.W. van der Eijken[2], J.H. van Bockel[1], M.R. Sobotka[2], W.R. Obermann[1], and W.K. Taconis[2]

Summary. In this study, the role of vascular resection and popliteofemoral reconstruction in rotationplasty for primary malignant bone tumors is examined. In 29 patients with rotationplasty, 13 had vascular preservation and looping of the vessels and 16 vascular resection and reconstruction. Twenty-five patients were studied by means of Doppler-flow measurement and phlebography. All Doppler-flow measurements showed normal arterial hemodynamics; all phlebograms normal indicated open venous systems, except for one case of loop obliteration and extensive collateral circulation after vascular preservation. Two local recurrences were found in the preservation group but none have so far been found in the resection group. For malignant bone tumors of the femur with tumor extension into the popliteal fossa, rotationplasty is a more feasible procedure if the vascular structures are resected together with the specimen and vascular reconstruction is performed.

Key words: Rotationplasty—Vascular preservation—Vascular resection

Introduction

Limb salvage procedures are well accepted in the treatment of malignant bone tumors. The type of reconstructive procedure is mainly limited by the intraosseous and extraosseous extension of the tumor. Malignant bone tumors located in the distal femur frequently show involvement of the extensor mechanism and popliteal fossa. Limb salvage is then hard to achieve. In these cases of extracompartmental tumor extension, especially in children, rotationplasty is an alternative for above-knee amputation. In rotationplasty, the femoral artery and vein are dissected intact and looped together with the ischiadic nerve. Involvement of the neurovascular structures in the femoral and popliteal area is the limiting factor for this procedure. For this reason, we started in 1984 to resect the vessels en bloc with the tumor, preserve the ischiadic nerve, and, after fixation, perform popliteal-femoral vascular reconstruction. The purpose of this study is to establish the role of vascular resection and reconstruction in the management of patients with primary malignant bone tumors treated with rotationplasty.

---

[1] Department of Orthopaedics, University Hospital Leiden, Leiden, The Netherlands
[2] OLVG/EKZ/AVL, Amsterdam, The Netherlands

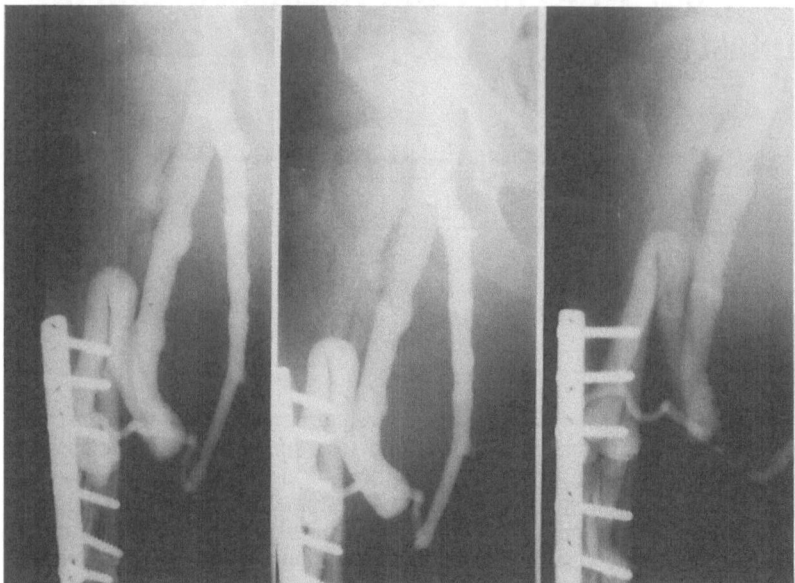

Fig. 1. Phlebogram after vascular preservation

Materials and Methods

All patients who underwent rotationplasty for malignant bone tumors treated in Leiden and Amsterdam between 1982 and 1987 were candidates for the study. Rotationplasty was performed in 29 patients. The age was 5–36 years (means 17.3 years). Histological diagnosis revealed the following: osteosarcoma in 24 cases, malignant fibrous histiocytoma in two, chondrosarcoma in one, clear cell sarcoma in one, and giant cell tumor in one. The surgical stage according to Enneking was stage 3 in one patient, IIB in 25, and IIIB in three. Three patients had metastatic disease at diagnosis (IIIB). Of the 29 patients, 13 had neurovascular dissection preservation and vascular looping (Fig. 1). Sixteen patients underwent dissection and preservation of the nerve and resection and popliteofemoral vascular reconstruction (Fig. 2). Four patients died due to tumor with related metastases—two in each group. Data for functional, vascular, and neurological results were collected in the remaining 25 patients by means of physical examination, Doppler-flow measurement, and phlebography.

Results

Between the group undergoing vascular preservation (11 patients) and the group undergoing vascular resection (14 patients), no differences were found in functional and neurological results. All except one patient have unrestricted ankle/knee motion with normal muscle strength. One patient has limited function and strength but is still recovering (8 months postoperation). No phantom-limb pain

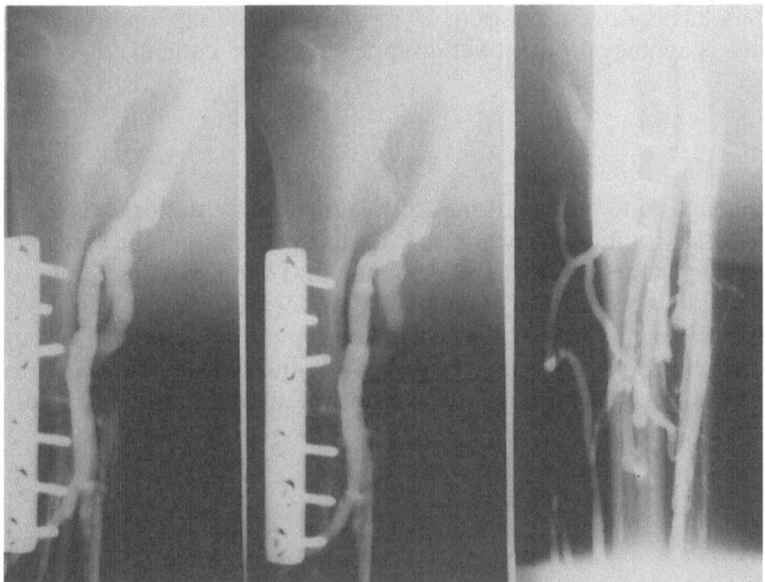

Fig. 2. Phlebogram after vascular resection and popliteal-femoral reconstruction

was reported in either group. In all patients, the affected limb showed normal arterial hemodynamics upon clinical examination and in Droppler-flow measurements. Arteriograms performed in two patients confirmed these findings. Study of the phlebograms of 25 patients who underwent rotationplasty showed normal open venous systems in all except one. One patient had extensive collateral circulation due to obliteration of the venous loop in a case of vascular preservation.

In two cases of vascular resection, some indentation was seen due to slight differences in diameter of the anastomosed vessels, but there were no clinical signs. Phlebography performed 10 months later in one patient showed a decrease of the indentation.

Following rotationplasty and vascular resection, two vascular reinterventions were performed due to technical errors in our first two cases. Kinking of the venous anastomosis with increased venous pressure was corrected.

There was one case of skin necrosis requiring muscle transfer of the latissimus dorsi muscle and one case of infection treated with gentamycin beats, both in the resected vessel group. There were two cases of local recurrence; both patients had undergone rotationplasty with vascular preservation and hindquarter amputation.

Pathological fractures were found preoperatively in six patients, all in the resection group. Of these, five (three in IIB, two in IIIB) had metastases but no local recurrences. So far, in the vascular resection reconstruction group, no local recurrences have been found, although rotationplasty was more frequently done in cases with large tumor extension, especially to the popliteal fossa.

The cosmetic disadvantage of rotationplasty is well accepted by all patients. Most of them can walk, ride a bicycle, and swim with and without a prothesis, and some can do sports. There are no problems with full weight bearing and phantom-limb pain has not been reported. Hypesthesia of the saphenous nerve after a few months is a minor problem but disappears in most patients.

Conclusions

For primary malignant bone tumors of the (distal) femur with tumor extension into the popliteal fossa, rotationplasty is a very feasible procedure if the vascular structures are resected together with the specimen and when popliteofemoral vascular reconstruction is performed. We think we will obtain safer margins and no contraindications for this procedure except for tumor infiltration into the nerves. Because of the good functional, neurological, and vascular results with vascular resection and reconstruction, we now perform this procedure in all our cases of rotationplasty.

References

1. Borggreve J (1930) Kniegelenkersatz durch das in der Beinachse um 180° gedrehte Fussgelenk. Archiv Orthop Unfall Chir 28: 175–8
2. van Nes CP (1950) Rotation-plasty for congenital defects of the femur, making use of the ankle of the shortened limb to control the knee joint of a prosthesis. J Bone Joint Surg 328: 12–6
3. Kotz R, Salzer M (1982) Rotation-plasty for childhood osteosarcoma of the distal part of the femur. J Bone Joint Surg 64A: 959–969
4. van der Eijken JW, Voûte PA, Slangen-Schotermans NR (1984) De behandeling van osteosarcoom van het distale femur door middel van rotatie plastiek van het onder-been. Nederlands Tijdschrift Geneeskunde 128: 1267–1272

Rotationplasty for Malignant Tumors of the Femur and Tibia

WINFRIED WINKELMANN[1]

Summary. Rotationplasty for malignant tumors of the femur or tibia is a good surgical alternative especially in patients who are still growing. The functional results are excellent; psychological problems due to the rotated limb are amazingly few and minor. Since 1981, I have performed 36 rotationplasties: 14 according to the technique first described by Salzer et al. [2] for distal femur lesions, three for malignant tumors in the proximal or proximomedial part of the tibia, and 19 according to my own technique for malignant lesions in the middle or proximal part of the femur. Seventeen patients had Ewing's sarcoma, 16 had osteosarcoma, and three had chondrosarcoma. All patients with Ewing's sarcoma and osteosarcoma received pre- and postoperative chemotherapy. The follow-up time is more than 5 years in four patients, more than 4 years in nine patients, and more than 2 years in 16 patients.

Of the 17 patients with type AI/AII rotationplasties the results were excellent in ten, good in five, fair in one, and poor in one. Of the 16 patients with types BI, BII, or BIII rotationplasties, the results were excellent in nine, good in eight, and fair in two patients. Three patients had superficial wound complications, one patient had a deep infection, one patient had transitory peroneal palsy, and one patient developed a compartment syndrome due to vascular complications and has still almost complete palsy of the sciatic nerve.

Thus far, there has been no local recurrence in any of the patients. One patient (with chondrosarcoma) developed a solitary pulmonary metastasis which was resected. Two patients died of their malignant disease. Rotationplasty should always be discussed with the patient as well as with his or her relatives when planning the treatment of a malignant tumor of the femur or tibia.

Key words: Rotationplasty type AI/II—Hip rotationplasty types BI, BII, and BIII—Malignant tumors of femur and tibia

Introduction

Limb saving operations in the treatment of malignant tumors of the femur or tibia are often not possible if at all effective. Local tumor resection has a high risk of local recurrence if there is extensive intra- and extraosseous tumor growth, especially if there is tumor contact to the major blood vessels and nerves

---

[1] Department of Orthopaedic Surgery, University of Düsseldorf, Düsseldorf, Federal Republic of Germany

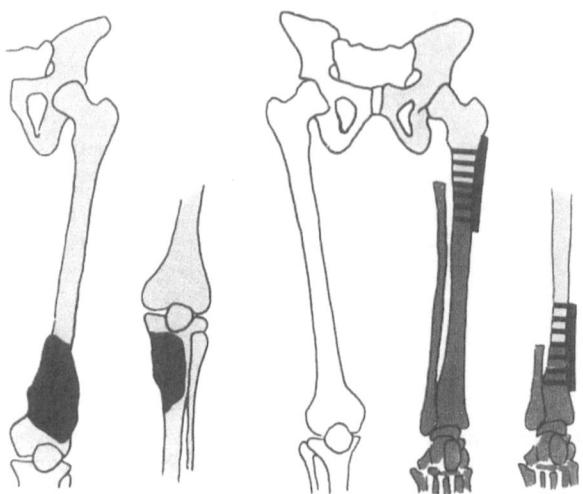

Fig. 1. Rotationplasty type
AI/AII

or if there are skip lesions. The same high risk of local recurrence is present in patients with a pathological fracture hematoma and contamination of the vascular system, as when biopsy is not done properly. In patients who respond poorly to preoperative chemotherapy, such risks have to be particularly considered.

It is also of importance that most patients with primary malignant bone tumors are children and adolescents, in whom a resection arthrodesis or implantation of a custom-made endoprosthesis, when possible, could be further complicated by nonunion of the transplanted bone, disturbances in growth, or loosening of the implant. For this reason, the question arises whether amputation should not be the treatment of choice in local therapy with an optimal tumor radical resection and a well-known speedy rehabilitation. The considerable functional deficits arising from an amputation have led to the development of rotationplasty as an alternative surgical procedure.

Indication and Technique of Rotationplasty

In all types of rotationplasty, the ankle and foot are used as a replacement for the knee joint. This technique is not new. It was first introduced by Borggreve [1] in 1927 for a patient with a shortened lower limb and a stiff knee following tuberculosis. Salzer et al. [2] in 1976 introduced rotationplasty to tumor surgery in the treatment of malignant tumors of the distal femur. In our classification, this type of rotationplasty is termed type AI (Fig. 1). It is different from our own modification—which we term type AII—for malignant tumors of the proximal part of the tibia (Fig. 1). In this technique, an osteosynthesis of the distal femur and the distal part of the tibia is performed. Again, the hip joint is anatomically and functionally normal, but the motion of the ankle joint and foot are done by the quadriceps and hamstring muscles.

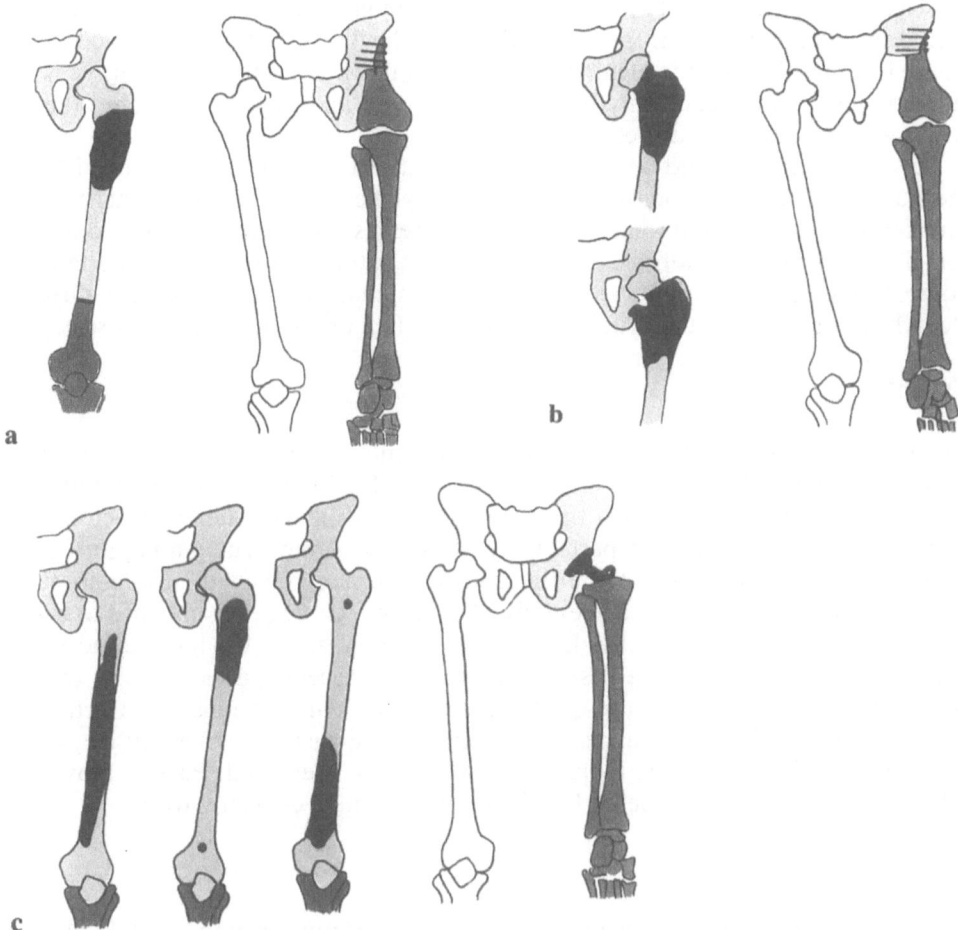

Fig. 2a–c. Rotationplasty **a** type BI; **b** type BII, **c** type BIII Type BI-III

The treatment of choice for malignant tumors of the proximal part of the femur, particularly in patients who are still growing, is disarticulation of the hip or hemipelvectomy. As a surgical alternative for these patients, it was my idea to use the 180° rotated knee joint as a hinge hip joint, and the ankle and foot functions as a knee joint [3–5].

In the meantime, based on the experience of 19 patients operated on by myself, three indications for hip rotationplasty have emerged—types BI, BII, and BIII (Fig. 2).

Type BI

The indication for a type BI hip rotationplasty is malignant tumors of the proximal part of the femur with maximal proximal extension to the intertrochanteric region, with no involvement of the hip joint and no infiltration of the gluteal muscle. For further security during operation, the gluteal muscle can be transsected approximately 1 in. from its insertion, and the iliopsoas muscle at the point where it comes through the inguinal ligament. At this point, the femoral nerve is cut too. The sciatic nerve only has to be preserved and dissected distally; the femoral artery and vein are resected segmentally.

The distal femur should be resected to such an extend that it can be fixed to the ala of the ileum with four to five screws. Active flexion of the knee joint, now functioning as a hinge hip joint, is effected by the gastrocnemius muscle and the remaining part of the iliopsoas muscle, which is sutured to the hamstring tendons. Active extension is effected through the remaining part of the gluteal muscle, which is sutured to the distal tendon-muscle flap of the quadriceps muscle.

Type BII

The indication for type BII hip rotationplasty is malignant tumors of the upper part of the proximal femur with involvement of the hip joint and the surrounding soft tissue. In this case, a similar operation to Bank-Colemann hemipelvectomy is performed, leaving only a part of the ala of the ileum. The whole gluteal muscle and the lower part of the iliopsoas muscle are removed; the femoral artery and vein are resected segmentally. Again, the sciatic nerve only has to be preserved and dissected distally. If possible, the branches of the femoral nerve which are distributed into the distal part of the quadriceps muscle are also dissected distally. This part of the quadriceps muscle then functions as an active extensor. Active flexion is carried out mainly by the gastrocnemius muscle, as often only small parts of the iliopsoas muscle can be preserved. Passive movement is comparable with type BI but active movement is distinctly worse.

Type BIII

Type BIII hip rotationplasty is indicated in malignant tumors in the middle part which require complete resection of the femur. It can also be applied in distal and proximal tumors of the femur with skip metastases. The sciatic nerve must be dissected totally, the femoral artery and vein resected segmentally; the femur is then disarticulated at the hip and knee joint. The tibia is attached to the pelvis with the help of an endoprosthesis.

Until the distal femur forms an osseous attachment to the ala of the ilium, patients with type BI and type BII hip rotationplasties receive postoperatively a synthetic cast, which allows active exercising. Patients with a type BIII hip rotationplasty can be immediately fitted with a prosthesis. A provisional prosthesis is fitted to all patients with rotationplasty within the 1st postoperative week, thus supporting the patient until standard care is possible. These prostheses are principally of cosmetic value but also allow for active and passive movements of the foot.

Furthermore, all of our patients are fitted with a waterproof prosthesis for swimming. This is of great importance for the patients, who are mostly children, in allowing them to go swimming. These swimming prostheses are adapted for each individual so that on entering the water the prosthesis fills up with water until it reaches the weight of the contralateral leg and, thus, does not float.

Material

Since 1981, I have performed 36 rotationplasties, 14 in the technique first described by Salzer et al. [2] for distal femur lesions (type AI), three of malignant tumors in the proximal or proximomedial part of the tibia (type AII), and 19 according to my own technique for malignant lesions in the middle or proximal part of the femur (types BI, BII, and BIII). Seventeen patients had Ewing's sarcoma, 16 had an osteosarcoma, and three patients had a chondrosarcoma. All patients with Ewing's sarcoma and osteosarcoma received pre- and postoperative chemotherapy according to the COSS- or CESS-protocol, respectively.

The follow-up time is more than 5 years in four patients, more than 4 years in nine patients, and more than 2 years in 16 patients.

Results

Of the 17 patients with type AI/AII rotationplasties, the results were excellent in ten, good in five, fair in one, and poor in one. Of the 19 patients with types BI, BII, or BIII rotationplasties, the results were excellent in nine, good in eight, and fair in two patients.

Complications

Three patients had superficial wound complications, one patient had a deep infection, one patient had transitory peroneal palsy, and one patient developed a compartment syndrome due to vascular complications and has still almost complete palsy of the sciatic nerve. Thus far, there has been no local recurrence in any of the patients. One patient (with chondrosacroma) developed a solitary pulmonary metastasis, which was resected. Two patients died of their malignant disease.

Discussion

Naturally, the shortened and, especially, the rotated lower limb is a cosmetic disfigurement and there is the question of psychological problems arising as a result. During a 3-day meeting with 29 patients with rotationplasty, our psychologists did detailed investigations. They reported that all patients with a rotationplasty are happy to have retained a part of their leg, particularly their foot even when it is rotated. All patients reported that thanks to preservation of the foot, being able to stand with two feet on the ground was of tremendous advantage; of course, the active mobility of the prosthesis itself, which functions as a replaced knee joint or a replaced hip and knee joint, is of great benefit. Due to the unrestricted participation in everyday life, this deformity is not noticeable even close-up (Fig. 3). At the beinning, patients with a rotationplasty express a psychological barrier, for example, in meeting new friends or taking part in school excursions. Once these barriers are overcome (this happens in all of the

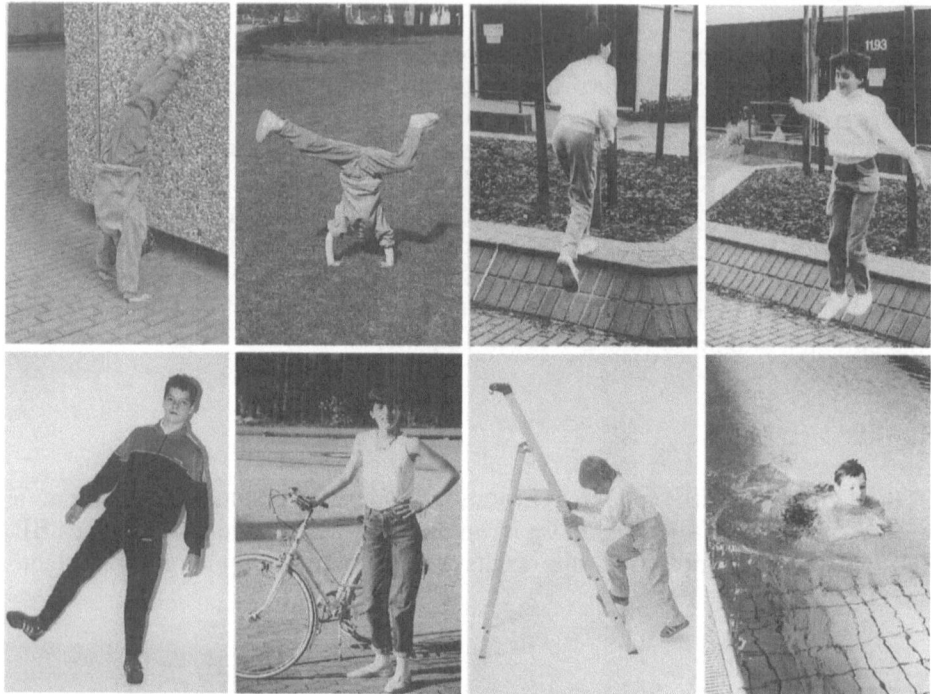

Fig. 3. Activities in daily life and sports in patients with rotationplasty

patients), they feel accepted and fully integrated. Relationships formed with the opposite sex have thus far been long-lasting in all patients, and in younger patients there have been no problems in forming new relationships.

Rotationplasty should always be discussed with the patient as well as his or her relatives when planning the treatment of a malignant tumor of the femur or tibia.

References

1. Borggreve J (1930) Kniegelenkersatz durch das in der Beinlängsachse um 180 Grad gedrehte Fußgelenk. Arch Orthop Unfall Chir 28: 175
2. Salzer M, Knahr K, Kotz R, Kristen H (1981) Treatment of osteosarcoma of the distal femur by rotation-plasty. Arch Orthop Traumat Surg 99: 131
3. Winkelmann W (1983) Die Umdrehplastik bei malignen proximalen Femurtumoren. Z Orthop 121: 547
4. Winkelmann W (1986) Hip rotationplasty for malignant tumors of the proximal part of the femur. J Bone Joint Surg 68-A: 362
5. Winkelmann W (1986) Eine Modifikation der Hüft-Umdrehplastik bei malignent Femurtumoren des mittleren/distalen Drittels. Z Orthop 124: 569

Chapter 4

Rationales of Adjuvant Therapies for Limb Salvage

Local Hyperthermia Reinforced by Thermotherapy As an Adjuvant Therapy for Limb Salvage

An Experimental Study

Yoshio Ogihara, Yasuhiko Tachi, and Tsuyoshi Naritani[1]

Summary. Local hyperthermia with chemotherapy is very attractive as a preoperative treatment for successful limb salvage. However, many problems still remain unsolved, such as its efficiency, its eligibility, selection of suitable drugs, determination of the route of administration of the drugs. In this report, such problems in local thermochemotherapy (with methotrexate, adriamycin, and *cis*-platinum) are discussed.

Sprague-Dawley rats, to which tibia MRMT-1 carcinoma had been implanted, underwent local hyperthermia with or without chemotherapy on day 10 after transplantation of the tumor (intratumoral temperature, 43°C; duration of heating, 1 h). The experimental animals were killed on day 30 after transplantation and the status of the local tumor and pulmonary metastasis were examined.

The tumor growth suppressive effect even in the local hyperthermia only group, was superior to that of the control group. In the thermochemotherapy groups (except for one group), a far better result in suppression of the tumor growth was shown. Especially with the method of intra-arterial infusion, the effect was remarkable regardless of the kind of drugs used. For suppression of pulmonary metastasis, intra-arterial infusion with thermotherapy also showed a superior result to that of the groups of other therapeutic regimens, and this tendency was again independent of the kind of drugs used.

Key words: Local thermochemotherapy—Local hyperthermia—Intra-arterial infusion

Introduction

Recently, many clinical or experimental studies about thermochemotherapy have been reported, and it is a focus of interest for many bone tumor surgeons as to whether hyperthermia with chemotherapy is reliable for successful limb salvage. However, with this treatment, especially in local hyperthermia to the extremities reinforced by chemotherapy, many problems still remain unsolved, such as its efficiency, its eligibility, which chemotherapeutic drugs should be used, and which method of administration should be employed.

In this report, we will discuss the problems of local hyperthermia combined with chemotherapy by the use of adriamycin (ADR), methotrexate (MTX), and *cis*-platinum (CDP).

---

[1]Department of Orthopaedic Surgery, Mie University School of Medicine, Mie, Japan

Materials and Methods

MRMT-1 rat mammary carcinoma was implanted as a 1-mm^3 tumor nodule in the left tibia of 4-week-old female Sprague-Dawley rats. Details of the character of this tumor have already been reported by Sato [1]. Ten days after transplantation, the tumor had grown to a palpable size and local hyperthermia to the tumor-implanted legs either with or without chemotherapy was undertaken.

Under anesthesia with sodium pentobarbital (28mg/kg, intraperitoneally), the tumor-bearing legs were heated in a hot water bath made of styrofoam, and chemotherapy was performed when the intratumor temperature had reached 43°C. The intralesional temperature was monitored by an electric thermometer with a thin needle inserted into the tumor (Analogical Thermometer).

The temperature of the tumor was kept at 43°C for 1 h. The temperature and duration of heating had been decided on the results of preparatory experiments.

The tumor-implanted rats were classified into three groups: a control group, a group receiving local hyperthermia only, and a chemotherapy group. The chemotherapy group was subdivided according to the type of chemotherapeutic treatment and the presence or absence of local hyperthermia (Table 1).

The one-shot arterial infusion was performed via the left-sided femoral artery with a Hamilton hypodermic needle, and the intravenous injection was undertaken through the tail vein with a thin 26-gauge needle. The host animals were killed on day 30 after transplantation, and the state of the local tumor and pulmonary metastasis was examined.

Results

Effect on Local Tumor

The size of the local tumors were expressed as the tumor volume index, which was calculated by: $\sqrt[3]{a \cdot b \cdot c}$, where a, b, and c signify the length of three axes of the tumor.

In the control group, the implanted tumor grew very rapidly. On the other hand, the group receiving hyperthermia even without chemotherapeutical reinforcement showed a significant suppression of the tumor growth, as shown in Figs. 1–3. The difference in growth suppressive effects between these two groups is statistically significant ($P < 0.01$). In the histological observation of the implanted tumors of the hyperthermia-alone group, more than 70% of tumor cells were necrotic or heavily degenerated in the examination of multiple specimens.

The tumor growth curves of the groups treated with MTX are shown in Fig. 1. The suppressive effect on the tumor growth in the animals treated by intravenous MTX without hyperthermia, namely, group 6, was inferior to that in the group receiving local hyperthermia alone. However, all the other groups showed a superior effect, both in the control group and the group treated by hyperthermia alone; the differences among these effects were all statistically significant. The growth suppression of the tumor in the group treated by local hyperthermia with intra-arterial infusion of MTX was prominent and the differences were also statistically significant (groups 9 vs. 8, $P < 0.02$; groups 9 vs. 7,

Table 1. Experimental animals

Group	Drug	Route	Local hyperthermia
1	None		+
2	ADR (2mg/kg)	IV	−
3		IA	−
4		IV	+
5		IA	+
6	MTX (50mg/kg)	IV	−
7		IA	−
8		IV	+
9		IA	+
10	CDDP (4mg/kg)	IV	−
11		IA	−
12		IV	+
13		IA	+
14	Control		

Number of animals in each group = 20
IA intra-arterial, *IV* intra-venous

$P < 0.001$). In the histological examination of group 9, necrosis of the tumor cells was more than 80% in multiple specimens.

In the ADR-treated group, the efficiency was more remarkable (Fig. 2). In this group also, intra-arterial infusion with local hyperthermia showed the most remarkable effect. Microscopically, the effectiveness was also confirmed. The superiority of effectiveness in the group receiving intra-arterial infusion of ADR with a hyperthermia was statistically significant in comparison with the effectiveness in all the other groups (groups 5 vs. 4, $P < 0.05$; groups 5 vs. 3, $P < 0.02$). The effect on tumor suppression by thermochemotherapy with CDP is shown in Fig. 3. In this group also, the most remarkable effect was observed in the animals treated by intra-arterial infusion of CDP with hyperthermia. The efficiency of intra-arterial infusion with hyperthermia was also statistically significant compared with that of all the other regimens in this groups (groups 13 vs. 12, $P < 0.02$; groups 13 vs. 11, $P < 0.02$).

As shown by these results, the effectiveness was rather more dependent on the method of administration of the drugs than on the kinds of drugs themselves. And no significant difference in effect on tumor growth suppression was observed among these three drugs when the intra-arterial route was employed.

Effect on Pulmonary Metastasis

With respect to the suppressive effect on pulmonary metastasis, a comparative study was made by estimation of the number and the size of the metastatic nodules which appeared at the lung surface, as reported by Wexler in 1966 [2]. Since these parameters correlated well with the incidence of metastasis, we present here the metastatic rates only in order to simplify the results. The metastatic rates were lower in the intra-arterial infusion groups than in the intravenous

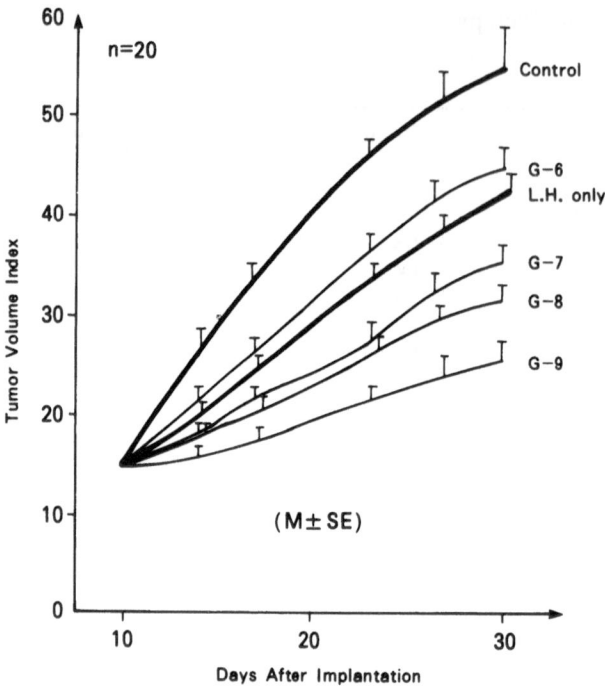

Fig. 1. Local tumor growth curve after treatment with MTX. *L.H.* local hyperthermia, *G* group. G-8 to G-6, $P < 0.001$; G-7 to G-6, $P < 0.01$; G-9 to G-7, $P < 0.001$; G-9 to G-8, $P < 0.02$

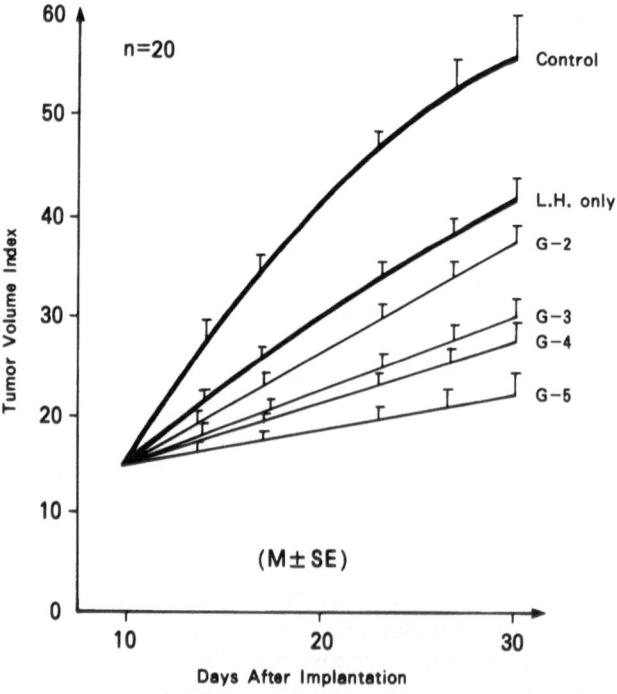

Fig. 2. Tumor growth curve after treatment with ADR *L.H.* local hyperthermia, *G* group. G-4 to G-2, $P < 0.01$; G-3 to G-2, $P < 0.01$; G-5 to G-3, $P < 0.02$; G-5 to G-4, $P < 0.05$

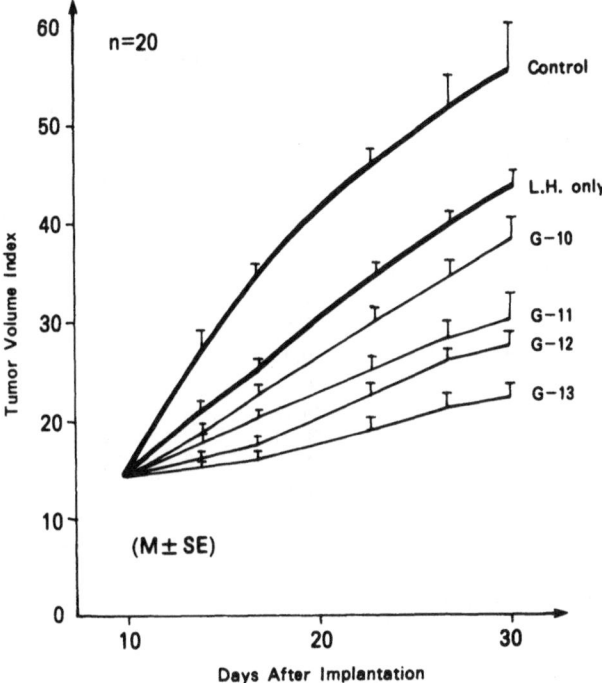

Fig. 3. Local tumor growth curve after treatment with CDP *L.H.* local hyperthermia, *G* group. G-12 to G-10, $P < 0.01$; G-11 to G-10, $P < 0.01$; G-13 to G-11, $P < 0.02$; G-13 to G-12, $P < 0.02$

injection groups regardless of the kind of chemotherapeutic drug used and combination or noncombination with hyperthermia.

In our pervious experimental study, which was not combined with thermotherapy, we found the same tendency; the results were reported when this symposium was held in Vienna [3]. Table 2 shows a comparison of the lung metastatic rates among the control group and the groups receiving various chemotherapeutic regimens both with and without hyperthermia.

Discussion

The result of our studies clearly indicate the remarkable effect of thermochemotherapy in the suppression of a tumor growth. In consideration of the intratumoral necrosis or degeneration, in addition to the suppression of the tumor volume index, hyperthermia combined with chemotherapy, especially by intra-arterial infusion, may have more than an additive effect.

As this result shows, thermochemotherapy appears to be a very attractive preoperative treatment for successful limb salvage. However, there are many points to be cleared before this method can be employed widely. Firstly, what kinds of drugs are most suited to the treatment in combination with hyperther-

Table 2. Pulmonary metastasis

Group	Treatment		Rate of metastasis	
	Drug	LH	No.	Percent
1	—	+	10/20	50
2	ADR	—	8/20	40
3		—	4/20	20[a]
4		+	7/20	35
5		+	3/20	15[a]
6	MTX	—	8/20	40
7		—	5/20	25[a]
8		+	7/20	35
9		+	4/20	20[a]
10	CDP	—	9/20	45
11		—	3/20	15[a]
12		+	7/20	35
13		+	4/20	20[a]
14[b]	—	—	14/20	70

[a] Control group
[b] Statistically significant compared with Group 14
LH Local hyperthermia

mia? In this study, local tumor suppression was not significantly influenced by the kinds of agents used as long as thermotherapy was used. Although the dose of MTX in the study was not as large as is usually used in clinical application, ADR or CDP appear to be more effective than MTX. But, when we take into account the nephrotoxic side effects of hyperthermia [4], CDP must be administered very carefully. From these points, would seen to be a more suitable agent in this kind of treatment. Secondly, in thermochemotherapy, it has been shown that the rates of uptake of chemotherapeutic drugs are strongly influenced by the length of heating according to the individual drug. This must be carefully considered in implementation of the treatment. However, in the presented data, the effectiveness of ADR, MTX, and CDP did not dwindle with hyperthermia of 1-h duration. Thirdly, with respect to pulmonary metastasis, some authors are seriously concerned that hyperthermia may have an enhancing effect. Our data did not show such a tendency (Table 2), but further meticulous and detailed research on this point must be carried out before a conclusion can be reached. Hei et al. [5] pointed out the possibility of a heightened risk of secondary malignancy induced by hyperthermia, and this problem must also be considered seriously.

As for the prominent tumor growth suppressive effect of thermotherapy combined with chemotherapy, the exact mechanism of the synergistic effect of this treatment has not yet been well explained. However, it may be relevant when considering the combination of these therapies and the indications that tumor cells in the S-phase, under low pH or anoxic conditions, are all susceptible to heat.

In conclusion, our experimental study shows that thermochemotherapy is very promising both in the controls of local tumors and lung metastasis. In terms of clinical significance, it is implied that local hyperthermia combined with intra-arterial infusion of chemotherapeutic drugs may become a very important key to successful limb salvage, especially in patients who show strong resistance toward ordinary preoperative treatment, such as chondrosarcoma or in some cases of osteosarcoma.

References

1. Sato M (1980) The experimental studies on lung metastasis of the malignant bone tumor: The influence by incisional biopsy on the development of lung metastasis. Cent Jap J Orthop Traumat 23: 961–972 (in Japanese)
2. Wexler H (1966) Accurate identification of experimental pulmonary metastasis. J Nat Cancer Inst 36: 641–645
3. Ogihara Y, Suzuki K, Sugiyama T, Tsuruta T (1983) Preoperative intraarterial infusion of adriamycin for limb-saving surgery. In: Kotz R (ed) Proceedings of 2nd international workshop on the design and application of tumor prostheses for bone and joint reconstruction, Vienna, Sept. 5–8, 1983. Egermann, Vienna, pp 49–52
4. Gerad H, Egorin MJ, Whitacre M, Van Echo DA, Aisner J (1983) Renal failure and platinum pharmacokinetics in three patients treated with cis-diamminedichloro-platinum (II) and whole-body hyperthermia. Cancer Chemother Pharmacol 11: 162–166
5. Hei TK, Hall EJ, Kushner S, Osmak PS (1986) Hyperthermia, chemotherapeutic agents and oncogenic transformation. Int J Hyperthermia 2: 311–320

Limb Salvage Treatment for Osteosarcoma Based on Clinicopathological Studies of Preoperative Chemotherapy

Kiyoo Furuse and Kichizo Yamamoto[1]

Summary. The effects of preoperative adjuvant chemotherapy were assessed with the ratio of decrease in serum alkaline phosphatase (ALP), radiographic improvement level, and tumor necrotic ratio. The subjects were 16 patients with nonmetastatic typical primary osteosarcoma (OS) of the limbs treated between March 1975 and November 1986. The patients were divided by response to therapy into three groups of good response (+R, eight patients), poor response (−R, eight patients), and total patients. The cumulative survival rate was in the total patient group 56% at 145 months, in the +R group 67% at 112 months, and in the −R group 38% at 145 months, showing a significant difference ($P < 0.005$) between the +R and −R groups. When any one of the three indices was determined to be good, we could expect the preoperative adjuvant chemotherapy to be effective. Prognosis was consistent with the serum ALP decrease ratio in 77% of patients, with the radiographic improvement level in 75%, and with the tumor necrotic ratio in 56%. Histopathologically, when the necrotic level exceeded 50%, necrosis extended from the central to peripheral part of the tumor rapidly; however, viable tumor tissues persisted in the peripheral part. Tumors penetrated the cortex and growth plate easily and rarely reached the joint cavity or capsular structures. Comparing the relation between periosteal and medullary tumors in 11 patients, the former were located more proximally than the latter in two patients, the latter were more proximal than the former in six patients, and the periosteal and medullary levels were the same in three patients. The gap between the tips of the former and the latter ranged from 2 to 3 cm. Two patients were involved with microthrombi in the vein, but there were no skip metastases.

Key words: Osteosarcoma—Preoperative chemotherapy—Clinicopathological evaluation

The advantages of neoadjuvant chemotherapy for osteosarcoma (OS) have been described in North America and Europe [1, 2]. In this study, we assessed the response of OS to preoperative chemotherapy and observed histopathological changes in OS caused by preoperative chemotherapy and the pattern of local extension of OS.

---

[1] Department of Orthopedic Surgery, Tottori University School of Medicine, Tottori, Japan

Subjects and Methods

The subjects were 16 patients with primary typical OS of the limbs who underwent radical surgery (en bloc resection in four and ablative surgery in 12) after preoperative adjuvant chemotherapy between March 1975 and November 1986. Eleven patients were males and five were females, aged from 9 to 74 years (mean 19.3 years). The primary lesion originated in the distal femur in seven, proximal tibia in five, distal tibia in two, and proximal humerus and proximal fibula in one each. Pulmonary metastasis was found in one patient at diagnosis, and postoperative chemotherapy was not applied in another patient age 74 years.

Tumor response to therapy was evaluated with the serum alkaline phosphatase (ALP) level, radiographic improvement level, and tumor necrotic ratio on the sectioned maximum cut surface of each tumor.

The ratio (percentage) of decrease in serum ALP was calculated as:

$$\frac{\text{level at diagnosis} - \text{level before operation}}{\text{level at diagnosis}} \times 100$$

Response was determined to be good for levels of 30% or more, and poor for less than 30%.

In evaluation by the radiographic improvement level, the response was determined to be effective when the tumor was reduced in size and/or sclerotic changes in the tumor were increased in combination with the clearly defined margin of extraosseous mass; the response was determined to be not effective when the tumor increased in size and/or there were no sclerotic changes in the tumor accompanied by a clearly defined margin of extraosseous mass.

In evaluation by the tumor necrotic ratio, the response was determined to be good for levels of 50% or more, and poor for less than 50%.

The 16 patients were classified by response into the good response (+R) group (eight patients) when any one or two or all three indices (available in all eight patients) were good and the poor response (−R) group (eight patients) when all the available indices were poor (all three indices were available in four patients).

Further, the distribution of tumor necrosis was mapped on the sectioned entire maximum cut surface of each tumor, and the pattern of local extension of OS was studied.

Results

As of April 1987, 10 of the 16 patients have survived and six have died because of the tumor. In the +R group, one of the eight died of multiple distant metastases 57 months after therapy was initiated. The mean survival period of the remaining seven patients was 48.7 months (5–112 months). Three of the seven had pulmonary metastasis, underwent thoracotomies, and have lived favorably 15 months, 22 months, and 82 months, respectively, since their last thoracotomy.

In the −R group, five of the eight died because of the tumor 15 months on average (8–30 months) after the beginning of treatment, and the remaining three have lived for 104.3 months on average (64–145 months).

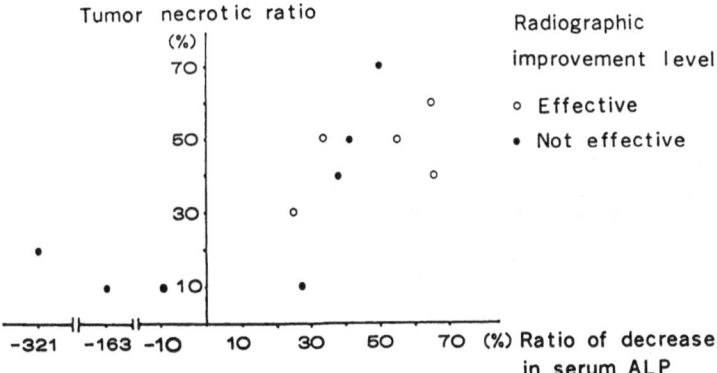

Fig. 1. Correlation among the ratio of decrease in serum ALP, radiographic improvement level, and tumor necrotic ratio. The ratio of decrease in serum ALP showed a tendency to correlate with the tumor necrotic ratio. Radiographic improvement was likely to be good in patients showed 30% or higher tumor necrotic ratio and 25% or higher ratio of decrease in serum ALP

The coincidence rate of the assessment by each index with prognosis in both (+R and −R) groups was studied. The coincidence was 76.9% (10/13) for the ratio of decrease in serum ALP, 75.0% (9/12) for the radiographic improvement level, and 56.3% (9/16) for the tumor necrotic ratio.

The correlation of each assessment among the three indices was analyzed in 12 patients (four patients of the −R group and eight of the +R group; Fig. 1). The serum ALP decrease ratio showed a relative tendency to correlate with the tumor necrotic ratio, but the difference was not significant. The degree of radiographic improvement was good in five (62.5%) of eight patients who showed a 30% or higher tumor necrotic ratio and 25% or higher ALP decrease ratio. However, the assessment with the three indices coincided with the prognosis in six (50.0%) of the twelve patients.

The cumulative survival rate was 55.6% in the total patient group at 145 months, 66.7% in the +R group at 112 months, and 37.5% in the −R group at 145 months (Fig. 2). The ratio differed significantly between the +R and −R groups ($P < 0.05$).

Histopathologically, the necrotic regions were diffuse and scattered. When the necrotic ratio exceeded 50%, necrosis extended from the central to the peripheral part of a tumor. However, in such a patient, viable tumor tissue persisted in the peripheral parts of the tumor, including the pseudocapsular area, distal end of the diaphysis, subchondral bone, areas in contact with the growth plate, within the cortex, and areas showing a telangiectatic OS-like pattern.

We observed patterns of local extension of OS in 16 patients (Fig. 3). The tumor penetrated the cortex in all patients.

The tumor penetrated through the growth plate in all seven evaluable patients, through the central portion of the growth plate in four of the seven patients, through the peripheral portion, perhaps the perichondral ring in two patients, and through both the central and peripheral portions of the physis in the remaining patient.

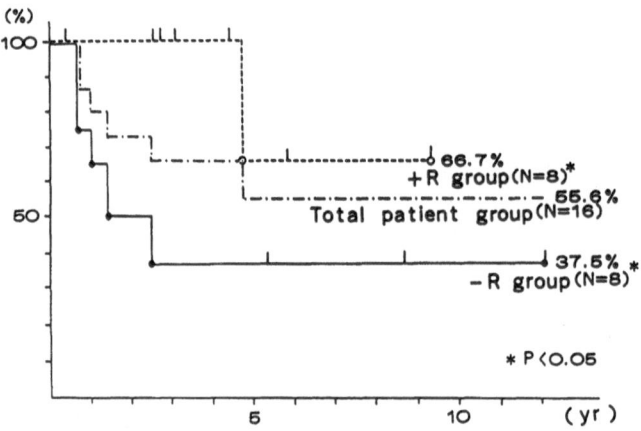

Fig. 2. Cumulative survival rates in the three groups of total patients, patients showing good response (+R), and patients showing poor response (−R) as of April 1987

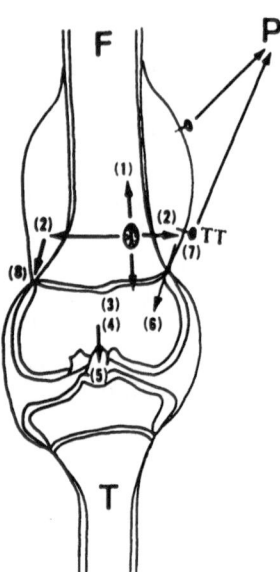

Fig. 3. Pattern of local extension of OS. A metaphyseal tumor (T) easily infiltrates the cortex and growth plate, and reaches the subperiosteal area (2) and epiphysis (3). A subperiosteal proliferating tumor appears to penetrate through the physis from the perichondral ring (6) to the epiphysis, or reaches the subsynovial area (8), pushing the capsular structure. A tumor proliferating in the periosteum forms tumor thrombi (TT, 7) in the vein beyond the periosteum, mostly resulting in pulmonary metastases (PM). A tumor reaching the epiphysis (4) rarely penetrates into the joint cavity (5) from the insertion of the cruciate ligament. A metaphyseal tumor (T) infiltrates into the diaphysis (1)

In one of ten patients with the tumor abutting against the articular cartilage, it penetrated into the joint cavity from an insertion of the anterior cruciate ligament.

In two patients, a subperiosteal proliferating tumor extended toward the joint cavity, pushing the capsular structures without penetrating the epiphysis. In one patient in particular, the tumor reached below the synovia.

Comparing the relation between the tumor in the periosteal region and the tumor in the bone marrow of 11 patients, the former was located more proximally than the latter in two patients, the latter was more proximal than the former in six patients, and the periosteal and medullary levels were the same in the remaining three patients. The gap between the tips of the subperiosteal and medullary involvement ranged from 2 to 3 cm.

Discussion

The effects of preoperative adjuvant chemotherapy for nonmetastatic primary OS of the limbs were assessed with three indices, and the correlation among the indices was studied. The serum ALP decrease ratio and the degree of radiographic improvement level are fully reliable as new assessment indices following the tumor necrotic ratio. The tumor necrotic ratio is accepted as a very reliable measure [4], but in this study showed the lowest level of coincidence with prognosis among the three indices. When any one of the three indices was determined to be good, we could expect the preoperative adjuvant chemotherapy to be effective. The prognosis for good responders appears to be better even if the postoperative protocol is the same as the preoperative one; conversely, the more aggressive regimen should be used postoperatively for poor responders. However, the effects of postoperative adjuvant chemotherapy and/or thoracotomy should be considered in this study.

This was a nonrandomized retrospective study. For higher accuracy in assessing therapeutic means, further studies should be performed under a logical and strategic regimen of preoperative adjuvant chemotherapy.

The histopathological findings were generally consistent with the hitherto reported results [5–8]. In the present study, we found that viable tumor tissue is likely to persist in the peripheral part of a primary tumor even when treated by preoperative adjuvant chemotherapy and that a primary tumor has a possibility of locally expanding to any part of the bone. Using various diagnostic imaging techniques in view of these facts, limb salvage treatment could be applied at minimum risk of local recurrence.

References

1. Roşen G (1986) Neoadjuvant chemotherapy for osteogenic sarcoma: a model for the treatment of other highly malignant neoplasms. Recent Results Cancer Res 103: 148–157
2. Winkler K, Beron G, Kotz R, Salzer-Kuntschik M for the COSS Study Group (1986) Adjuvant and neoadjuvant chemotherapy of osteosarcoma: experience of the German-Austrian cooperative osteosarcoma studies (COSS). In: van Oosterom AT, van Unnik JAM (eds) Management of soft tissue and bone sarcomas. Raven, New York, pp 275–288
3. Enneking WF, Kagan A (1975) "Skip" metastases in osteosarcoma. Cancer 36: 2192–2205
4. Simon MA, Nachman J (1986) Current concepts review. The clinical utility of preoperative therapy for sarcomas. J Bone Joint Surg 68-A: 1458–1463
5. Enneking WF, Kagan A Jr (1978) Transepiphyseal extension of osteosarcoma: incidence, mechanism and implications. Cancer 41: 1526–1537
6. Enneking WF (1983) Musculoskeletal tumors surgery. Churchill Livingstone, New York, pp 1054–1075

7. Usui M, Sasaki T, Minami A, Yagi T, Kobayashi M, Matsuno T (1985) A histological study on osteosarcoma: II. The mode of local extension of osteosarcoma. Nippon Seikeigeka Gakkai Zasshi 59: 45–53 (in Japanese)
8. Picci P, Bacci G, Campanacci M Gasparini M, Pilotti S, Cerasoli S, Bertoni F, Guerra A, Capanna R, Albisinni U, Galletti S, Gherlinzo F, Calderoni P, Sudanese A, Baldini N, Bernini M, Jaffe N (1985) Histologic evaluation of necrosis in osteosarcoma induced by chemotherapy. Regional mapping of viable and nonviable tumor. Cancer 56: 1515–1521

Results of Combination Treatment of Osteogenic Sarcoma Patients

N.N. Trapeznikov, L.A. Yeremina, A.T. Amiraslanov, and P.A. Sinukov[1]

Summary. Experience in the management of 142 patients with local osteogenic sarcoma who received intra-arterial adriamycin infusion followed by en bloc resection of an affected bone and irradiation (20–36 Gy) is presented here. Various modalities of adjuvant chemotherapy (not randomized) were also applied. With surgery alone, only 7.0% of patients survived free of disease 5 years from the primary treatment Adjuvant chemotherapy (adriamycin + vincristine + melphalan + cyclophosphamide) increased this rate to 35.5%; in patients with grade 4 tumor damage, the rate increased to 57.9%. In adjuvant monochemotherapy with adriamycin, 73.0% of patients survived free of metastases for 2 years. The third regimen of adjuvant chemotherapy (cisplatin + adriamycin + cyclophosphamide) gives 76.0% of patients 2 years disease-free survival.

A correlation between the grade of tumor damage in the course of preoperative treatment and survival rate was noted. The toxic manifestations of the chemotherapy regimens used are moderate.

Key words: Osteogenic sarcoma—Adjuvant chemotherapy

Introduction

Osteogenic sarcoma is the basic nosological form in the array of primary malignant skeleton tumors. Until quite recently, prognosis in the disease was extremely unfavorable, and the 5-year survival rate, regardless of the therapy modality directed at the primary tumor site, did not exceed 7.0%–18.0% [1–3]. Progress over the last decade in the treatment of patients with local osteogenic sarcoma has been brought about by the application of adjuvant chemotherapy directed at the suppression of clinically undetectable metastases. Its application has been in three main regimens: (a) adriamycin as monochemotherapy; (b) vincristine and high methotrexate doses with leukovorin rescue; (c) multicomponent complex regimens including the above-mentioned agents have made it possible to improve substantially long-term results [2–4]. Such an approach has enabled the survival rate to be increased and new programs o be developed toward sparing the function limb.

The All-Union Cancer Research Center of the USSR AMS has experience in

---

[1] All-Union Cancer Research Center of the USSR AMS, Moscow, USSR

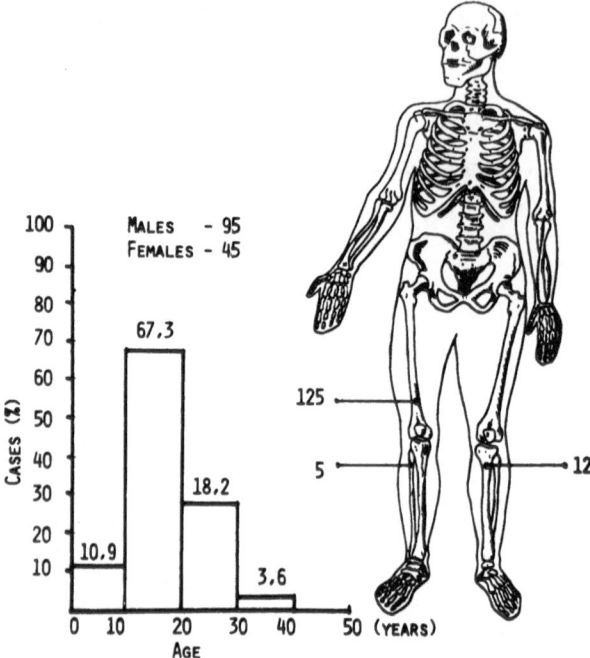

Fig. 1. Distribution of patients with combination therapy by sex, age, site

the treatment of 480 patients with osteogenic sarcoma. For 35 years, there has been an ongoing quest for more effective therapy methods for the tumor. This report presents data on, in our opinion, promising trends in the management of osteogenic sarcoma deserving consideration and further development. Of primary concern are multiple modalities in the treatment of local tumors with the use of preoperative chemo- and radiotherapy en bloc resection, and various regimens of adjuvant chemotherapy.

Material and Methods

Presented here are 142 local osteogenic sarcomas, characterized by the absence of previous special therapy (surgery, radio-, or chemotherapy) and any clinical or roentgenological manifestations of dissemination. In the considered group, there were 96 males (67.7%) and 46 females (32.3%), ranged in age from 15 to 42 years; 67.3% of patients were under the age of 20 years. This series included patients with bone tumors about the knee: in 125 cases, distal epiphysometaphysis of the femur was affected; in 12 cases, the proximal part of the tibia; and in five cases proximal epiphysometaphysis of the fibula (Fig. 1).

All the cases were confirmed histologically and had a typical morphological structure for osteogenic sarcoma (there were no cases of parosteal sarcoma, osteogenic sarcoma developed from Paget's disease, postirradiation osteogenic sarcoma, etc.).

Osteogenic sarcoma was diagnosed on the basis of biopsy and, finally, following histological examination of the whole removed tumor. In addition, the grade of tumor damage as a result of preoperative chemo- and radiotherapy was considered. The morphological criteria of Lavnikova [5] were used.

In grade 1 tumor damage, a general tumor structure is maintained, there are dystrophic changes in the tumor cells, signs of damage to tumor vessels, and surrounding tissues are noted, and cells with mitotic figures are observed.

In grade 2 tumor damage, a focal "disappearance" of parenchyma is noted. There are dystrophic changes in the remaining tumor cells, "curative forms," damage to the vascular wall in the form of plasmorrhagia, and perivascular sclerosis appears. Mitoses are seldom encountered.

In grade 3 tumor damage, there are marked signs of vascular hyperpermeability manifested as plasmorrhagia, perivascular hemorrhage, and perivascular sclerosis is noted in some areas.

In grade 4 tumor damage, tumor cells are not found upon examination of a great number of sections.

Therapy

In all patients, the combination treatment was initiated with intra-arterial adriamycin infusion at 30 mg/m^2 for 3 days. On the 4th day, radiotherapy was initiated, checking the tumor itself and all along the length of the affected bone. It was performed with middle fractions with 2.0–3.6 Gy per treatment, from two oncoming fields. The cumulative focal dose was 20–36 Gy over 10 days. If there were no complications the day following the completion of radiotherapy, operation in the form of a wide en bloc resection was performed.

After wound adhesion, adjuvant chemotherapy was utilized according to three regimens. In group 1 (106 cases), it contained the drug combination adriamycin—0.75 mg/kg on days 1, 3, 6, 18, 21, and 24, and 0.5 mg/kg on days 35, 36, 54, and 55; cyclophosphamide—5 mg/kg/day for 7 days, on days 12–18, 45–51, and 66–72; vincristine—0.025 mg/kg every 7th day in a total of 12 administrations; melphalan—0.3 mg/kg on days 30, 42, 60, and 72. All the agents were administered intravenously. The treatment was continued for 76 days. In a course, patients received an average 390–580 mg adriamycin, 12–20 mg vin-cristine, 3700–5900 mg cyclophosphamide, and 60–80 mg melphalan. Chemotherapy was interrupted for a leukocyte content of below 3000, a thrombocyte content below 100 000, and was resumed with normalized parameters.

In group 2 (15 cases), adjuvant chemotherapy was applied with adriamycin. The drug was administered at 30 mg/m^2 for 3 days. Patients received six courses with 3–4 week intervals.

In group 3 (21 patients), the adjuvant chemotherapy contained an intra-arterial cisplatin infusion—30–40 mg/m^2 on days 1, 2, 3 following previous hyperhydration; adriamycin 40–50 mg/m^2 intravenously; and cyclophosphamide 500–600 mg/m^2 on the 2nd day. Considering tolerance, patients received six to nine courses with 3–4 week intervals. The regimen is remarkable not only for cisplatin application but higher cumulative adriamycin doses too—350–540 mg/m^2.

The treatment effect was evaluated by disease-free survival. The starting point

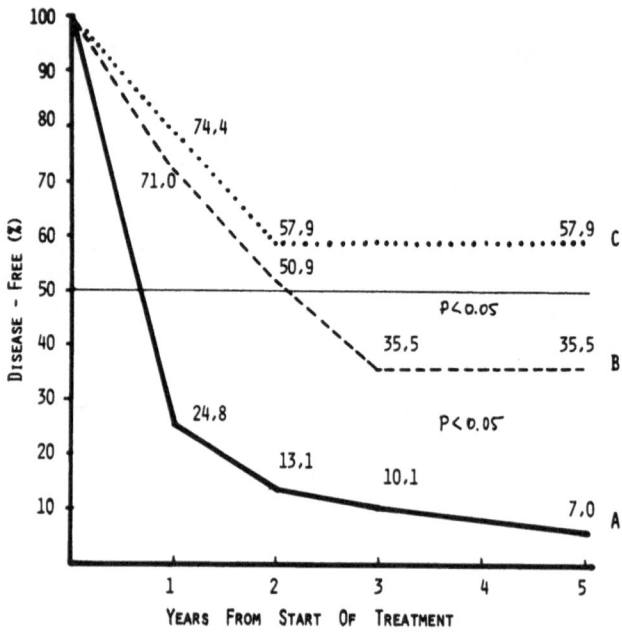

Fig. 2. Disease-free survival in osteogenic sarcoma patients. Historical control group (*A*), group of combination treatment with adjuvant polychemotherapy (*B*), group of patients with grade 4 tumor damage after preoperative chemo- and radiotherapy (*c*)

for calculating the survival rate was the time of intra-arterial adriamycin infusion. To evaluate the above-mentioned parameter in the group of more than 50 patients the Cutler and Ederer [6] technique was used, and the parameter in smaller groups was estimated by the Kaplan and Meier [7] method. Statistical difference was estimated by either Student's t-test or the Wilcoxon test, with the approximation not less than 95% ($P < 0.05$).

Results

The chief parameter of adjuvant chemotherapy effect is disease-free survival rate. Figure 2 presents the disease-free survival rate of 106 patients in group 1. The analysis of the presented data shows that within the 1st year 71.0% of patients survived free of disease; within 2 years 50.9% survived; at the 5-year level 34.0% survived. It should be emphasized that there were no recurrences in any case.

The morphological examination of 106 removed tumors demonstrated that in the majority of cases the grade of tumor damage in the course of preoperative chemo- and radiotherapy was marked differently. The distribution of patients in relation to tumor size and grade of tumor damage after preoperative therapy is presented in Table 1. In 55 (51.9%) cases, grade 3 tumor damage was recognized. In 21 cases (19.8%), upon examination of a large number of sections, tumor cells were not recognized at all—grade 4 tumor damage. In 26 cases,

Table 1. Tumor size and grade of damage after preoperative therapy

Tumor size	Grade of tumor damage				
	1	2	3	4	Total
Less than 10 cm	1	4	29	19	53
11–15 cm	1	10	23	1	35
More than 15 cm	2	12	3	1	18
Total	4	26	55	21	106

there was grade 2 tumor damage, and in four cases grade 1. For the present, it is difficult to correlate statistically the probability of tumor damage of any grade with some objective facts; however, the following objective trends laws are evident. Therapeutic pathomorphism was noted in all 53 cases with tumor dissemination of not more than 10 cm along the bone; moreover, these changes corresponded to grade 4 tumor damage in 19 cases. A similar picture was noted in 35 cases, with tumor size fluctuating from 11 to 15 cm. Of these, in 24 cases, posttherapy changes in tumor tissues corresponded to grade 3–4 tumor damage. Of 18 cases with tumor dissemination of more than 15 cm, only in four cases was therapeutic pathomorphism noted.

To evaluate the relation between the grade the morphological changes in the course of preoperative chemo- and radiotherapy and prognosis, the time of metastasis manifestation was studied in 21 patients with grade 4 tumor damage (Fig. 2). The analysis of results of treatment in this group showed that within the 1st year 74.4% of patients survived free of metastases; and 57.9% of patients survived 1–5 years. Therefore, there is an objective correlation between the grade of tumor damage in the course of preoperative therapy and disease-free survival rate—the more aggressive the tumor damage, the higher the long-term results.

The study of long-term results of treatment in group 2, receiving adjuvant monochemotherapy with adriamycin, demonstrated that 73.0% of patients survived 2 years free of disease. In group 3, with adjuvant chemotherapy by CAP regimen, this parameter was 76.0% (Fig. 3).

Toxic Manifestations of Chemotherapy

Toxic manifestations of chemotherapy in groups 1 and 2 were evaluated in 121 patients. The most common effects noted were nausea and vomiting (75.0%), suppression of hemopoiesis (82.5%), which in most cases manifested as leukopenia above $1500–2000/mm^3$, and alopecia (90.2%). Moreover, there were no registered cases of serious cardiotoxicity; ECG changes noted in 10% of patients were of temporary character. It should be noted that of 121 patients who underwent intra-arterial adriamycin infusion, nine had focal changes on the skin in the tumor field accompanied by marked hyperthermia and edema, skin pruritus, and sharp pains. In five of these patients, the changes resulted in superficial necrosis of the skin and subcutaneous fat.

The side effects of chemotherapy with platinum derivatives were evaluated in

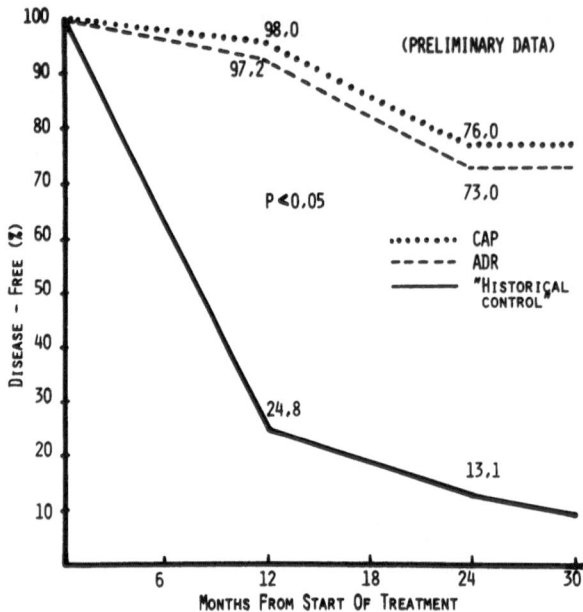

Fig. 3. Disease-free survival in osteogenic sarcoma patients. *CAP* cisplatin + adriamycin + cyclophosphamide, *ADR* adriamycin

21 patients. Most often seen were nausea and vomiting (87.1%), suppression of hemopoiesis (52.8%), nephrotoxicity (48.6%), and alopecia (75.7%). The suppression of hemopoiesis was manifested in leukopenia and more seldom in thrombocytopenia. The duration of leukopenia was from 3 days to 1.5 months.

The gastrointestinal disorders most frequently encountered were nausea and vomiting; in ten patients this was moderated and occurred only once; in eight cases it was marked and repeated, and in three cases it was intolerable and needed special medication. In two of those three patients, it was accompanied by neurotoxicity, which proved to be the main cause of nausea and vomiting from the use of platinum derivatives. The increase of transaminase was noted in three patients, two of them having an increase of alkaline phosphatase at the same time, and one showing increased bilirubin as well. In two patients chemotherapy was continued when these conditions were normalized; in one patient, we had to stop chemotherapy as a result of toxic hepatitis.

Nephrotoxicity was noted in ten patients and manifested mainly as different degrees of proteinuria. Deterioration of renal function was revealed radioisotopically in two cases.

The rate of neurotoxicity was rather high (10%), which as a rule was symptomatically characterized by a headache, vertigo, changes in arterial pressure, and convulsions.

Analysis of the side effects of chemotherapy with platinum derivatives in patients with osteogenic sarcoma, therefore, demonstrated that the most serious of these is hemopoiesis suppression.

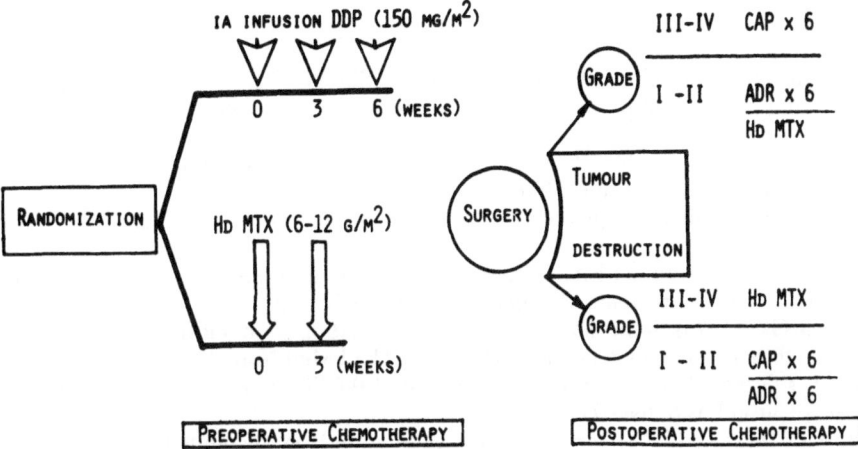

Fig. 4. General schedule for choice of adjuvant chemotherapy for osteogenic sarcoma in relation to preoperative primary tumor damage

Discussion

Study of the long-term results of various regimens of chemotherapy demonstrated that in any regimen the rate of disease-free survival was statistically higher than in surgery alone (Fig. 2, 3).

The outlook for further improvement of results in the management of patients with local osteogenic sarcoma is related to the extent of our knowledge on the role of preoperative chemotherapy. Its utilization as adriamycin intra-arterial infusion or high-dose methotrexate provided a certain local control only and avoided amputation of the limb and performing a limb salvage operation. This has been demonstrated by the data of the All-Union Cancer Research Center of the USSR AMS, where after intra-arterial adriamycin infusion there were no recurrences. However, upon analysis of the long-term results, a certain correlation between grade of tumor damage in the course of preoperative treatment and effect of adjuvant chemotherapy was noted. The tendency is graphically presented in Fig. 2 and it may be briefly formulated as follows—the higher the grade of tumor damage, the better the long-term results of treatment. Therefore, an attempt to apply preoperative (regional or systemic) chemotherapy as an initial prognostic test, preventing a reaction of the primary tumor to postoperative adjuvant chemotherapy and the development of subclinical tumor metastases, should be considered justifiable.

For reasons, in the All-Union Cancer Research Center of the USSR AMS, a study of the efficacy of intra-arterial cisplatin infusion for the treatment of bones of the lower limbs was initiated. The treatment was given at a course dose of 150 mg/m^2 for 2-h infusion. Considering a response of tumor which is tested clinically and roentgenologically (angiography, computed tomography) patients received two–three courses every 2–3 weeks, followed by surgery. If the grade of tumor damage is above 50% the adjuvant chemotherapy with cisplatin is continued; alternatively, postoperative therapy is applied with other drugs (Fig. 4).

References

1. Trapeznikov NN, Yeremina LA, Amiraslanov AT, Sinukov PA (1982) Role and place of radio- and chemotherapy in the management of bone sarcomas. Vopr Onkol 5: 57–66
2. Rosen G, Nirenberg A (1982) Chemotherapy for osteogenic sarcoma: An investigative method, not a recipe. Cancer Treat Repts 66, 9: 1687–1697
3. Sutow W (1978) Primary adjuvant chemotherapy in osteosarcoma. Cancer Bull 30: 178–181
4. Trapeznikov NN, Yeremina LA, Amiraslanov AT, Sinukov PA (1986) Management of osteogenic sarcoma patients. Seminars Surg Oncol 2: 1–16
5. Lavnikova GA (1976) Some objective laws of irradiation pathomorphism of human tumours and their preventive application. Vestn Akad Med Nauk SSSR 6: 12–19
6. Cutler SJ, Ederer F (1958) Maximum utilization of the life-table method in analysing survival. J Chron Dis 8: 699–712
7. Kaplan EL, Meier P (1958) Nonparametric estimation from incomplete observation. J Am Atat Assoc 53: 457–481

Neoadjuvant Chemotherapy for Osteosarcoma

Results in 126 Consecutive Patients

P. Picci[1], G. Bacci[1], R. Capanna[1], E. Madon[2], G. Paolucci[3], M. Avella[1], N. Baldini[1], M. Mercuri[1], and M. Campanacci[1]

Summary. From March 1983 to September 1986, 126 patients with localized high-grade osteosarcoma of the extremities were treated with neoadjuvant chemotherapy. Preoperative treatment consisted of two cycles of i.v. methotrexate (MTX; 7.5 g/m^2 randomized vs. 750 mg/m^2) and two cycles of i.a. cis-diammine dichloroplatinum (CDDP; 120–150 mg/m^2). Conservative surgery was performed in 91 cases (72%). Postoperatively, until December 1983, the patients with a necrosis greater than 90% were treated with two cycles of MTX and CDDP at the same doses used preoperatively. Of the 15 patients treated in this arm, ten (67%) developed distant metastases. The remaining 111 patients were treated postoperatively with three cycles of MTX, CDDP, and adriamycin (ADM) if necrosis was greater than 60% and with five cycles of ADM plus bleomycin (BCD) if necrosis was lower than 60%. At a medium follow-up of 30 months, 68 patients have been continuously disease free (61%), three had a local recurrence (3%), and 43 had distant metastasis (39%). Analyzing the results in terms of the dose of MTX, the percentage of continuously disease-free patients is higher for those treated with 7.5 mg/m^2 (70%) than for those treated with lower doses (52%). Regarding the grade of necrosis, 82% of the patients with a good response have been continuously disease-free compared with 47% for the patients with a fair response and 33% for patients with a response lower than 60%.

Key words: Osteosarcoma—Neoadjuvant chemotherapy—Necrosis

In March 1983, the Bone Tumor Center of the Istituto Ortopedico Rizzoli of Bologna, in collaboration with the department of Pediatric Oncology of the University of Turin and the 3rd Pediatric Clinic of the University of Bologna, started a new study of preoperative chemotherapy in patients with localized osteosarcoma of the extremities.

Design of Study

Preoperative chemotherapy consisted of two cycles of methotrexate (MTX) and two cycles of cis-diamminedichloroplatinum (CDDP). MTX was given on day 1

[1] Bone Tumor Center Istituto Ortopedico Rizzoli, Bologna, Italy
[2] Pediatric Clinic, University of Turin, Turin, Italy
[3] 3rd Pediatric Clinic, University of Bologna, Bologna, Italy

intravenously at two different doses on a randomized basis: 750 mg/m² in a 30-min and 7.5 g/m² in a 1-h infusion. In both cases, citrovorum factor rescue was started 24 h after the beginning of MTX. CDDP was given intra-arterially in all patients and at the same dose of 120–150 mg/m² in a 72-h infusion starting on day 6. A second cycle of both drugs was given starting on day 21. Surgery was usually performed 3 weeks after the end of chemotherapy.

Surgery was always performed at the same institution by the same surgeons with great expertise in the treatment of bone tumors. The choice between limb salvage procedures and ablative surgery was taken considering the size of the tumor, the involvement of major neurovascular structures, the efficacy of preoperative treatment in delimiting the tumor, and the residual expected functional activity. In other words, the choice was determined by considering, on the one hand, the risk of a local recurrence and, on the other, the residual functional activity remaining to the patient. After surgery, all the specimens were studied by the same pathologist and the necrosis was evaluated on at least two entire sections on the two major diameters of the tumor. Necrosis was graded as "good" if it was greater than 90%, as "fair" if it was between 60% and 90%, and "poor" if it was less than 60%. Postoperatively, the treatment was chosen according to the grade of necrosis observed: (a) For a "good" necrosis, the same preoperative treatment at the same dose was given, intravenously, for two cycles. (b) For a "fair" necrosis, adriamycin (ADM) at the dose of 90 mg/m² over 2 or 3 days was added to the two drugs employed preoperatively. The treatment started with ADM followed after 21 days by MTX and CDDP at the same doses used preoperatively for three complete cycles. Another cycle of ADM was given at the end of the treatment. In this way, 360 mg/m² ADM were given over about 6 months. (c) For a "poor" necrosis, the treatment consisted of five cycles of ADM with the same modalities used for fair responders, alternated with five cycles of 20 mg/m² belomycin, 750 mg/m² cyclophosphamide, and 0.6 mg/m² actinomycin-D (BCD) for about 9 months.

In December 1983, after four early metastases observed in the good responders where ADM had not been used, this arm was closed; so after this, the good responders were treated with the same schema employed for "fair" responders.

Patients

Until September 1986, 224 patients with osteosarcoma were observed. Eighty patients were excluded, being considered ineligible for the study for several reasons: metastases, histological variety, previous tumor (two retinoblastomas and one leukemia), site not in an extremity, age over 45 years, refusal of the protocol. The remaining 144 patients entered the study and were randomized to receive high or moderate doses of MTX. Preoperative investigations included computed tomographic (CT) scan of the lesion, and bone scan before and after preoperative treatment. Lung tomograms were performed after preoperative treatment, before surgery. Angiograms were performed before each infusion of CDDP.

Of the 144 randomized patients, 18 were not evaluable for several reasons: Ten patients after the end of preoperative treatment refused surgery and were, therefore, sent to other institutions for other treatment; three patients, all randomized to receive high doses of MTX, developed after the first MTX a severe toxicity and, therefore, received a change of treatment; three patients received postoperative treatment 50 days after surgery due to surgical complications and another one, for the same reasons, was not given any postoperative treatment other than one cycle of ADM. Another patient was excluded following sudden death due to unknown causes.

The remaining 126 patients are the object of this report. Sixty-six were randomized to receive high doses of MTX, and 60 to receive low doses.

Results

Ninety-one patients (72%) were surgically treated with limb salvage procedures, and 35 (28%) with amputation or disarticulation. In spite of this high number of limb salvage procedures, only four local recurrences were observed (three in resected patients and one in an amputated patient). Necrosis was evaluated in all 126 specimens. In total, 52% of the patients showed a good necrosis, 36 a fair necrosis, and 12 a poor necrosis. Differences were noted between the patients treated with high or moderate doses of MTX, but these were not statistically significant; in fact, good responders were 62% with higher doses vs. 42% with lower doses; fair responders were 29% and 43% and poor responders 9% and 15%, respectively.

Fifteen patients, all "good" responders (nine treated with high doses of MTX and six with lower doses), were postoperatively treated without ADM. At present, at a median follow-up of 48 months (range 45–54) only four (27%) have been continuously disease-free (two in each of the two groups of MTX), ten of the remaining eleven patients developed lung metastases after 4–18 months (average = 11 months), and another patient developed a local recurrence after 29 months due to a skip metastasis not detected preoperative. In December 1983, after four of these patients developed early lung metastases, this arm was closed, and the good responders were treated with the same postoperative schema employed for fair responders. The remaining 111 patients were, therefore, all treated postoperatively with ADM; these patients are described in the following. At a median follow-up of 30 months (range 12–54), 68 patients (61%) have been continuously disease-free; 43 (39%) developed distant metastases. Three of these patients developed a contemporary local recurrence (3%). Regarding the doses of MTX, 70% (40/57) of the patients treated with high doses have been continuously disease-free versus 52% (28/54) of the patients treated with lower doses. This difference is statistically significant ($P < 0.05$). Evaluating the same data with Kaplan and Meier disease-free survival curves, the figures become 68% and 51%, respectively (Fig. 1).

Analyzing the results in terms of necrosis induced by preoperative chemotherapy, 82% (42/51) of good responders have been continuously disease-free versus 47% (21/45) of the fair responders and 33% (5/15) of the poor responders. The difference between good and fair responders is statistically highly significant ($P < 0.001$), while the difference between fair and poor responders is not statistically significant. Evaluating the same data with Kaplan and Meier disease-free

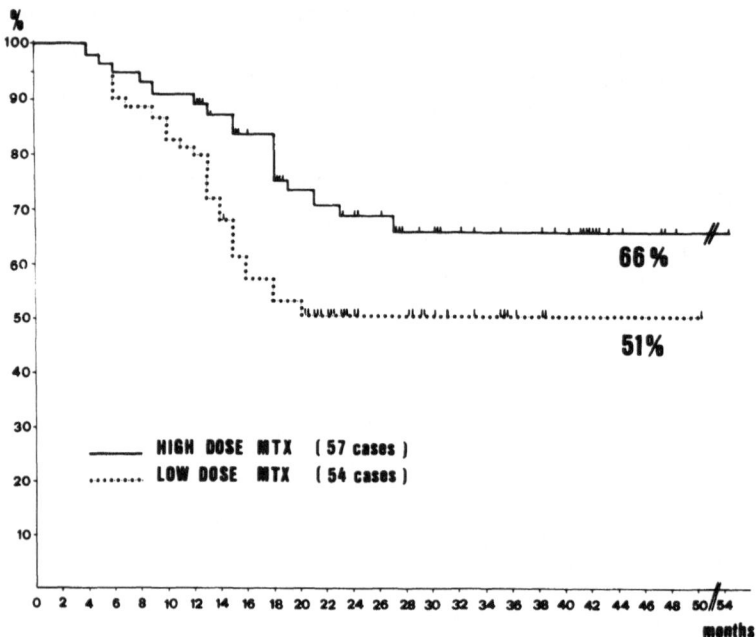

Fig. 1. Disease-free survival and dose of methotrexate (*MTX*)

survival curves, the figures become 81% for good responders, 44% for fair responders, and 22% for poor responders (Fig. 2).

Our study involves pediatric and adult patients and it is thus appropriate to evaluate the prognosis with regard to age. Of our patients, 50 were 14 years or younger and 34 (68%) of these have been continuously disease-free versus 56% (34/61) of the older patients, ranging from 15 to 45 years. Finally, again no difference in disease-free survival was observed between patients treated by amputation (64%, 21/33) and patients treated by limb salvage surgery (60%, 47/78).

Conclusions

In our study, with the multidrug association and doses we employed, ADM is absolutely necessary. Our attempt to avoid this drug for its cardiotoxicity was evaluated in 15 patients only. This attempt revealed to be prognostically nega-tive, only four have been disease-free, and this arm of the treatment was sudden-ly closed.

Limb salvage is possible and safe. In spite of the very high percentage of limb salvage procedures (73%), only four patients experienced a local recurrence. It is to be noted that one of these local recurrences was observed after a hindquar-ter amputation and that another was due to a skip metastasis not detected during the preoperative staging, but subsequently revealed by careful examination of the preoperative radio and angiograms. Our study confirms that good respon-

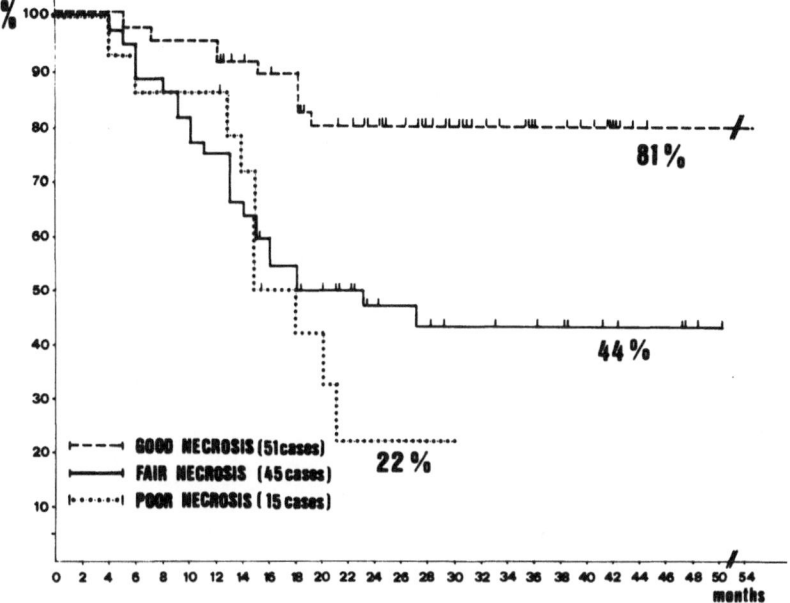

Fig. 2. Disease-free survival and grade of necrosis

ders have a very good prognosis (more than 80%). In our experience, to change postoperative treatment after a poor necrosis, does not increase the disease-free survival.

From our experience, the "breaking point" for the choice of postoperative treatment is 90% necrosis. Our data in fact underline that below this percentage of necrosis, postoperative treatment should be changed or increased, and these variations should not be limited to poor responders only.

The comparison between high and low doses of MTX seems to indicate a better prognosis using higher doses. Although our results indicate a statistically significant difference, a longer follow-up is necessary to confirm this fact.

Acknowledgments. Supported in part by a grant from National Council for Research, project Oncology n. 88.02679.44 and by a grant from Regione Emilia Romagna, law n. 1970 of 13 May 1986.

The Effects of Preoperative *Cis*-Platinum (CDDP) Therapy for the Purpose of Limb Salvage of Osteosarcoma Evaluated by Multifactor Evaluation Method

Japanese Intergroup Study of Osteosarcoma

Akio Tateishi, Hiroshi Miki, Shinsei Takeyama, Seiichi Ishii, Shinya Yamawaki, Tomonori Yagi, Hiroshi Kakizaki, Masaki Chigira, Norihiko Takada, Fujinori Endo, Hisashi Kawano, Shunzo Osaka, Shozo Higaki, Yoshiki Hamada, Shoji Takeuchi, Katsuro Tomita, Hisao Matsui, Kiyoshi Shinjo, Hirokazu Daisaku, and Osamu Inoue[1]

Summary. The effects of preoperative *cis*-platinum (CDDP) therapy against the primary tumor of osteosarcoma are evaluated. The cases consist of 48 patients treated between July 1984 and December 1986 at the 19 cooperative institutions. The regular dose of CDDP was 3.0 mg/kg/day and it was administered intra-arterially as far as possible. The drug was administered twice to 23 patients, three times to 24 patients, and four times to one. A multifactor evaluation method was used, which consisted of four primary factors—clinical, graphic, biochemical, and histological findings. The final evaluation was done by synthesizing the evaluation results of these four primary factors. Definite effects were observed in seven cases, and moderate effects in 18 cases. If definite and moderate cases are assumed to be effective, 25 of 48 cases showed a therapeutic effect (52%). The effective ratio was higher in the intra-arterial administration group (68%) than in the intravenous groups (18%). At the time of follow-up (8–37 months), the survival rate of effective cases was 69.6%, whereas in noneffective cases it was 43.1%.

Key words: Preoperative chemotherapy—*Cis*-platinum (CDDP)—Osteosarcoma—Multi-institutional study

Introduction

For the purpose of functional limb salvage without local recurrence in the treatment of osteosarcoma, it is important to perform aggressive preoperative chemotherapy. Although the effectiveness of *cis*-platinum (CDDP) in the treatment of osteosarcoma has been reported [1–3], the effects of the drug as a preoperative chemotherapeutic agent have not been assessed. A multi-institutional group study was, therefore, performed to assess the effectiveness of preoperative CDDP chemotherapy. In this study, the effects are evaluated by a multifactor evaluation method.

---

[1] Department of Orthopaedic Surgery, School of Medicine, University of Teikyo, Tokyo, Japan

Material and Methods

Cases

Our cases consists of 54 osteosarcomas treated between July 1984 and December 1986 at the 19 cooperative institutions. Six cases were eliminated from the study because of side effects of the drug. Therefore, we evaluated 48 cases to which two or more courses of CDDP were administered as the initial treatment agent for primary tumor. They were 34 males and 14 females and the age ranged from 5 to 66 years with an average age of 18.4 year. Tumors occurred on the femur in 24 cases, on the tibia in nine, on the humerus in nine, on the pelvis in three, on the fibula in two, and on the rib in one.

Administration of CDDP

The regular dose of CDDP was 3.0 mg/kg body weight/day, but it was reduced to 2.5 mg/kg according to the general status of the patient. The maximum dose per day was limted to 180 mg. The second administration was done 2 weeks later, and the third was done 3 weeks after the second. The drug was administered through the regional artery as far as possible, but in difficult cases it was administered intravenously. The drug was administered through the regional artery in 28 cases, through the artery and vein in nine cases, and through the vein in 11 cases. The drug was administered twice in 23 cases, three times in 24 cases, and four times in one.

Evaluation Method

Our evaluation method consisted of four primary factors—clinical, graphic, biochemical, and histological findings.

With regard to the clinical findings, the degree of pain and degree of disturbance of jount motion were divided into three grades, and improvement after chemotherapy was evaluated using certain criteria. The tumor size in the extremities was represented by the maximum circumference above the tumor. The reduction rate of the circumference was calculated in each case. From synthesis of these findings, the clinical findings were evaluated.

Concerning the graphic findings, we assessed repair of bony destruction, regression, and sclerotic changes in the extraskeletal tumor masses on plain X-ray film. At the same time, the decreasing or disappearing rate of the abnormal tumor vessels was evaluated on the angiograms, which were taken at 2 or 3 weeks' interval.

As for the biochemical findings, the decrease in the serum alkaline phosphatase level was evaluated. Since in this study, cases where the initial level was higher than 150% of the normal adult level were evaluated, 16 cases were omitted. Histological findings were evaluated in the tumor specimens, which were taken after at least 4 weeks after the initial administration of CDDP. Detailed histological analysis was done in 25 cases on the entire cut surface of the specimen, and the necrotic ratio of the tumor cells was calculated. The histological effects of the preoperative chemotherapy were classified into four

Table 1. Results of evaluation of primary factors

	Clinical findings	Graphic findings	Biochemical findings[a]	Histological findings[b]
Grade IV	8 ⎫ 46%	4 ⎫ 43%	13 ⎫ 88%	4 ⎫ 48%
Grade III	14 ⎭	16 ⎭	15 ⎭	7 ⎭
Grade II	18	9	0	7
Grade I	8	17	4	7

[a] If the initial level of the serum alkaline phosphatase was not higher than 150% of normal adult level, this factor was not evaluated
[b] Twenty-three cases were not fully analyzed.

grades according to the necrotic ratio of the tumor cells. In grade IV, the necrotic ratio was more than 95%, in grade III 80%–94%, in grade II 50%–79%, and grade I less than 50%.

Results and Discussion

From the clinical findings of 48 cases, we evaluated the preoperative CDDP therapy as grade IV in eight cases and grade III in 14 cases. From the graphic findings of 46 cases, it was evaluated as grade IV in four cases and grade III in 16 cases. From the biochemical findings of 32 cases, it was evaluated grade IV in 13 and grade III in 15 cases. From the histological findings of 25 cases, it was evaluated as grade IV in four and grade III in seven cases (Table 1).

The final evaluation was done by synthesizing the results of these four primary factors. When two or more factors were evaluated as grade IV, the final evaluation was "definite effect." The final evaluation was made in each case according to the following criteria:
Definite effect—two or more grade VI
Moderate effect—two or more grades IV, III
Minor effect—two or more grades IV, III, II
No effect—less than two grade IV, III, II

A definite effect was observed in seven cases, and a moderate effect in 18 cases. If definite and moderate cases are assumed to be effective, the effective cases were 25 of 48 cases; the effective ratio, therefore, was 52%. In our cases, the effective ratio was higher in the group where the drug was administrated via the intra-arterial route. Of 28 intra-arterial administration cases, 19 (68%) were evaluated as effective, whereas two (18%) were effective out of 11 cases in the intravenous administration group. These results suggest that for the purpose of local tumor control, intra-arterial administration of the drug is more effective than intravenous administration.

With regard to the operative treatment of our cases, the limb salvage operation was done in 27 cases, whereas amputation was done in 18 cases. Local recurrence was observed in one noneffective case.

The relation between the effectiveness of the preoperative chemotherapy on the primary tumor and the prognosis of the cases is interesting. At the time of

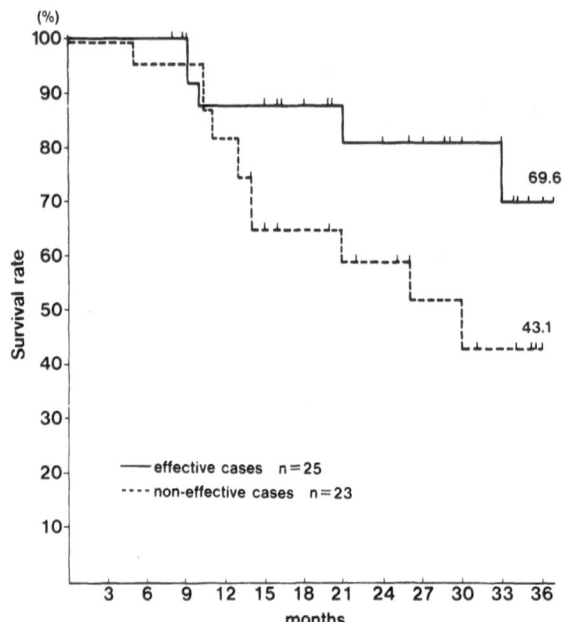

Fig. 1. Cumulative survival by Kaplan-Meier method

follow-up, in 21 of 25 effective cases the patient was alive, while four had died because of the tumor. Of 23 noneffective cases, 12 patients were alive, while 11 had died because of the tumor. The follow-up perioid was 8–37 months, which is short for evaluation; however, as shown in Fig. 1, when compared by the Kaplan-Meier method, the effective cases appear to show a good prognosis.

Acknowledgements. The cooperative Institutions were: Teikyo University, Mizonokuchi Hospital of Teikyo University, Sapporo Medical College, Sapporo National Hospital, Hokkaido University, Hirosaki University, Gunma University, Chiba Cancer Center Hospital, Chiba University, Nihon University, Surugadai Hospital of Nihon University, Tokyo University, Osaka University, Gifu University, Kanazawa University, Toyama Medical and Pharmaceutical University, National Nagoya Hospital, Hiroshima University, and Ryukyu University.

References

1. Ettinger LJ et al. (1981) Adjuvant adriamycin and cis-diamminedichloroplatin (cisplatin) in primary osteosarcoma. Cancer 47: 248–254
2. Jaffe N et al. (1983) Osteosarcoma: intra-arterial treatment of the primary tumor with cis-diamminedichloroplatin (II) CDP. Cancer 51: 402–407
3. Gasparini M et al. (1985) Phase II study of cisplatin in advanced osteogenic sarcoma. Cancer Treatment Reports 69: 211–213

The Influence of Intra-Arterial Chemotherapy on Local Control of Bone Sarcoma

William W. Marsden, Frederick O. Stephens, Martin H.N. Tattersall, Stanley W. McCarthy, and Richard Waugh[1]

Summary. We have used pre-operative intra-arterial chemotherapy (adriamycin and cis-platin) over the last 5 years in order to obtain better local control in a small series of patients with tumours where local control appeared to be difficult to achieve by surgery alone. The results in a series of 11 cases with treatment completed by mid-1986 using this method are reviewed. The series includes six cases of osteosarcoma, two of chondrosarcoma, one each of fibrosarcoma, malignant fibrous histiocytoma and Ewing's sarcoma. Four patients in this series have subsequently died, one is alive with metastatic disease and the remainder are alive with no evidence of disease. Minimal response to this treatment has resulted in pain relief and temporary palliation. Maximal response has resulted in complete local control with limb salvage possible. The clinical, radiological and histological responses to pre-operative intra-arterial chemotherapy are discussed.

Key words: Intra-arterial—Chemotherapy—Sarcoma

The influence of adjuvant chemotherapy on improved survival in the treatment of bone sarcoma is now established. It remains doubtful, however, that this treatment modality influences local control and, in particular, local tumour recurrence. An adequate surgical margin is essential and long-term survival is dependent upon complete local control. Any beneficial effect from systemic post-operative chemotherapy is totally negated if there is local recurrence of the tumour after primary resection. Pre-operative chemotherapy may have some influence on local control but not to the degree where the principle of a wide excision can be relaxed. The early reports of improved local response to pre-operative intra-arterial chemotherapy are encouraging [1–3], but if survival with limb salvage is to be achieved the principle of tumour resection with a wide margin of uninvolved tissue remains unaltered. Rosen and colleagues [4] have shown that complete tumour necrosis can be achieved in a significantly high proportion of cases with systemic chemotherapy and that this correlates well with long-term survival. Assessment of this response has been based on the total cell population of the primary tumour [5]. The elegant study of Picci et al. [6] showed that this cell response is not uniform throughout the tumour mass but did not differentiate between response to either systemic or intra-arterial che-

[1] Royal Prince Alfred Hospital, Sydney, Australia

motherapy. It has been our observation that intra-arterial chemotherapy has a significant clinical influence at the periphery of the tumour and in the surrounding reactive zone. It is this area which is of maximum interest to the surgeon because it is here that the safety of resection surgery is determined. It is also our observation that intra-arterial chemotherapy has been of singificant benefit where local control was not feasible surgically in advanced disease or where the surgery would have been unacceptably radical for large proximally placed tumours.

The purpose of this paper is to demonstrate how we used intra-arterial chemotherapy at first in a small group of difficult cases where local control seemed to be an impossibility by conventional surgical methods.

Material and Methods

The programme began in 1983. Intra-arterial chemotherapy was used in 11 cases over the ensuing 3 years to May 1986. Follow-up then, in this group of patients, ranges from 53 to 20 months from the time of presentation.

Our first case presenting in early 1983 was a 16-year-old male with a large proximal humeral telangiectatic osteosarcoma, staged IIB. It was close to the root of the limb extending into the axilla and there was significant doubt as to whether any form of local control would be effective even with radical amputation. The patient was treated with five cycles of intermittent cisplatin and adriamycin at 3-week intervals. Marked dminution of the tumour mass resulted and the progress computed tomography (CT) scans revealed peripheral as well as intra-lesional calcification. It was possible to resect this with a clear margin and a tumour prosthesis was used for reconstruction. Post-operative histological study showed complete obliteration of all viable tumour with replacement fibrosis. No viable tumour was found in the resection specimen. The patient is currently disease-free and exhibits excellent hand and arm function. Initially, this therapy was restricted to large proximally placed lesions and then latterly to more distal lesions in association with limb salvage procedures.

By May 1986, 11 cases in all had completed their treatment. Distribution of tumour type is shown in Table 1. This is out of 56 cases of malignant bone tumours presenting over the same period.

All cases of high-grade sarcoma received adjuvant systemic chemotherapy. Intra-arterial chemotherapy was used as neo-adjuvant therapy prior to surgery or as initial palliative treatment prior to radiotherapy.

Two early cases were treated with cisplatin only (100 mg/m^2 to a maximum dose of 200 mg). The one case of fibrosarcoma was referred after incomplete local excision. This was treated by continuous intra-arterial infusion chemotherapy as used in our unit for soft tissue sarcoma [7]. This regime consists of 15 mg/m^2 adriamycin intra-arterially on day 1 with 800 mg/m^2 hydroxyurea and cyclophosphamide 150 mg/m^2 orally on day 2, 0.3 mg/m^2 actinomycin D intra-arterially on day 3 and 0.7 mg/m^2 vincristine intra-arterially on day 4. Three days with heparin in saline only follows before recommencing the programme the following week. This treatment is complete within 1 month but the disadvantage is that the patient has to be managed as an inpatient totally through this time.

Table 1. Distribution of tumour type and site, response to treatment and follow-up in 11 cases treated by intra-arterial chemotherapy between May 1983 and May 1986

Case no.	Condition	Age (years)	Treatment	Result
Osteosarcoma				
1	Proximal humerus	16	Local control complete resection, prosthesis	NED at 53 months
2	Proximal pelvis and sacrum	23	Initial local control Partial pelvectomy, local recurrence, hemipelvectomy	Metastases at 34 months Died at 39 months
3	Distal femur	13	Good local control, above-knee amputation	NED at 36 months
4	Distal femur	13	Good local control, resection prosthesis	NED at 22 months
5	Proximal femur	24	Good local control, resection, prosthesis	Metastases at 20 months
6	Pelvis	42	Palliation only, pain control	Pulmonary metastases, died at 11 months
Malignant fibrous histiocytoma				
1	Distal femur	52	Complete local control, resection, prosthesis	NED at 28 months
Fibrosarcoma of bone				
1	Metacarpal	18	Good local control, local resection and graft	NED at 22 months
Chondrosarcoma				
1	Pelvis	42	Dedifferentiated local recurrence after resection, temporary control of pain	Died at 6 months
2	Pelvis	36	Improved local control, partial pelvectomy	NED at 23 months
Ewing's sarcoma				
1	Thigh ? extraosseous ? femur	28	Temporary local control, local resection	Widespread metastases died at 8 months

NED no evidence of disease

The remainder were treated with intermittent cycles of cisplatin and adriamycin given over a 2-day admission at 3-weekly intervals [8]; this consists of adriamycin (35 mg/m^2 over 24 h to a maximum dose of 70 mg) on day 1 and cisplatin (100 mg/m^2 over 4 h to a maximum of 200 mg) on day 2. Our current practice is to review response after three cycles, extending to a maximum of five if judged appropriate. These patients experience all the inconveniences and side effects of systemic chemotherapy. They are nauseated, they vomit and they are ill throughout the infusion. They lose their hair. Temporary neutropaenia occurs and this needs close monitoring. Adriamycin can cause skin staining and tissue hyperaemia. Two cases in this series experienced some superficial necrosis, but there was no deep necrosis or ulceration. Subsequent to this series, we have had one patient develop an area of deep necrosis, which required resection and grafting prior to limb salvage surgery.

In large lesions, it has proved to be essential to define all feeder vessel supply. Large lesions within the pelvis or at the root of the limb, for instance, may be supplied by major branches from both internal and external iliac vessels. Catheters are placed by the Seldinger technique prior to each cycle. Insertion can be varied from cycle to cycle, ensuring that all areas are, indeed, perfused. This can be checked either by local dye infusion or by isotope scan techniques. Serial biopsies using a Tru-cut needle defined response by demonstrating necrotic tumour. Management planning, by mapping the response is possible using this technique.

Results and Discussion

Our interest in this series of patients has been local control and the influence of the intra-arterial chemotherapy on this and, consequently, on management. All patients had some response to this treatment.

The objective clinical response can be graded as:
a) Reduction of pain
b) Reduction of tumour bulk
c) Resolution of extra-osseous tumour mass

Minimal response is reduction in pain. This can be immediate following the first cycle of treatment. Diminution of tumour bulk generally occurs with a significant number of patients demonstrating resolution of all extra-osseous tumour mass.

The degree of influence on management can be graded as follows:
0. No response
1. Temporary palliation; control of pain
2. Temporary palliation; surgery feasible
3. Improved local control; amputation more distal
4. Good local control; limb salvage possible

We believe that it is important to define these treatment goals, not only with this method of treatment, but in all cases of malignant disease. It is significant to differentiate at the outset whether or not any treatment protocol aims at producing palliation in advanced disease with pain control at one end of the scale or whether complete local control with limb salvage is possible at the other.

Serial responses seen radiologically include reduction of the soft tissue mass, encapsulation with high-density material and intra-lesional calcification. The arteriogram is an excellent monitor of progress and this can be performed without inconvenience to the patient at the time of drug delivery. Marked reduction in feeder supply and tumour blush can occur as early as after the first treatment.

Table 2. Influence on management

Grade		No. of patients
0 No response		0
1 Temporary palliation	Control of pain	2
2 Temporary palliation	Surgery feasible	2
3 Improved local control	Amputation more distal	1
4 Good local control	Limb salvage possible	6

These responses can be monitored along with the subjective clinical response and, in general, these have lived up to the expectations of the original management plan.

Histological response varies from fibrous encapsulation at the periphery right up to complete tumour necrosis with fibrous replacement through the whole tumour mass.

The response to this treatment in the 11 patients under review is shown in Tables 1 and 2.

These six cases of osteosarcoma demonstrate a wide range of response. In all cases, the response expected in the initial management plan was achieved. Considerable help has been given to patients with late disease at one end of the scale and, at the other, there has been the ability to perform limb salvage procedures for more accessible lesions. The response in the one case of malignant fibrous histiocytoma and the one case of fibrosarcoma has been equally encouraging.

Chondrosarcoma, as might be expected, responded minimally, although palliative help was gained in one case of explosive local recurrence of dedifferentiated chondrosarcoma, which had been referred after inadequate excision. The second case of chondrosarcoma was also referred with local recurrence after prior inadequate excision. Reduction of the reactive zone with peripheral necrosis made a marginal excision possible.

The peculiar circumstance of the one case of Ewing's sarcoma demanded an attempt at local control of a massive lesion in a massive leg. Although local control was achieved, this patient died of widespread metastatic disease within months of the surgery.

Conclusion

No case gained no help from this treatment. Review of influence on management (Table 2) shows that two cases had good pain control with temporary palliation. Two cases had sufficient local response to allow for local palliative surgery. One case had improved local control, allowing a more distal amputation and six cases have shown good to excellent local control, making limb salvage possible.

The follow-up on these patients is that six of these eleven patients were alive and free of disease, although it must be conceded that this is meaningless at this stage and that the treatment method must be judged on the early response, which has allowed us local control in a number of otherwise very difficult situations. It cannot be recommended that intra-arterial chemotherapy be used to change currently acceptable surgical margins. However, in most of these cases, such margins were either not feasible or unacceptable.

it is very encouraging to see patients brought into a situation where survival and limb salvage becomes feasible. It is equally important, however, that this form of treatment gives some help to patients with more advanced disease not amenable to standard surgical resections.

References

1. Eilber FR Mirra JJ, Grant TT, Weisenburger T, Morton DL (1980) Is amputation necessary for sarcomas? A seven-year experience with limb salvage. Ann Surg 192: 431–438
2. Jaffe N, Knapp J, Chuang VP, Wallace S, Ayala A, Murray J, Cangir A, Wang A, Benjamin RS (1983) Osteosarcoma: Intra-arterial treatment of the primary tumor with cis-diammine-dicholoroplatinum II (CDDP). Angiographic, pathologic and pharmacologic studies. Cancer 51: 402–407
3. Ogihara Y, Suzuki K, Tsurata T, (1983) Arterial infusion of adriamycin as a preoperative treatment in limb-saving surgery. In: Chao EYS, Ivins JC (eds) Tumour prostheses for bone and joint reconstruction—The design and application. Thieme-Stratton, New York, pp 61–81
4. Rosen G, Marcove RC, Huvos AG, Caparros BI, Lane JM, Nirenberg AM, Cacavio A, Groshen S (1983) Primary osteogenic sarcoma: eight years experience with adjuvant chemotherapy. J Cancer Res Clin Oncol 106: 55–67
5. Rosen G, Caparros B, Huvos AG, Kosloff C, Nirenberg A, Cacavio A, Marcove RC, Lane JM, Mehta B, Urban C (1982) Preoperative chemotherapy for osteogenic sarcoma: selection of postoperative adjuvant chemotherapy based on the response of the primary tumor to preoperative chemotherapy. Cancer 49: 1221–1230
6. Picci P, Bacci G, Campanacci M, Casparini M, Gherlinzoni F, Calderoni P, Pilotti S, Cerasoli S, Capanna R (1986) Evaluation of necrosis in 42 patients with osteosarcoma of the extremities created by preoperative chemotherapy. In: van Oosteron AT, van Unnik JAM (eds) Management of soft tissue and bone sarcomas. Raven, New York, pp 245–251
7. Stephens FO, Stevens MM , McCarthy SW, Johnson N, Packham NA, Ritchie JD (1987) Treatment of advanced and inaccessible sarcomas with continuous intra-arterial chemotherapy prior to definitive surgery or radiotherapy. Aust NZ J Surg 57: 435–440
8. Stephens FO, Marsden FW, Tattersall MHN (1987) Regional chemotherapy with the use of cisplatin and doxorubicin as primary treatment for advanced sarcomas in limbs. Cancer 60: 624–735

Osteosarcoma in Children

Preoperative Chemotherapy with Intra-Arterial Cis-Diamminedichloroplatinum-II (CDP) Followed by Tumor Resection, Biological Reconstruction and Postoperative Adjuvant Chemotherapy

NORMAN JAFFE[1], JOHN MURRAY[2], KUNIAKI SASAKI[1], HUBERTO CARRASCO[3], SIDNEY WALLACE[3], A. KEVIN RAYMOND[4], and ALBERTO AYALA[4]

Summary. Biological reconstruction of an extremity was performed in seven children undergoing treatment with chemotherapy and tumor resection for osteosarcoma. An allograft was utilized in six patients and an autograft in one. One patient had a local recurrence at 6 months and was treated by hemipelvectomy. Healing at the distal site of the autograft was present prior to the operation. Among the remaining six patients, union occurred in 11 of 12 potential sites of osteosynthesis. Two patients required secondary procedures. All patients have remained free of pulmonary metastases. The patient treated with an autograft developed a secondary (? metastatic) osteosarcoma in the allograft and at other bony sites. Biological reconstruction deserves further investigation as a means of accomplishing limb salvage.

Key words: Osteosarcoma—Chemotherapy—Biological reconstruction

Introduction

Intra-arterial *cis*-diamminedichloroplatinum-II (CDP) in osteosarcoma has emerged as a major therapeutic modality for the treatment of the primary tumor [1–3]. At the M.D. Anderson Hospital and Tumor Institute it is utilized as preparatory therapy for limb salvage [4]. The procedure is generally accomplished by local resection and reconstruction by means of a metallic or ceramic prosthesis [4–6]. We report our experience with biological material for reconstruction. The results are updated to September 1987.

Materials and Methods

Seven patients with high-grade osteosarcoma were treated initially with chemotherapy followed by extirpation of tumor and insertion of an allograft or autograft. The patients were $8–14\frac{1}{2}$ years old at the time of diagnosis and surgery was performed 4 months to 3 years later. Eligibility for biological reconstruction was similar to that for limb salvage with a metallic prosthesis (Table 1); additionally, selection was influenced by an attempt to preserve the integrity and

Divisions of Pediatrics[1], Surgery (Orthopedics)[2], Diagnostic Radiology[3], and Pathology[4], Anderson Hospital and Tumor Institute, Houston, TX, USA

Table 1. Eligibility for limb salvage

Factor	
Medullary osteosarcoma of the extremities	
Lesion safely resectable	Acceptable anatomical site Neurovascular bundle intact Small lesion preferable
Lower extremity lesion	Attainment of complete/nearly complete linear growth (exoprosthesis preferred if predicted limb length descrepancy will be in excess of 8 cm)
Upper extremity lesion	Less restriction on linear growth
Biopsy	Properly placed (needle biopsy preferred)
Pathological fracture	Not a contraindication
Pulmonary metastases	Not a contraindication

viability of the adjacent joint. Accordingly, lesions had to be located in the metaphyseal or diaphyseal region, permitting intercalary resection. Patients requiring osteoarticular grafts were excluded.

The protocol called for initial treatment with intra-arterial CDP at 2-weekly intervals for seven courses. Thereafter, provided an adequate response was obtained, radical resection of the tumor and replacement by an allograft was performed. Patients were generally hospitalized for 10 days, during which antibiotics were administered for the first 3 days. They were then discharged and followed on an outpatient basis. This involved clinical and radiographic examination of the allograft and host bone at 2- to 3-monthly intervals and monthly chest radiographs. Additional monthly evaluation comprised a full clinical examination and routine studies for administration of chemotherapy. A computed axial tomography (CAT) scan of the chest and a radionuclide bone scan were also performed at 6-monthly intervals for 4 years. All patients were free of metastases as determined by a CAT scan of the chest and a radionuclide bone scan at initiation of treatment.

The therapeutic efficacy of intra-arterial CDP was determined by clinical radiographic, angiographic, and pathological criteria [1–4]. Patients who demonstrated a complete or partial response (tumor necrosis above 60%) were treated postoperatively with intravenous CDP, adriamycin (ADR), and high-dose methotrexate with citrovorum factor rescue (MTX-CF). More recently, patients exhibiting a complete response (over 90% necrosis) have been treated only with ADR. Lesions were staged according to the Musculoskeletal Tumor Society grading system [7].

Results

The sites of tumor, histological subtype, stage, and age at presentation are presented in Table 2. Six patients were stage IIB and one IIA. Initially, only pa-

Table 2. Patient Characteristics and results of therapy

No.	Site	Stage	Age at diagnosis (yrs)	CDP courses	Other Chemotherapy	Preoperative histological subtype	Interval (yrs)	Necrosis (%)	Time to union (mos)		Secondary procedure	Survival (yrs)	Comment
									Proximal site	Distal site			
1	Distal femur	IIB	14 1/2	16	MTX-CF ADR (Preop)	Chrondroblastic	3 1 1/4 off chemotherapy	100	2	2		5 1/3	Full weight bearing
2	Proximal tibia	IIB	11 1/2	14	MTX-CF ADR (Preop)	Chrondroblastic	3 1 1/2 off chemotherapy	100	25	7	Autograft to proximal end of allograft × 2	5 1/3	Full weight bearing
3	Midfemur	IIB	14	13	MTX-CF ADR (Pre- and Postup)	Osteoblastic	1	100	3	3		3 1/2	Full weight bearing
4	Midfemur	IIB	15	7	MTX-CF ADR (Postop)	Osteoblastic	1/3	80–90		4		3	Modified hemipelvectomy for recurrence, union present at distal site
5	Proximal tibia	IIB	13 1/2	7	MTX-CF ADR (Preop)	Fibroblastic	1/2	100	9	16		3/4	Full weight bearing
6	Distal radius	IIB	9	7	ADR (Postop)	Osteoblastic	1/3	95	13	7	Pins removed, autograft to pseudoarthrosis left wrist	3/4	Recurrence of osteosaroma autograft and other bones
7	Midtibia	IIA	13	6	ADR (Postop)	fibroblastic	1/2	94		11		1/2	Full weight bearing with brace, secondary procedure contemplated for proximal site

tients 4 and 7 were considered eligible for the procedure. In patients 1–3, the lesions were considered too extensive for limb salvage and they had not attained maximum or near-maximum skeletal maturity. They achieved an initial dramatic response to intra-arterial CDP and at the patients' request surgery was deferred and an experimental chemotherapy program was implemented. This comprised an additional seven to nine courses of intra-arterial CDP and MTX-CF and ADR. Limb salvage was performed in patients 3–7 after intra-arterial CDP during "adjuvant" chemotherapy and in patients 1 and 2 approximately $1\frac{1}{2}$–2 years after discontinuation of chemotherapy. The patients requested a surgical procedure in view of the possibility of local recurrence despite the fact that chemotherapy appeared to have induced a complete response by clinical, radiographic, and pathological (needle biopsy) criteria.

Local en bloc resection, biological reconstruction, and restoration of the integrity of the limb were successfully accomplished in all patients. An allograft was utilized for all patients except patient 6, who was treated with a fibular interpositional autograft to the left distal radius. Pathological examination revealed 95%–100% destruction in six patients and 80%–90% in the seventh. Preoperative chemotherapy, therefore, downstaged the primary tumors from IIB to IIA in six patients who initially presented with IIB lesions. Local recurrence was detected 6 months after the surgical procedure in patient 4 and was successfully treated with a modified hemipelvectomy. In retrospect, this patient probably had a proximal skip metastasis in the host bone.

The possibility of union was eliminated in the patient who underwent the modified hemipelvectomy. However, it appeared that at the distal site, union was nonetheless present. In the remaining six patients, at 12 sites of potential osteosynthesis between allo- or autograft and host bone, radiological evidence of union was noted in 11. Ten occurred between 2 and 16 months in five patients receiving various forms of postoperative chemotherapy (CDP, MTX-CF, and ADR), and at the 11th 25 months after two secondary procedures (see below). Chemotherapy in the latter had been discontinued 12 months earlier. An example of healing with preoperative treatment, tumor resection, allograft insertion, and successful union is presented in Fig. 1.

Secondary procedures were performed at two nonunion sites. Autograft bone chips on two occasions were inserted into the proximal end of the allograft of the tibia in patients 2, and on one occasion in patient 6 to repair an autograft pseudoarthodesis of the wrist. It is anticipated that autograft bone chips will also be required to achieve union of the proximal end of the allograft of patient 7 if this is not observed within the next 6 months.

No patient has developed pulmonary metastases. The follow-up period ranges from $1\frac{1}{4}$ to $2\frac{1}{2}$ years from surgery and $1\frac{1}{2}$ to $5\frac{1}{3}$ years from diagnosis. Patient 6 with the radial autograft developed a secondary osteosarcoma at the distal end of the graft $1\frac{3}{4}$ years from diagnosis ($1\frac{1}{3}$ years from the operative procedure). Concurrently, tumor was detected in several other sites (vertebra, femur, and skull). The lungs were free of pulmonary metastases and the patient remains alive with disease. The other patients are disease-free with excellent allograft function from $1\frac{1}{2}$ to $5\frac{1}{3}$ years. All patients with lower extremity lesions are fully weight bearing. This includes patient 7, who uses a brace because of apparent nonunion at the proximal site.

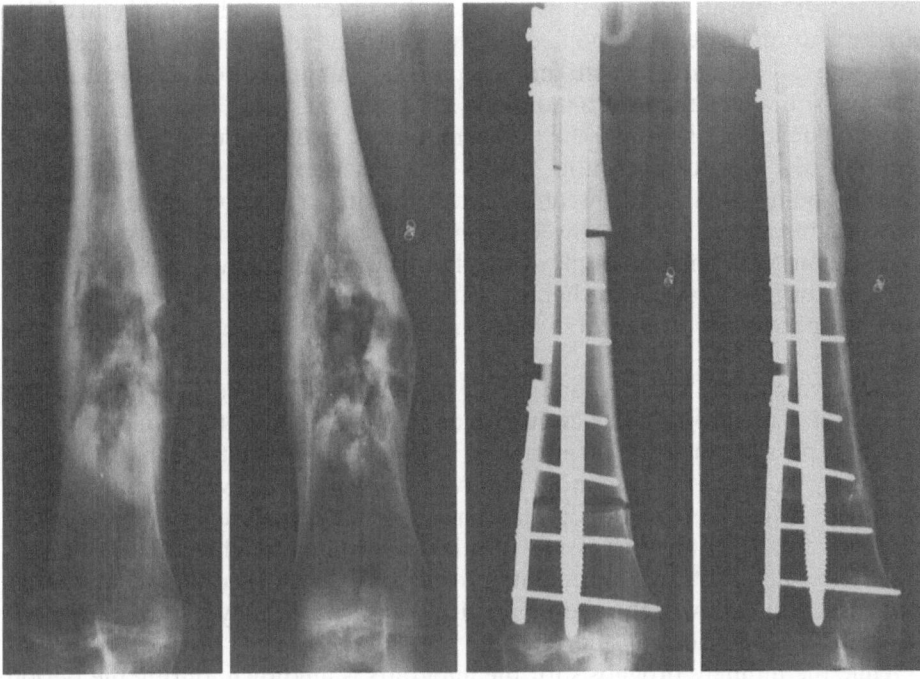

a, b   c, d

Fig. 1. a Osteosarcoma, diaphysis of right femur in patient 4 (Table 2). Extensive destruction with mixed lytic and blastic areas is evident. Moderate periosteal reaction and a soft tissue component is also present. **b** Following treatment with intra-arterial CDP, MTX-CF, and ADR, tumor destruction and healing of bone was achieved. This is particularly evident with reconstitution of the cortex and a layered periosteal reaction. A stainless steel coil at the site of occlusion of the right superficial femoral artery is present. **c** Postoperative appearance following tumor resection with insertion of allograft. Allograft is held in position by two metallic plates and intramedullary rod. Note the small gap between allograft and host bone at the superior and inferior region. **d** Union of allograft with host bone. A moderate amount of callus is present at each site of osteosynthesis

Discussion

All patients undergoing limb salvage in our previous reports were subjected to reconstruction with a metallic prosthesis [1–5]. However, the ultimate benefit of the metallic implant remains to be determined. Late potential complications include mechanical failure, loss of fixation, fracture, and stress shielding. Some of these may also be applicable to biological reconstruction, since most human grafts have no viable bone and generally function in the capacity of a "trellis" or lattice upon which host bone can be laid down [9, 10]. In fact, studies suggest that foreign bone can be slowly revascularized and replaced with host bone.

The above factors rekindled our interest in the possible use of biological reconstruction for limb salvage. It appeared particularly attractive for tumors where attempts could be made to retain the integrity of a joint. Among the 12 potential sites of osteosynthesis between allo- and autograft and host bone, union was eventually accomplished in 11 although three secondary procedures in two patients were also required. Union was also observed at the distal end of the patient who underwent a modified hemipelvectomy at 6 months. A secondary procedure is contemplated for the last patient if union is not achieved in the proximal site within the next 6 months.

The influence of chemotherapy in promoting or retarding union of biological materials deserves consideration. Grafts were inserted during treatment in five patients and in two after its discontinuation. Failure to incorporate was noted in both circumstances. Further, three secondary procedures were performed after discontinuation of chemotherapy and only two were successful. This limited experience suggests that chemotherapy, either during or after its administration, does not necessarily prevent biological incorporation of donor graft into host bone.

The development of osteosarcoma in the autograft and several parts of the skeleton in patient 6 suggests an innate or genetic potential to develop the disease. It is possible that the phenomenon may have been due to micrometastases originating in the primary tumor; however, there was no evidence of lung involvement. Nonetheless, tumor may have originated at the primary site and surfaced after a finite suppression of micrometastases by chemotherapy. This experience demonstrates a potential drawback to autograft for biological reconstruction. Conversely, the possibility that allograft may harbor tumor (or infection) must also be considered.

While the ultimate prognosis for the allografts is unknown, during the period of observation, no metastases, degenerative changes, immune reactions, rejection, infection, or fractures have been observed. Healing has been excellent in most patients and the possibility that all grafts may ultimately become vascularized is a serious consideration. Many of the documented complications encountered with metallic or plastic prostheses have been avoided. This experience encourages further investigation in the use of biological materials for reconstruction and functional rehabilitation.

References

1. Jaffe N, Knapp J, Chuang VP, Wallace S, Ayala A, Murray J, Cangir A, Wang Y-M, Benjamin RS (1983) Osteosarcoma: Intra-arterial treatment of the primary tumor with cis-diamminedichloroplatinum II (CDP). Angiographic, pathologic and pharmacologic studies. Cancer 51: 402–407
2. Jaffe N, Robertson R, Ayala A, Wallace S, Chuang V, Anzai T, Cangir A, Wang Y-M, Chen T (1985) Comparison of intra-arterial cis-diamminedichloroplatinum-II with high dose methotrexate and citrovorum factor rescue in the treatment of primary osteosarcoma. J Clin Oncol 3: 1101–1104
3. Jaffe N, Spears R, Eftakhari F, Robertson R, Cangir A, Takaue Y, Raymond K, Wang Y-M (1987) Pathologic fracture in osteosarcoma. Impact of chemotherapy on primary tumor and survival. Cancer 59: 701–709
4. Jaffe N, Murray J, Ayala A, Wallace S, Raymond K, Carrasco H, Robertson R (1987) Limb salvage using cis-diamminedichloroplatinum-II as preoperative treatment and in the design of post-operative adjuvant treatment in children with osteosarcoma. In: Enneking WF (ed) Limb salvage in musculoskeletal oncology. Churchill Livingstone, New York, pp 333–341

5. Sim EH, Ivins JC, Douglas DJ (1978) Surgical treatment of osteogenic sarcoma at the Mayo Clinic. Cancer Treat Rep. 62: 205–211
6. Burrows HJ, Wilson JN, Scales JT (1975) Excision of tumours of humerus and femur, with restoration by internal prosthesis. J Bone Joint Surg (Br) 57: 148–159
7. Enneking WF, Spanier SS, Goodman MA (1980) A system for the surgical staging of musculoskeletal sarcoma. Clin Orthop 153: 106–120
8. Pallor RM (1983) Use of biologic fixation in tumor prosthesis development. In: Chao EYS, Ivins JC (eds) Tumor prosthesis for bone and joint reconstruction—The design and application. Thieme-Stratton, New York, pp 429–435
9. Herrdon CH, Chase JW (1954) The fate of autogenous and homogenous bone grafts including articular surfaces. Surg Gynec Obstet 98: 273–290
10. Bonfiglio M, Jeter WS, Smith CL (1955) The immune concept: Its relation to bone transplantation. Ann NY Acad 59: 417

Neoadjuvant Chemotherapy by Intra-Arterial Infusion for Osteosarcoma

HISASHI KAWANO and SADAYOSHI TORIYAMA[1]

Summary. Forty-seven patients with malignant bone and soft tissue tumors were treated with two kinds of intra-arterial infusion chemotherapy prior to surgery. These chemotherapeutic regimens were divided into two groups according to the infusional technique. Both techniques aimed to obtain a higher concentration of infused drug in the tumor tissue than conventional continuous intra-arterial infusion. Group A consisted of 35 cases, including 12 Osteosarcomas, treated with intra-arterial infusion under arterial blockade; group B consisted of 12 cases, including seven osteosarcomas, treated with balloon-occluded intra-arterial infusion (BOAI). The effect of preoperative chemotherapy was evaluated in the primary lesions of 22 patients with osteosarcoma. A better objective response was recognized in group B in all the monitored points. In clinical studies on *cis*-platinum (CDDP), it was also proved that BOAI is effective in administering the drugs at a higher concentration in the tumor tissue. It is believed that BOAI is a very useful technique for preoperative chemotherapy when planning limb salvage to obtain local control of the tumor.

Key words: Osteosarcoma—Intra-arterial infusion—Chemotherapy

Introduction

In recent years, limb salvage has been employed by an increasing number of institutions as surgical treatment of osteosarcoma. The progress in preoperative treatment of malignant tumors in bone and soft tissue has enabled us to preserve safely the affected limb for which amputation would have been indicated otherwise. One of the contributory factors is the potent preoperative chemotherapy and radiotherapy, which can effectively control the condition of the effected area. Any limb salvage procedure requires effective control of the primary tumor lesions, unless local control of the tumor is accomplished, wide excision may be immpossible [1].

However, when anticancer agents are systemically administered, the resulting side effects sometimes prevent increasing the dose as much as desired. Intra-arterial administration of cytostatic drugs for the treatment of malignant bone and soft tissue tumors is a very effevtive method of introducing drugs into the tumor site in high concentrations [2]. The present paper presents the efficacy and rationale of a special method of intra-arterial infusion chemotherapy for osteosarcoma in particular.

---

[1]Department of Orthopaedic Surgery, Nihon University, School of Medicine, Tokyo, Japan

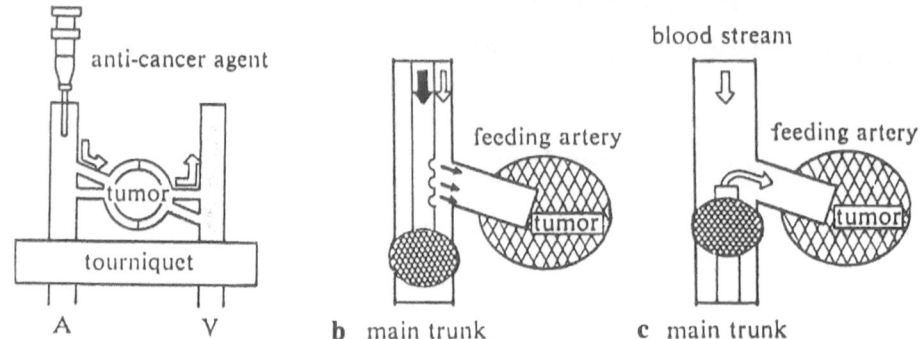

Fig. 1a–c. The rationales of the two kinds of infusional chemotherapy. **a** Intra-arterial infusion under arterial blockade. **b, c** Balloon-occluded arterial infusion. **b** Berman catheter; **c** Wedge pressure catheter

Material and Methods

Intra-arterial infusion under arterial blockade techniques that produce hemostasis at the periphery of the tumor to accelerate penetration and adherence of the drug in the tumor has been adopted as a pilot study at the Nihon University Hospital since 1980; the patients treated under this study are classified as group A.

The rationale of this method (Fig. 1), consisting of blocking the distal blood flow by tourniquet, is that natural arterial blood pressure is enough to thrust the drug into the tumor in high concentrations. The tourniquet is usually applied for 30 min without any anesthesia. When the tumor is located around the knee, an infusion tube is inserted from the femoral artery percutaneously and placed in the proximal blood supply to the tumor visualized by angiography. A bolus shot infusion with hemostasis is then usually carried out once a week for 3 weeks prior to surgery. Before 1984, this procedure combined a bolus shot of a multiple drug regimen consisting of mainly adriamycin, but *cis*-platinum as a single agent replaced this in 1984. This method was applied for 15 cases of osteosarcoma from 1980 to 1985 [3].

From 1986, we have adopted balloon-occluded arterial infusion (BOAI) as neoadjuvant chemotherapy for 12 patients, including seven osteosarcomas. These patients are classified as group B. This new method involves two kinds of balloon catheter used inside the artery to block the arterial flow just distal to the tumor-nourishing arteries. The rationale of this new approach consists of introducing a catheter with a balloon into an artery, inflating the balloon at the appropriate site to block the main bloodstream, and thrusting the infused drugs selectively into the feeding artery of the tumor from the hole in the catheter head. For the tumor developing around the knee, a Berman catheter, which has a hole just below the balloon, is introduced descendingly into the femoral artery. The balloon is inflated several times before it is fixed where the tumor is most clearly demonstrated with the contrast medium, and the drug is released. When the cathether had to be inserted ascendingly into the artery, a wedge pressure catheter, with a hole in the catheter head, was used. Under general or epidural

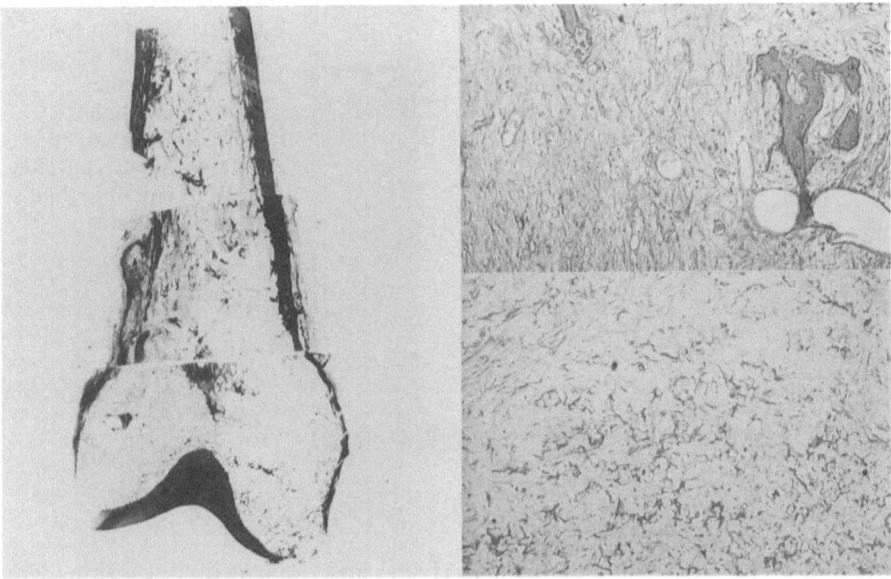

Fig. 2. Total cross section obtained by wide resection of osteosarcoma in 16-year-old male

anesthesia, the drug was infused with an automatic infusor over a period of 1 h while the balloon was inflated. The agent used was *cis*-platinum at a dose of 3 mg/kg weekly for three courses prior to surgery.

A total of 47 cases of malignant bone and soft tissue tumors including 22 osteosarcomas were treated with these treatment protocols. The effectiveness of the treatment was determined in terms of reduction in tumor size, angiogram, and patho-histological examinations.

Results and Discussion

The reduction of tumor size was calculated using a special formula and in more than 60% of cases there was a reduction of tumor size. The reduction rate was less significant in the osteosarcoma cases than in those with a soft tissue tumor. All the cases where hypervascularity had been demonstrated before chemotherapy showed a decrease or loss of the feeding arteries. These results were not significantly different between groups A and B. Histological evaluation was carried out on the basis of pathohistological criteria established by Ohoshi et al. Most patients revealed marked destruction and damage in the tumor area and two patients treated as group A showed more than 90% tumor necrosis. In group B, complete necrosis was noted in two cases and the remainder showed more than grade 3 (Fig. 2). The local necrosis rate recognized in group B was much higher than that in group A.

The non-protein binding *cis*-platinum level in peripheral blood was determined 11 times in five cases. Figure 3 shows a comparison of the blood *cis*-

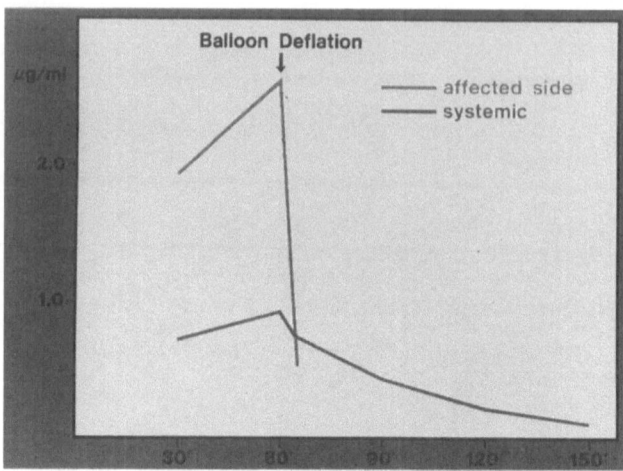

Fig. 3. Comparison of free *cis*-platinum concentration with affected side and systemic circulation. Higher concentration can be obtained in affected side by BOAI method than contralateral side

platinum concentration between the BOAI side and the contralateral side. The concentration on the BOAI side was two to three times higher than that on the contralateral side. Thus, it is speculated that the tumor received the drug at an even higher concentration. From the result that the contralateral blood concentration was almost as high as that obtained with systemic administration of *cis*-platinum, it is inferred that the agent is maintained in the systemic circulation, after passing the tumor, at a drug concentration is still effective enough to eradicate micrometastases [4].

Local control of the tumor involves increasing the tumor necrosis in the lesion and shelling out the tumor so that reduction surgery or safely marginal resection may become possible [5]. Such techniques, especially the BOAI method, could deliver a large amount of the anticancer agent directly to the tumor. The remainder of the drug in the systemic circulation proved to the effective against micrometastases. This is, thus, considered to be a very promising type of neoadjuvant chemotherapy.

References

1. Eilber FR, Mirra JJ, Grant TT, Weisenburger T, Morton D (1978) Is amputation necessary for sarcomas? Ann Surg 192: 431–438
2. Takagi M, Ishikawa G. Akahoshi Y, Takeuchi S, Nishimoto T, Chen S (1974) Pathologic study of the therapeutic effects in the osteosarcoma treated with continuous intra-arterial infusion. J Jpn Soc Cancer Ther 9: 109–121
3. Kawano H, Toriyama S (1983) Intra-arterial chemotherapy under arterial blockade for sarcoma. Orthop Traum Surg 26: 77–83
4. Matsumoto S (1987) A study of cisplatinum dosage regimen with particular reference to its pharmacokinetics. J Jpn Soc Cancer Ther 22: 621–631
5. Kawano H (1987) Recent concept of treatment for osteosarcoma. Nihon Univ J Med 46: 107–113

Clinical Experience with Preoperative Continuous Intra-Arterial Chemotherapy As Part of a Combined Modality Treatment for Osteosarcoma of the Extremities

Shoji Takeuchi, A.C. W. Wong, Chiaki Kasai, Yoshiteru Kushida, Masao Satoh, Yutaka Nishimoto, and Yoshihiko Akahoshi[1]

Summary. Fifty-three patients with osteosarcoma of the extremities were managed by combined modality treatment, which included preoperative intra-arterial infusion chemotherapy, surgery, and postoperative adjuvant chemotherapy between 1968 and 1986. Fifteen of these cases underwent limb salvage procedures. Enneking's surgical staging system was used for preoperative evaluation. Radio-isotope (RI) angiography was performed to estimate the effect of intra-arterial chemotherapy and the possibility of reduction surgery. There were three intralesional cases, ten marginal resections, and two wide resections. There were only two cases of local recurrence. Histologically, we found the formation of a fibrous capsule along the tumor margin and also observed a correlation between this capsule and tumor necrosis. The 5-year cumulative survial rate for limb salvage cases was 60.0%, as compared with 46.4% of the amputation cases.

Key words: Osteosarcoma—Limb salvage surgery—Preoperative continuous intra-arterial infusion

Introduction

Limb salvage procedures for osteosarcoma have been frequently performed in recent years because of the many advances achieved in the development of a multimodal treatment regimen, which includes preoperative and postoperative adjuvant chemotherapy [1, 5–7]. Enneking's surgical staging system [2] announced in 1980 received much attention and is an accepted means of evaluation of the surgical margin and reduction surgery.

We report here our clinical experience on 15 slected cases of limb salvage procedures done at our clinic between 1968 and 1986. Emphasis is placed on the usefulness of preoperative intra-arterial infusion chemotherapy and the results of our series of limb salvage procedures.

---

[1]Department of Orthopaedic Surgery, Gifu University School of Medicine, Gifu, Japan

Table 1. Limb salvage for osteosarcoma of the extremities in 15 cases (1968–1986)

	No. of cases
Site	
Prox. tibia	4
Prox. humerus	3
Dist. femur	2
Prox. fibula	2
Dist. fibula	2
Dist. radius	1
Prox. femur	1
Radiological features	
Osteoblastic	9
Osteolytic	4
Mixed	2
Therapy[a]	
Resection only	4
Resection—massive bank bone grafting	6
Resection—Prosthesis replacement	5

[a] Preoperative i.a. infusion for 10–82 days (av. 49.3 days)
Prox. proximal, *Dist.* distal

Methods and Materials

Patients

Between 1968 and 1986, 64 cases of osteosarcoma were treated at the Department of Orthopardic Surgery, Gifu University Hosptial. Among them, 53 patients had lesions in the extremities. Fifteen cases underwent limb salvage procedures (28%) and 38 cases (72%) had amputation. There were ten males and five females in the limb salvage group; the age ranged from 10 to 47 years (average 17.9 years). The minimum intra-arterial infusion time was 10 days and the maximum 82 days (average 49.3 days) preoperatively (Table 1).

Staging

According to Enneking's staging system, there were two IIA cases, 12 IIB cases, and one III case. Stage IIB was further classified according to the criteria of Takada and Umeda for extraosseous involvement; there were one IIB-I case, four IIB-II cases, and seven IIB-III cases. Of our cases, 80% involved bilateral cortical destruction of the affected bone (Table 2).

Surgical Procedures

There were three intralesional cases, ten marginal resections, and two wide resections. Of the cases, 67% had marginal resection.

Table 2. Method of operation and staging according to Enneking

Stage	Method	
	Limb salvage	Amputation
IIA	2	—
IIB-I	1 (1)[a]	—
II	4 (1)	6 (2)
III	7 (2)	28 (14)
III	1 (1)	4 (2)
Total	15 (5)	38 (18)

[a] Figures in *parentheses* refer to number of deceased patients
IIB-I extraosseous involvement, unilateral; *IIB-II* extraosseous involvement, unilateral with >1/2 diameter of intraosseous involvement; *IIB-III* extraosseous involvement, bilateral

Planning

Biopsy was done and specimens taken subject to a drug sensitivity test. Continuous preoperative intra-arterial infusion followed and the antitumor effects were monitored. Radical surgery was performed when sufficient local tumor control was achieved. After surgery, systemic adjuvant chemotherapy was administered in order to prevent pulmonary metastasis.

Preoperative Continuous Intra-Arterial Infusion

Earlier reports [1, 9, 10] have recognized the usefulness of preoperative intra-arterial infusion [3, 7]. The tumor-feeding artery was primarily detected by angiography. This artery was catherized before performing biopsy. The catheter used was radiopaque and made of Teflon. The tip of the Teflon tube was placed in an appropriate position depending on the location of the tumor. 5-FU and urokinase are infused continuously. Adriamycin (ADR), *cis*-platinum (CDDP), and mitomycin (MMC) were used either independently or in combination according to the results of the sensitivity test (succinic dehydrogenase inhibition; SDI test). Intermittent administration was done twice/week in a single shot. We monitored the total period of infusion to exceed the doubling time of the tumor. Adverse effects and systemic immunocompetence of the host were carefully checked throughout the course. The ideal period was 4–8 weeks of infusion.

RI Angoigraphy Using Tc 99m Macroaggregated Albumin

To achieve maximum effect of the anticancer agents against a tumor, it is an imperative to maintain a constant and even flow of drugs to the tumor. This can be monitored by infusing Tc 99m macroaggregated albumin into the catheter and tracing its flow immediately afterward by a scintillation camera. This maneuver was performed every 2 weeks.

Results and Discussion

Improved results of preoperative intra-arterial infusion against the local tumor enabled us to perform wide resection as limb salvage surgery in a number of cases. The success of intra-arterial infusion was attributed to the ability to achieve high concentration and tumor penetration. Other factors affecting indications for limb salvage surgery included age, lesion site, stage, and local recurrence. The latter factor is important when considering reduction surgery for the purpose of function preservation. Correct interpretation of the antitumor effect is thus essential since it influences the entire prognosis.

Clinical Results

A significant reduction in pain and slight diminution in swelling were usually seen 2–3 days after infusion started. Marked reduction in extraosseous involvement was not often seen in osteosarcoma; however, diminution in swelling and circumference of the affected limb over the lesion was observed. In the majority of cases, significant lowering of the alkaline phosphatase titer was noted.

Angiography

Disappearance or reduction in tumor vascularity was seen in cases when intra-arterial infusion achieved good results. Angiography was done every 4 weeks to estimate the effect of intra-arterial infusion.

Bone Scintigraphy

As intra-arterial infusion become effective, there was a reduction in abnormal accumulation. Bone scintilation was useful in determining the extent of resection.

Computed Tomography Scanning

In effective cases, a high-density area was represented. This was similar to the sclerotic change as revealed by plain X-ray. A low-density area was noted peripheral to the tumor margin as the margin became sharp. This layer was the reactive zone induced by effective intra-arterial infusion.

Local Effect Observed When Monitoring Intra-Arterial Infusion

On histological examination of the specimen from resected samples, we found the dynamic image of RI angiography provided us with information pertaining to the effectiveness of intra-arterial infusion. Sites with a high degree of degeneration were revealed by high accumulation; complete necrosis was revealed by low accumulation, which was usually found in the core of the tumor. Sites with unclear margins and low accumlation represented in most cases the presence of viable cells. Thus, we could predict the effect of intra-arterial infusion especially on the tumor margin.

Table 3. Limb salvage cases in osteosarcoma

Case	Sex	Age (yrs)	Location	Radiological features	Surgical stage	Intra-arterial infusion	Surgical procedures	Operation	Prognosis
1. M.S.	F	21	R. dist. fibula	Osteoblastic	IIB	22 days / 24 mg MMC, 2000 rad ^{60}Co	Marginal	Massive allograft	18 yr. 10 mons., *alive*
2. C.S.	F	15	l. prox. tibia	Osteoblastic	IIB	10 days / 36 mg MMC, 180 mg CA, 4000 mg 5-FU	Intralesional	Massive allograft	3 yr. 2 mons., *dead*
3. T.S.	M	17	R. prox. tibia	Osteoblastic	IIB	51 days / 36 mg MMC, 100 mg MTX, 2000 mg 5-FU	Marginal	Massive allograft	11 yr. 8 mons., *alive*
4. Y.S.	F	16	R. dist. femur	Mixed	IIA	28 days / 130 mg ADR, 750 mg 5-FU	Wide	Massive allograft	10 yr. 7 mons., *alive*
5. K.T.	M	10	l. dist. femur	Osteoblastic	IIB	67 days / 120 mg ADR	Marginal	Prosthesis	2 yr. 7 mons., *dead*
6. H.N.	F	13	l. prox. fibula	Osteolytic	IIB	41 days / 120 mg ADR, 2 mg MMC, 9.6 mg VCR, 3750 mg 5-FU	Intralesional	Resection only	1 yr. 1 mons., *dead*
7. Y.N.	M	16	R. prox. humerus	Osteolytic	IIB	32 days / 30 mg ADR, 16 mg MMC, 3 mg VCR, 10 g Ifos, 3500 mg 5-FU	Marginal	Resection only	7 yr. 3 mons., *alive*
8. K.Y.	M	14	R. dist. radius	Osteoblastic	IIB	42 days / 52 mg ADR, 2 mg VCR, 1250 mg 5-FU	Intralesional	Resection, bone cement	5 yr. 7 mons., *alive*
9. T.M.	F	47	R. prox. humerus	Osteolytic	IIB		Marginal	Prosthesis	4 yr. 2 mons., *alive*
10. K.T.	M	13	R. prox. tibia	Osteoblastic	IIB	48 days / 130 mg ADR, 4 mg MMC, 11 mg VCR, 2375 mg 5-FU	Marginal	Massive allograft	2 yr. 4 mons., *dead*
11. K.I.	M	37	l. prox. femur	Mixed	IIA	43 days / 70 mg ADR, 140 mg CDDP, 4 mg MMC, 6 mg VCR, 3250 mg 5-Fu	Wide	Prosthesis	4 yr. 1 mons., *alive*
12. M.T.	M	9	l. prox. humerus	Osteoblastic	III	79 days / 150 mg ADR, 275 mg CDDP, 2 mg MMC, 11 mg VCR, 7625 mg 5-FU	Marginal	Prosthesis	4 mons., *dead*
13. T.M.	M	11	l. prox. tibia	Osteoblastic	IIB	63 days / 60 mg ADR, 2.5 mg VCR, 30 mg CDDP, 4000 mg 5-FU	Marginal	Massive allograft	2 yr. 3 mons., *alive*
14. K.N.	M	14	R. dist. fibula	Osteolytic	IIB	82 days / 140 mg ADR, 6 mg VCR, 310 mg CDDP, 5750 mg 5-FU, 30 Gy microtron	Marginal	Resection only	1 yr. 4 mons., *alive*
15. K.K.	M	17	l. prox. fibula	Osteoblastic	IIB	63 days / 60 mg ADR, 40 mg CDDP, 15 mg VDS, 5250 mg 5-Fu	Marginal	Resection only	1 yr. 0 mons., *alive*

Table 4. Five-year cumulative survival rate of osteosarcoma using Cutler's method (1968–1986)

Years after diagnosis	Alive at beginning of interval (lx)	Died during interval (dx)	Withdrawn alive during interval (wx)	5-year cumulative survival rate (%)
A. Amputation group (38 cases)				
0–1	38	6	0	84.2
1–2	32	9	3	59.3
2–3	20	3	2	49.9
3–4	15	0	0	49.9
4–5	15	1	0	46.4
5	14			
B. Limb-salvage group (15 cases)				
0–1	15	1	1	93.1
1–2	13	1	1	85.6
2–3	11	2	1	69.3
3–4	8	1	1	60.0
4–5	6	0	1	60.0
5	5			

Concomittant screening of the lung gave information concerning the relative change in of arteriovenous (A-V) shunt on the primary lesion. A decrease in accumulation of the lung indicated a reduced A-V shunt due to the effectiveness of intra-arterial infusion.

Pathological Features

Significant hemorrhagic necrosis was seen scattered over a large area macroscopically. In the intramedullary region, there was marked demarcation between the lumen and the tumor. A fibrous capsule was seen adjacent to the tumor parenchyma. Histologically, atypical mitosis and disappearence on reduction of viable cells could be noted extensively; especially in sites approaching the tumor tissues, there is a high degree of degeneration or necrosis.

Surgical Procedures and Prognosis

We experienced one case of local recurrence among three intralesional cases, and one case among 12 marginal resection cases. Metastasis was found in all three intralesional cases and in only two marginal resection cases. In ten other cases, where the follow-up period ranged from 1 to 18 years 10 months (average 4 years 1 month), no evidence of disease was achieved (Table 3). As mentioned above, in cases where an intra-arterial infusion-induced fibrous capsule occurred, marginal resection was possible and no local recurrences have been reported. This is an important observation on which much emphasis must be placed when contemplating surgery.

Five-Year Cumulative Survival Rate

Superior results were obtained in our clinic with the limb salvage group (60.0%) compared with the amputation group (46.4%; Table 4). Cases with over 4 weeks' preoperative intra-arterial infusion had a comparably better prognosis than those with less than 4 weeks' preoperative chemotherapy. We suggest that as long as the host immunocompetence can be well maintained throughout the course, a period of over 4 weeks of preoperative intra-arterial infusion will give a better prognostic result.

References

1. Akahoshi Y, Takeuchi S, Chen SH, Nishimoto T, Kikuike A, Yonezawa H, Yamamuro T (1976) The results of surgical treatment combined with intra-arterial infusion of anticancer agents in osteosarcoma. Clin Orthop 120: 103–109
2. Enneking WF, Spantier SS, Goodman MA (1980) A system for the surgical staging of musculoskeletal sarcoma. Clin Orthop 153: 106–120
3. Jaffe N, Knapp J, Chuang VP (1983) Osteosarcoma: Intra-arterial treatment of the primary tumour with cis-diamminedichloroplatinum II (CDP). Angiographic, pathologic and pharmacologic studies. Cancer 51: 402–407
4. Kantarjian HM (1983) Arterial perfusion with TC-99m macroaggregated albumin in monitoring intra-arterial chemotherapy of sarcoma. J Nucl Med 24: 297–301
5. Morton DL, Eilber FR, Townsend CM, Grant TT, Mirra J, Weisenburger TH (1976) Limb salvage from a multidisciplinary treatment approach for skeletal and soft tissue sarcomas of the extremity. Ann Surg 184: 268–278
6. Rosen G, Marcove R, Caparros B, Nirenburg A, Kosloff C, Huvos AG (1979) Primary osteogenic sarcoma: the rationale for preoperative chemotherapy and delayed surgery. Cancer 43: 2163–2177
7. Rosen G, Caparros B, Huvos AG (1982) Preoperative chemotherapy for osteogenic sarcoma. Selection of postoperative adjuvant chemotherapy based on response of the primary tumour to preoperative chemotherapy. Cancer 49: 1221–1230
8. Takeuchi S (1980) Studies on the sensitivity test of anticancer agents in malignant bone tumor. J Jpn Orthop Asso 54: 1497–1512
9. Takeuchi S, Akahoshi Y (1986) Preoperative intra-arterial infusion chemotherapy in the treatment of osteosarcoma. Jpn J Cancer Chemotherapy 14: 402–415
10. Wong ACW, Akahoshi Y, Takeuchi S (1986) Limb-salvage procedures for osteosarcoma: An alternative to amputation. International Orthopaedics 10: 245–251

A Monoclonal Antibody Against a Subgroup of Malignant Round Cell Tumors

Cytochemical, Immunological Findings and Chromosomal Analysis

Erich J. Fellinger[1], Gerhard Hamilton[2], Ingeborg Schratter[3], Peter F. Ambros[4], Peter Ritschl[1], Rainer Kotz[1], and Mechthild Salzer-Kuntschik[3]

Summary. Characterization of Ewing's sarcoma (ES) and primitive neuroectodermal tumor (PNET)-derived cells may be achieved by combined analysis of studies of secretion of specific cellular products, surface antigen analysis by monoclonal antibodies, and cytogenetic investigation. We have developed a new monoclonal antibody HBA-7/1, which was produced by immunization with a PNET-derived cell line ESIM-1. The HBA-7/1 antibody exhibits unique cell membrane reactivity with ES and PNET-derived cell lines and no reactivity with neuroblastoma or other malignant small round cell tumors. The epitope recognized by HBA-7/1 is preserved in paraffin-embedded tumor material in a highly reactive form. HBA-7/1 is directed to an as yet uncharacterized protein determinant expressed exclusively on cells of PNET orgin. Our results show common traits of neuroectoderm and ES-derived cells. Further study of HBA-7/1 and previously described antigens my contribute to the histological diagnosis of malignant small round cell tumors.

Key words: Ewing's sarcoma—Neuroectodermal tumors—Monoclonal antibodies

Introduction

The denotation of the term " small round cell tumor" leads to inexactitude in diagnosis. The difficulties in the differential diagnosis of these tumors have been extensively reported in the literature [1, 2]. Morphological, cytogenetic, immunohistochemical, and biochemical studies have established phenotypic similarities among a group of small round cell tumors in the central and sympathetic nervous system, soft tissues, and bone—the so-called primitive neuroectodermal tumors (PNET) [2–5]. That these various clinicopathological entities are histogenetically related is still an unproven hypothesis [2]. The second most frequent primary bone tumor of childhood and adolescence, Ewing's sarcoma (ES), morphologically belongs to the group of small round cell tumors, but due to the absence of unequivocal features of differentiation the histogenesis of ES is

[1] Orthopaedic University Clinic of Vienna, Vienna, Austria
[2] I University Clinic of Surgery of Vienna, Vienna, Austria
[3] Pathological Anatomical Institute, University of Vienna, Vienna Bone Tumor Registry, Vienna, Austria
[4] St. Anna Kinderspital, Vienna, Austria

still debated. Most authors consider it to be derived from mesenchymal cells. Neuroectoderm-associated antigens have been found to be expressed by ES-derived cell lines (ganglioside GD-2, HKN-1 antigen, N-CAM antigen) [3, 4]. These antigens are not specific markers and can be detected on other tissues and various tumors. Antibodies against these antigens were not raised primarily using ES or PNET cells as immunogen but for other purposes like the search for neuroblastoma differentation markers or natural killer-cell characterization. We have collected tumor cells from fresh biopsy specimens of patients with a histologically proven diagnosis of PNET or ES to raise monoclonal antibodies.

In this study, we report results from primary characterization of a very promising monoclonal antibody, termed HBA-7/1

Material and Methods

Cell lines were cultured in 10% fetal bovine serum (FBS/RPMI (Rosswell Park Memorial Institute)/1640 supplemented with glutamine and gentamycin). A cell line from tumor tissue was established from a single-cell suspension in 10% FBS/ DMEM (Dulbecco Modified Eagle Medium). The ESIM-1 cell line has been kept in tissue culture for approximately 70 passages since its initialization. Several cell lines classified as ES-derived were obtained from culture collections and were used for the tests.

Production of Monoclonal HBA-7/1 Antibody

The ESIM-1 cell line, established from tumor material of a patient with a diagnosis of PNET was used to immunize (i.p. and i.v. booster) Balb/c mice. Spleen cells were fused with P3X63.Ag8.653 cells and the resulting hydridomas were screened for positive membrane immunofluorescence (MIF) with ESMI-1 cells and negative reactivity with different neuroblastoma cell lines by fluorescence activated cell sorter (FACS) analysis (Fig. 1). The selected hybridomas were further characterized by their reactivity pattern with ES lines, carcinoma cell lines, and normal blood cells. A hybridoma with the desired specifity was obtained and termed HBA-7/1.

Neuron-Specific Enolase

Determination of NSE either in serum or fixed tissue specimens can be used to detect tumors with neuroendocrine properties [5]. Elevated concentrations of NSE can be found in patients with neuroblastoma [5] and small cell lung carcinoma [6]. In our study, NSE was measured in tissue culture supernatants from different cell lines (0.5 million/ml, 18-h incubation) using a commercially available RIA method (NSE RIA 100, Pharmacia, Sweden).

Histology

Formalin-fixed, paraffin-embedded tissue sections were dewaxed and stained by immunoperoxidase with the HBA-7/1 antibody according to standard methods.

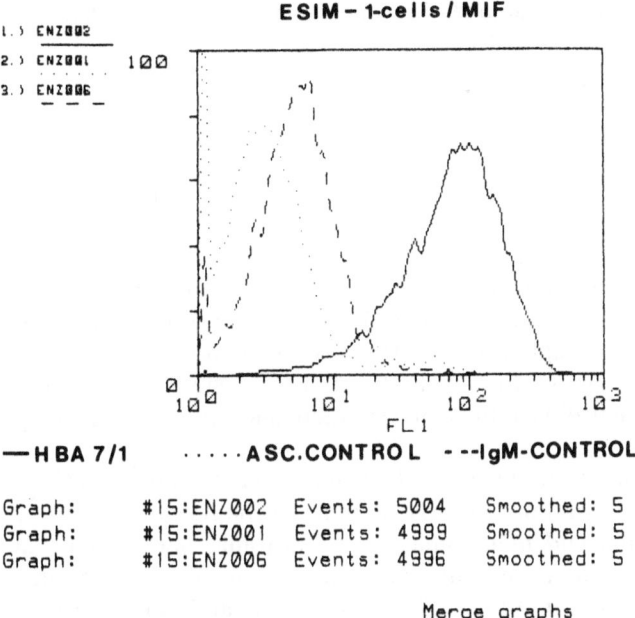

Fig. 1. Fluorescence activated cell sorter analysis of ESIM-1 cells with HBA-7/1 antibody and controls

Cytogenetic Investigation

Cytogenetic analysis of the tumor material was performed after short-term culture according to standard conditions. An R-banding pattern was enabled by a modified chromomycin/distamycin/DAPI (4,6 Diamidino-2 phenylindole) (CDD) banding technique [6, 7].

Results

The HBA-7/1 monoclonal antibody belongs to the mouse IgM subclass and shows bright MIF with different ES cell lines (SK-ES-1, EW-2, EW-7, EW-11, and ESIM-1). The epitope recognized by HBA-7/1 is preserved in paraffin-embedded tumor material in a highly reactive form. The antigen is protease-sensitive and insensitive to periodate oxidation. Binding of HBA-7/1 is not inhibited by a mixture of gangliosides or by an antibody (Leu 7, Becton-Dickinson) directed to the HNK-1 antigen. So HBA-7/1 is directed to an as yet uncharacterized protein determinant expressed exclusively on cells of PNET origin, as far as its reactivity pattern has been tested.

All neuroblastoma cell lines had significant amounts of NSE in their culture supernatants (5.0–18.6 μg/ml), whereas a panel of controls showed NSE concentrations below the RIA detection limit. Three of five ES cell lines (SK-ES-1, EW-2, and EW-7) secrete large amounts of NSE. Two other lines (RD-ES and EW-11), which were also recognized by the HBA-7/1 antibody, were NSE negative. The patient line ESIM-1 exhibited an intermediate NSE production rate

Table 1. Tissue specificity of HBA-7/1 antibody by indirect immunoperoxidase staining

Classification of tumor	++	+	−	Total
Ewing's sarcoma	4	3	1	8
PNET	6	—	—	6
Neuroblastoma	—	—	13	13

(8.3 μg/l) in tissue culture.

Immunohistochemical stains showed that the epitope recognized by HBA-7/1 was mainly associated with the cell membrane of positive tumor cells. Four of eight cases with ES reacted strongly positive, three of eight were positive, and one of eight was negative. All of the six PNET tumors tested were strongly positive. None of 13 neuroblastomas investigated showed any reactivity (Table 1).

Forty different type of tumors studied so far have not reacted at all with HBA-7/1 antibody; in particular, we did not observe staining in small cell lung cancer (SCLC), pheochromocytoma and melanoma, retinoblastoma, neurinoma and meningeoma, Wilms' tumor, and rhabdomyosarcoma. Tumors of the lymphoma group were also negative. Further studies of human tumors and normal tissues are under way; especially, reactivity testing with tumors of the central nervous system needs to be done.

Cytogenetic analysis

Constant aberrations were deletions on chromosomes 1 (p33) and 22 (q11–q12). In more than 50% of the cells, we observed additional material on chromosome 1 (pter). The cytogenetic investigations are in accordance with other findings, where more than 90% of the analyzed ES and PNETs, with the exception of neuroblastomas, display a deleted chromosome 22 (q11–q12) or a reciprocal translocation between chromosomes 11 and 22 (q23–24; q11–q12).

Discussion

Characterization of malignant round cell tumor cells (ES and PNET derived) may be achieved by combined analysis of chromosomal abnormalities, studies of secretion of specific cellular products, and surface antigen analysis by specific monoclonal antibodies [2–5].

In this study, we have developed a new monoclonal antibody showing different reactivities in FACS analysis of ES and neuroblastoma cell lines.

HBA-7/1, which was produced by immunization with ESIM-1 cells, exhibits unique cell membrane reactivity with ES and PNET-derived cell lines and no reactivity with neuroblastoma or other round cell tumors.

In conclusion, the results show common traits of neuroectoderm and ES-derived cells. The further study of HBA-7/1 and previously described antigens may contribute to the histological diagnosis of ES. Determination of effector mechanisms mediated by the antibody in vitro and definition of its imaging characteristics and antitumor activity in vivo are objectives of present investigations [8].

References

1. Reynolds CP, Smith RG, Frenkel EP (1981) The diagnostic dilemma of the "small round cell neoplasm". Cancer 48: 2088–2094
2. Dehner LP (1986) Peripheral and central primitive neuroectodermal tumors. Arch Pathol Lab Med 110: 997–1005
3. Lipinski M, Braham K, Philip I, Wiels J, Philip T, Goridis C, Lenoir GM, Tursz T (1987) Neuroectoderm-associated antigens on Ewing's sarcoma cell lines. Cancer Res 47: 183–187
4. Mujoo K, Cheresh DA, Yang HM, Reisfeld RA (1987) Disialoganglioside GD-2 on human neuroblastoma cells: Target antigen for monoclonal antibody-mediated cytolysis and suppression of tumor growth. Cancer Res 47: 1098–1104
5. Vinores SA, Bonnin JM, Rubinstein LJ, Marangos PJ (1984) Immunohistochemical demonstration of neuron-specific enolase in neoplasms of the CNS and Other tissues. Arch Pathol Lab Med 108: 536–540
6. Van Kessel AG, Turc-Carel C, de Klein A, Grosveld G, Lenoir G, Bootsma D (1985) Translocation of oncogene c-sis from chromosome 22 to chromosome 11 in a Ewing sarcoma-derived cell line. Mol Cell Biol 5: 427–429
7. Ambros PF, Schratter I, Hamilton G, Strehl S, Fellinger E, Salzer-Kuntschik M, Gadner H (1987) Neuroectodermal tumor with Del 1 (p33) and Del 22 (q11–q12). SIOP, XIX Meeting, Abstract 97, Jerusalem, Israel
8. Embleton MJ (1987) Drug-targeting by monoclonal antibodies; Editorial. Br J Cancer 55: 227–231

Chapter 5

Biomaterial and Biomechanical Evaluation of Tumor Prostheses

Histomorphological Evaluation of the Diaphyseal Anchorage in KMFTR-Type Tumor Prostheses

FLORIAN GOTTSAUNER-WOLF[1], HANNS PLENK, JR.[2], KARL KNAHR[3], and RAINER KOTZ[1]

Summary. The diaphyseal anchorage of the Kotz Modular Femur and Tibia Reconstruction (KMFTR) System, made of cobalt base alloy with integrally cast beads upon the intramedullary shaft and two paracortical flanges for screw fixation, can be stabilized on long bones without using cement. Implants retrieved up to 36 months after implantation in a clinically stable or loosened condition were investigated histomorphologically. The primary stability is based upon an intramedullary press-fit and screw fixation of the flanges. Secondarily, bone ongrowth to the implant and ingrowth occurred at many locations. Nevertheless, vascular damage, adverse cellular reactions to the implant material, and nonphysiological stress distribution must be regarded as risk factors for long-term anchorage.

Key words: Tumor endoprostheses—Cobalt base alloy—Integrally cast beads—Microscopic investigation—Long-term anchorage

Introduction

The reconstruction of large bone defects after tumor surgery can be achieved with endoprostheses, thus salvaging the limb without decreasing the patient's survival prognosis. Problems with artificial joints as widely used in orthopedic surgery, e.g., cementless or cemented fixation, stress distribution, bone reaction, and compatibility, are even increased in tumor endoprostheses. We are often dealing with very young patients with a long life expectation, large bone defects with high lever arm forces, and the patients' intention of fully using their limbs under dynamic loading conditions. However, young patients offer a better bone healing capacity and physiological reactivity to changing biomechanical conditions, which favor biological fixation and could make it superior to cemented systems [1, 2].

Skeletal anchorage through bone on- and ingrowth to the implant is only possible under mechanically stable conditions. This primary fixation, however,

[1] Orthopaedic University Clinic of Vienna, Austria
[2] Bone and Biomaterials Research Laboratory, Histological Institute, University of Vienna, Vienna, Austria
[3] Orthop. Hospital Gersthof, Vienna, Austria

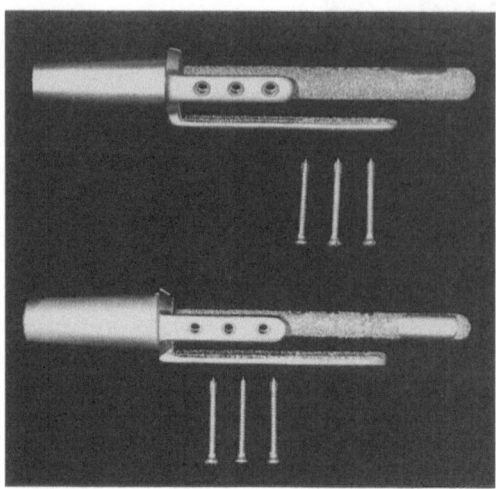

Fig. 1. KMFTR-diaphyseal anchoring element with two screw-fixated flanges and an intramedullary stem. The surface is structured with integrally cast beads

has to resist full load bearing without allowing relative movements over relatively long periods of time in tumor patients until secondary bone healing takes place. Adequate stability without using bone cement can be achieved by intramedullary or extracortical press-fit of a stem and/or screw fixation of paracortical flanges. Surface structures not only improve the primary fit, but also allow for on- and ingrowth of bone, thus providing a three-dimensional mechanical interlocking through new bone formation. It has to be kept in mind that a porous coating causes mechanical weakening of the material and decreases its corrosion resistance due to surface enlargement [3].

Different structures can be achieved by sintering or casting procedures with so-called madreporic surfaces in cobalt basic alloys [4]. Titanium alloys with better corrosion resistance do not allow similar structures, but alternatives like Titanium-Fibermetal are in use [5, 6]. The KMFTR system (manufactured by Howmedica GmbH, Kiel, Federal Republic of Germany) allows bridging of large tumor resection defects and exclusively uses cementless methods of primary fixation: The diaphyseal anchorage element consists of an intramedullary stem augmented by two paracortical flanges fixed with three screws (Fig. 1). All bone-contacting surfaces are structured with integrally cast beads. The prosthesis consists of Vitallium R, a highly corrosion-resistant cobalt base alloy [7].

From retrieved prostheses, which were evaluated histomorphologically, we could compare our findings with clinical phenomena and it is intended in this study to draw general conclusions for cementless fixation.

Material and Methods

The tumor prostheses were retrieved from patients of the Orthopaedic University Clinic of Vienna and the Gersthof Orthopaedic Hospital. Implantation periods ranged from one prosthesis retrieved 2 days postoperatively to a loosened implant investigated 36 months after implantation. In our laboratory,

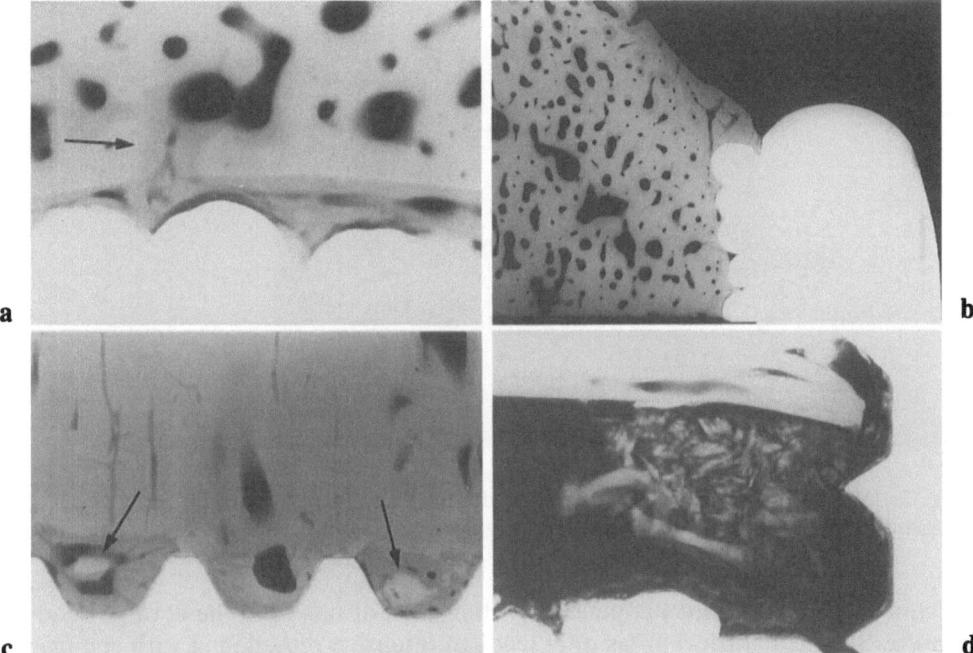

Fig. 2 a–d. Microradiograph enlargements from Fig. 4 demonstrating different bone-implant contacts. **a** Endosteal bone in growth, transverse haversian canal in direction of load transmission (*arrow*); ×15. **b** Periosteal osseointegration of the paracortical flange; ×5. **c** Cortical bone ingrowth into the spiral turns of a screw. *Arrows* indicate necrotic bone particles embedded into new bone; ×15. **d** Bone debris, No sign of resorption of remodeling; × 15

as a routine histological procedure, embedding in ploymethylmethacrylate (PMMA) is performed and then ground sections are made with the implant in situ. From implant-free undecalcified specimens, hard tissue microtome sections were also prepared. Light-microscopic techniques as well as microradiographs were used for the evaluation [8].

Results and Discussion

Bone Implant Contact—Osseointegration

Long-term anchorage without the use of bone cement depends on direct contact of the implant with bone. Usually, after implantation, a granulation tissue including osteoprogenitor cells develops, filling up the distance to the implant, and then woven bone is formed. Normally, in the course of time, this reactive bone formation matures into lamellar, fully loadable bone (Fig. 2). The mechanism of this remodeling is not yet completely understood [10]. Nevertheless, we know that it is also dependent on mechanical stability and adequate load transmission through the surface structures of the implant. Cortical biological interlocking

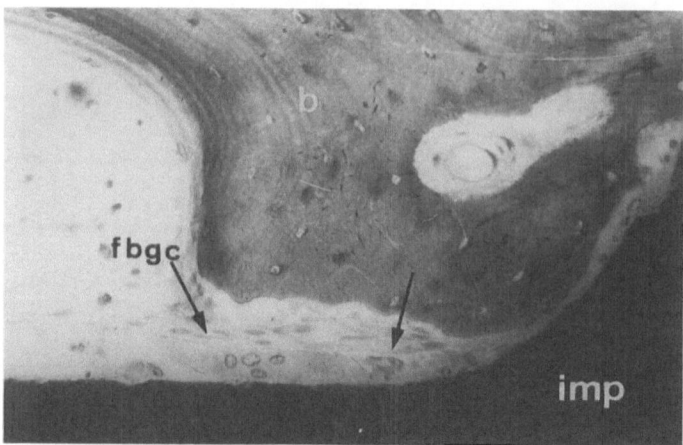

Fig. 3. Foreign body giant cells (*fbgc*) on the interface (*arrows*), no direct bone (*b*)-implant (*imp*) contact, Ground section, Paragon surface staining, ×20

occurs only through direct contact or within small distances to the cortex. Load transfer to small cortical areas only leads to intensive remodeling with spongification and periosteal reactions. The desired maximal cortical contact can be achieved by a functional design of the implant and by exact operative techniques. The alternative spongy bone fixation seems to offer a better stress distribution but is highly endangered by the fracture of load-bearing trabeculae through unphysiological stresses. Unfortunately, the secondary fixation of implants by new bone structure is by its nature only partly cortical, which would be preferable because of the higher stress resistance and slower adaptability of cortical bone to changes in loading conditions [11].

The diaphyseal anchorage of the KMFTR type provides stable primary fixation by the development of multiple direct bone contacts. Incongruencies between bone and implant are filled up to a certain extent, preferably at the screws and increasing from the distal end of the stump to the proximal. A large amount of bone debris was found in intramedullary areas, neither remodeling nor inducting new bone formation. These bone particles originate from intramedullary reaming and drilling and are devitalized through beat and mechanical trauma. Thus, intervening debris can even disturb the approach of bone to the implant.

Adverse Cellular Reactions

Areas of the implant which are not connected to bone are covered with a fibrous membrane, containing macrophages and foreign body giant cells. This tissue is found in the neighborhood of all foreign bodies, indicating a slightly chronic inflammation (Fig. 3). These reactions may partly be due also to corrosion phenomena, which are increased by the enlarged surface. There are materials which are more resistant to corrosion than cobalt base alloys, such as titanium, tantalum, or niobium, but only from the latter material can globular structures be manufactured which have proved to be effective for mechanical interlocking and osteointegration [3].

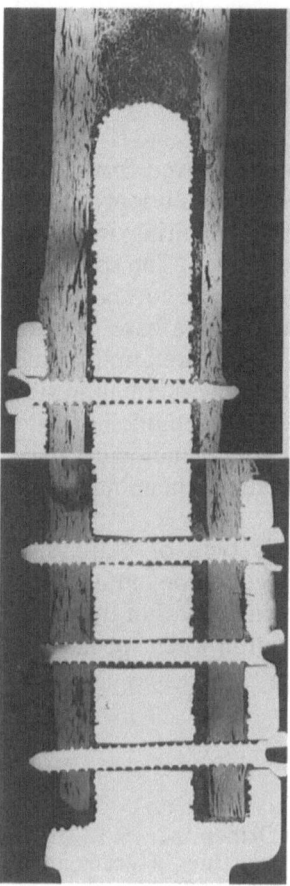

Fig. 4. Longitudinal section through a KMFTR anchorage element retrieved 13 months postoperatively (Patient DB, female, 22 years old malignant fibrous histiocytoma distal femur, death). The right cortex beyond the paracortical flange shows no remodeling because of vascular damage. Compare with the oppositional cortical bone with intensive remodeling. Screws are very well integrated, periosteal bone integration at the paracortical flanges; no bone ingrowth apparent into the medullary stem

Stress Distribution

The primary fixation to a cortical bone stump with an intramedullary stem press-fit and two screwed-on paracortical flanges seems to be sufficient for full load bearing over longer periods of time. Careful operative techniques can avoid incongruencies between bone and implant but cause necrosis through vascular damage (Fig. 4)

There seem to be two types of reaction in this bone stump area. On the one hand, we find dense bone with very little remodeling activity and large areas of necrosis in specimens after up to 13 months of implantation. Mechanically, the stability fully depends on the screws and flanges. On the other hand, intensive remodeling can be seen with new bone formation, integration the flanges, screws, and the intramedullary stem, but the cortex seems to change in terms of spongification. The preparation of the bone stump always causes vascular damage. This leads to bone necrosis that can stay unremodeled for a long period of time but still preserving stability through the screw fixation. Revascularization leads to remodeling and if the load is transmitted a new secondary bone will develop with further osseointegration of the implant. If this area is stress protected, however, resorption apparently leads to disuse atrophy, as observed clinically.

Aseptic Loosening

One specimen from a loosened diaphyseal anchorage was retrieved from a 20-year-old patient with knee exarticulation on the left side and an endoprosthesis in the right distal femur after two primary osteosarcomas. During intensive sporting activity, aseptic loosening with only slight pain occurred. The specimen showed intensive remodeling with extensive spongification of the cortex. In the endosteum, we found new lamellar bone, which is unusual in a case of pure mechanical loosening. There was a great deal of new bone formation in the former cortex beside necrotic areas. Loosening can be due to overloading, which certainly occurred in this case. Nevertheless, this extensive remodeling with atypical bone formation resembles our histological and roentgenological findings in stable implants and could be due to revascularization phenomena discussed above and thus be responsible for loosening.

Long-term anchorage seems to be possible with this type of diaphyseal anchorage. The advantages of stable primary fixation and good bony integration are obvious. Nevertheless, we have to consider long-term influences of the cellular reaction to the material and the extreme stress distribution when speculating on the future of this type of prosthesis.

References

1. Morscher E (1983) Cementless total hip arthroplasty. Clin Orthop 181: 76–91
2. Zweymüller K, Semlitsch M (1982) Concept and material properties of a cementless hip prosthesis system with Al203 ceramic ballheads and wrought Ti-6Al-4V stems. Arch Orthop Traumatol Surg 100: 229
3. Semlitsch M (1983) Metallische Implantatwerkstoffe für zementierte und zementfrei verankerte Hüftendoprothesen. In: Morscher E (ed) Die zementlose Fixation von Hüftendoprothesen. Spinger, Berlin Heidelberg New York, pp 58–69
4. Hungerford DS, Kenna RV, Krakcow KA (1982) The porous coated anatomic (PCA) total knee. Orthop Clin North Am 13: 12
5. Galante J, Rostoker W, Lueck-Ray RD (1971) Sintered fiber metal composite as a basis for attachment of implants to bone. J Bone Joint Surg (Am) 53: 101
6. Chao EYS, Sim FH (1987) Modular types of endoprostheses for limbs salvage. In: Enneking WF (ed) Limb salvage in musculoskeletal oncology. Churchill Livingstone, New York, pp 198–206
7. Kotz R, Engel A (1983) Cementfree design of a tumor posthesis for osteosarcoma of the distal femur and proximal tibia with a new fixation technique for the ligamentum patellae. In: Chao EY, Ivins JC (eds) Tumor prostheses for bone and joint reconstruction—the design and application. Thieme-Stratton, New York, p 187
8. Plenk H Jr (1986) The microscopic evaluation of hard tissue implants. In: Williams DF (ed) CRC series in biocompatibility. CRC Press, Boca Raton, pp 35–81
9. Salzer M, Zweymüller K, Locke H, Plenk H Jr, Punzet G (1975) Biokeramische Endoprothesen. Med Orthop Techn 95: 40–45
10. Urist MR (1980) Fundamental and clinical bone physiology. Lippincott, Philadelphia
11. Gottsauner-Wolf F, Plenk H Jr (1987) Knochenverankerung mit Kügelchen aus Kobalt Basislegierung. Orthopädie 16: 252–257

The HSS Modular Linked System for Segmental Replacement

James C. Otis[1,2], Albert H. Burstein[1,2], Joseph M. Lane[2], Timothy M. Wright[1], and Robert W. Klein[1]

Summary. A modular linked system for segmental replacement has been developed at the Hospital for Special Surgery (HSS). Its evolution from the original custom endoprosthesis is discussed and the analysis of retrieved components is presented.

Key words: Endoprosthesis—Segmental replacement

Introduction

A modular linked system for segmental replacement (Fig. 1) has evolved from the earlier Hospital for Special Surgery design of a custom segmental knee replacement presented previously at the 1985 Limb Salvage Symposium [1]. The purposes of this paper are: (a) to discuss the original design and its evolution into the present modular system; and (b) to present our analysis of retrieved components.

Materials and Methods

The original design incorporated a ball and socket joint with a transverse medial-lateral axle, which permits 130° of flexion, 3.5° of hyperextension, and minimal rotational and varus/valgus motions. The femoral component consists of a titanium alloy stem with a 28-mm titanium alloy sphere, which articulates against an ultra-high molecular weight (UHMW) polyethylene spherical socket contained in the tibial component. An UHMW polyethylene extension stop limits hyperextension which, combined with the posteriorly located flexion axis, enhances knee stability during stance. Femoral fixation at the femoral stem was initially designed for a press-fit using a self-broaching fluted rod system. The titanium alloy tibial component has a plateau and stem, which engage the tibia and are usually interfaced with polymethylmethacrylate. The tibial component holds three

---

[1] Biomechanics Department, Hospital for Special Surgery, New York Hospital, Cornell University Medical Center, New York, NY, USA
[2] Bone Tumor Service, Memorial Sloan Kettering Cancer Center, New York, NY, USA

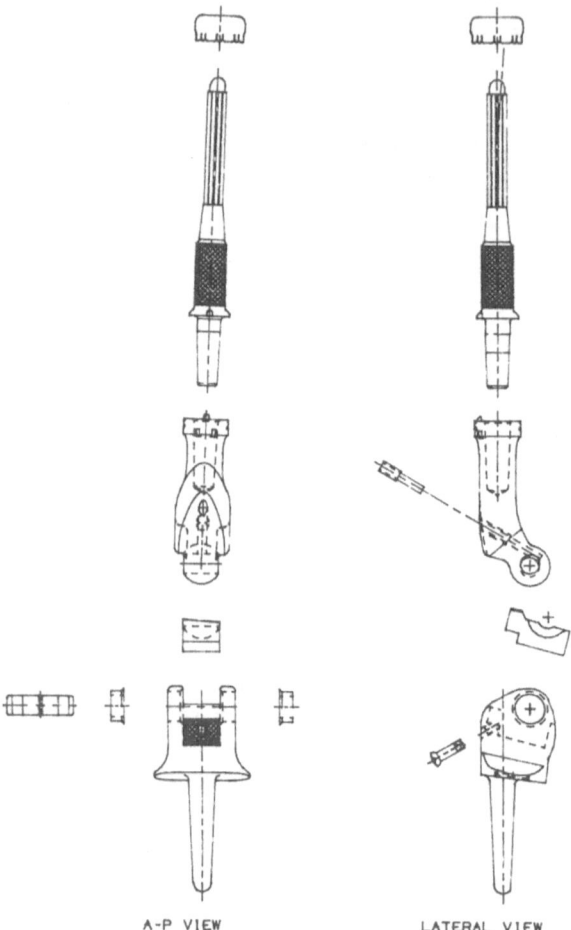

A-P VIEW   LATERAL VIEW

Fig. 1. Assembly drawing of the HSS modular linked system for segmental replacement following resection of distal femoral tumors

polyethylene inserts, which serve as articulating surfaces: the weight-bearing spherical socket, which accepts the ball of the femur and extends anteriorly to provide the extension stop, and two bushings, which fit into lateral and medial cylindrical recesses and articulate with the transverse axle.

The articulation at the knee has undergone several modifications. Initially, valgus angulation was incorporated in the distal femur 6 cm proximal to the flexion axis and was individually matched to the valgus angle of the patient's contralateral knee. It was realized that the contralateral valgus angle was not always compatible with the desired goals of the segmental replacement, in that excessive valgus angulation could result, which would negatively affect gait. Subsequently, a nominal valgus position of 5° (at 41° of flexion) was used for all patients and it was relocated at the flexion axis for easier manufacturing and a more anatomical appearances. At full extension, the nominal valgus angulation is 3.7°. This eliminated the need for right and left femoral segments and permitted the side to be determined when press-fitting the ball into the distal femoral segment. More recently, the original allowable varus/valgus motion and internal/external rotation of $\pm 5°$ was reduced to $\pm 2\frac{1}{2}°$. This reduced the laxity of the knee joint, which was felt by patients with minimal soft tissue to be in excess. The trade-off, however, was in giving up some of the capability for energy dissipation into the soft tissue surrounding the knee.

The mechanical performance of the segmental replacement has been determined in part from examination of retrieved component. To date, components from nine knee replacements have been retrieved. Five were removed due to loosening of the femoral component, two were removed because of fracture of the femoral component, one was removed due to wound closure problems, and one was removed at autopsy from a patient who had expired from complications due to his disease. The average length of time the components were implanted was 38 months (range 3–81 months).

Each component was thoroughly examined using a $\times 10$ eye loop. Articulating surfaces and the fracture surfaces of the two failed femoral components were further examined in the light and the scanning electron microscopes. In addition, carbon-coated acetate replicas were made of portions of the fracture surfaces for examination in the transmission electron microscope.

Results and Discussion

The polyethylene components did not show excessive damage. The bushings showed some wear damage in the form of scratches and burnishing on the interior surface where they articulated with the transverse axle. The polyethylene socket also showed evidence of wear with parallel scratches consistent with articulation of the titanium alloy ball in flexion-extension. In general, more wear damage was seen in those components implanted for longer periods of time. The polyethylene extension stop often showed considerable deformation and burnishing, consistent with impact loading against the femoral component in hyperextension. The surface of the titanium alloy ball showed severe scratching in most cases. Scratches were again parallel, consistent with articulation with the polyethylene socket in flexion-extension.

The two failed femoral components fractural by quite different mechanisms. One fracture was the direct result of trauma. The patient was in a vehicular accident in which her knee impacted against the dashboard. Examination of the fracture surfaces showed evidence of fast fracture. The second fracture was associated with a fall, but the fracture surface showed evidence of fatigue, with areas of fatigue striations and the presence of two secondary cracks.

Based on the observations of the retrieved components, two further design modifications have been introduced. The titanium alloy ball is currently ion-implanted with nitrogen in an effort to increase surface hardness and wear resistance. The junction between the ball and the remainder of the femoral component has been strengthened by increasing the sizes of the components in this region.

The techniques employed for femoral fixation have included press-fitting using a self-broaching fluted stem and cemented stems. Both methods have recently been combined an extramedullary porous collar, which is located on the segmental portion adjacent to the cut end of the bone. Several years ago, we attempted using a porous intramedullary titanium mesh, which was sintered onto the distal stem of the femoral component; however, technical problems in assembling were encountered and additional difficulties in obtaining good bone apposition led to our discontinuing those attempts especially in light of a trade-off in strength. Recently, porous ingrowth has been incorporated for patellar attachment to the tibial component, initial fixation being made by a screw, which passes through the patella and is threaded into the tibial component. In early attempts, we experienced screw failure, which was corrected by increasing the screw diameter and also by directing the screw in a more upward direction, such that the tension by the quadriceps pulled the patella against the porous anterior surfaces of the tibia. None of the porous devices have been retrieved at this time to evaluate them for porous ingrowth.

During the past 2 years, we have converted to a modular system, which has the obvious advantages of custom-fitting in the operating room and immediate availability. the modular system will include segmental knees for distal femoral and proximal tibial resections, hips for proximal femoral resections, and a saddle prosthesis for pelvic resections.

Acknowledgment. The authors gratefully acknowledge the support of the Clark Foundation.

Reference

1. Burstein AH, Otis JC, Lane JM, Wright TM (1983) The B-L knee en bloc total knee prosthesis—Design and performance. In: Kotz R (ed) Proceedings of 2nd international workshop on the design and application of tumor prostheses for bone and joint reconstruction, Vienna, Sept. 5–8, 1983. Egermann, Vienna, pp 200–212

Biological and Biomechanical Justification of Porous-Coated Modular Segmental Bone/Joint Prostheses

EDMUND Y.S. CHAO and FRANKLIN H. SIM[1]

Summary. The concept of extracortical bone bridging and ingrowth as a means of achieving long-term biological fixation of porous-coated modular segmental bone/joint prostheses has been validated using experimental bench tests, theoretical modeling, and animal experiments. Aside from being available at the time of surgery, other potential advantages of such an implant system include: (a) allowing optimal dimensional match to the bone defect; (b) minimizing stem fracture, loosening, or bone resorption; (c) enhancing initial implant stability; and (d) facilitating easier implant removal. Additional studies and continuous clinical follow-up are necessary to ensure long-term success of the present porous-coated modular segmental bone/joint prosthetic devices.

Key words: Modular system—Extracortical bone bridging—Porous coating

Introduction

Two important factors responsible for permitting ready amalgamation of a limb salvage program to treat malignant and aggressive benign bone and soft tissue tumors were the introduction of adjuvant therapy and a classification scheme to stage surgically musculoskeletal sarcomas [4]. A variety of surgical techniques was used to resolve these problems, ranging from leaving the limb flail and replacing the defect with an autogenous graft or allograft to using a custom-designed prosthetic device [1, 2, 5, 8, 9]. Each method had advantages and disadvantages, but all were more or less experimental in nature. Among these, resecting the bone ends and leaving the major joints flail was only minimally effective in special cases where weight bearing and limb function were less demanding. Allograft replacement continues to have many enthusiasts but, currently, is still regarded as another experimental procedure.

Custom-designed segmental bone/joint prostheses to restore skeletal continuity and maintain limb function have a long medical history. Anatomical areas of replacement have included the proximal femur and hip joint, distal femur or proximal tibia and knee joint, proximal humerus, and the diaphyseal sections of the three major long bones. Although early clinical results were encouraging,

[1] Biomechanics Laboratory, Department of Orthopedics, Mayo Clinic/Mayo Foundation, Rochester, MN, USA

the common biomechanical problems of stem loosening, fracture, and joint dislocation were encountered. In addition, custom implant fabrication is time-consuming, and the finished product sometimes does not match the skeletal defect. A two-stage operation appears undesirable because of the additional risk of infection and rehabilitation problems.

Primary bone and soft tissue tumors usually occur in younger and more active patients. Consequently, prostheses with sufficient strength are required to sustain long periods of utilization. Massive bone and soft tissue resection tends to alter normal joint mechanics and thus cause severe stress distribution on the prosthetic system. These concerns prompted the development of better implant systems for segmental bone and joint replacement following tumor resection.

Design and Application of First-Generation Prosthetic System

In 1978, two segmental bone/joint prosthetic systems were developed and tested clinically. The first system consisted of cast Co-Cr-Mo prostheses of various segmental lengths and constant stem dimensions. Design configurations of the proximal femur and proximal humerus prostheses were similar to previous custom devices. The bone segmental prosthesis including the knee was changed to the kinematic rotating hinge, which allowed axial rotation with a metal-to-polyethylene hinge design. Prefabricated prostheses of incremental lengths and dimensions were available to allow immediate utilization.

The second system used Ti-6Al-4V alloy with a Ti-fibermetal coating for bony ingrowth fixation. A modular design concept was first adopted for these interchangeable implant components so that they could be used to replace regions of the proximal femur, proximal humerus, and diaphyseal bone segments, including knee fusion. A self-locking conical coupling with offset screws was used to join the components. Porous-coated stems of different diameters and lengths were available to accommodate various margins of replacement, and fixation was achieved by press-fit.

Our initial clinical experience and experimental study results revealed several important problems associated with the first generation implant design. These included: (a) the Co-Cr-Mo system could not cover all necessary ranges of surgical variation; (b) the Ti fibermetal sintering process appeared to weaken the fatigue strength of the substrate, thereby causing stem fracture; (c) the press-fit stem did not produce the required implant stability to enhance extracortical bone bridging and ingrowth; (d) different types of adjuvant therapy appeared to affect bone tissue incorporation into the porous-coated prosthesis; and (e) soft tissue attachment to the prostheses was still ineffective. Thus, additional developmental efforts were devoted to improving implant design in the hope of resolving these problems.

New Modular System Design

Based on long-bone geometrical data and past clinical experience, a Co-Cr-Mo modular system was developed. Components of appropriate dimension can be joined securely for segmental replacement of specific anatomical regions. Hip joint diameters will be compatible with existing acetabular and universal endo-prosthetic cup sizes. Dimensions of Knee joint widths and humeral head diameters were determined from anatomical data from the normal population. The knee joint still adopts the kinematic rotating hinge design, with left/right variation. Prosthetic fixation relies on bone cement. Porous coating can be added to the shoulder region of the prosthetic segment to achieve extracortical bone bridging and ingrowth biological fixation [3]. This system is expected to accommodate 95% of the clinical needs, with the remaining cases dependent upon custom design.

The second prosthetic system is similar in joint design and modular composition, except that it will be made of Ti-6Al-4V alloy with a different conical coupling locking mechanism and solid stems without porous coating. The porous-coated sections at the segmental shoulder region and near the conical coupling joint area allow extracortical bone bridging. Soft tissue attachment features at the femoral neck, humeral neck, and anterior proximal tibial region are also available (Fig. 1). Initial prosthetic fixation depends on bone cement, but the long-term implant stability will be achieved through extracortical bone bridging at the porous shoulder region of the segmental component. Biological fusion across the conical coupling joint is expected to secure the components permanently.

The new design has several advantages compared with the previous system. First, initial stem fixation will be more secure and thus allow bony incorporation over the cortical region of the bone/segment junction. This type of prosthetic fixation to bone (extracortical bridging) is superior to intramedullary fixation since the transfer of bone stress is more physiological, and the stem's role in sharing load will be reduced significantly after bone bridging is accomplished (Fig. 2). Second, the number of segmental components will be reduced because press-fitting the stem to the bone cortex is no longer necessary. Third, the stem can be made stronger without the porous layer. Stem fatigue strength reduction due to notch effects or grain growth created by the sintering process can also be avoided. Finally, prosthetic implant removal will be easier with the cemented stem as opposed to bony ingrowth. Review of 16 cases with this type of prosthetic implant shows promising results thus far [7].

Biomechanical and Biological Analyses of the New Modular Prosthetic System

The strength of the conical coupling was examined both statically and under cyclic load using experimental models. In static compression and torsion tests, a smaller cone angle in the conical coupling joint improved its locking strength, and titanium provided stronger fixation than stainless steel. During fatigue testing, the distraction force ratio increased as the number of compressive loading cycles increased. Distraction force at the conical joint under zero compression was not significantly affected by repeated torsional loading. The cyclic bending load applied to the joint appeared significantly to decrease distraction initially, but as the number of cycles increased, the distraction force ratio approached 1.0.

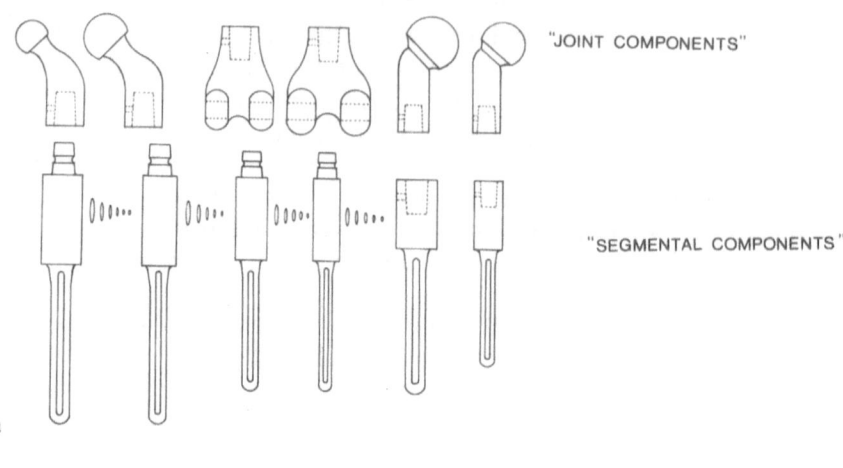

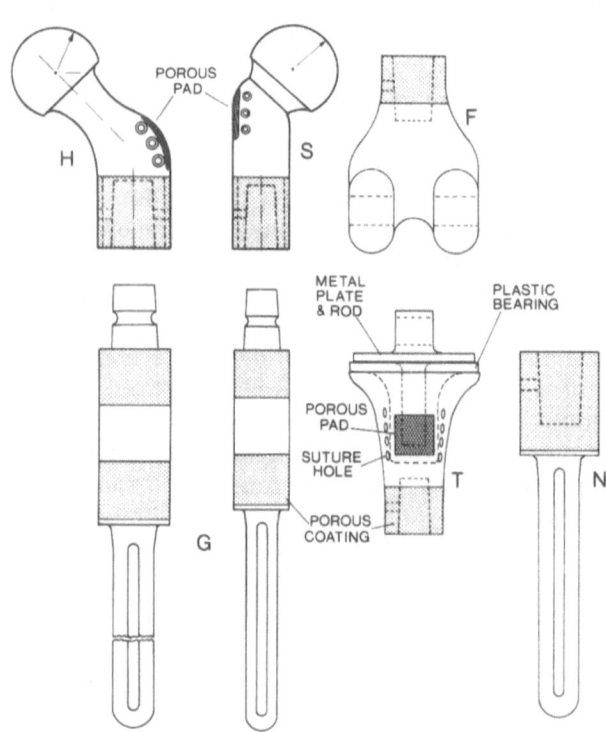

Fig. 1. a The "joint components" and the "segmental components" used in the modular segmental bone/joint replacement prosthesis design. **b** Basic design configuration for the porous-coated modular prosthetic system for tumor replacement with soft tissue attachment feature. Proximal femoral head component (*H*) proximal humeral component (*S*), distal femoral component in the Kinematic Rotating Hinge Knee joint (*F*), proximal tibial component in the Kinematic Rotating Hinge knee joint (*T*), segmental bone component with cone (*G*), segmental bone component with conical sleeve (*N*). The segmental length increments, segment diameters, stem diameters, and other geometric dimensions are identical to those of the nonporous modular prosthetic system for tumor replacement

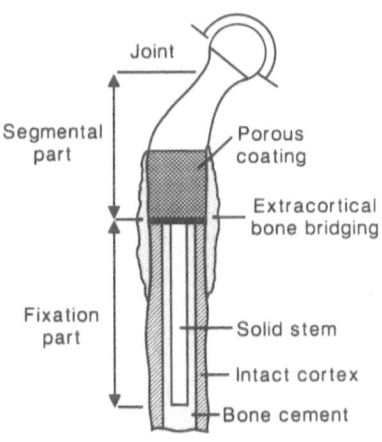

Fig. 2. Schematic diagram illustrating the concept of extracortical bone bridging and ingrowth with cemented stem to achieve a "composite" implant fixation.

Table 1. Maximum stresses in the conical coupling joint with a 2° cone angle under axial compression and bending loads

Loading mode	Critical[c] region	Stress (n)	Magnitude (p)	(psi)
Axial Compression	1	−7.48	−2.06	−3.54
(1 lb)	2	−20.06	0.90	−23.35
	3	−7.48	0.58	18.90
	4	−20.06	−4.52	10.06
Bending movement[a]	1	−29.65	−46.36	−33.74
(1 in-lb)	2	—[b]	−0.16	—[b]
	3	−36.69	0.65	32.93
	4	—[b]	−2.78	—[b]

[a] Stresses are on the compressive side
[b] Assumed zero stress due to interface separation
[c] See the right diagram for the location of these critical regions

Set screws further improved the locking strength of the conical coupling joint. The Co-Cr-Mo alloy with proper machining tolerance and surface finish should be able to provide a similar mechanical performance.

Since the conical coupling joint constitutes the key element in the modular prosthetic design for tumor replacement, it must have the mechanical strength to withstand a long period of loading without failure. The effect of biological ingrowth into the porous layer and across the joint on stress augmentation was investigated. Three-dimensional finite element analysis was used based on an axisymmetric model. High stresses occurred at the tip and base of the inner cone and outer sleeve under both compressive and bending loads (Table 1). Based on current modular system design, the maximum principal stress in the conical coupling joint reached only half of the material fatigue stress. However, such stress will increase significantly under a smaller cone angle (<4°). The effect of conical sleeve wall thickness on stress was minimal. The presence of interface friction reduced the magnitude of critical stress.

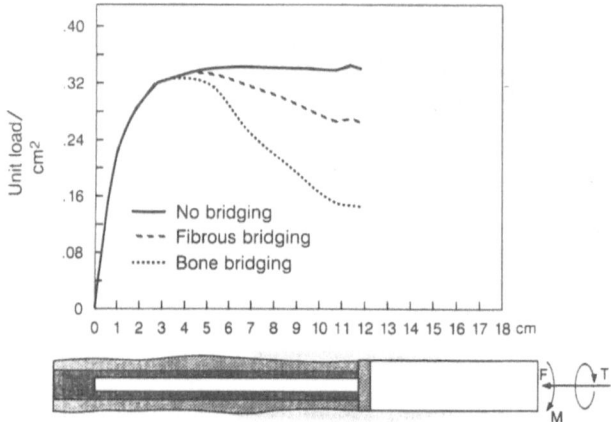

Fig. 3. Distribution of stem normal stress alone its length under unit bending load (*M*) with and without tissue bridging at the prosthetic stem shoulder region. The stress is expressed in normalized units of unit load/cm²

With tissue ingrowth into the porous layer, critical stresses in the conical coupling joint were significantly reduced. Maximum reductions in equivalent stress were 31 times and 7 times respectively, for bone and fibrous tissue ingrowth, as compared with the noningrowth state. The maximum reduction in stress under bending load was less. Thus, the design concept adopted for the modular prosthetic system with a porous-ingrowth surface appears effective and advantageous.

With cemented custom prostheses, it is important to provide an optimal stem design to avoid stem fracture and loosening under high interface stress conditions. Stress analysis using the finite element method and compound beam theory was performed to determine the optimal stem length and corss-sectional geometry. Results showed that a longer stem length may not improve implant fixation and the optimal cement thickness should be 2–3 mm. Based on stress distributions in the bone, cement, and stem as a function of stem thickness, an optimal stem design was proposed. The present stress analysis model was also used to determine the effect of extracortical bone bridging and ingrowth on stem/cement stress reduction. With successful bone incorporation, the normal stress in the stem due to bending was significantly reduced as compared with cement fixation without bone sleeve formation at the shoulder region (Fig. 3).

A segmental prosthesis coupled by a conical joint was developed for experimental studies in canine femur models (Fig. 4). Research studies were conducted to investigate the effects of limb immobilization, types of porous coating, animal age, and the use of bone cement for initial fixation on bone bridging and ingrowth. Quantitative histological study of the bone/prosthetic stem system, torsional strength of the conical coupling joint, and the push-out strength of the implant/bone interface were performed.

Initial immobilization was found to have a significant effect on organized fibrous tissue ingrowth in the porous layer rather than on bone ingrowth. Such

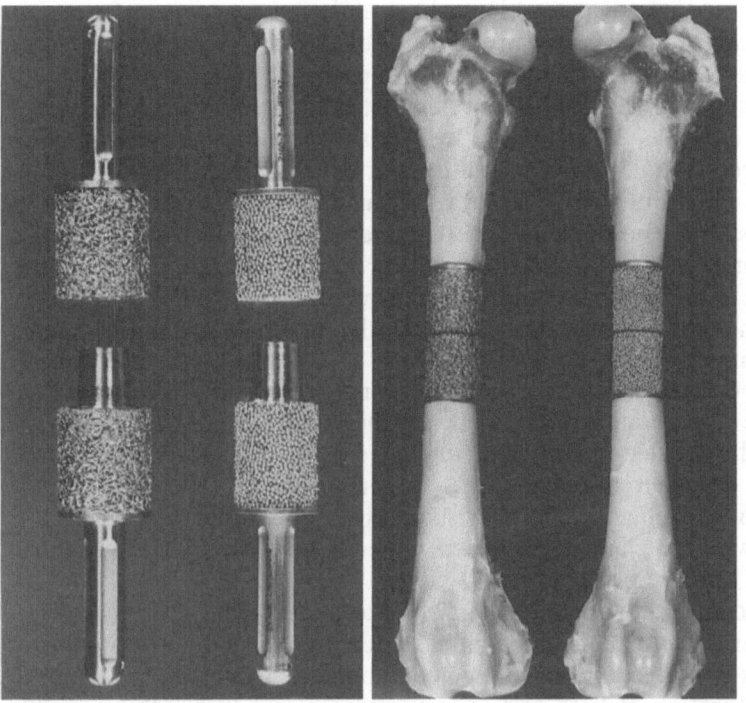

a   b

Fig. 4a, b. Canine segmental bone prostheses used to study the effects of limb immobilization, age, types of porous coating, and bone cement fixation on tissue incorporation extracortically with autogenous bone graft application. **a** Disassembled implant with Co-Cr-Mo beaded surface and the Ti-6AI-4V fibermetal coating. **b** The assembled and implanted prostheses in canine femora

tissue apepeared to be strong against interface shear load. Therefore, at the early stages of prosthetic incorporation, organized fibrous tissue ingrowth can provide adequate fixation strength. Whether this fibrous tissue will remodel and become bone must be studied under a longer followed-up period. Successful bone ingrowth appears to occur, regardless of the animal's age. In addition, better fixation internally through press-fit or proper application of cement appears to be beneficial to the enhancement of bony incorporation. The types of porous coating did not affect the results for achieving bone bridging and ingrowth at the bone segmental shoulder junction. Initial implant stability and sufficient autogenous grafts with bone marrow were identified as the two key factors in achieving successful extracortical bone bridging and ingrowth.

Discussion

Emerging advances in adjuvant therapies for malignant bone and soft tissue tumors and introduction of a surgical staging system to rationalize the extent and margin of tissue resection have renewed interest in limb saving procedures. Prosthetic implants based on advanced biomechanical design concepts and new implant materials appear to be very promising, not only to provide useful limb function for curable cancer patients but also as palliative treatments to benefit patients with metastatic lesions. Two systems of metallic prosthesis for tumor replacement were developed. Although preliminary results are promising, additional investigation is indicated on: (a) effects of adjuvant therapy on tissue incorporation into the porous implant; (b) experiments to validate the efficacy of attaching soft tissue to the prosthesis; (c) autogenous bone graft substitutes to enhance extracortical bone bridging and ingrowth; (d) correlation of patients' clinical assessment results with their biomechanical functions; and (e) development of guidelines for patient selection, surgical technique, and patient home care instruction involving these prostheses.

The study of bone geometry, and theoretical and experimental stress analyses should continue to optimize the design of the present modular prosthetic systems. Animal experiments must be conducted to investigate the biological, functional, and adjuvant therapy effects on prosthetic fixation. Established objective functional evaluation methods should be used to study patient results for correlation with the clinical assessment criteria proposed by the American Musculoskeletal Tumor Society [5].

Multi-institutional trials should be conducted to evaluate the short- and long-term results after the prosthetic systems have been developed and tested. Our long-term goal is to perfect these two segmental bone/joint prosthetic systems to provide safe restoration of limb and joint function in patients with resectable tumors and in those with metastasis for palliative treatment. These devices could also be used effectively in general orthopedics for bone and joint reconstruction after severe trauma, prolonged infection, metabolic bone disease, and failed joint arthroplasty cases with extensive bone loss. We hope that such an option will be safer and more effective than other alternative methods.

Acknowledgement. This investigation was supported by PHS Grant Number CA23751, awarded by the National Cancer Institute, DHHS

References

1. Bradish CF, Kemp HBS, Scales JT, Wilson JN (1987) Distal femoral replacement by custom-made prostheses J Bone Joint Surg 69B: 2: 276–284
2. Chao EY, Ivins JC (eds) (1983) Tumor prostheses for bone and joint reconstruction: The design and application. Thieme-Stratton, New York
3. Chao EY, Okada Y, Hein T, Sim FH, Pritchard DJ, Shives TC (1987) Extracortical bone Bridging: A new concept for implant fixation. Transactions of the 33rd Annual Meeting of the Orthopedic Research Society, January 19–22, San Francisco, p 435
4. Enneking WF, Spanier SS, Goodman MA (1980) A system for the surgical staging of musculoskeletal sarcoma. Clin Orthop 153: 106–120
5. Enneking WF (ed) (1987) Limb salvage in musculoskeletal oncology. Proceedings of Bristol-Myers/Zimmer orthopaedic symposium. Churchill-Livingstone, New York
6. Heck DA, Nakajima I, Kelly PJ, Chao EY (1986) The effect of immobilization on biologic ingrowth into porous titanium fibermetal prostheses. J Bone Joint Surg 68A: 1: 118–125

7. Heck DA, Chao, EYS, Sim FH, Pritchard DJ, Shives TC (1986) A roentgenographic analysis of patients with titanium fibermetal segmental bone and joint prostheses. Clin Orth Rel Res 204: 166–185
8. Langlais F, Aubriot JH, Postel M, Tomeno B, Vielpeau C (1986) Prosthese de reconstruction de l'extremite superieure du femur. Resultat a moyen terme de 20 resection pour tumeurs. Revue de Chirurgie Orthopaedique 72: 415–525
9. Mankin HJ (1983) Complications of allograft surgery. In: Friedlaender GE, Mankin HJ, Sell KW (eds) Osteochondral allografts: Biology, banking and clinical applications. Little Brown, Boston, pp 259–274
10. Mooz A (1980) Mechanical properties of a surgical grade titanium alloy. Master's Thesis, University of Toronto

Porous-Coated Segmental Prosthesis for Large Tumor Defects

A Prosthesis Based upon Immediate Fixation (PMMA) and Extracortical Bone Fixation

MARTIN M. MALAWER, DANIEL CANFIELD, and ISSAC MELLER[1]

Summary. Twenty patients with custom-designed Co-Cr-Mo (Vitalium) porous-coated segmental bone and joint protheses of the lower limbs were reviewed. The minimum follow-up period was 6 months (range 6–30 months). The stems were cemented in the medullary canal and autogenous bone grafts were laid upon the porous surface of the protheses in order to achieve extracortical bone bridging. The series includes 11 men and nine women with an average age of 29 years. The histological diagnoses were nine osteosarcomas, two periosteal osteosarcomas, two parosteal osteosarcomas, two chondrosarcomas, four giant cell tumors (two recurrent and two stage III), and one nonunion. The locations of the lesions were distal femur (14 cases), proximal tibia (three), femoral shaft (two), and proximal femur (one). The surgical stages were 13 stage IIB, four stage IB, two stage IA and one stage IIA. Zonal and sequential radiographic analyses of plain X-ray films and bone scan of the prothesis-bone junction area were performed. Extracortical bone bridging was achieved in 60% (12) of these patients; in the remainder, the bone graft resorbed. There was no evidence of hypertrophy. The fate of the grafts was obvious within 6–12 months of surgery. The amount of graft and the technique of its fixation to the surface are major determinants of outcome. Chemotherapy and tumor type had no effect on graft incorporation. Better methods of evaluating bone graft incorporation are needed. This preliminary clinical trial leads us to conclude that extracortical fixation is a useful technique; however, further experimental and clinical data are needed in order to improve results.

Key words: Bone tumor—Prosthesis—Porous coating—Extracortical fixation

Introduction

After several decades of cementless fixation, followed by 25 years of virtually exclusive use of cement, there is renewed interest in fixing implants directly to bone without an interposed grouting medium. Loosening was the major problem in cemented or press-fitted implants; today, porous implants or porous implant surfaces that permit a "biological" fixation with host bone to develop tissue in-

[1] Children's Hospital National Medical Center, George Washington University School of Medicine and Health Sciences, and The Washington Hospital Center, Washington DC, USA

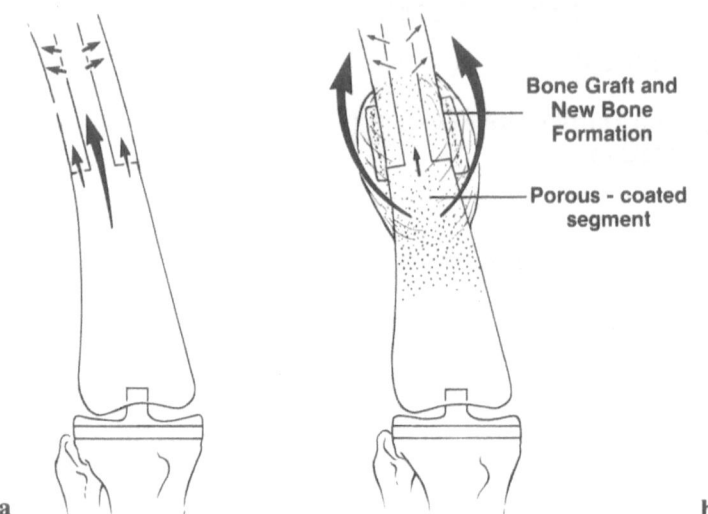

Bone Graft and
New Bone
Formation

Porous - coated
segment

a   b

Fig. 1a, b. Extracortical fixation: relation to stress transmission. **a** Intramedullary fixation; **b** intramedullary and extracortical fixation

growth are a viable alternative [1]. The basic assumptions are that a large number of fixation points can be achieved by bone ingrowth and that loads transmitted from the implant to bone can be distributed over a large surface, thereby minimizing stress to the bone-implant interface. The creation of a "living" bone implant interface that can potentially remodel or adjust to changing loads or stress (Wolf's law) for an indefinite period of time may be the ultimate solution to the problem of loosening in implant fixation [1].

The concept of fixing implants by bony ingrowth into porous surfaces has been applied in tumor prostheses in two ways: (a) porous coating of the stem that will be located in the medullary canal, analogous to fixation of the femoral component in a conventional hip replacement as represented by the Kotz system of tumor protheses [2, 3]; and (b) extracortical fixation, a technique developed by Chao and co-workers [4–6], in which the stem is fixed by cement into the medullary canal and in addition the segmental component is porous coated and supplemented by bone graft in order to create a bony bridge from the adjacent cortex to the segment (across the bone-prothesis junction). This latter method has several advantages over intramedullary "biological" stem fixation, according to Chao et al.: it allows more effective transfer of stress from the implant to the bone; it reduces proximal stem and cement interface stresses; it minimizes stem failure due to smaller size of the substrate and weakening effect caused by sintering process; it provides immediate stability to achieve bone ingrowth; and it allows easier implant removal (See Fig. 1) [6].

The purpose of this presentation is to report the results of a detailed clinical and radiological analysis of our first 20 cases of segmental bone and joint replacements using extracortical fixation.

Materials and Methods

Between November 1984 and November 1986, 20 patients were treated by implantation with a variety of porous-coated segmental protheses in the lower limbs. Serial radiographs and bone scans were performed at 3-month intervals. The minimum follow-up period was 6 months, the maximum 30 months. The average follow-up time was 16 months. All 20 patients are alive with no evidence of disease.

Sex and Age

There were 11 men and nine women. Their mean age was 29 years (range 12–59 years).

Diagnosis

The histological diagnoses included nine osteosarcomas (classic), two periosteal osteosarcomas, two parosteal osteosarcomas, two chondrosarcomas, four giant cell tumors (GCT; two recurrent and two stage III), and one nonunion (distal femur).

Stage

The surgical stages (Musculoskeletal Tumor Society System) of the 20 patients were 13 stage IIB, four stage IB, two stage IA, and one stage IIA. Two GCTs (stages IB and IA) progressed to stage III due to benign pulmonary metastases.

Sites

The locations of the lesions were distal femur (14 cases), proximal tibia (three), whole femoral shaft (two), and proximal femur (one).

Four types of surgical procedure were done: distal femoral and total knee replacement (14 cases), proximal tibial and total knee replacement (three), proximal femoral replacement with hip hemiarthroplasty (three, including one total femur). No cases of intercalary segmental replacement or arthrodesis are included in this study.

No patient received radiotherapy. Ten of the twenty patients received chemotherapy. Of these, five received preoperative intravenous chemotherapy and three received preoperative intra-arterial chemotherapy (IAC); two patients did not receive preoperative chemotherapy. All ten patients received postoperative i.v. chemotherapy, beginning approximately 6 weeks after the operation (range 3–8 weeks) and lasting for 6–9 months, according to the specific oncological protocol.

Prosthetic Design and Specifications

All protheses were custom-designed from cast Co-Cr-Mo. The hip component (three cases) was of the Bicentric design and the knee joint (17 cases) was of the

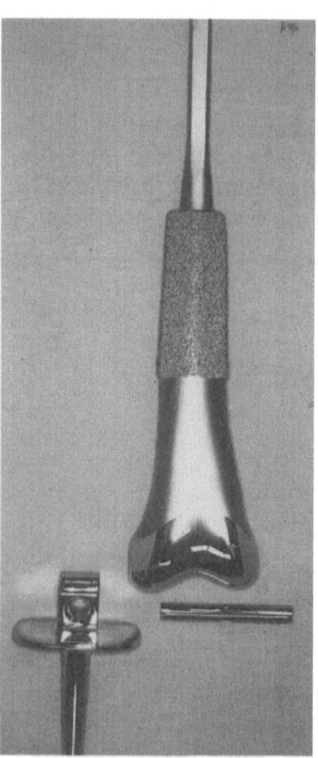

Fig. 2. The Kinematic rotating hinge segmental prosthesis with porous coating on the extramedullary component. This prosthesis allows immediate fixation by intramedullary cementation of the stem and extra-cortical fixation by ingrowth into the segmental component. Courtesy of Howmedica Inc. Rutherford, NJ, USA

Kinematic rotating hinge design (both by Howmedica Inc., Rutherford, NJ, USA; Fig. 2). The average length of the replacement segment (except the total femoral prostheses) was 17 cm (range 10–25 cm). The average length of the intramedullary stem was 15 cm (range 11–22 cm). The stem was solid and quadrant-shaped with an average diameter of 11 mm (range 9–13 mm). It was always cemented after reaming of the canal using cements restrictors and pressurized cement injection techniques. All distal femoral and proximal tibial replacement segments had a porous-coated section at the segmental shoulder region. This section consisted of a circumferential sleeve of beads sintered on the solid substrate. The porous surface had a mean pore diameter of 425 μm and a density of 35% [7]. The porous coating was not applied to the undersurface of the shoulder region. The average length of the porous-coated portion was 8 cm (range 4.5–13 cm). In the proximal femur region, an area corresponding to the major trochanter was similarly porous-coated. The anterior aspect of the proximal tibial segment also contained soft tissue attachment features in the form of loops.

Bone Graft Characteristics

Two types of bone graft (BG) were used: (a) local, which usually consisted of cancellous strips in limited amounts from the proximal tibia, distal femur, and major trochanter areas; and (b) corticocancellous strips from the iliac crest. In nine patients, only local BG was applied, and in nine others iliac crest BG + local BG were used. In two patients, no BG was used. The BG was placed on the bone-prothesis junction without fixation. In the last five patients, the cortex was roughened near the junction routinely with a burr, and in the last case the BG was fixed to the underlying surface using circumferential Dacron tape.

Radiographic Analysis

The cemented stems were assessed for the presence or absence of radiolucent lines at the bone-cement interface and reactive cortical changes.

The outcome of the segmental bone grafted bridging process was evaluated specifically using a zonal and sequential analysis of the radiographs. The following criteria were used:
(a) Length of BG contact with porous-coated section
(b) Percentage of porous-coated portion's total length in contact with BG
(c) Length of BG in contact with cortex above the bone-prothesis junction
(d) Function and appearance (lucency and cortical resorption or hypertrophy)
(e) General amount of bone in width and length in the bridge relative to the immediate postoperative radiograph
(f) Presence and width (1 mm) of a lucent interval and/or sclerotic line between the bone bridge and porous-coated area
(g) Appearance and sequential changes of oriented trabeculation and remodeling of the bony bridge

Bone Scintigraphy

The scans were evaluated qualitatively for the presence or absence (intensity) of activity in the bony bridge area relative to previous bone scans and the ipsilateral and contralateral cortical areas.

Results

Stem/Bone Appearance

No stem showed clinical or radiographic evidence of loosening. No cortical porosis was noted. In three cases, radiolucent lines less than I mm wide appeared at the bone-cement interface in some projections.

Gone Graft

An average of 68% of the porous-coated portion (range 22%–100%) was in contact with the BG on initial postoperative X-ray film. An average of 3.4 cm of the cortex (range 0–6 cm) above the bone-prothesis junction was in contact with the BG on the same initial radiographs.

In almost all instances a union between the BG and cortex was achieved in 3–6 months. Of 17 patients, 10 showed definite bone bridging in zones II and III. Two of the remaining patients had no bone grafting and one developed infection. The bony bridge became established approximately 6 months after surgery.

No significant changes were seen in established bridges beyond 12 months after surgery. There was a general trend toward diminution of the amount of the BG in the bridge with time. A steady state was eventually reached after which the bridge remained stable. There was one case of hypertrophy of the bone bridge in the bone around the proximal femur due to myositis ossificans after surgery.

In seven patients, the BG was resorbed within 12 months of surgery. In seven cases, radiolucent intervals and sclerotic lines appeared between the porous-coated surface and the BG, usually between 3 and 6 months after surgery. In five of these seven cases, the BG eventually resorbed.

Relation of BG Resorption to Amount of Bone and Site

In the seven cases with BG resorption, the initial percentage of the porous-coated portion's length that was in contact with the BG was 32%, in the low range of average (range 22%–50%). In five of these seven cases, the origin of the BG was local, and in the other two it was from the iliac crest but in young and small children.

Among the three cases of proximal tibial replacement, one BG resorbed, one BG was removed immediately after surgery due to vascular complications, and one became an established bridge. The bone bridge was well established in all three cases where the proximal femur was involved.

Analysis of Bone Scans

There was a good correlation between scintigraphic activity and the establishment of a bony bridge. Conversely, whenever the BG resorbed the activity disappeared.

Chemotherapy vs. BG Healing

No correlation was found between pre- or postoperative chemotherapy and BG incorporation or resorption.

Discussion

This report is the first description of patients treated with segmental bone and joint replacements utilizing extracortical fixation.

Our series does not include histological data since no autopsies, second-look operations, regrafting procedures, or revisions were performed. No correlation with the radiological and clinical data is available. It should be remembered that the histology of the bone-implant interface is the only valid proof of bony ingrowth into porous materials as a technique of permanent implant fixation. This information is crucial and should be obtained in the future using experimental models in animals, second-look biopsies in patients, and, if possible, autopsy specimens.

We noted that no extracortical bone bridge will develop without BG. The amounts of BG were higher in the cases of iliac crest + local graft than with local graft only, suggesting that a certain minimal critical mass of BG is a prerequisite

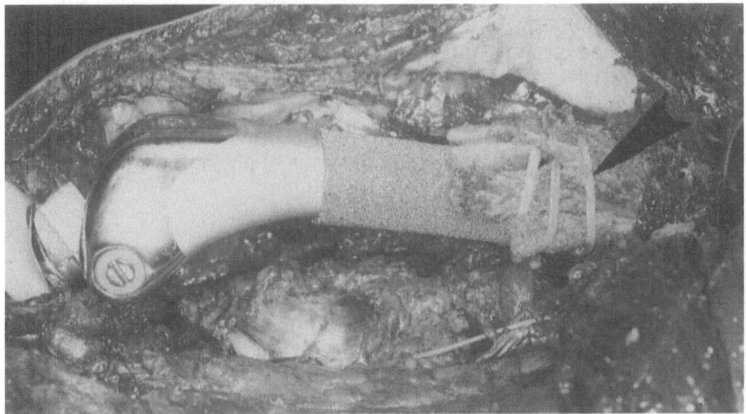

Fig. 3. Intraoperative photograph following resection of a high-grade osteosarcoma of the distal femur and reconstruction with a Kinematic rotating hinge prosthesis (Howmedica, Rutherford, NJ, USA). Note the porous-coated segment and the strips of corticocancellous bone graft surrounding the prosthesis, which are held in place by Dacron tape. Bone graft is necessary to create an extracortical bone bridge. Dacron tape (*arrow*) prevents the graft from floating in the adjacent muscle and increases the rate of graft incorporation

for the development of a bony bridge. The size of this mass is not known. The use of bone formation and promoting/inducing agents, such as hydroxyapatite, tricalcium phosphate, collagen, or BMP coating [8], may increase the rate of bone production. Another major difference between local BG and iliac crest BG is the relative amounts of cancellous vs. cortical bone. Local BGs taken from the distal femur or proximal tibia or major trochanter are almost purely cancellous, while the BG taken from the iliac crest contains a fair amount of cortical bone from at least one iliac table.

What is the optimal amount and/or location of the BG around the prosthesis-bone junction? What is the optimal thickness of the layer of BG? How much of the cortex and the porous-coated segment should be covered by BG? The answers to these questions depend upon laboratory studies and cannot be answered from our study.

At the beginning of the series, the BG was put on the surface without any fixation. It soon became obvious that in spite of relative immobility of the patients during the first 2–3 weeks after surgery, pieces of BG moved and floated in the surrounding soft tissues and eventually resorbed in most cases where contact was lost. It is well known that the initial bony growth into a porous surface is totally dependent on the stability of the area and maximal contact between graft and surface [9, 10]. These two observations emphasize the importance of graft fixation, which we do now with Dacron tape placed circumferentially around the grafts (Fig. 3); they also emphasize the importance of postoperative immobilization. An apparent problem arises: It seems that the optimal conditions for achievement of soft tissue and joint mobility (early mobilization) contradict the basic requirement for bony ingrowth (immobilization and delayed mobilization). It is, therefore, not surprising to find that in five cases flexion of the knee is

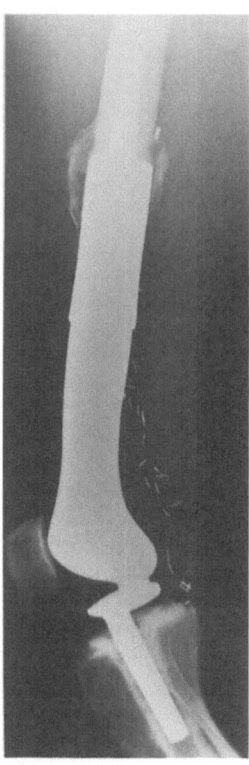

Fig. 4. Radiograph following resection of 6 inches of the distal femur for a high grade sarcoma and replacement with a segmental porous coated prosthesis and autogeneous bone graft. Note the incorporation of the bone graft into the porous component of the prosthesis and the adjacent segment of femur. There is maturation of the peripheral portion of the graft along the lines of physiological stress, analogous to that of fracture callus

limited to 30°–50°, probably due to quadriceps muscle adhesion.

Although the number of proximal tibial or proximal femoral resections vs. distal femoral resections is low, the effects of anatomy on the outcome of the BG can be estimated. Relatively small amounts of BG in the proximal femoral area achieved tremendous bone formation, including a myositis ossificans phenomenon, which resulted in good bony ingrowth of the porous-coasted segment. Poorer results were found in the proximal tibial area. The distal femoral area is intermediate. The proximal femur, which consists of a large soft tissue mass, demonstrated the well-known tendency of heterotopic bone formation. While the proximal tibia is poor in soft tissue mass, it has very tight compartments, can accommodate a small volume of BG than the proximal femur, and demonstrated the least extracortical incorporation.

Conclusion

This early study substantiates the value of extracortical bone fixation of large tumor implants. Many technical aspects remain to be evaluated, including the amount and type of BG methods of fixation, length and rigidity of postoperative immobilization, and choice of bone-enhancing material. Biomechanical data are essential.

References

1. Engh CA, Bobyn JD (eds) (1985) Biological fixation in total hip orthoplasty. Slack, Thorofare, NJ, pp 5–16
2. Kotz R, Engel A (1983) Cement-free design of a tumor prosthesis for osteosarcoma of the distal femur and proximal tibia with a new fixation technique for the ligamentum patellae. In: Chao EY, Ivins JC (eds) Tumor prostheses for bone and joint reconstruction. Thieme-Stratton, New York, p 399
3. Kotz R, Ritschl P, Trachtenbrodt J (1986) The modular femur-tibia reconstruction system. Orthopedics 9: 1639–1652
4. Chao EY, Sim FH (1983) Modular design and system for tumor prostheses. In: Kotz R (ed) Proceedings of 2nd international workshop on the design and application of tumor prostheses for bone and joint reconstruction, Vienna, Sept. 5–8, 1983. Egermann, Vienna, pp 207–213
5. Chao EY, Sim FH (1985) Modular prosthetic system for segmental bone and joint replacement after tumor resection. Orthopedics 8 (5): 641–651
6. Chao EY, Okada Y, Hein T, Sim FH, Pritchard DJ, Shives TC (1987) Extracortical bone bridging: a new concept for implant fixation. Presented at the 33rd annual meeting of the orthopedic research society, San Francisco
7. Bobyn JD, Pilliar RM, Cameron HU, Weatherby GC, Kent GM (1980) The effect of porous surface configuration on the tensile strength of fixation of implants by bone ingrowth. Clin Orthop 149: 291–298
8. Eschenroder HC, McLaughlin RE, Reger SI (1987) Enhanced stabilization of porous-coated metal implants with tricalcium phosphate granules. Clin Orthop 216: 234–246
9. Anderson GBJ, Lereim P, Galante JO, Rostoker W (1982) Segmental replacement of the femur in baboons with fiber-metal implants and autologous bone grafts of different particle size. Acta Orthop Scand 53: 349–354
10. Cameron HU, Pilliar RM, Macnab I (1973) The effect of movement on the bonding of porous metal to bone. J Biomed Mater Res 7: 301–311

The Use of Extracortical Implant Fixation to Reconstruct Large Bony Defects

BURKHARD W. WIPPERMANN, FRANKLIN H. SIM, DOUGLAS J. PRITCHARD, THOMAS C. SHIVES, and EDMUND Y.S. CHAO[1]

Summary. To improve the long-term prognosis of custom-designed implants for the reconstruction of large bony defects after tumor resection or failed total joint arthroplasty, the concept of extracortical bone bridging was developed at the Mayo Clinic. This report summarizes the results of 24 operations with a minimum of 2 years' follow-up (mean 56 months). The mean length of resection or bone loss was 163 mm. Eight knee joint arthrodeses and seven segmental diaphyseal resections of either the femur or the tibia were performed. Five and three resections of the ends of the femur were performed with replacement of the hip and knee joint, respectively. There was also one proximal humeral resection which involved the shoulder joint. Two implants had to be removed because of infection or stem fracture. Two cases of implant loosening could be salvaged by refixation and bone grafting. Extracortical bone bridging was uniformly achieved with a 70% coverage of the effective zones of bone bridging. Overall functional results were good or excellent in 70%, fair in 10%, and poor in 20%. For the evaluation of the devices, 75% were classified as good and excellent, whereas 12.5% each were classified as fair and poor.

Key words: Extracortical bone bridging—Custom implant—Limb salvage

Introduction

One of the most significant limitations of custom-designed or modular prostheses for the reconstruction of large bony defects is the failure of implant fixation after longer periods of follow-up. With today's improvement in patient survival, even after the resection of high-grade malignancies, there is definitely a need for improved techniques for the fixation of such implants. The concept of extracortical bone bridging (Fig. 1) as a means to enhance the long-term fixation of custom-designed implants has, therefore, been developed at the Mayo Clinic [1]. This is the first report of long-term clinical results for prostheses that utilize this concept for fixation.

[1] Orthopedic Biomechanics Laboratory, Department of Orthopedics, Mayo Clinic/Mayo Foundation, Rochester, MN, USA

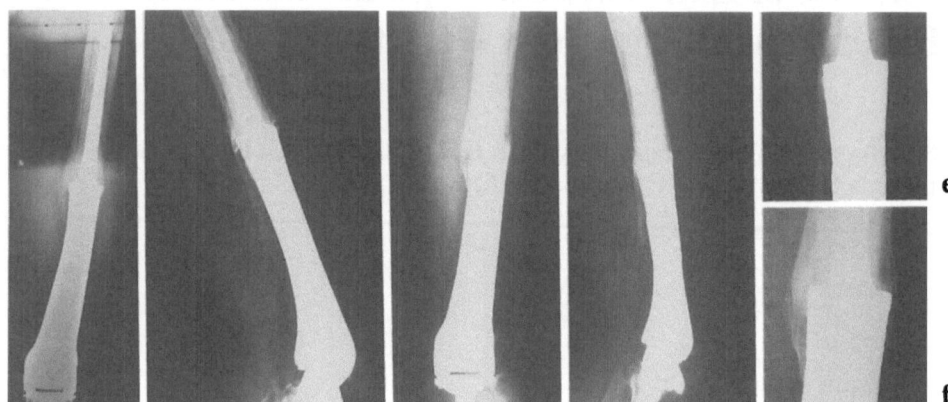

a–d   **e**

f

Fig. 1. a, b A 31-year-old male with loose custom knee prosthesis 3 years after implantation. **c, d** Final follow-up 3 years 7 months postoperation **e, f** Close-up of the shoulder region showing extracortical bone bridging

Materials and Methods

A total of 24 procedures in 23 patients with a minimum follow-up of 24 months was reviewed. Also included in this review were patients whose procedures were performed before May 1985 and who have subsequently died of their disease even if the follow-up was shorter than 24 months. Follow-up by telephone interview, chart review, and radiographic analysis was available on all patients. The procedures were performed between December 1976 and May 1985, which resulted in an average follow-up of 56 months, ranging from 9 to 129 months. The average patient age at operation was 31.9 years, ranging from 15 to 71 years. There were 13 females and 10 males in the study population. The majority of the procedures (83%) were done for limb salvage in the reconstruction of malignant bone tumors, whereas the remainder of the operations were performed to reconstruct bony defects after failed total joint arthroplasty. Eight operations were performed as arthrodesis of the knee joint; there were seven segmental diaphyseal resections of the femur and the tibia. Five and three procedures were done for resection of the ends of the femur with replacement of the hip and knee, respectively. There was also one proximal humeral resection which involved the shoulder joint. The average length of resection or bone loss was 163 mm, ranging from 60 to 330 mm. Fixation of the implants to the remaining bone was achieved with cement or press-fitting of porous-coated stems in 12 cases each.

For the clinical assessment, the rating system of the Musculoskeletal Tumor Society was used [2]. The performance of the devices was analyzed separately by a similar form, which evaluates the following parameters: availability of the device, anatomical restoration, morbidity, tissue reaction, loosening or migration, and device failure [3]. The overall device performance is evaluated with the same scheme as used for the clinical assessment.

For the radiographic analysis of the amount of extracortical bone bridging, three zones were analyzed on plain anteroposterior (AP) and lateral radio-

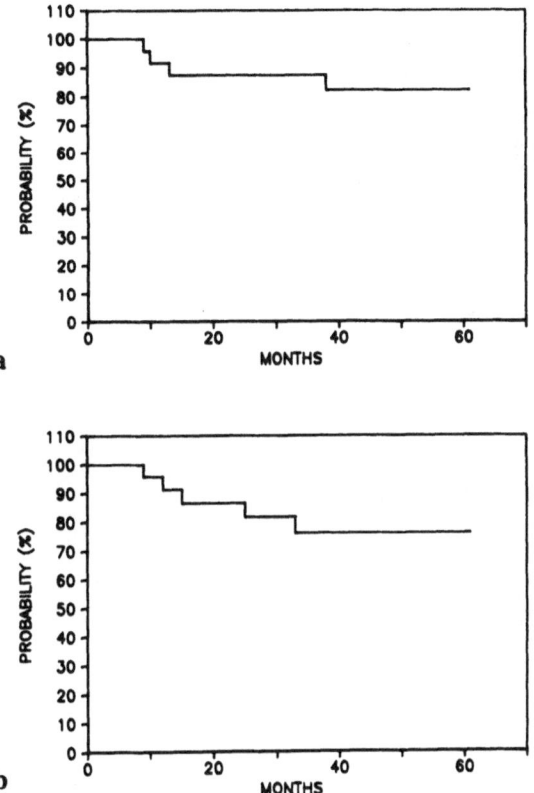

Fig. 2. a Survival curve for patients. **b** Implant performance. Probability of being free of revision for implants

graphs. These zones included the proximal 25 mm of the porous-coated implant body, the central 50 mm which included the conical coupling joint, and the distal 25 mm of the implant body. These zones were considered the effective zones of bone bridging. All results were expressed as percentage of available implant length in the effective zone covered by bone. All extracortical bone which on radiographs appeared to have a lucent line between the extracortical bone and the implant itself was not included in the analysis.

Results and Discussion

The average operation time was 3 h 47 min (2 h 15 min to 8 h 35 min), with a mean estimated blood loss of 1340 ml (350 ml–2500 ml). Four patients with high-grade malignant tumors died of their disease after an average of 18 months postoperatively. Survival analysis of the patients after the Kaplan-Meier method revealed an 82% probability of survival at 60 months follow-up (Fig. 2a). There were no local recurrences. Two of the original implants had to be removed because of stem fracture and infection in one case each. There is one further case of stem fracture with a revision pending. These three cases were counted as failures in all evaluations, regardless of the patients' current status. Four other complications were encountered in the series. There were two cases of stem

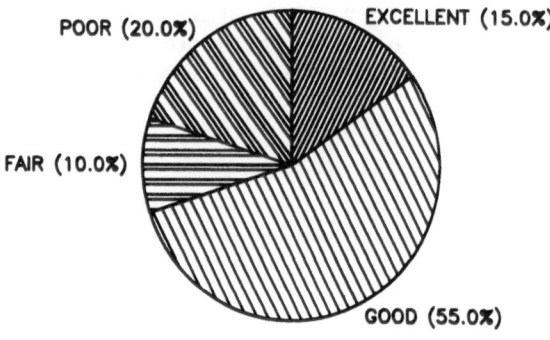

a

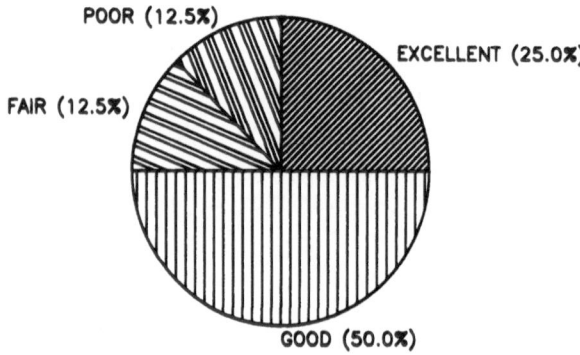

b

Fig. 3. a Overall results for functional evaluation. b Overall results for implant evaluation

loosening, which required revision with refixation and regrafting of bone of the
implants. One femoral shaft fracture occurred 8 months after a distal femoral
replacement with total knee arthroplasty. One radial nerve palsy was observed
after the proximal humeral replacement. Kaplan-Meier analysis performed on
the implants showed a 78% probability of being free of revision after 60 months
(Fig. 2b).

Radiographic analysis of the effective zones of bone bridging at final roentgenographic follow-up was determined after an average of 48.8 months postoperatively. The overall coverage of these zones was 68.8%, with a standard
deviation of 28.1%. Separate analysis of the medial, lateral, anterior, and
posterior aspects of the implants showed significantly less coverage on the
anterior aspect of the implants when compared with the other areas ($P < 0.05$,
Kruskal-Wallis test). Statistical analysis also revealed that the administration
of chemotherapy had a significant influence on the amount of bone formation
($P < 0.05$, Mann-Whitney U-test). The type of fixation (cement versus press-fit),
length of follow-up, the patient's age, and length of resection did not have an
influence on bone formation. Neither of the factors mentioned above had an
influence on the overall results as determined by the evaluation proposed by the

Musculoskeletal Tumor Society. Overall, 70% of the patients in this group were rated as good or excellent, 10% were rated as fair, and 20% as poor (Fig. 3a). For the evaluation of the devices, 75% were classified as good and excellent, whereas 12.5% each were classified as fair and poor (Fig. 3b).

The results presented here compare favorably with those obtained for similar patient populations using standard fixation techniques for custom-designed implants [4]. When these results are compared with those obtained by allograft [5] or autograft [6] replacement, the decreased morbidity and low rate of complications in this patient population become evident, especially when cement is used for the initial implant fixation. Since biological fixation was uniformly achieved in all the patients who thus far have not exhibited implant loosening, we anticipate that these patients will continue to do well. Extracortical bone bridging combines the advantages of prosthetic replacement, namely absolute sterility and early functional recovery, with the advantages of allograft replacement, namely the potential for biological implant fixation.

Acknowledgment. This study was supported by grant number CA 23751, awarded by the National Cancer Institute, DHHS.

References

1. Heck DA, Chao EYS, Sim FH, Pritchard DJ, Shives TC (1986) Titanium fibermetal segmental replacement prosthesis. A radiographic analysis and review of current status. Clin Orthop 204: 266–285
2. Enneking WF (1987) A system for evaluation of the materials used in musculoskeletal reconstruction. In: Enneking WF (ed) Limb salvage in musculoskeletal oncology. Churchill Livingston, New York, pp 16–19
3. Enneking WF (1987) A system for functional evaluation of the surgical management of musculoskeletal tumors. In: Enneking WF (ed) Limb salvage in musculoskeletal oncology. Churchill-Livingston New York, pp 5–16
4. Bradish CF, Kemp HB, Scales JT, Wilson JN (1987) Distal femoral replacement by custom-made prosthesis. Clinical follow-up and survivorship analysis. J Bone Joint Surg 69-B: 276–284
5. Mankin HJ, Gebhardt MC, Tomford WW (1987) The use of frozen cadaveric allografts in the management of patients with bone tumors of the extremities. Orthop Clin North Am 18: 275–289
6. Enneking WF, Eady JL, Burchardt H (1980) Autogenous cortical bone grafts in the reconstruction of segmental skeletal defects. J Bone Joint Surg 62-A: 1039–1958

Experience in the Use of a Custom Modular Titanium Intramedullary Rod in Resection/Arthrodesis of the Knee

JAMES R. NEFF[1]

Summary. A modular titanium intramedullary rod has been designed for resection/arthrodesis of the knee using a curved femoral and straight tibial rod joined together with a conical press-fit taper joint. Rods of 11-mm, 13-mm, and 15-mm diameter can be joined in any combination to accommodate the dissimilar intramedullary canal diameters. The conical press-fit joint is designed with a 4° taper with equilaterally spaced locking screws to prevent distraction and rotation. Titanium was selected for construction because of its favorable modulus of elasticity and fatigue characteristics.

The rod has been used in 42 patients selected for resection/arthrodesis or arthrodesis of the knee. Twenty-three patients have been followed for a minimum of 2 years without evidence of mechanical failure of either the rod or the conical press-fit couple. The use of a modular titanium intramedullary rod system for internal fixation of the knee would appear to provide adequate fixation and superior flexibility of application, offering an attractive option to a one-piece stainless steel design.

Key words: Intramedullary rod—Modular prosthetic implant—Resection/arthrodesis

Introduction

The concept of modular prosthetic design provides an attractive alternative to individual custom prosthetic fabrication. In 1983 at the Second International Workshop on Design and Application of Tumor Prostheses in Vienna, a modular titanium mesh intercalary prosthesis using intramedullary fixation was reported to achieve a resection/arthrodesis of the knee [5]. The system as designed continued to provide unprotected fixation of the arthrodesed lower extremity until the patient's death from pulmonary metastases 22 months later. The modular design using a press-fit coupled taper provided the necessary background and design concept for the development of a modular titanium intramedullary rod designed and developed at the University of Kansas.

The role of resection/arthrodesis remains a standard for reconstruction after resection of bone and soft-tissue tumors about the knee [3]. Rigid intramedullary fixation provides the foundation on which reconstruction using either large conventional autogenous grafts or an intercalary allograft can be achieved. Re-

---

[1] University of Kansas Medical Center, Kansas City, KS, USA

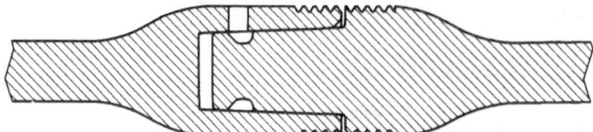

Fig. 1. A cross-section engineering drawing through the conical couple. Note that the locking screws as designed are to seat the taper further and prevent distraction and rotation

trograde insertion of a one-piece nail requires penetration and dissection of the buttock tissues, where potential contamination can occur either from a tumor margin or an unrecognized "skip" lesion. The commonly dissimilar intramedullary canal diameters of the femur and tibia make fixation by a one-piece, one-diameter intramedullary nail less than optimal. Also, deformities of rotation are encountered because of the difficulty in estimating appropriate rotation of the tibia upon antegrade insertion of a one-piece nail [1].

In response to these potential disadvantages, a custom modular two-piece titanium alloy (Ti-6Al-4V) intramedullary rod was developed [6]. This curved femoral nail, designed with a 60-in. radius of curvature, could be introduced in a retrograde fashion through an incision in and about the knee and coupled to a straight tibial nail of appropriate diameter. Splines were machined into the surface of a solid uniform cross-section titanium rod to enhance rotation control. The nails were produced with 11-mm, 13-mm, and 15-mm diameters to accommodate the variability in size of femoral and tibial intramedullary canals. All nails were 400 mm long and were designed to be cut to the appropriate length intraoperatively.

The femoral and tibial intramedullary rods, often of different diameters, were designed to be coupled together within the metaphyseal portion of the distal femur or proximal tibia using a conical coupling joint (Fig. 1). This joint has a 4° press-fit taper and three equilaterally spaced locking screws used to secure the taper and resist rotation (Figs. 2–4). A titanium alloy was selected because of the modulus of elasticity of titanium (16.5×10^6 psi), about one-half that of stainless steel (30×10^6 psi), and because of its superior fatigue characteristics.

Materials and Methods

Since January 1984, 42 modular intramedullary rod combinations have been inserted. Nine selected surgeons at nine separate educational centers in the United States agreed to provide data on patients in whom the nails were used. Each participating surgeon responded to a questionnaire that provided retrospective data on: (a) ease of selection and insertion of the nails; (b) intraoperative complications; (c) postoperative or late complications; (d) failure of the device or loss of fixation. The data were then compiled and analyzed.

Of the 42 modular intramedullary nail combinations inserted, 27 were used to achieve arthrodesis after major tumor resections involving the distal femur or

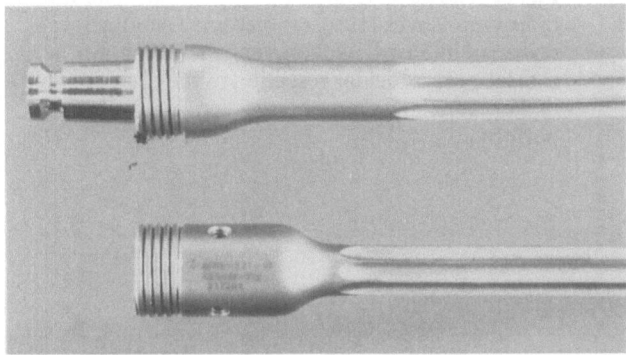

Fig. 2. The conical couple of the femoral (upper) and tibial portion of the modular intramedullary nail. Two of the three equilaterally spaced locking screw holes can be identified in the tibial (female) portion of the couple

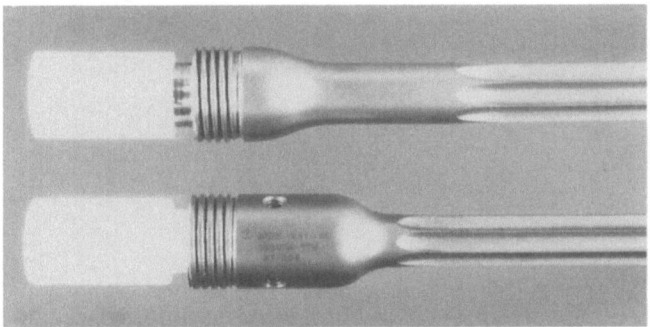

Fig. 3. Two delrin plastic taper protectors in place, designed to protect the press-fit conical couple during driving and extraction procedures

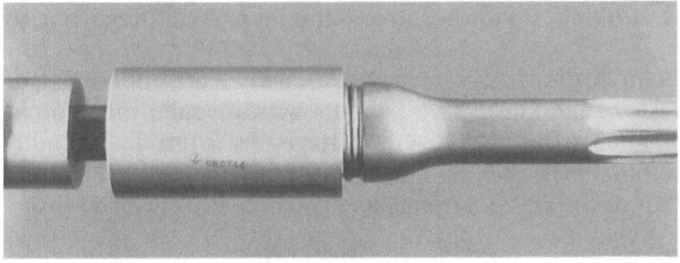

Fig. 4. The driver/extractor placed over the delrin protector and secured to the femoral portion of the nail by threads machined into the conical couple

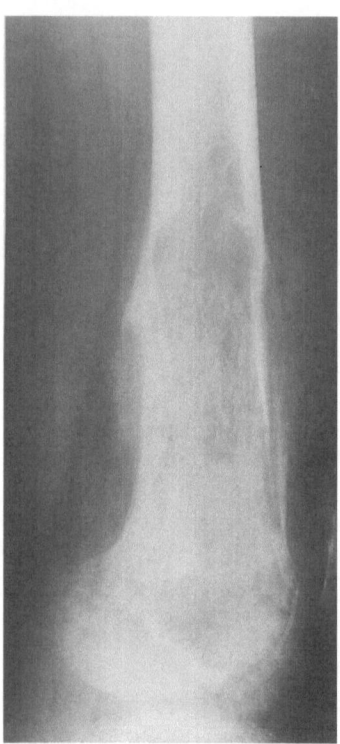

Fig. 5. The distal femur of a 27-year-old male with a biopsy-proven classic osteosarcoma. After a 6-week course of intensive neoadjuvant chemotherapy, a radical extra-articular resection of the distal femur and proximal tibia measuring 22 cm in length was performed

proximal tibia. Four of these involved reconstruction using an intercalary allograft and the other 23 were used for reconstruction with conventional autogenous rotation graft techniques (Figs. 5–7).

Four patients sustaining major trauma in and about the knee were managed by intramedullary fixation and arthrodesis of the knee. Two of these patients had established osteomyelitis prior to insertion of the nail and were managed extensively with intravenous antibiotics with negative bone biopsy cultures prior to insertion of the nail.

Seven patients with complications associated with total knee arthroplasty were managed with arthrodesis of the knee. Two patients with juvenile rheumatoid arthritis and failed total knee arthroplasty were managed by arthrodesis requiring construction of custom tibial nails (8 mm and 9 mm) to fit the small intramedullary canals. Two of the seven patients had osteomyelitis prior to insertion of the tibial nail.

There were two patients in whom the device was used to achieve fixation of pathological fractures. One of them had multiple complications associated with a proximal tibial fracture complicated by chronic renal failure and the other had a pathological fracture associated with metastatic adenocarcinoma.

Of the two remaining patients, the one with severe degenerative osteoarthritis, a previous patellectomy, and failed high tibial osteotomy was treated with a primary arthrodesis of the knee. The other patient sustained failure of a Samp-

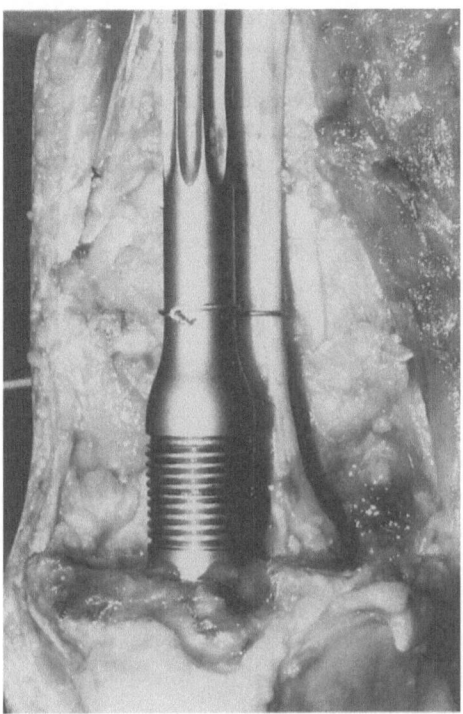

Fig. 6. A 15-mm femoral and a 13-mm tibial modular nail in place with the expanded conical couple positioned within the metaphyseal portion of the proximal tibia to accommodate the larger diameter portion of the nail. The fibula has been secured to the femoral portion of the nail; however, the tibial turn-back graft has been removed to illustrate the correct position of the nail

son rod through a nonunion of the conventional grafts used in an extra-articular epiphysiodiaphyseal resection of the distal femur for giant cell tumor.

Results

The femoral nails selected for internal fixation of the femur ranged from 15 to 11 mm in diameter. A 15-mm rod was most commonly selected for adult males and 13 mm for adult females and adolescents. No complications were reported upon retrograde insertion into the femur. In most instances, attempts were made to introduce the rod to the level of the lesser trochanter in patients with a significant portion of the distal femur absent or resected. Insertion to only 5–6 cm above the isthmus was required for arthrodesis where sufficient distal bone was available to share the axial load-bearing forces.

The diameter of rods chosen for the tibia ranged from 15 to 8 mm, with 13 mm most commonly selected in adult stature males and 11 mm in females. As notes, two custom rods (8 and 9 mm) were used to accommodate the small intramedullary canal diameters of the tibia in two patients with juvenile rheumatoid arthritis. No ankle joint penetration was reported either upon insertion or as a late complication.

Two surgeons reported intraoperative difficulties in accommodating the expanded conical couple portion of the rod. Both procedures were associated with

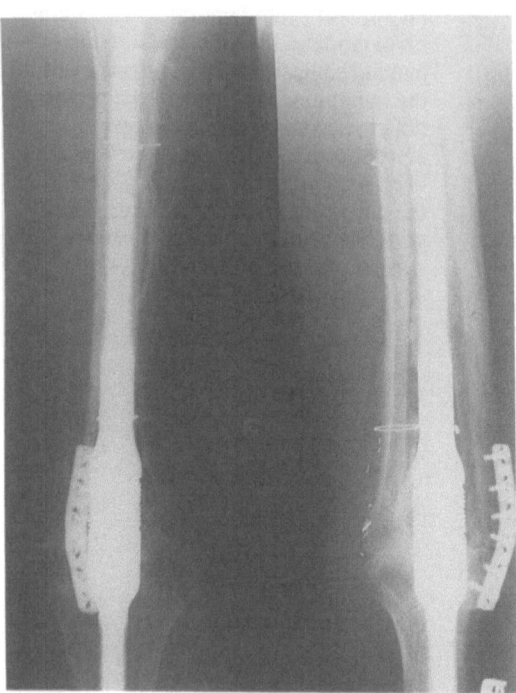

Fig. 7. Evidence of radiographic union at 6 months of the conventional resection/arthrodesis. The patient was full weight-bearing on the extremity at 6 months in a long-leg brace

tumor resections where intercalary allografts were used for reconstruction. One procedure required windowing of the allograft, resulting in 4 cm of shortening. A persistent nonunion at the proximal allograft/host juncture remained 2 years after the definitive procedure.

Four surgeons reported difficulty driving and extracting the nails when using a prototype design. The drive/extractor encircled the conical couple, achieving purchase over ridges formed on the outer surface of the couple. These difficulties were resolved by redesigning the driver/extractor with threads added to achieve a secure purchase on the rod.

In two instances, intramedullary fixation was chosen by the operating surgeon as the preferred method of fixation in patients with active drainage from previously infected open fractures or failed knee arthroplasty. Four other patients had prior drainage or osteomyelitis but were believed adequately treated at the time of nail insertion. Two of the six patients reactivated their chronic osteomyelitis, but the limbs remain stable. The surgeons caring for these patients elected to continue oral antibiotic management and await solid union before removing the implant. One patient with a resection/arthrodesis for tumor sustained a full-thickness ulcer through insensate skin over his grafts and developed a deep infection about the implant. This patient is being managed with oral antibiotics until osseous union is well-established when the rob is removed.

No mechanical failures of the rod have been reported to date. Only one patient has persistent shortening related to a nonunion of allograft/host bone at 28 months. This patient clearly has a poor overall result and is the only one reported in whom the operative constraints placed upon the surgeon requiring the accommodation of the expanded conical couple resulted in a less than optimal result. The average time for clinical union for conventional autogenous grafts used in resection/arthrodesis patients was 8 months with radiographic union occurring at 14 months. Those patients undergoing arthrodesis for failed total knee arthrodesis (TKA) or trauma clinically united in 6 months with evidence of radiographic union at 8 months. At present, 23 patients have been followed for a minimum of 2 years without evidence of mechanical failure of either the rod or the conical press-fit couple.

Discussion

A biomechanical analysis of the conical couple has been tested and reported previously [2]. To test the modular nail in a resection/arthrodesis configuration, the right and left lower extremities of an adult male cadaver were instrumented and tested using static loading conditions. The right lower extremity was reconstructed after resection of 20 cm of the proximal tibia with a 13-mm femoral rod and an 11-mm tibial rod in a femoral turn-down configuration. The left lower extremity was reconstructed in the same manner with a 15-mm femoral and a 13-mm tibial nail. The femoral nail was instrumented with appropriate strain gauges in the region of maximum eccentricity (the anterior surface of the femoral nail) and in regions of anticipated hoop stresses about the conical couple. Results of these studies suggest that maximum bending stresses, observed in the anterior aspect of the femoral nail in a region 8 cm proximal to the conical couple, were well below loads that could result in failure of the nail. The bone appeared to share a significant portion of the load even beyond the point of osseous failure. Bending stresses were observed across the conical couple and only minimal hoop stresses were noted to measurement [4].

A finite element model of the conical couple was developed, differing only slightly from the previous analysis [4]. Results of finite element modeling and testing suggest that the conical couple as designed has a safety factor of approximately 1.5 when using a 13-mm-diameter femoral and tibial rod.

Potential advantages of the modular intramedullary rod include the use of a superior material (titanium) and the ability to couple intramedullary rods of different diameters to accommodate the frequently dissimilar intramedullary canal diameters. Also, the retrograde insertion of the device through the resection incision avoids potential contamination of buttock tissues, which could result in a radical salvage procedure (modified hemipelvectomy) if a local recurrence occurred as a result of a tumor implant.

Potential disadvantages include the difficulty in removing the nail. Because of the need to provide a nearly continuous strength design, the larger diameter expanded conical couple would require its removal prior to removal of the tibial and femoral portions of the nail. The femoral portion could be removed either in segments through an incision in the region of the knee or, once the expanded portion of the nail has been removed, the femoral portion could be removed through an approach to the greater trochanter, followed by retrograde removal of the femoral portion if indicated. The remaining tibial segment requires removal in multiple segments through the knee once solid arthrodesis has been achieved.

Presently, the cost of materials and manufacturing is approximately twice that of a one-piece stainless steel design nail. However, with increased usage and the resultant mass production of the nail, it is anticipated that the cost will decrease. Because of the superior qualities of titanium and the flexibility of the application and design of the system, it is believed that the advantages outweigh the potential disadvantages. The system as designed offers the surgeon the freedom to reconstruct the extremity tailored to the needs of the patient heretofore not available when using a custom one-piece intramedullary rod.

References

1. Allen WC, Heiple KC, Burstein AH (1978) A fluted femoral intramedullary rod. J Bone Joint Surg 60–4: 506–515
2. Chao EY, Kwak BM, Kasman D (1984) Stress analysis of conical coupling joint in modular prosthetic system design. Ortho Res Soc 9: 103
3. Enneking WR, Eady JL, Brochardt H (1980) Autogenous cortical bone grafts in reconstruction of segmental skeletal defects. J Bone Joint Surg 62–7: 1039–1057
4. Gruenberg S (1987) The structural analysis of the femoro-tibial intramedullary nail using finite element and experiment analysis. Dissertation, Michigan Technological University
5. Neff JR (1983) The use of a custom modular titanium mesh intramedullary rod to reconstruct intercalary defects in the lower extremity in a patient undergoing resection for sarcoma. In: Kotz R (ed) Proceedings of 2nd international workshop on the design and application of tumor prosthesis for bone and joint reconstruction. Vienna, Sept. 5–8, 1983. Egermann, Vienna, pp 239–242
6. Schmidt RG, Dalinka MK, Schwamm HA, Black J, Neff JR (1985) Clinical pathologic conference. Univ Pa Ortho J 1: 46–54

Demineralized Bone Powder

Use in Bone Tumor Surgery

R.M. WILKINS[1]

Summary. Demineralized bone powder (DBP) was prepared from human cortical bone using methods to preserve its osteoinductive properties. The DBP was then used in 100 consecutive patients in whom autologous grafts would normally be used. Thirty-eight of these patients had bone tumors and underwent 40 grafting procedures. There were 15 sarcomas and 23 benign conditions. Various procedures were applied to these groups of patients: massive allografts (16 cases), porous-coated custom prostheses (three), curettage and bone graft (21). Patients were followed long enough to establish whether or not radiographic union had been achieved. In the allograft group the average tie to union was 8.5 weeks (range 4–19 weeks). There were two nonunions in the same patient. There were also two infections in this group, which necessitated allograft removal. In the prosthesis group, the average time to radiographic union between the host and the prosthesis was 4 weeks. The curettage group had radiographic evidence of incorporation at an average of 4.1 weeks (range 2–6 weeks). There were no complications in this group. DBP showed efficacy in the treatment of space-occupying lesions of bone when curettage was used as the treatment modality. Furthermore, DBP shows promise in the induction of bony union between host bone and porous-coated prostheses. While DBP appeared effective in promoting union between the host and large allografts (union rate 86%), a higher union rate would be desirable.

Key words: Demineralized bone powder—Bone tumor—Allograft

Introduction

Autograft bone has been used in the treatment of bone neoplasms for many years; however, in very large space-occupying lesions or tumors which require massive cortical grafts there is rarely enough autograft available. Allograft bone has been used alone or to augment autograft successfully [1]. These techniques involve osteoconduction, but little if any osteogenesis or osteoinduction [1, 2]. Demineralized bone matrix used as particulate powder has been effective in a clinical setting as an inductive agent [2]. This prospective study was undertaken to investigate the effect of the exclusive use of allogenic bone materials in bone tumor surgery with augmentation with an osteoinductive material, demineralized bone power (DBP).

---

[1] The Institute for Limb Preservation and Mile High Transplant Bank, Denver, CO, USA

Materials and Methods

Preparation of DBP

Demineralized bone power was prepared according to the methods developed by other investigators [3, 4]. DBP is prepared from cortical diaphyseal specimens removed from appropriate human donors (age 15–50 years). The marrow and soft tissue are removed from the bone and the bone is sectioned and placed in a mechanical crusher, which produces 3- to 5-mm chips. These chips are then placed in a water-cooled bone mill to reduce their size further, resulting in a powder, which is then placed through a sieve, allowing particles 250–500 μm to pass through (average size 400 nm). This material is then demineralized in 0.6 M hydrochloric acid at 4° C for 12 h. The powder is washed with a phosphate buffer (pH 7.4) and distilled water. The powder is further treated in ethanol, then ether. The powder is place in glass containers and undergoes lyophilization and ethylene oxide sterilization. The glass containers are vacuum-sealed at the end of this procedure and then stored at room temperature until utilized.

Patient Selection

One hundred consecutive patients who would have ordinarily needed autologous bone grafts comprised the original study group. All procedures were performed by the author. Of these 100 patients, 38 had tumorous conditions requiring 40 grafting procedure. The patients were followed clinically with physical and X-ray examination at regular intervals. When both clinical the X-ray examinations confirmed bony bridging and graft incorporation, union was judged present. The patients were followed at least 6 months after union to assess further progression of healing.

Results

There were 38 patients who had various benign or malignant primary processes involving bone. There were 15 sarcomas and 23 benign conditions. The majority of patients were in the third or fourth decade of life. The patients were grouped according to the type of surgical procedure performed: massive allografts (16 cases), porous coated custom prosthesis (three), curettage and bone graft (21).

Massive allograft procedures were defined as those requiring fresh frozen sterile cortical grafts greater than 5 cm in their largest dimension. Both intercalary and osteochondral grafts were included. Once the lesion was resected and rigid internal fixation of the replacement graft was obtained, DBP was meticulously inserted in and about the graft—host junctions. Additional powder was placed upon the surface of the cortical bone several millimeters in thickness. Whenever possible, local muscle was wrapped about the graft area. In two cases, a free fibular transfer was performed to augment the reconstruction. Four of the massive graft patients had chemotherapy preoperatively and at least 6 months postoperatively for either Ewing's sarcoma (one case) or osteosarcoma (three cases). In the massive allograft group, the average time to union was 8.5 weeks (range

4–19 weeks). The time for union for the three patients on chemotherapy was 4, 12, and 19 weeks. One patient who received chemotherapy had loosening of the internal fixation and developed a nonunion, which needed an additional grafting procedure. This graft was also unsuccessful due to loss of fixation and the patient was converted later to a custom prosthesis (not included in this study). There were two proximal humerus grafts which developed infection and were treated by removal with no subsequent reconstruction. There were no other complications, major or minor, in this group.

Three patients had design and insertion of a custom titanium hip (one) or distal femoral (two) prosthesis with a porous-coated collar at the bone—prosthesis junction. All three patients had sarcomas and underwent preoperative and postoperative chemotherapy. The intramedullary stem was cemented and DBP was used to graft from the host bone onto the porous mesh collar. "Union" was judged to be present when the decalcified graft mass became ossified and little or no radiological gap could be appreciated between the graft mass and the porous areas of the prosthesis. In all three of the prosthesis patients, the graft had ossified and appeared to be opposed to the mesh at 4 weeks. With additional time, the graft mass appeared to remodel along lines of weight-bearing stresses. There were no complications in this group.

The curettage and bone graft group consisted of 20 patients who had 21 grafting procedures. One patient had two separate lesions. All of these lesions were benign and included giant cell tumors (four), aneurysmal bone cysts (three), fibrous dysplasia (three), large nonossifying fibromas (four), and other miscellaneous lesions (seven). In all cases, the lesional area was widely exposed through a large cortical window and a meticulous curettage was performed, using traditional techniques as well as a high-speed burr to ensure complete removal of the lesion. No topical agent was used. The areas were then packed with a mixture of DBP and demineralized cancellous chips (5 mm × 5 mm × 5 mm). In no instance was cortical bone replaced over the window throughwhich the graft had been inserted.

The average time of graft incorporation of the curettage group was 4.1 weeks (range 2–6 weeks). There were no complications or local tumor recurrences in the 6 months' period following graft incorporation in this group.

Discussion

Ever since a basic understanding of fracture healing was first established, scientists and clinicians have endeavored to augment and stimulate the process. it became evident that the use of autologous grafting materials could assist in the healing and in many cases change the local milieu in such a way as to promote bone formation that had been previously inhibited. However, problems with harvesting of autologous grafts have been identified and complications reported [1].

The use of allograft bone is becoming accepted practice because it eliminates site morbidity and is readily available. It has been established that standard allograft material has little or no bone induction properties, but serves as a bone conductor [1]. Urist and others [1, 2, 3, 5] have demonstrated that demineralized bone matrix has inductive properties, which are associated with proteins present in the matrix. Urist has gone on to isolate a specific protein (bone morphogenetic protein) which shows bone inductive paracrine function in specific situations. Reddi and others [3, 6, 7] have shown that many factors are necessary for the phenotypic conversion of multipotential cells into bone-producing tissues. In using a powdered, particulate bone matrix material, which is deantigenized, we are able to place a highly concentrated inductive material in and about the area of bone healing. Animal studies have demonstrated the inductive property of DBP [8], but human studies are few [2]. The present study consists of a group of patients with major grafting problems who have been treated exclusively with allograft materials and DBP. Presumably, we are furnishing many of the necessary induction factors in the crude powder as well as bone morphogenic protein.

This study included 38 patients and 40 grafting procedures, involving tumorous conditions of bone. There were four complications—two nonunions in the same patient and two infections. All of these complications involved massive allografts. The average time of union was comparable and in some cases less than that seen in similar cases using autograft [9]. DBP has been shown to be more effective than autologous chips or inlays when used to bridge large defects in an animal model [8]. Several theories have been developed. The particulate nature of the powder allows a very large surface area of the matrix to be exposed and thus have its inductive effect. Also, histological studies have demonstrated that unlike autologous bone grafts the demineralized bone matrix induces a cartilaginous anlage prior to osteogenesis [1, 8]. This is a more physiological situation (endochondral bone formation) and may allow earlier bone growth.

Demineralized bone powder appears to be useful as a bone-inductive agent when used with other allograft materials in bone tumor situations. There is early animal evidence that inductive materials may hasten graft incorporation and assist in bony ingrowth into porous prostheses [4, 6]. It is not clear at present which factors (i.e., marrow, plasma, fibronectin, or other growth factors) are needed in addition to demineralized bone matrix to obtain maximum paracrine bone formation [3, 6, 7, 10]. Additional studies are underway to investigate the induction properties and incorporation of allogeneic bone.

References

1. Prolo DJ, Rodrigo JJ (1985) Contemporary bone graft physiology and surgery. Clin Orthop 200: 322–342
2. Glowacki J, Kaban LB, Murray JB, Folkman J, Mulliken JB (1981) Application of the biological principle of induced osteogenesis for cranial facial defects. Lancet 1: 959–963
3. Muthukumaran N, Reddi AH (1985) Bone matrix-induced local bone formation. Clin Orthop 200: 159–164
4. Kohler P (1986) Reimplantation of bone after autoclaving: Reconstruction of large diaphyseal defects in the rabbit. Karolinska Institute (unpublished)
5. Sato K, Urist MR (1985) Induced regeneration of calvaria by bone morphogenetic protein (BMP) in dogs. Clin Orthop 197: 301–311
6. Ronnigen H, Solheim LF, Langeland N (1985) Bone formation enhanced by induction. Acta Orthop Scand 56: 67–71
7. Wittbjer J, Palmer B, Rohlin M, Thorngren K (1983) Osteogenic activity in compo-

site grafts of demineralized compact bone and marrow. Clin Orthop 173: 229–238

8. Gepstein R, Weiss RE, Saba K, Hallel T (1987) Bridging large defects in bone by demineralized bone matrix in the form of a powder. J Bone Joint Surg 69A: 984–992

9. Enneking W (1983) Musculoskeletal tumor surgery. Churchill Livingston, New York, pp 1233–1235

10. Delloye C, Hebrant A, Munting E, Piret L, Contelier L (1985) The osteoinductive capacity of differently HCI-decalcified bone alloimplants. Acta Orthop Scand 56: 318–322

Thermal Aspects of the Use of Polymethylmethacrylate in Large Metaphyseal Defects in Bone

A Clinical Review and Laboratory Study

Mark C. Leeson[1], Steven B. Lippitt[2], and John T. Makley[3]

Summary. The technique of aggressive local resection and reconstruction of defects with methylmethacrylate is an excellent alternative to resection, which compromise the joint. Forty consecutive patients with a varity of diagnoses (giant cell tumor, aneurysmal bone cyst (ABC), chondromyxoid fibroma, low-grade chondrosarcoma, myeloma, metastases) underwent this treatment. The advantages of this are: (a) immediate stability and early function, (b) early radiographic diagnosis of local recurrence, (c) increased "tumor kill" secondary to thermal necrosis. Local recurrence in these patients was less than that recorded in the literature. The technique of this procedure is demonstrated. A graphic demonstration of laboratory work documenting aspects of thermal necrosis at the bone-cement interface is included.

Key words: Bone tumor—Hyperthermia–Polymethylmethacrylate

Introduction

Neoplasms of bone occur commonly in the metaphyseal area. In an attempt to obtain an adequate surgical margin, the condyle must often be sacrificed. Because this usually necessitates a large reconstruction, it is advantageous to the patient if the tumor can be removed and the patient's own joint preserved. This type of surgery results in a large defect that must then be "filled" in. We performed this type of "joint sparing" procedure in 40 patients, using polymethymethacrylate cement (PMMA) to fill the surgical defect.

The use of bone cement as a "filler" is not new. Charnley introduced self-curing PMMA to orthopedic surgery for use in total joint replacements [2]. Acrylic cementation has also provided for the fixation of pathological fractures and increased stability to large bone defects following bone tumor excision [7, 10, 19–21, 24, 27].

This extensive experience with PMMA in reconstructive surgery has raised

---

[1] Northeast Ohio University College of Medicine and Akron General Medical Center and Department of Biomedical Engineering, Akron University, Akron, OH, USA

[2] Department of Orthopaedic Surgery, Akron General Medical Center, OH, USA

[3] Department of Orthopaedic Surgery, Case Western Reserve University, Cleveland, OH, USA

questions regarding the potential effects of the heat produced during the exothermic polymerization process [1, 8, 9]. Charnley, in 1970, demonstrated that golf-ball size masses of PMMA produced temperatures in the range of 90°C [2]. A temperature range of 42°–47°C is necessary to kill several types of cells, including gonadal, embryonal, blood, cartilage, and carcinoma cells [13, 17, 23].

The purpose of the laboratory portion of this study is to analyze the amplitude and distribution of heat in cadaver bone when large metaphyseal bone defects (simulating tumor excision) are filled with polymerizing PMMA. We will demonstrate how this generated heat radiates in bone, the effect of mass on temperature, and whether significant necrotizing temperatures can be reached. From a clinical standpoint, we performed this type of procedure on 40 patients and will discuss these cases with regard to diagnosis and results.

Methods and Materials

Clinical

Forty patients with primary and metastatic osseous neoplasm were treated at Case Western Reserve University and Akron General Hospital Medical Center from 1978 to 1984 with local tumor extirpation (curettage), high-speed burring of the tumor cavity, and insertion of PMMA. These cases were all followed to conclusion and have been reviewed with attention to local recurrence, mobility of the surgical procedure, and function of the extremity.

Laboratory

In the laboratory, two groups of five cadaver distal femora, which were sectioned at the midshaft level and stripped of all soft tissue, were selected as the experimental bone model (Fig. 1). The lateral epicondylar region was chosen as the site for placement of the standard bone defect in an attempt to mimic an area which could result from curettage of a bone tumor in this region (e.g., giant cell tumor, ABC, chondroblastoma).

In the first set of femora, a 3.2-cm-diameter, 1.85-cm-deep hole was carefully drilled in the center of the lateral epicondylar region. In the second group, a larger bore defect was made in the same region using a 3.75-cm auger bit to a depth of 2.5 cm. These small-bore and large-bore defects correspond to the volume occupied by one and two packets of acrylic cement (Zimmer low viscosity, respectively.

Next, several 2-mm-diameter drill holes were precisely placed parallel to the vertical wall of the bore defect at 1-, 2-, 3-, or 5-mm intervals (Fig. 1). The depth of these drill holes stopped 3 mm short of the corresponding depth of the bore defect (Figs. 2, 3), and their purpose was to accommodate 2-mm-diameter thermistor probes (Omega RTD temperature elements), which measure temperature accurately to ±0.1°C. Temperature probes were also placed in the core of the cement and at the bone/cement interface when the PMMA had been placed in the bone defect.

To simulate a physiological fluid environment and temperature, the femor specimens were initially warmed to 37°C by suspending them in a thermostat-

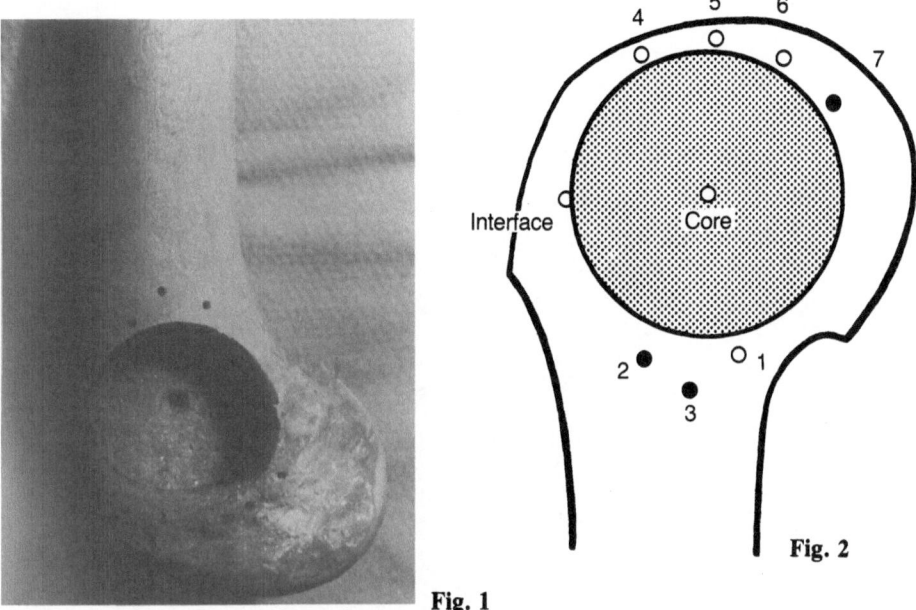

Fig. 1

Fig. 2

Fig. 1. Cadaver femur with large bore defect

Fig. 2. Schema of bone model. Probes are: core, *int* interface, leads *1, 5* (distance 1 mm), leads *4, 6* (2 mm), *2, 7* (3 mm), and *3* (5 *mm*)

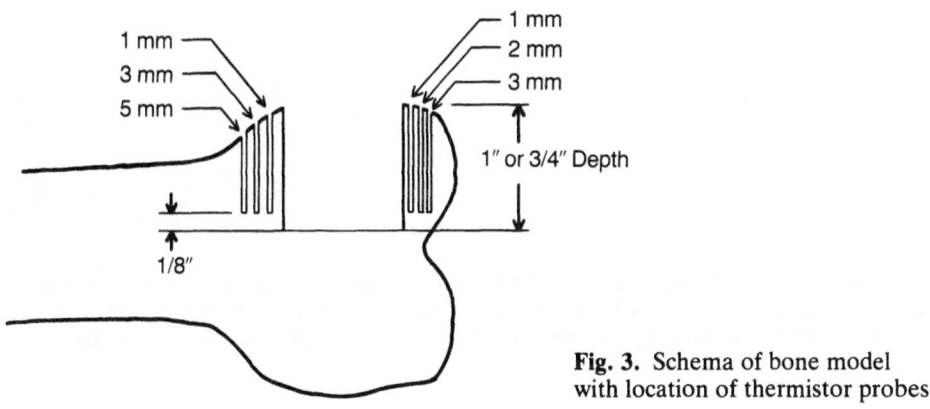

Fig. 3. Schema of bone model with location of thermistor probes

controlled 20-l normal saline bath. The thermistor probes were placed at their respective positions, including two 1-, two 2-, two 3-, and one 5-mm drill holes (Fig. 2).

The experiment was then conducted by preparing the acrylic cement dough (Zimmer low viscosity) by a standardized mixing technique at room temperature (25°C) and injecting this via a 50-cm^3 syringe into the bone defect. This step required lifting the bone specimen from the 37°C bath only long enough to empty the fluid from the defect and to inject the cement. After this, the bone was

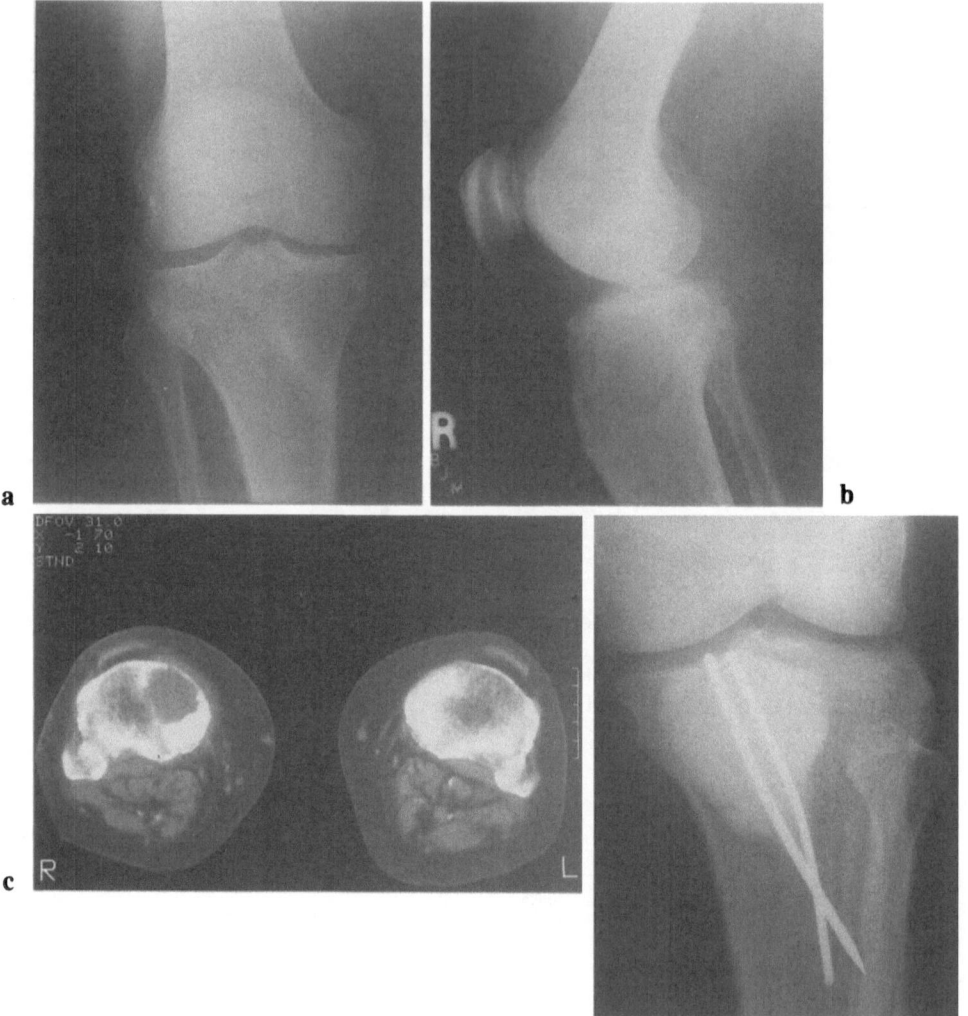

Fig. 4a–d. A 46-year-old male with giant cell tumor of bone. **a** Anteroposterior radiograph. **b** Lateral radiograph. **c** Computed tomography demonstrating tumor and adjacent subchondral bone. **d** Anteroposterior radiograph, postoperative at 4 years' follow-up

resuspended in the 37°C bath flush with the surface level; the core and bone cement interface probes were placed, and individual monitors were utilized to display the temperature changes at each of the nine probes before, during, and after the polymerization process. These temperature data were recorded with the corresponding time every 15 s continually throughout the experiment until all probe temperatures returned below 40°C

This procedure was repeated for each of the five small-bore and each of the five large-bore cadaver femora. As mentioned, above the small-bore defect group were each filled with one packet of cement while the large-bore defect group each required two packets.

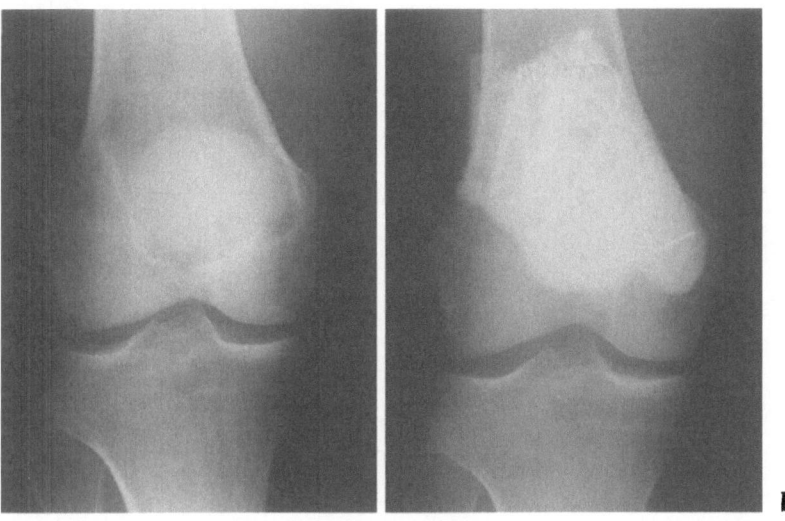

a   b

Fig. 5a, b. A 31-year-old male with aneurysmal bone cyst. **a** Anteroposterior radiograph. **b** Postoperative radiograph at 5 years' follow-up

Results

Clinical

Forty patients underwent the operative procedure of excisional curettage through a large bone window, followed by the use of a high-speed burr and cementation of the cavity in an attempt to excise the tumor and to preserve the joint and a fully functioning extremity. There were 18 males and 22 females in the study. The ages ranged from 11 to 82 years with an average of 36.

Giant cell tumor of bone and aneurysmal bone cysts were the two most common tumors treated in this fashion: giant cell tumor, 21 cases; aneurysmal bone cyst, ten cases; metastases, three cases; citondroblastoma, two cases; plasmacytoma, two cases; chondrosarcoma (low grade), two cases. (Figs. 4–6) The distal femur was the most commonly affected bone: femur, 23 cases; tibia, 12 cases; fibula two cases; humerus, one case; radius, one case; os cakis, one case.

There were two local recurrences. One in a 16-year-old male with giant cell tumor of bone (1/21, 5%), and the other in an 11-year-old, male with aneurysmal bone cyst of the proximal fibula (1/10, 10%; Fig. 7).

The most common complaint at the time of follow-up was that of persistent pain. This was present in five cases, two of which indicated local recurrence. These were treated with a wide surgical margin and reconstruction as necessary. In two of the other three cases, the cement was removed, the cavity again curetted and biopsied and then grafted with autogenous bone graft. This relieved the pain in these two patients. The last patient continues to complain of pain without any evidence of local recurrence but refuses any further surgical procedures. There was one patient who developed a fracture at the bone-cement interface and this was treated with cement removal, bone grafting, and conventional fracture management.

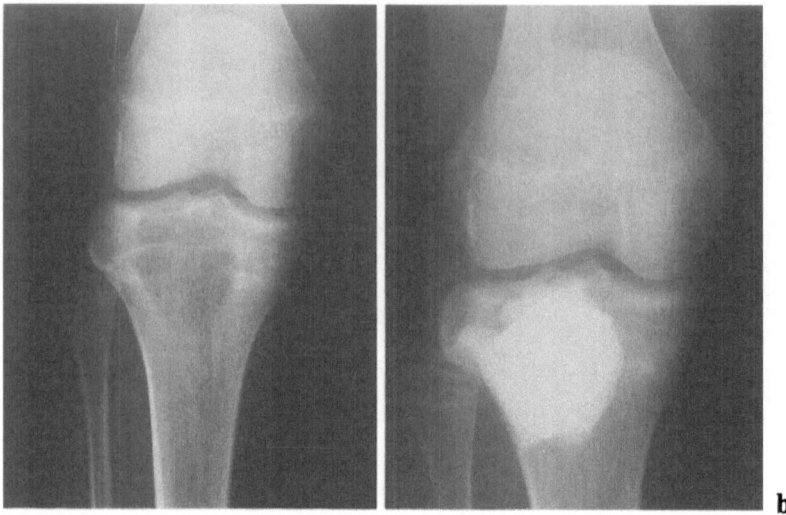

Fig. 6a, b. A 15-year-old female with a chondroblastoma. **a** Anteroposterior radiograph. **b** Anteroposterior radiograph, 3 years' follow-up

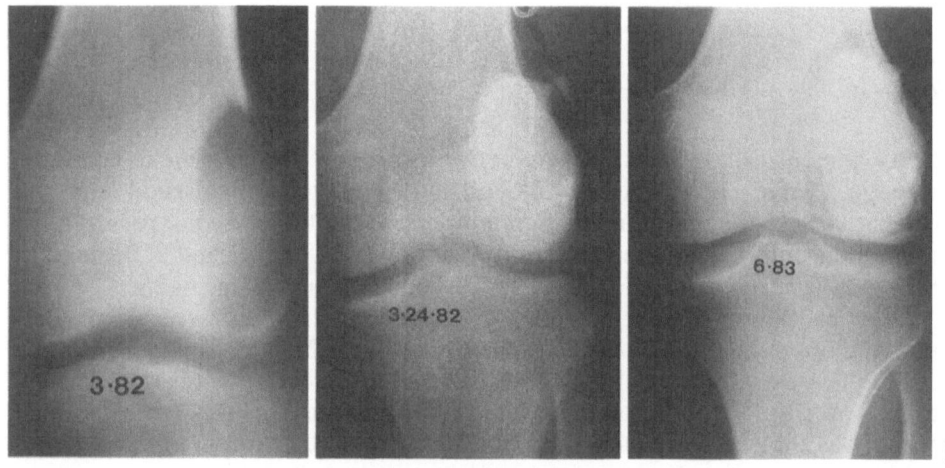

Fig. 7a–c. A 17-year-old male with giant cell tumor of bone. **a** Anteroposterior (AP) tomogram, preoperative. **b** AP radiograph, postoperative. **c** AP radiograph, 15 months after operation. Note radiolucency demonstrative of early recurrence

Laboratory

The temperature versus time data could be plotted graphically for each experiment as illustrated by a typical small-bore case (Fig. 8) and typical large-bore case (Fig. 9). For each experiment, the peak temperature was selected from these data. These peak temperatures for each probe (core, interface, and leads 1–7) for the five small-bore experiments are recorded in Table 1. The "average"

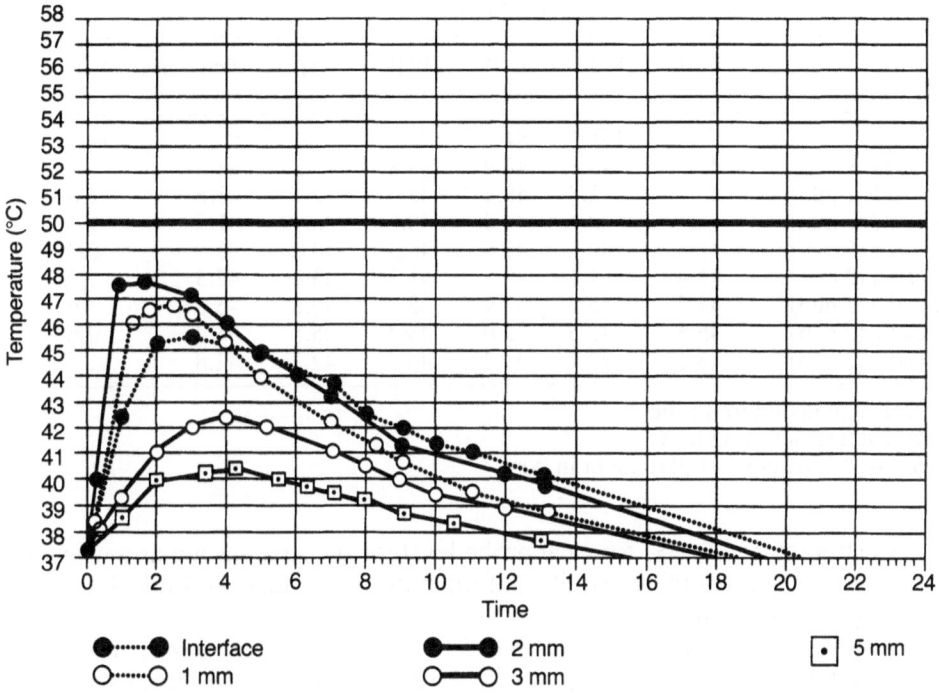

Fig. 8. Temperature-time graph for small-bore defect

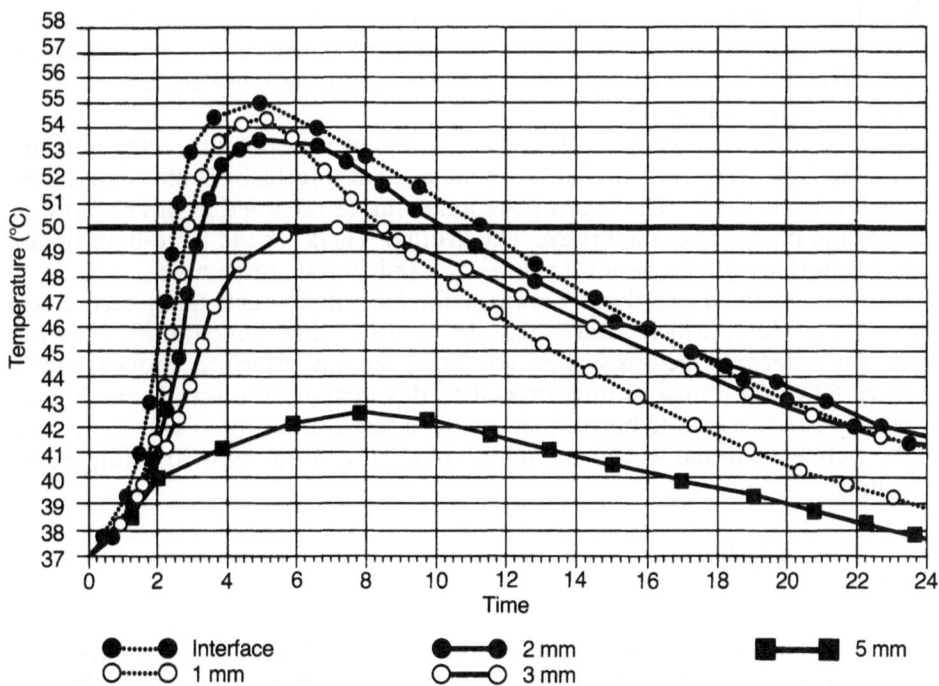

Fig. 9. Temperature-time graph for large-bore defect

Table 1. Peak temperatures (°C) for small-bore defects

	Exp. 1	Exp. 2	Exp. 3	Exp. 4	Exp. 5	Average	SD
Core	89.6	101.8	84.1	72.2	0[a]	86.9	12.0
Interface	47.7	46.8	47.9	43.8	47.8	46.8	1.7
Lead 1 (1 mm)	40.8	42.8	48.2	43.6	42.4	43.6	2.8
Lead 2 (3 mm)	41.4	40.4	45.0	40.6	40.9	41.7	1.9
Lead 3 (5 mm)	41.6	40.8	41.6	40.3	40.3	40.9	0.7
Lead 4 (2 mm)	41.4	44.1	42.5	41.1	43.2	42.5	1.3
Lead 5 (1 mm)	45.5	45.2	43.9	45.1	46.8	45.3	1.0
Lead 6 (2 mm)	45.5	45.5	45.0	44.4	45.8	45.2	0.6
Lead 7 (3 mm)	43.1	43.7	44.2	40.9	42.3	42.8	1.3

[a] Broken temperature probe
SD standard deviation in °C
See Fig. 1 for leads 1–7 placement in bone

peak temperature (Tmax) for each probe level for the small group as a whole is also indicated in this table. Similar information is provided in Table 2 for the large-bore experiments.

These data easily demonstrate that for each probe level (core, interface, 1 mm, 2 mm, 3 mm, and 5 mm), the peak temperatures in the large-bore two-pack cement group were consistently higher than the corresponding level in the small-bore one-pack cement group. The average core Tmax for the small-bore group was 86.9°C.

The highest temperature recorded in the bone in any of the individual small-bore experiments was 46.8°C at the bone-cement interface. No temperatures greater than 50°C were encountered in the bone during these small-bore (one pack) cement experiments.

However, in the large-bore (two packs) cement experiments, temperatures exceeding 50°C were recorded at the bone-cement interface, 1-mm, and 2-mm probe levels (Table 2). The higest peak temperature recorded in this group was 57.2° at the bone-cement interface. The average Tmax for the large-bore bone-cement interface and 1-mm level was 53.5°C and 50.9°C, respectively (Fig. 9).

All leads in the Large-bore group maintained their peak temperature for greater than 30 s, which establishes the reported time-temperature requirement for osteocyte necrosis. For the bone-cement interface probes which reached 50°C, the range of time exceeding this temperature was 8 min 30 s to 9 min 45 s. In these large-bore experiments, a few 2-mm probes and one 3-mm probe were even found to have temperature of 50°C for at least 30 s (range 30 s to 2 min).

Discussion

Since the initial use of PMMA in orthopedic surgery over 30 years ago, the potential adverse affects of the heat released during polymerization have been a

Table 2. Peak temperatures (°C) for large-bore defects

	Exp. 6[a]	Exp. 7	Exp. 8	Exp. 9	Exp. 10[a]	Average	SD
Core	108.8	0[b]	114.9	104.1	102.4	107.6	5.6
Interface	49.0	57.2	56.6	55.0	49.7	53.5	3.9
Lead 1 (1 mm)	47.1	53.5	56.8	46.1	48.4	50.4	4.6
Lead 2 (3 mm)	41.7	45.6	46.9	43.5	43.6	44.3	2.0
Lead 3 (5 mm)	40.0	47.4	48.1	42.7	41.9	44.0	3.6
Lead 4 (2 mm)	42.2	50.6	43.7	47.2	45.9	45.9	3.2
Lead 5 (1 mm)	45.5	56.0	49.6	54.9	51.2	51.4	4.2
Lead 6 (2 mm)	45.7	47.4	51.3	53.7	54.1	50.4	3.8
Lead 7 (3 mm)	42.2	49.8	47.8	50.0	49.0	47.8	3.2

[a] Slightly less than full two packets of PMMA cement used because of spillage
[b] Broken temperature probe
SD standard deviation in °C
See Fig. 1 for leads 1–7 placement in bone

subject of concern. Several variables help determine the peak temperatures reached by polymerizing PMMA including the amount of reacting monomer, the rate at which heat is released, the surface area over which the heat is dissipated, and the thermal physically properties of PMMA such as the heat capacity and thermal conductivity. Perhaps most important in determining the peak temperature of cement is the amount (mass) used. Since the total heat content is fixed by the weight of the reacting monomer, the maximum temperature tends to increase with increasing mass [9, 26]. The sizes of defects in bone (small and large) made in this experiment exemplify this point. Also of significant importance is the surface area over which the heat is dissipated. All things being equal, a sphere of PMMA (small surface to volume ratio) will become much hotter than a flat sheet (high surface area to volume ratio) of equal mass [12]. We chose a cylindrical bore defect because it best simulated a cavity after tumor curettage.

The rate of temperature rise within any substance depends primarily upon two physical factors—the heat capacity of the substance and the ability to transport heat [16]. These thermal properties of cement (when mixed appropriately) are fairly constant [12, 26]. However, these same properties vary considerably when comparing dry bone and hydrated bone specimens. The hydrated bone closely resembles vital bone tissue in respect of both thermal conductivity and heat capacity [16]; thus, we chose to perform this experiment in a saline environment. In addition, we chose to maintain the bath at the physiological temperature of 37°C rather than at room temperature since the absolute temperature rise in a substance being heated is dependent on its initial temperature [9, 16].

Another factor which theoretically could influence the thermal properties of bone tissue is the circulation of blood [4]. Since the usual tumor curettage and cementation procedure utilizes a proximally inflated tourniquet, causing hemostasis of the operative field, a static fluid environment was justified for this experiment.

The average peak PMMA core temperatures for the small- and large-bore groups were 86.9°C and 107.6°C, respectively, which correspond to the figures from previous reports [9, 26, 30]. The variation of reported core temperatures in these previous experiments is due to the use of different volumes of PMMA. Swenson and Schurman revealed increases in the peak temperature of 33°–80°C as the diameter of the mold containing the cement increased from 0.75 to 2.0 cm [26]. Another experimental model demonstrated that a cement thickness of 1 cm generated a core temperature of 70°C, while a 3-cm thickness of PMMA generated a 124°C core temperature [9]. The consistently higher core temperatures observed in our large-bore two-pack cement versus the small-bore one-pack cement experiments further support the finding that increasing amounts of polymerizing PMMA yield higher peak temperatures [16].

The use of PMMA in these types of tumors has three important advantages: (a) It provides for immediate stability of the reconstructed defect; (b) it allows for close monitoring of the lesion and early diagnosis of local recurrence (Fig. 7); (c) it provides the potential to increase the surgical margin, while continuing to spare the adjacent joint.

A 50% reduction in the recurrence rate of giant cell tumors (from 20% to 10%) has been reported when comparing curettage followed by PMMA cementation to curettage and bone grafting alone [11, 15, 19, 20]. The authors of these studies have accounced for this decrease in recurrence rate by suggesting that the heat of PMMA polymerization may adversely affect tumor cells remaining in the curetted cavity. Others have suggested that mechanical or chemical trauma is associated with the use of PMMA, rather than the thermal mechanism of injury [9, 14]. For example, the forcible extrusion of the polymer dough into trabecular bone may disrupt vascular channels. Jefferiss [9] describes free radicals generated during the polymerization reaction as chemically highly reactive and potentially toxic to lipid constituents of cell membranes. He suggested that these free radicals could also cause protein coagulation.

The heat from large amounts of PMMA could have similar effects on other tumor tissues as well. Certainly, the concept of hyperthermia having an antitumor effect is by no means new [4, 5]. Hyperthermic temperatures in the range of 42°–47°C are now recognized by experimentalists and clinicians alike as having definite, yet ill-defined, potential in the treatment of certain solid tumors. A study by Dickson [5] demonstrated significant regression of large solid tumors (rabbit VX2 intramuscular carcinoma, which behaves in a similar manner to human cancer) when heated at temperature of 47°C–50°C [4, 13, 16].

PMMA-related thermal necrosis can extend the surgical margins 1–2 mm and decrease the recurrence rate in patients treated by curettage and cementation.

From a clinical standpoint, the ability to preserve a functioning extremity and joint while eradicating the tumor is the surgeon's main goal. While allograft joints and custom prostheses have marked a tremendous advance in the treatment of tumors in the extremities, nothing functions as well as the patient's own joint.

In patients with aggressive benign and low-grade malignancies, this type of procedure may allow the surgeon to preserve the joint and still exact a marginal to wide margin of tumor removal.

Conclusion

Based on an experimental model with polymerizing PMMA and metaphyseal defects in cadaver bone, thermal necrosis adjacent to polymerizing PMMA occurs when two or more packs of cement are utilized. The zone of necrosis when this amount of cement is used reaches a radius of 1–2 mm and occasionally more. However, the heat from one pack of cement will not, under normal clinical circumstances, reach significant necrotic temperatures.

The use of aggressive curettage and methacrylate cementation clinically reduces the percentage of recurrences previously reported for these types of tumors treated in a more conventional curettage and grafting fashion.

What remains to be answered is the effect of a large mass of PMMA adjacent to an active joint. The long-term laboratory and clinical studies on this situation have yet to be performed.

Based on both clinical and laboratory evidence, we can then recommend the use of aggressive curettage and methacrylate cementation in patients with benign, benign aggressive, and low-grade malignant tumors involving the metaphyseal portion of bone in an attempt to eradicate the tumor and preserve a functioning joint.

Acknowledgments. The authors express special thanks to Ms Dana Smith-Evans for her clerical assistance and to the Biomedical Communications Department at Akron General Medical Center.

References

1. Andersson GBJ, Freeman MAR, Swanson SAV (1972) Loosening of cemented acetabular cup in total hip replacement. J Bone Jt Surg 54-B: 590–599
2. Charnley J (1970) Acrylic cement in orthopaedic surgery. Williams and Wilkins, Baltimore
3. Charnley J (1970) The reaction of bone to self-curing acrylic cement. J Bone Jt Surg 52-B: 340–353
4. Clattenberg R, Cohn J (1975) Thermal properties of cancellous bone. J Biomed Mater Res 9: 169–182
5. Dickson JA, Shah SA (1977) Technology for the hyperthermic treatment of large solid tumours at 50°C. Clin Oncol 3: 301–318
6. Flory PJ, Garrett RR (1958) Phase transitions in collagen and gelatin systems. J Am Chem Soc 80: 4836
7. Harrington KD, Johnston OJ, Turner RH, Green DL (1972) The use of methyl-methacrylate as an adjunct in the internal fixation of malignant neoplastic fractures. J Bone Jt Surg Am 54: 1665–1676
8. Homsy CA, Tullos HS, Anderson MS, Differante NM, King JW (1972) Some physiological aspects of prosthesis stabilization with acrylic polymer. Clin Orthop Related Research 83: 317–328
9. Jefferiss CD, Lee AJC, Ling RSM (1975) Thermal aspects of self-curing polymethyl-methacrylate. J Bone Jt Surg 57B: 511–518
10. Kiviluoto O, Salenius P, Santavirta S (1981) Acrylic comentation in treatment of benign bone tumors. Acta Orthop Scand 52: 443
11. Larsson SE, Lorentzon R, Boquist L (1975) Giant cell tumor of bone. J Bone Jt Surg 57-A: 161–173

12. Lautenschlager EP, Stupp SI, Keller JC (1984) Functional behavior of orthopaedic biomaterials, vol 2. CRC Press, Clemson, SC, pp 88–119
13. Leach EH, Peters RA, Rossiter RJ (1943) Experimental thermal burns, especially the moderate temperature burn. Quart J Exp Physiol 32: 67
14. Linder L (1977) Reaction of bone to the acute chemical trauma of bone cement. J Bone Jt Surg Am 59: 82–87
15. Lorentzon R (1978) Genuine giant cell tumor of bone. Umea University Medical Dissertations no. 33
16. Lundskog J (1972) Heat and bone tissue—an experimental investigation of the thermal properties of bone tissue and threshold levels for thermal injury. Scand J Plast Reconstr Surg (Suppl 9) 6: 63–71
17. Mendelssohn K, Rossiter RJ (1944) Subcutaneous temperatures in moderate temperature burns. Quart J Exp Physiol 32: 201
18. Meyer PR, Lautenschlager EP, Moore BK (1973) On the setting properties of acrylic bone cement. J Bone Jt Surg 55A: 149–156
19. Persson BM, Ekelund L, Lovdahl R, Gunterberg B (1984) Favourable results of acrylic cementation for giant cell tumors. Acta Orthop Scand 55: 209–214
20. Persson BM, Wouters HW (1976) Curettage and acrylic cementation in surgery of giant cell tumors of bone. Clin Orthop 120: 125–133
21. Ray AK, Romine JS, Pankovich AM (1974) Stabilization of pathogenic fractures with acrylic cement. Clin Orthop 202: 182–185
22. Reckling FW, Dillon WL (1977) The bone-cement interface temperature during total joint replacement. J Bone Jt Surg Am 59: 80–82
23. Sevitt S (1949) Local Blood flow changes in experimental burns. J Pathol Bact 61: 427
24. Singh SH (1966) Use of plastic cement in the treatment of pathological fractures due to malignancy. Proc R Soc Med 59: 121–122
25. Spengler DM, Iida M, Burstein A, Frankel V (1975) Efficacy of methylmethacrylate in the re-establishment of bone structural strength in experimentally produced di-aphyseal defects. An in-vitro biomedical analysis. J Bone Jt Surg Am 57: 580
26. Swenson L, Schurman D (1981) Finite element temperature analysis of a total hip replacement and measurement of PMMA curing temperatures. J Biomed Mater Res 15: 83–96
27. Vidal I, Mimran R, Allieu Y, Jamne M, Goalard G (1969) Plastic de comblement par metacrylate de methyle traitement de certaines tumeours osseuses benignes. Mont-pelliers vol 15, no 4
28. Willert HG, Ludwig J, Semlitsh M (1974) Reaction of bone to methacrylate after hip arthroplasty. J Bone Jt Surg 56A: 1368–1382
29. Kuhl PR, Sheline GE, Alpen EL (1954) Blister formation and tissue temperature in radiant energy and contact burns. Am J Pathol 30: 695
30. Kusy RP (1978) Characterization of self curing acrylic bone cement. J Biomed Mater Res 12: 271–305
31. Moritz AR, Henriques FC Jr (1947) Studies on thermal injury: II. Am J Pathol 23: 695

The Use of Methylmethacrylate As a Hyperthermia Agent for the Treatment of Giant Cell Tumors

Experience of 78 Cases in a Long-Term Appraisal (1974–1987)

OLAVO PIRES DE CAMARGO[1]

Summary. Since 1974, we have employed acrylic cementation for the treatment of giant cell tumors as hyperthermia agent and to achieve complete filling of the cavity. Local recurrence with preservation of the joint function occurred only in four cases. In cases of extensive bone lesion, we used a polyethylene prosthesis molded according to the size of the tumor. This did not require postoperative immobilization and we did not observe osteoarthrosis even in the long term. We did not remove the cement after complete stability had achieved.

Key words: Acrylates—Bone neoplasms—Giant cell tumors

Introduction

The use of acrylic cementation in reconstructive surgery is not a new procedure. It was first employed for the treatment of giant cell tumors in 1969 by Vidal to create stability after curettage of the lesion

We started employing methylmethacrylate cement in the treatment of giant cell tumors in 1974 because it fills the cavity completely after curettage and also because of its effect against the neoplastic cells, leading to an accentuated decrease of local recurrence, which is otherwise frequent with the classic procedure of curettage and bone grafting. Many experimental studies, including those of Strube and Komitowski [6] and Malawer et al. [4], demonstrated the hyperthermal and cytotoxic effect of the methylmethacrylate cement against the neoplastic cell, making this procedure an effective form of adjuvant therapy for benign cavity bone lesions, particulary giant cell tumors. This method is in accordance with Enneking's staging for the margin of control of benign tumors (IIB or IIIB), such as giant cell tumor, where an intracapsular or marginal resection with an effective adjuvant therapy, i.e., acrylic cement, is recommended.

We have already operated on 78 cases of giant cell tumors with this method and after a long-term appraisal we obtained a very low incidence of local recurrence, infection, and pathological fracture. Furthermore, in those cases reeval-

[1] Musculoskeletal Tumors Group, Department of Orthopaedics, Faculty of Medicine, University of São Paulo, São Paulo, Brazil

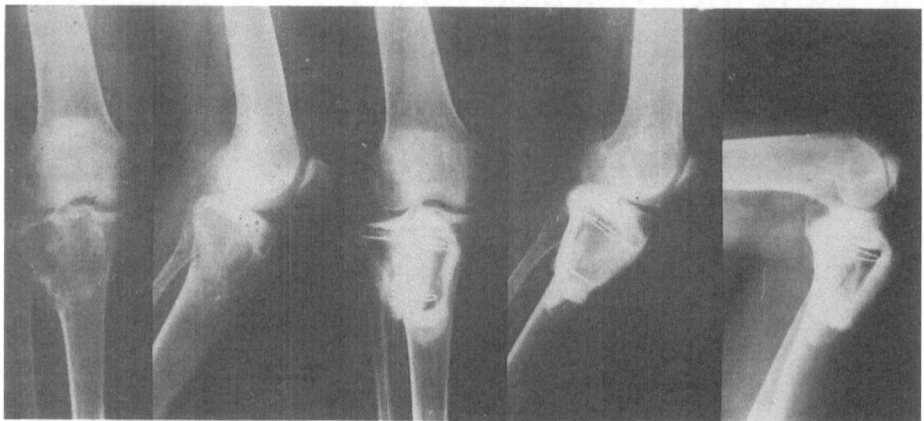

Fig. 1. Giant cell tumor. Anteroposterior and lateral radiographs of a 32-year-old man. Postoperative radiographs taken 13 years after curettage and cementation showing a good functional result

uated 10 years or more after surgery no clinical or radiological evidence of osteoarthrosis was noted in the joint involved with preservation of the articular mobility. In cases of large bone lesions where a considerable amount of cement was employed, we used a polyethylene prosthesis molded according to the radiographic form of the lesion.

This prosthesis reduces the amount of cement used, avoiding the risk of excessive cortical destruction. This aspect may also explain the absence of osteoarthrosis of the knee in our cases when compared with the results of other authors [5] who use only acrylic cement.

This procedure has been effective in preserving the joint function, which is an important point to be considered as the giant cell tumor affects mainly young adults. Only in cases of great involvement and destruction of the articular cartilage do we perform a wide local en bloc resection of the giant cell and a custom-made endoprosthesis

Material and Methods

This study consisted of 78 cases of giant cell tumors of bone with the histological diagnosis confirmed by biopsy. The first patient was operated upon in 1974. Of these cases, 41 were considered histologically aggressive (grade II). The mean age was 28 years. There were 38 males and 40 females in the study. The site most commonly affected was near the knee joint (61 cases).

Those cases in which the articular cartilage was greatly involved were not eligible for this method and underwent a nonconventional endoprosthesis or an arthrodesis.

The surgery must be performed in a bloodless field and it is important to make a wide opening of the tumor walls to permit good visualization and to allow digital palpation of the inner walls. After meticulous curettage, mainly in the

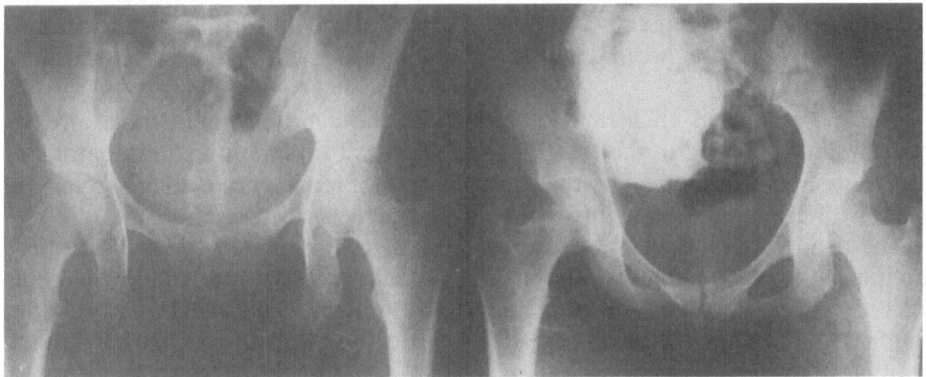

Fig. 2. Preoperative and postoperative radigraphs of a giant cell tumor of the sacrum with 8 years of follow-up

areas of cortical penetration, the medullary canal that is frequently obliterated is opened and the cavity is rinsed with saline solution. The cavity is then dried and cauterization is performed on the inner walls by means of an electric cautery. The acrylic cement with barium contrast is introduced with digital pressure so that the filling can reach all the corners of the inner surface. In cases of a giant cell tumor attaining great proportions, we use a polyethylene prosthesis molded according to the size of the lesion. The prosthesis is introduced against the wall that is in contact with the articular cartilage. If the tumor is small, cementation only is employed to fill the cavity

The tourniquet is then released and a careful hemostasis is performed. After closure and soft dressing of the wound, immediate mobilization is permitted. Two weeks after surgery, ambulation and weight bearing as normally allowed.

Results and Discussion

The results obtained in 78 cases, most of them with a long follow-up, may be considered good with a low incidence of local recurrence, infection, or pathological fracture. Furthermore, the articular movements were preserved without clinical or radiological evidence of osteoarthrosis.

There were only four cases of local recurrence and three cases of infection. These cases underwent reoperation with new local cementation or with en bloc resection of the lesion and a nonconventional endoprosthesis with a good end result. In those patients where the knee joint was greatly affected due to an aggressive giant cell tumor, limitation in the last degrees of flexion was noted, without pain or knee effusion. Our patients were submitted to Enneking's functional evaluation system and the results were 67 excellent, eight good, and three fair, with no poor result.

No complications were observed concerning the use of methylmethacrylate cement even in those patients reevaluated after a long period of time and for this reason we think that is not necessary to remove it 2 or 3 years after the surgery

(Fig. 1), a procedure recommended by Wilert [7]. Progressive remodeling of the cortex involving the cement was noted in some cases by means of periodic radiographs. Furthermore, we did not have any case of pathological fracture postoperatively.

The hyperthermal effect and cytotoxity of the acrylic cement have already been well established in the treatment of giant cell tumors in experimental studies [4, 6, 8] and as evident by the low incidence of recurrence even in aggressive cases with great bone tissue involvement and cortical destruction (Fig. 2).

The use of a polyethylene prosthesis together with cement in cases of huge cavities is helpful to stabilize the wall in contact with the articular cartilage as well as decrease the amount of cement to be utilized. This aspect may explain the fact we did not observe any occurrence of osteoarthrosis even in the patients with more than 10 years of follow-up.

After 13 years, this seems to be a reliable method as is also demonstrated in other publications [1–3, 5] with preservation of the joint function and without any immediate or late complications.

References

1. Kiviluoto O, Salenius PS, Santavirta S (1981) Acrylic cementation in treatment of benign bone tumors. Acta Orthop Scand 52: 443
2. Camargo FP, Camargo OP (1985) Surgical treatment of benign cavitary bone lesions employing methylmethacrylate cement and polyethylene prosthesis—An experience with 135 cases. In: Proceedings of international symposium on limb salvage in musculoskeletal oncology, Orlando, Oct. 1985
3. Conrad EU, Enneking WF, Springfield OS (1985) Giant cell tumor treated with curettage and cementation. In: Proceedings of international symposium on limb salvage in musculoskeletal oncology, Orlando, Oct. 1985
4. Malawer MM, Marta M, McChesney D, Shmookler BM, Gunter S (1985) A dog model for the study of criosurgery and PMNA on a tumor cavity—Evaluation of bone necrosis and bone graft incorporation. In: Proceedings of international symposium on limb salvage in musculoskeletal oncology, Orlando, Oct. 1985
5. Persson BM, Rydholm A, Berlin O, Gutemberg B (1985) Curettage and acrylic cementation in surgery of giant cell tumors of bone. In: Proceedings of international symposium on limb salvage in musculoskeletal oncology, Orlando, Oct. 1985
6. Strube HD, Komitowski (1985) Experimental studies on the use of bone cement in the treatment of malignant bone tumors. In: Proceedings of international symposium on limb salvage in musculoskeletal oncology, Orlando, Oct. 1985
7. Willert HG (1985) Clinical results of the temporary acrylic cement plug in the treatment of bone tumors: A multicentric study. In: Proceedings of international symposium on limb salvage in musculoskeletal oncology, Orlando, Oct. 1985
8. Wilkins RM, Okada Y, Gonski JP, Sin FH, Chao EY (1985) Methylmethacrylate replacement of subcondral bone. A biomechanical and morphologic analysis. In: Proceedings of international symposium on limb salvage in musculoskeletal oncology, Orlando, Oct. 1985

Chapter 6

The Use of Ceramic Prostheses for Replacement of Bone Tumors

Long-Term Results with Ceramic Tumor Prostheses

K. Knahr[1], M. Salzer[1], H. Plenk, Jr.[2], and M. Böhler[1]

Summary. Between 1973 and 1979, ceramic tumor endoprostheses were used in 40 patients treated at the Orthopedic Hospital Wien-Gersthof. The main localization was the proximal humerus, where 25 ceramic endoprostheses were implanted, followed by the proximal femur with ten implants. Elongation of a femoral stump after high amputation was performed in three cases, while in two cases after above-knee amputation and disarticulation of the femur a special disarticulation endoprosthesis was implanted.

We now have experience with 15 patients having a ceramic implant for more than 5 years. The clinical results of these limb-salvage procedures are analyzed and a special study of the results concerning the fixation between ceramic and bone is made.

All the tumor prostheses of the proximal femur were combined with a cement-free acetabular component, which was also used in patients with osteoarthritis. Results are also presented of 46 cement-free ceramic sockets with a follow-up observation period of 6–10 years.

Key words: Alumina ceramic—Tumor endoprosthesis—Ceramic hip socket

Introduction

At the beginning of the 1970s, the first failures were encountered with cemented total hip endoprostheses. Normally, these total endoprostheses consisted of a polyethylene socket and a metal stem. As a result of these failures, a search for new implant materials was started. The prerequisites for these new materials were good biocompatibility, minimal wear, and the possibility of biological attachment to the bone. These requirements led to the introduction of aluminum oxide ceramic, since this material met all these conditions: (a) Aluminum oxide ceramic displays good tissue compatibility, a fact confirmed by our own animal experiments [5]. There are no clinically or histologically detectable indications of irritation in the tissue, and there is no bone resorption. On the contrary, newly formed bone grows into the grooves provided in the ceramic implant. (b) With regard to compression, the mechanical properties of aluminum oxide ceramic are superior to those of metals, and its tensile strength is sufficient for the likely

---

[1] Orthopedic Hospital Wien-Gersthof, Vienna, Austria
[2] Institute of Histology, University of Vienna, Vienna, Austria

Table 1. Bioceramic implants at Wien-Gersthof Orthopedic Hospital, 1974–1983 ($n = 112$)

	No. of patients	Died of disease: prosthesis in function	Complication with endo-prosthesis	Long-term follow-up
Proximal humerus	28	12	4	12
Proximal femur	11	8	1	2
Femur stump elongation	4	—	1	3
Hip enucleation prosthesis	2	1	1	—
Acetabular sockets in THA	67	10	2	55
Total	112	31	9	72

loading of an endoprosthesis. However, only suitable design allows the material to withstand adequate bending loads [2]. (c) Tribological investigations of the ceramic-to-ceramic surface produced results superior to those of the conventional combination of polyethylene and metal [1].

To take advantage of the good biocompatibility of this material, bone cement was not used for the anchorage of the ceramic prostheses. This necessitated the development of a fixation system that allowed direct contact between the implant and bone. Instead of an intramedullary stem, the principle of a conical sleeve was selected for fixation to long bones. This also made it possible to achieve adequate bending strength. The sleeve is placed over the bone, which is shaped into a conical stump using a special milling cutter after resection.

This form of attachment permits stable primary anchorage of the implant. The inside surface of the sleeve is provided with indentations into which the new bony tissue can grow for long-term anchorage. The maximum width and depth of these grooves is 1 mm, and the distance between the grooves is also 1 mm.

Material

A total of 112 bioceramic implants were inserted at the General Orthopedic Department of Wien-Gersthof Hospital (Table 1). This involved 28 patients with resections of the proximal humerus and 11 patients with resections of the proximal femur. Elongation of the femoral stump was carried out in four patients, and in two cases a special implant was inserted after enucleation of the hip. In 67 cases, bioceramic socket prostheses were used in combination with conventional total hip joint endoprostheses.

Thirty-one of the total number of patients have since died. In nine cases (8%), there were loosening complications which necessitated removal of the implant. Thus, a total of 72 patients were available for a long-term follow-up investigation. A survival analysis of the ceramic implants, for which the definition of failure was taken as reoperation as a result of loosening, indicated a survival rate of 88.9% ±3.7% after 8 years (Fig. 1).

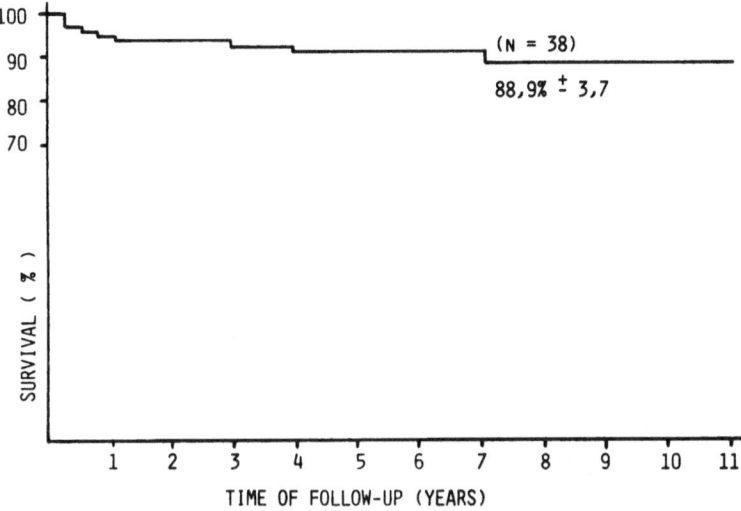

Fig. 1. Survival analysis of bioceramic implants ($n = 112$)

Humerus Endoprosthesis

The bioceramic humerus endoprosthesis is used to bridge defects after resection of tumors of the proximal humerus. It consists of three parts—a conical sleeve, a distance, piece, and a ball. The three components of the prosthesis are selected during the operation and joined intraoperatively using polymethyl methacrylate. A sterilizable container holding all operating tools and a set of implants was developed for this prosthesis [6]. This humerus prosthesis was implanted in a total of 18 patients with primary malignant bone tumors and ten patients with bone metastases. The survival curve for the implants shows that 78% ±1% of these endoprostheses are still functioning after a period of 5 years.

In an ideal case of stable anchorage there is complete incorporation of the implant, with a smooth transition between bone and implant (Fig. 2a). Very frequently, new periosteal bone formation develops in addition to the conical anchorage in the sleeve, functioning as a further stabilizing factor (Fig. 2b).

Traumatic fracture in the area of the anchorage occurred in two patients after 54 and 128 months. In one patient, this resulted in a loosening of the implant, which had to be replaced by a metal prosthesis; in the second patient, however, the anchorage was so stable that the fracture occurred just below the prosthesis. The fracture healed without complications, and the patient is still able to pursue his profession as a dental surgeon.

In two cases, the implant had to be removed as a result of local infection after 1 and 5 months. In another patient, there were clear indications of loosening of the prosthesis after 5 years. However, clinically, the patient was largely free of pain and did not want to undergo revision surgery. After 9 years, a fracture occurred in the vicinity of the conical stump. The patient is still satisfied with the functional result and does not want another operation.

Radiological signs of instability of the conical sleeve connection were encoun-

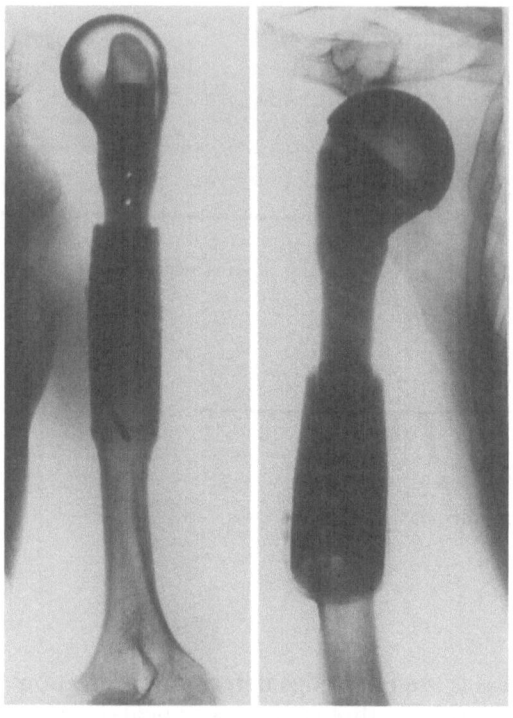

a   b

Fig. 2. a B.W., 29 years old, male, resection of a reticulosarcoma of the left proximal humerus. Twelve years postoperatively, the X-ray shows a stable anchorage with "incorporation" of the implants. **b** P.H., 58 years old, male, resection of a chondrosarcoma of the right proximal humerus. X-ray control 10 years postoperatively shows stable anchorage and slight malpositioning of the axis with periosteal bone formation for additional stabilization of the prosthesis

tered in two patients after only 4 months. There was slight malpositioning of the axis and a high degree of extracortical bone formation providing support. In neither case was there a deterioration of this radiological loosening. On the contrary, there was subsequently marked stabilization of the osseous connection. Although radiologically the anchorage is not optimal in either of these cases, the patients are very satisfied with the clinical result. They are completely free from pain, have absolutely no symptoms of loosening, and have free mobility in the area of the elbow joint and hand.

Femoral Shaft Endoprosthesis

This prosthesis, shaped like the proximal femur, was used to bridge defects after the resection of tumors in the area of the proximal femur. The one-piece implant consisted of a ball with a diameter of 32 mm and a shaft ending in a conical sleeve, which was connected to the bone extracortically as described above. The prosthesis was combined with a hemispherical ceramic socket, on the outer surface of which there were three pegs to provide stable anchorage in the pelvic

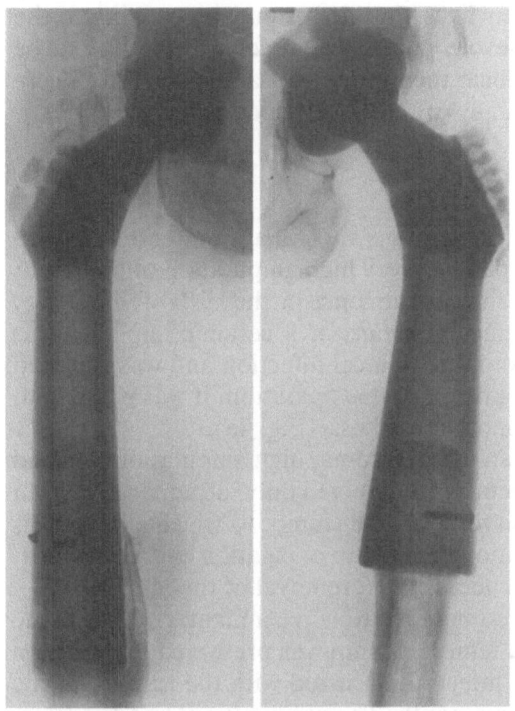

a   b

Fig. 3. a B.S., 66 years old, female, resection of a chondrosarcoma of the right proximal femur. Secondary stabilization of the implant by subsiding of the prosthesis and massive extracortical bone formation. **b** D.M., 60 years old, male, resection of an osteosarcoma of the left proximal femur. Ten years postoperatively, stable anchorage with full weight-bearing capacity of extremity

bone. The femoral shaft prosthesis was available in three different lengths with four different cone sizes. The socket prosthesis was available in four different sizes.

Implantation of the femoral part was similar to that of the humerus prosthesis. After milling the proximal femur to shape, the prosthesis was attached with a firm push fit and secured with a cortical screw for rotational stability. After milling the roof of the acetabulum with a special hemispherical milling cutter, a template was inserted, through which the three anchoring holes for the pegs could be drilled in the roof of the acetabulum. The socket was then inserted using a special instrument, which was used to knock the socket firmly into place.

The femoral prosthesis was used in three patients with primary bone tumors and eight with bone metastases. Two patients have now been followed up for more than 10 years. Whereas in one case stable incorporation of the implant occurred (Fig. 3b), another patient displayed clear signs of irritation in the area of attachment, with the formation of an extensive reactive osseous sleeve. Nevertheless, this anchorage was still sufficient to offer the patient satisfactory loadability of the lower extremities for the next 10 years (Fig. 3a). The third patient died after 4 years as a result of generalized metastases.

Seven of the eight patients with metastases had a functional lower extremity for the remaining short period of their lives. In one instance, loosening of the implant occurred, accompanied by severe pain. A hemipelvectomy had to be carried out in view of the fact that local recurrence had also occurred. There were no loosening complications with any of the 12 ceramic sockets.

Stump Elongation and Hip Enucleation Prosthesis

Three of the four patients with stump elongations are still alive after a follow-up period of more than 10 years. In one patient, very high amputation of the femur had to be carried out as a result of an osteosarcoma in the distal femur. We, therefore, decided to extend the stump by means of a ceramic implant. This implant had to be temporarily removed due to local infection and was replaced again after a period of 6 months. As a result of this operation, it was possible to fit this patient with a conventional femoral prosthesis (Fig. 4a).

In the case of another patient with an osteosarcoma, high amputation also had to be carried out as a result of skip metastases detected only intraoperatively. In this case, it was also possible to preserve a femoral stump, to which a prosthesis could be fitted thanks to the implantation of a stump elongation endoprosthesis. One patient suffered infection, which necessitated removal of the implant.

In the case of two patients, it proved possible to leave a mantle of soft tissue after enucleation of the femur, and a femoral stump was preserved by insertion of a ceramic prosthesis. In one case, infection occurred with the result that the implant had to be removed again after a month. The other patient had an actively mobile femoral stump up until his death 2 years postoperatively. In this case, very good rehabilitation results were obtained with a conventional above-knee prosthesis (Fig. 4b).

Ceramic Socket Implants for Total Hip Arthroplasty

The hemispherical pegged ceramic socket was implanted in the course of total hip arthroplasty in 67 patients with degenerative diseases of the hip joint [2]. Most of these patients were old, and ten have since died. Reoperation was necessary in only two cases due to isolated loosening of the socket implant. In nine cases, the implants had to be removed because of breakage of the ceramic head. This was due to an insufficient connection between the ceramic ball and the metal cone of the femoral stem endoprosthesis. At the time of reoperation, all nine sockets removed were still firmly anchored in the roof of the acetabulum.

In 40 of the 46 sockets that could be followed up over a period of 6–11 years, the clinical picture was one of a radiologically stable socket, i.e., the position had not changed in the course of the years (Fig. 5).

In six patients, there was a radiologically detectable change in the position of the socket with a slowly increasing valgus migration and protrusion of the implant. However, so far, these radiological changes have not produced any clinical symptoms.

If removal of the implant as a result of aseptic loosening is taken as the criterion for failure, after a follow-up period of 8 years the survival rate for ceramic sockets is 94.4% ±4.0%.

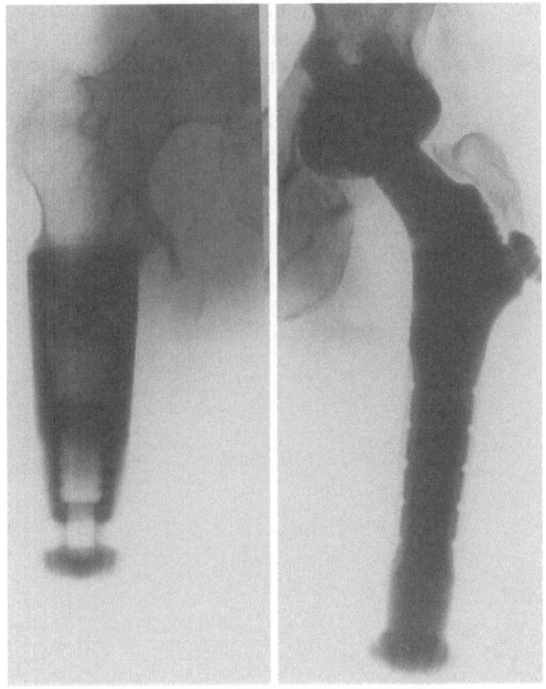

a   b

Fig. 4. a L.G., 24 years old, male, high amputation of an osteosarcoma of the right femur. Stable stump elongation endoprosthesis permits the fitting of a conventional above-knee prosthesis. **b** K.A., 34 years old, male, hip disarticulation of the left thigh due to recurrent malignant fibrous histiocytoma. Preservation of an active movable femur stump by implantation of a special endoprosthesis

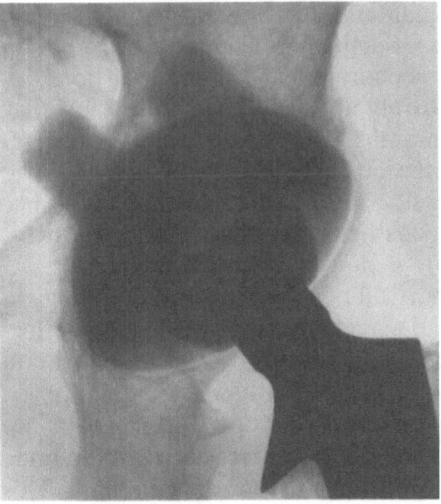

Fig. 5. S.H., 77 years old, female, osteoarthritis of left hip joint. Nine years postoperatively, sufficient anchorage of the acetabular socket

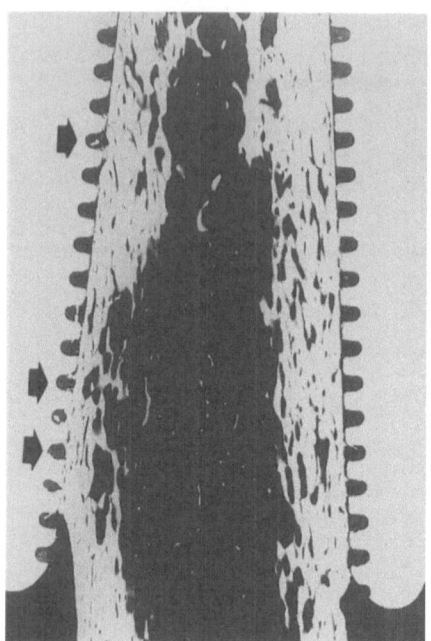

Fig. 6. G.M., 58 years old, female, micro-radiograph of a longitudinal ground section through the conical sleeve of an alumina ceramic humerus endoprosthesis, 28 months after implantation. Partial spongification of the cortical bone stump, but also local bone ingrowth into the ceramic grooves can be observed (arrows). × 2

Histological Results

Seven tumor endoprostheses and two reoperated socket implants from conventional hip endoprostheses were available for histological investigation. Six tumor implants were clinically stable, and only in one case was a loose humerus endoprosthesis encountered 12 months after implantation.

All the stable implants showed that bone tissue had grown into the grooves in the ceramic, resulting in stable long-term anchorage. The process of bone ingrowth started in the 1st month postoperatively and new bone with a lamellar osseous structure was evident after only 3 months. Microradiographic investigation of a stable humerus implant 28 months postoperatively showed that the cortex layer had become spongy in areas not subjected to loading. In other areas, there was clear ingrowth of the osseous tissue into the ceramic grooves, providing stable implant anchorage (Fig. 6).

In the case of the unstable implant, the cortical bone was extremely spongy in the entire area of the cone and distally it had even been partly resorbed. Periosteal reactions at the base of the bone stump would appear to be an indication that the bone had attempted to start providing support around the implant.

During the reoperation of the two ceramic sockets with conventional total hip endoprostheses, it was found that there was no direct contact between the bone and implant; there was alway a thin film of connective tissue between them. This layer also contained small quantities of wear particles, which prevented direct contact between the implant and bone (Fig. 7).

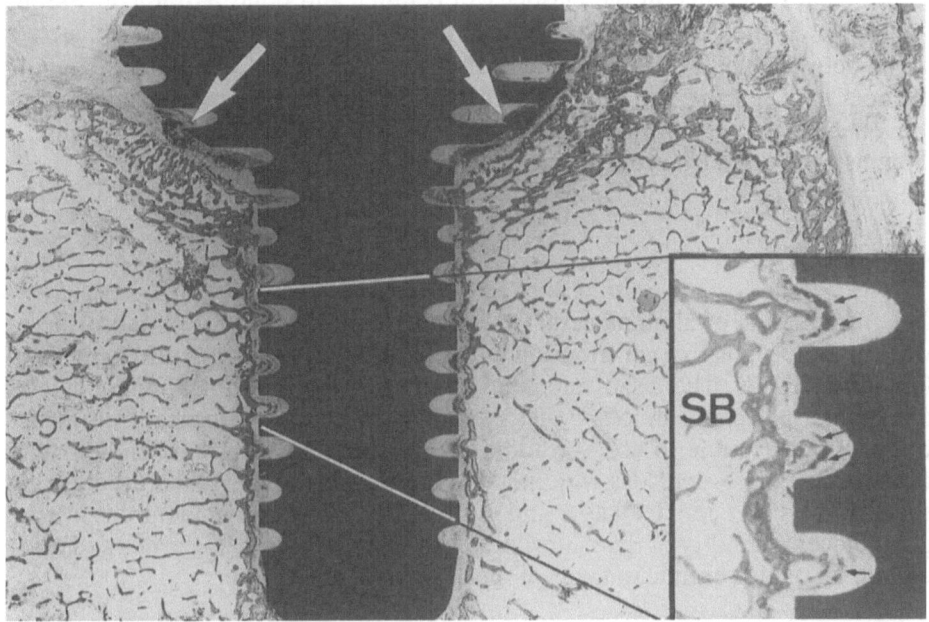

Fig. 7. A.M., 68 years old, female, ground section through one peg of an alumina ceramic hip socket, 12 months after implantation. Distinct ingrowth of pelvic spongy bone into the grooves, but always with a fibrous connective tissue in interlayer containing wear particles (*insert*, see *arrows*). × 2

Discussion

Our own experience confirms the good biocompatibility of aluminum oxide ceramic, which was one of the reasons for selecting this material for the manufacture of endoprostheses. Excellent primary stability between the implant and long bones can be achieved with the principle of the conical sleeve.

If mechanical loading of the connection between the bone and prosthesis is not too great (reduced lever arm with a rather short length of resection), stable long-term anchorage of the prosthesis is obtained by ingrowth of bone tissue into the grooves provided for this purpose. Histologically, there is direct contact between the bone and ceramic without an intervening membrane of connective tissue.

If loading is too great—especially the bending load—there is bone resorption in the area of the conical sleeve, leading to loosening of the implant. In some patients, an osseous mantle formed on the outer surface of the ceramic sleeve as a result of periosteal new bone formation. This sometimes resulted in spontaneous refixation of the prosthesis.

The design of the pegged socket has proved a clinical success. Implantation is technically simple, and it was always possible to achieve stable primary fixation. Nevertheless, in contrast to the conical anchorage, we found no direct contact between the ceramic and bone in the socket implants. This is apparently due to the great difference in the elasticity of ceramic and bone. Although osseous tissue grows into the ceramic grooves, there is always a layer of connective tissue between the implant and the roof of the acetabulum, forming a damping element between the two materials of different hardness. The constant micro-movements that result also produce slight wear of the surface of the ceramic, a circumstance that also prevents intimate bone-implant connection.

Conclusion

The introduction of alumina ceramic as an implant material for endoprostheses was certainly a positive contribution in the field of joint surgery with many good long-term results. The disadvantage in its use as a material for bridging defects after tumor resections in long bones lies in its low bending strength. This means that it is not possible to use any additional securing aids (intramedullary stem, extracortical plates, etc.) as with metallic tumor prostheses. When used for hip sockets, no direct contact was found between the bone and implant despite the good biocompatibility of the material. For these reasons, we again stopped using aluminum oxide ceramic in favor of metal implants.

Acknowledgment. The authors are indebted to the Verein für orthopädische Forschung und Rehabilitation for its support in the preparation of this paper.

References

1. Boutin P (1972) Arthroplastie totale de la hanche par prothese en alumine frittee. Rev Chir Orthop 58: 229
2. Knahr K, Böhler M, Frank P, Plenk H, Salzer M (1987) Survival analysis of an un-cemented ceramic acetabular component in total hip replacement. Arch Orthop Traumat Surg 106: 297–300
3. Plenk H Jr (1982) Biocompatibility of ceramics in joint prostheses. In: Williams DF (ed) Biocompatibility of orthopedic implants, vol I. CRC, Boca Raton, pp 269–295
4. Salzer M, Locke H, Engelhardt H, Zweymüller K (1975) Keramische Endoprothesen der oberen Extremität. Z Orthop 113: 458–61
5. Salzer M, Zweymüller K, Locke H, Zeibig A, Stärk N, Plenk H Jr, Punzet G (1976) Further experimental and clinical experience with aluminum oxide endoprostheses. J Biomed Mater Res 10: 847
6. Salzer M, Knahr K, Locke H, Stärk N, Matejovsky Z, Plenk H Jr, Punzet G, Zweymüller K (1979) A bioceramic endoprosthesis for the replacement of the proxi-mal humerus. Arch Orthop Traumat Surg 93: 169–184

New Technique for Providing Ligamentous Stability in Prosthetic Replacement of the Knee for Tumors

YOSHIAKI YANASE, SEISUKE TANAKA, MITSUO TOMIHARA, SATOSHI SOEN, and
HARUHIKO YAMASAKI[1]

Summary. The follow-up results of patients treated by limb preserving resection of the tumor and reconstruction with prosthesis are described. The main problem with our procedure was reattachment of the soft tissue to provide ligamentous stability. In recent cases, we have applied a new technique using the Leeds-Keio artificial ligament for ligamentous stability in replacemental surgery, and satisfactory results have been gained in joint stability and motion.

Key words: Bone neoplasms—Knee prosthesis—Articular ligaments

Introduction

Recent improvements in clinical staging and adjuvant chemotherapy for malignant bone tumor have increased the potential for limb salvage. A large defect of the osseous and soft tissues produced by the resection surgery poses a complex reconstructive problem. The custom-made protheses or total prostheses we used did not guarantee stability of the reconstructed joint. In this paper, we give details of a new technique for providing ligamentous stability.

Materials and Methods

Between 1980 and 1986, a total of ten patients with bone tumor of the distal femur or proximal tibia were treated by limb salvage and adjuvant therapy in Kinki University Hospital. One to two weeks following preoperative chemotherapy, the patients underwent en bloc resection of all the tumor. The affected bone was removed 5 cm proximal or distal to positive tumor evidence in ^{99m}Tc-phosphate scan and ^{67}Ga-citrate scan. Tumor-free margins were confirmed by microscopic sections.

No major nerves or blood vessels were sacrificed. Following excision of the primary skeletal tumors, bony replacement was accomplished with endopros-

---
[1]Department of Orthopaedic Surgery, Kinki University School of Medicine, Osaka, Japan

Table 1. Tumors treated by surgery and chemotherapy (1980–1986)

Case	Age (yrs)	Sex	Site	Diagnosis	Stage	Metastasis	Reoperation	Status
1	20	F	L-DF	OS	IIB	5 yrs	Hemi-pel.	DOD 6 yrs
2	20	M	L-PT	CS	IIA	3 mos	AK amp	DOD 6 mos
3	47	M	L-PT	RCS	IIB	None	AK amp	NED 6 yrs
4	14	F	R-DF	GCT	IIA	None	None	NED 5 yrs
5	16	M	L-DF	OS	IIB	None	AK amp	NED 5 yrs
6	38	M	R-PT	CMF	IC	None	None	NED 4 yrs
7	14	F	L-DF	OS	IIB	2 yrs	Lobectomy	NED 2.5 yrs
8	41	M	L-DF	PVS	IC	None	AK amp	NED 2.3 yrs
9	68	M	L-DF	MFH	IIB	None	AK amp	Post-op. 1 mo
10	36	F	R-DF	SCS	IIA	None	None	NED 1 yr

DF distal femur, *PT* proximal tibia, *OS* osteosarcoma, *CS* chondrosarcoma, *RCS* reticulum cell sarcoma, *GCT* giant cell sarcoma, *CMF* chondromyxoid fibroma, *PVS* pigmented villondular synovitis, *MFH* malignant fibrous histiocytoma, *SCS* secondary chondrosarcoma, *AK amp* above-knee amputation, *DOD* died of disease, *NED* no evidence of disease

Table 2. Follow-up results of our cases

	Case no.						
	4	5	6	7	8	9	10
Age (yrs)/sex	19/F	21/M	38/M	16/F	41/M	68/M	36/F
Motion	F	P	F	G	P	G	E
Pain	E	E	E	E	E	E	E
Stability	E	E	F	G	E	E	E
Deformity	E	E	E	E	E	E	E
Strength	G	G	G	G	G	G	G
F. activity	F	F	G	G	F	E	E
E. acceptance	G	G	G	G	G	E	E
Status	NED	AKamp	NED	NED	AKamp	AKamp	NED
Follow-up	6 yrs	3.5 yrs	5 yrs	2.5 yrs	14 mos	12 mos	13 mos

E excellent, *G* good, *F* fair, *P* poor, *NED* no evidence of disease, *AKamp* above knee amputation

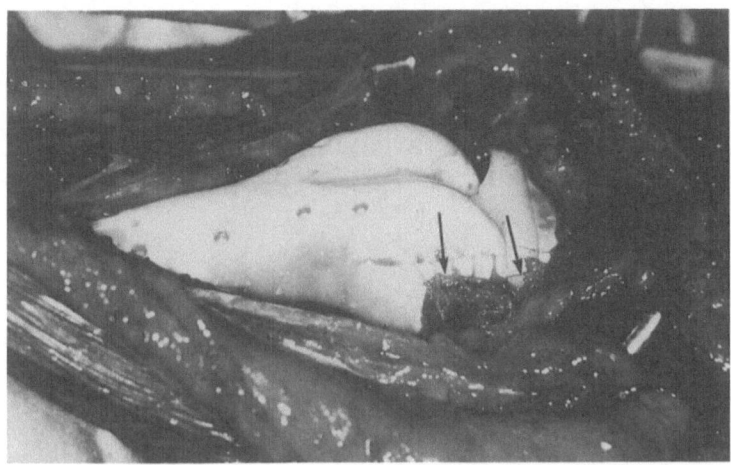

Fig. 1. Case 10. Leeds-Keio artificial ligament was sutured to a femoral component

thesis or nonhinged-type ceramic total knee prosthesis: custom-made Vitallium and high density polyethylene (HDP) endoprosthesis in two, custom-made ceramic endoprosthesis in one, custom-made ceramic total knee prosthesis in five, and ready-made total knee prosthesis in two cases. The diagnosis was osteosarcoma in three patients, chondrosarcoma in two, and giant cell tumor, malignant fibrous histiocytoma, reticulum cell sarcoma, pigmented villondular synovitis (PVS), and chondromyxoid fibroma in one case each.

Results and Discussion

Table 1 lists the clinicopathological features [1]. Five of these patients required amputation because of prosthetic or skin trouble or local recurrence. Two of them died from lung metastasis. Eight of ten patients are currently still alive and free of disease, four of them beyond 5 years. Table 2 shows the follow-up results of seven of our ten patients. The functional result is unsatisfactory in five patients because of limited range of motion and instability. The main problem with our procedure was reattachment of soft tissue to provide ligamentous stability.

Previously, the dissected tendons and ligaments were reattached via holes in the prosthesis provided for this purpose, and postoperative exercise was started after a long period of immobilization. It was not then possible to obtain satisfactory stability or range of motion. Furthermore, the problem of lateral instability of the knee joint occurred over a range of 5°–15°. This problem was due to two reasons: one was that the attachment of the collateral ligament was removed, the other was that the prosthesis was not of the hinged type. So, recently, we have applied a new technique using the Leeds-Keio artificial ligament for ligamentous stability in replacement surgery. Satisfactory results were gained in stability and motion.

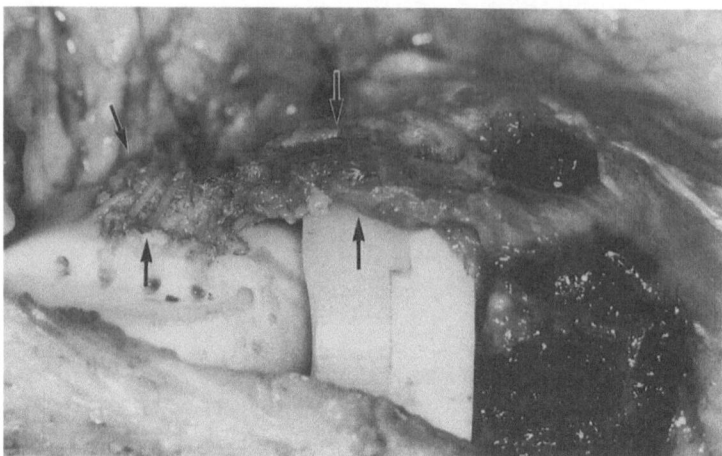

Fig. 2. Case 9. Twelve months postoperatively, artificial ligament was firmly bridged between femoral and tibial component

Case Reports

A 35-year-old woman was examined in July 1986 after a history of a steadily growing swelling at the suprapatellar region of 20 years' duration. Knee flexion was difficult and increased steadily in the grade of limitation. Preoperative examination suggested a malignant bone tumor. After excising the entire involved bone with the adjacent muscle, the bony defect was replaced with a nonhinged-type total knee ceramic prosthesis. At that time, a Leeds-Keio artificial ligament was laid underneath the tibial component and both sides were sutured to the hole of the femoral component using silk sutures to stabilize a lateral instability (Fig. 1). Two weeks postoperatively, active and passive range of motion exercises of the knee joint were started streneously. One year after surgery, the patient gained 90° flexion and was satisfied the results.

However, the other case treated by the same procedure developed local tumor recurrence at 12 months. The histological diagnosis was malignant fibrous histiocytoma. After amputation was carried out at the level of the proximal femur, the reconstructed area was explored. The artificial ligament was firmly bridged between two components and covered by connective tissue, as shown in Fig. 2.

We conclude that our new procedure has the following advantages: (a) It is technically very easy to perform; (b) early range of motion exercise is possible; (c) stability is easy to obtain.

Reference

1. Enneking WF (1986) A system of staging musculoskeletal neoplasms. Clin Orthop 204: 9–24

Results of Alumina-Ceramic Endoprostheses Used for Bone Tumor Cases

Seiichi Matsumoto[1], Noriyoshi Kawaguchi[1], Katsuhisa Amino[1],
Jun Manabe[1], Kohtaro Furuya[2], and Yasushi Isobe[2]

Summary. Alumina-ceramic endoprostheses were applied to ten cases of bone tumors in the following categories: osteosarcomas (four cases), malignant fibrous histiocytomas (two), parosteal osteosarcomas (two), chondrosarcoma (one), and extended giant cell tumor (one). Of these, three cases were evaluated as excellent and one as good. In three cases, revision occurred because of breakage and loosening of the prosthesis. Additionally, three cases were lost due to patient death or local recurrence. The alumina-ceramic showed fragility and less affinity to the bone than had been expected. From these results, we conclude that alumina-ceramic endoprostheses have a limited indication for use with low-malignant bone tumors that only require small amounts of bone and soft tissue resection.

Key word: Alumina-ceramic endoprosthesis

Introduction

Alumina-ceramic is a new material which was expected to have a good affinity to bone. From 1983 to 1984, alumina-ceramic endoprostheses were applied after removal of bone tumors (Fig. 1). We evaluated these cases.

Materials and Methods

Ten patients underwent reconstructive surgery; four of the ten had osteosarcoma and two had parosteal osteosarcoma. The sites of the tumors were the distal femur in nine cases and distal tibia in one case. With regard to the operative procedures, wide resection was applied to the parosteal osteosarcoma, chondrosarcoma, and extended giant cell tumors. Transcapsular resection was applied to osteosarcoma and malignant fibrous histiocytoma (MFH). Incomplete extracapsular resection was applied to osteosarcoma, and marginal resection was applied to tibial MFH. For fixation of the prosthesis, bone cement was not used except in one case (Table 1).

[1] Department of Orthopedic Surgery, Cancer Institute Hospital, Tokyo, Japan
[2] Department of Orthopedic Surgery, Tokyo Medical and Dental University, Tokyo Japan

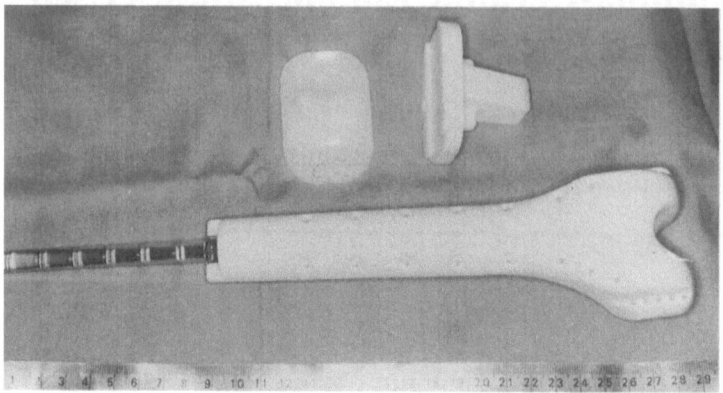

Fig. 1. Custom-made alumina-ceramic prosthesis for distal femur lesion

Results and Discussion

According to the functional evaluation, three cases were excellent and one was good. The follow-up period of these cases was from 39 months to 4 years. Of these, three cases underwent revision, two required amputation following local recurrence, and in one case the patient died [1].

Excellent Group

The cases of chondrosarcoma, parosteal osteosarcoma, and extended giant cell tumor belong to this group. For the primary chondrosarcoma and giant cell tumor, bone cement was not used. But in these cases, the femoral component were relatively short. The size of the femoral component was 9 cm and 13 cm, respectively. In the third case, the femoral component was 18.5 cm, which was rather long. Only in this case was bone cement used to fix the femoral component. To summarize the results of the excellent group, the operative procedure was wide resection. The femoral component was well fixed to the bone because of the short femoral component size or use of bone cement. These factors were thought to contribute to joint stability and component fixation.

Good Group

The only case of osteosarcoma that underwent incomplete extracapsular resection belongs to this group. At 3 years 3 months after the operation, the patient was evaluated as good in functional activity and motion. With respect to the other factors, the patient was evaluated as excellent. However, in X-ray findings, slight bone resorption and implant loosening were detectable. Revision in the near future is anticipated for this case.

Table 1. Patient data

Patient	Age	Site, histology	Operation	Result
I.N.	16	Femur OS	Incomplete extracaps.	3 yrs 3 mos good
I.T.	22	Femur OS	Incomplete extracaps.	1 yrs 8 mos revision
Y.K.	27	Femur OS	Trascaps.	1 yrs 1 mos dead
K.M.	27	Femur OS		3 yrs revision
T.S	27	Femur MFH		4 yrs 5 mos recurrence, amputation
T.K.	30	Femur Paro. OS	Wide	4 yrs 4 mos revision
K.K.	34	Femur Paro. OS		3 yrs 3 mos excellent
M.Y.	34	Femur Chondro Sa		4 yrs excellent
M.T.	53	Femur GCT	Wide	3 yrs 5 mos excellent
G.J.	30	Tibia MFH	Marginal	2 yrs 3 mos recurrence, amputation

OS osteosarcoma, *MFH* malignant fibrous histiocytoma, *Paro. OS* parosteal osteosarcoma, *Chondro* Sa chondrosarcoma, *GCT* giant cell tumor

Revision Group

Two patients with osteosarcoma and one patient with parosteal osteosarcoma underwent replacement of the alumina-ceramic endoprosthesis by a titanium-alloy endoprosthesis. The cause of revision was breakage and loosening. In one case, the joint was easily broken. This patient had osteosarcoma of the distal femur. A year after the operation, the patient had flexion of only 20° because of severe joint instability, which required a brace for an extended period.

In X-ray findings, reactive bone formation around the proximal end of the prosthetic shaft was seen. Subsequently, 1 year 5 months after the operation, the patient had a fall at home and the prosthesis broke easily (Fig. 2). The prosthesis was replaced by a hinged prosthesis. Instability was lessened and the patient was able to walk better than before. In the other two cases, severe implant loosening and bone resorption occurred. The patients consequently had their prostheses replaced by a titanium-alloy prosthesis.

Two primary problems occurred with the alumina-ceramic endoprosthesis. The first involved the decision not to use bone cement in order to make the most use of the material. During the early period after the operation, the femoral component migrated easily. The patients complained of instability of the knee joint and sometimes felt abnormal motion between the femoral component and the femur. Consequently, the start of an exercise program was delayed and joint function stayed poor. The second problem concerned the material itself. Alumina-ceramic showed less affinity to the bone than had been expected. So, it

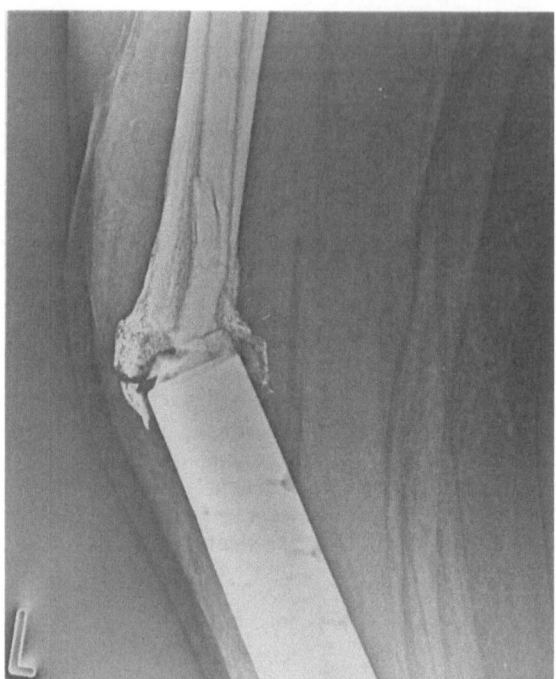

Fig. 2. Xerography of femoral component which broke in a minor trauma

took a long time to fix the component [2]. A more serious difficulty was its fragilty. As was seen , it can easily break in a minor accdient. Thus, the alumina-ceramic endoprosthesis is not free from breakage and loosening.

Conclusion

Ten cases with alumina-ceramic endoprosthetic replacement were reviewed. Three cases underwent revision because of breakage and loosening. Alumina-ceramic endoprosthesis has a limited indication in low-malignant bone tumors which only require small amounts of bone and soft tissue resection.

References

1. Kawaguchi N, Amino K, Matsumoto S, Manabe J, Furuya K, Isobe Y (1987) Limb salvage operation of osteosarcoma. Rinsho Seikei Geka 22: 1189–1197
2. Oonishi H, Okabe N, Nabeshima T, Kushitani S, Tsuyama K, Masaoka S, Ootuki S, Yamamoto T, Wakimoto Y (1984) Some problems of cementless alumina ceramic total knee prosthesis and its solutions. Orthopedic Ceramic Implants 4: 275–288

Results of Replacement with Ceramic Prostheses for Bone Tumors

HIDEKI HAYASHI[1], YASUAKI AOKI[2], and YOSHIO KOMATSUBARA[2]

Summary. A ceramic prosthesis consisting of a polycrystal-alumina body and mono-crystal-alumina stem was inserted for tumors of long tubular bone. Twenty-five patients who had bone tumors underwent replacement by a ceramic prosthesis with a cementless technique and were followed for 3–65 months. The replaced sites were the proximal femur (14 cases), distal femur (five), proximal tibia (two), proximal humerus (two), and two others. Of the 21 patients who underwent replacement of the lower extremity, 18 could walk with or without a cane, two ambulated on a walker. Three patients with a distal femur prosthesis needed a brace to compensate for the instability. The specially designed prostheses on which the tibial tuberosity was preserved were used for the prox-imal tibias, and two patients obtained a well-functioning knee. Both patients with a proximal humerus prosthesis obtained a satisfactorily functioning arm. In functional eval-uation, 16 (67%) sites were rated as good, seven (28%) fair, and two (8%) poor in overall grade. Stability was the main parameter that lowered this grade. Radiographic follow-up study in the patients who were observed after 2 years revealed sinking of the prosthesis in 33% of cases, clear zone around the stem portion in 89%, linear new bone around this clear zone in 67%, and sclerotic change at the junction to the prosthesis in 56%. The clear zone did not progressover 1 mm and no clinical loosening was observed if the prosthesis was fixed accurately without cement during the operation.

Key words: Bone tumor—Ceramic prosthesis—Noncement fixation

Introduction

Alumina ceramics is one of the best materials for tumor prosthesis because of its high tissue compatibility and strength [1, 2]. In alumina ceramics, monocrystal alumina has the advantage of strength against compression and bending but has the disadvantage of shaping difficulty. On the other hand, polycrystal alumina has the reverse features. The Kyocera Bioceram prosthesis is ideal as it is a composite of polycrystal alumina for the resected part and monocrystal alumina for the stem portion. As the procedure for intramedullary fixation, a noncement technique is needed to take the advantage of the tissue compatibility. This paper

[1] Hayashi Hospital, Osaka, Japan
[2] Department of Orthopaedic Surgery, The Center for Adult Diseases, Osaka, Japan

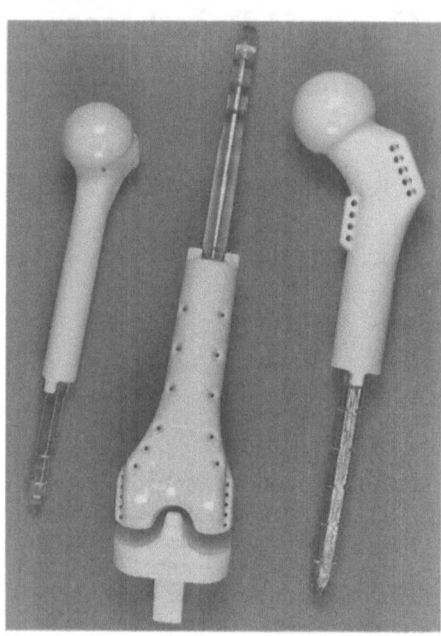

Fig. 1. Tumor prostheses make of alumina ceramic for the proximal humerus, distal and proximal femur

presents the results of ceramic prosthetic replacements which have been performed for bone tumors since 1980.

Materials and Methods

Twenty-five patients were studied, including 12 males and 13 females, ranging in age from 8 to 73 years. They were observed for 3–65 months. There were five osteosarcomas, four chondrosarcomas, two giant cell tumors, one myeloma, leukemia, fibrous dysplasia, enchondroma, eight metastatic carcinomas, and two metastatic sarcomas.

The prostheses for the proximal femur and proximal humerus were the head type without an artificial joint, and those for the distal femur and proximal tibia had the kinematic-stabilizer type knee joint (Fig. 1). A channel was made at the anterior side of the tibial prosthesis to fix the tibial tuberosity for preserving function of the quadriceps. A custom-made implant, which consisted entirely of polycrystal alumina, was used for the metacarpal and sternoclavicular replacements.

The treatment of the bone lesion was simple resection for 16 benign and metastatic lesions and radical en bloc resection for nine primary malignancies. The most important point of the replacement with ceramic prosthesis is the stable intramedullary fixation without cement. Straight reamers of graduated size (0.5-mm steps) were made to create accurately a hole with just the same size as the monocrystal stem. For soft tissue reconstruction, a joint capsule was created using the contralateral tensor fascia latae in the cases subjected to en bloc resection. A Teflon mesh was used as a periost, to which the insertion and origin of the muscles were attached for cases requring a long prosthesis of over 150 mm.

Results

Clinical Results

Of 14 patients who had the replacement of the proximal femur, 11 could walk with a cane while two ambulated on a walker as the maximum ability. Four patients survived for over 3 years with a stable gait function (Table 1), but one case had infection and revision was performed using a long-stem total hip replacement (THR) after the irrigation and filling with cement beads containing antibiotics. Among the five patients who had replacement of the distal femur, three required a knee brace for walking to compensate for the instability caused by extensive soft tissue resection for osteosarcoma. Four patients are now free from disease without complication. Both patients who underwent replacement of the proximal tibia could walk freely without a brace or a cane, as the instability did not appear when the quadriceps muscles were tensed. The range of motion in the knee joint was also satisfactory (0°–100°) to them. Both patients who had replacement of the proximal humerus obtained satisfactory function of the shoulder joint with a range of motion (ROM) of 90° in anterior and lateral and 30° in posterior elevation. Sinking of the implant occurred in one case because the diameter of the stem was too small. In the patients who underwent replacement of the metacarpal and sternoclavicula, the implants become dislocated and were finally removed.

Functional Evaluation

Sixteen (67%) sites were rated as good, seven (28%) as fair, and two (8%) as poor in overall grade. With respect to the sites, 100% were in the proximal tibia and proximal humerus, 71% in the proximal femur, 40% in the distal femur, and none at other sites were rated as good. With regard to each parameter, 76% in motion, 96% in pain, 40% in stability, 92% in deformity, 80% in strength, 76% in functional activity, and 64% in emotional acceptance were rated as excellent or good.

Radiographic Analysis

In the nine patients who were observed over 2 years, radiographic analysis was performed (Fig. 2). There were four major findings, which were sinking of the prosthesis, clear zone around the stem, linear new bone formation around this clear zone, and sclerotic change at the junction and the stem end (Table 2). Sinking over 1 mm was observed in 33% of cases, clear zone in 89%, linear new bone formation in 67%, and sclerotic change in 56%. The sinking progressed time-dependently, but the width of the clear zone did not progress over 1 mm except in one case in which the size of the stem was inadequate. The clinical stability of the prosthesis was maintained in the remaining eight cases.

Table 1. Demographic, clinical, surgical and functional data of the patients with ceramic prostheses

Site replaced	Case no.	Age (yrs)	Sex	Diagnosis	Surgical staging	Pathological fracture	Length of prosthesis (mm)	Surgical procedure	Functional evaluation	Follow-up (months), final status
Proximal femur	1	42	M	Giant cell tumor	I B	−	120	Resection	Good	65 disease-free
	2	58	F	Myeloma		+	125	Resection	Good	45 dead
	3	73	M	Chondrosarcoma	I A	−	150	En bloc resection	Good	41 disease-free
	4	66	F	Fibrous dysplasia		+	150	Resection	Good	32 disease-free
	5	25	M	Osteosarcoma	III B	−	250	En bloc resection	Good	14 alive with disease
	6	8	M	Osteosarcoma	II B	+	200	En bloc resection	Poor	13 dead
	7	65	M	Metastatic carcinoma		−	175	Resection	Good	39 dead
	8	47	M	Metastatic carcinoma		−	125	Resection	Good	13 dead
	9	65	M	Metastatic carcinoma		−	125	Resection	Good	9 dead
	10	49	M	Leukemia		+	125	Resection	Good	9 dead
	11	30	F	Metastatic sarcoma		+	175	Resection	Good	4 dead (chemotherapy induced)
	12	76	F	Metastatic carcinoma		+	175	Resection	Fair	4 dead
	13	51	M	Metastatic carcinoma		−	150	Resection	Fair	3 dead
	14	57	F	Metastatic sarcoma		+	120 (with hemipelvis)	Resection	Poor	3 dead (chemotherapy induced)
Distal femur	15	21	M	Osteosarcoma	II A	−	150	En bloc resection	Fair	56 disease-free
	16	65	F	Osteosarcoma	II B	+	185	En bloc resection	Fair	29 disease-free
	17	13	M	Osteosarcoma	II B	−	180	En bloc resection	Fair	12 dead
	18	67	F	Giant cell tumor	I A	−	110	En bloc resection	Good	29 disease-free
	19	73	F	Chondrosarcoma	I B	−	110	En bloc resection	Good	16 disease-free
Proximal tibia	20	43	F	Metastatic carcinoma		−	70	Resection	Good	36 alive with disease
	21	60	M	Chondrosarcoma	IB	−	90	En bloc resection	Good	14 dead (with other cancer)
Proximal humerus	22	66	M	Metastatic carcinoma		+	110	Resection	Good	33 alive with disease
	23	61	M	Metastatic carcinoma		−	120	Resection	Good	6 dead
Others	24	52	F	Enchondroma + lipoma		−	Metacarpal	Resection	Fair	21 disease-free
	25	55	F	Chondrosarcoma	I B	−	Sterno clavicular	En bloc resection	Fair	28 dead

Table 2. Radiographic analysis of bone in which ceramic prosthesis was inserted

Site replaced	Case no.	Radiographic follow-up (months)	Length of sinking (mm)	Width of clear zone (mm)		Linear new bone formation	Appearance of sclerotic change		Clinical stem stability
				Near	Far		Junction	Stem end	
Proximal femur	1	12	<1[a]	<1	<1	+	−	−	Stable
		24	<1	<1	<1	+	+	+	Stable
		36	<1	<1	<1	+	+	+	Stable
		48	<1	<1	<1	+	+	+	Stable
		60	<1	<1	<1	+	+	+	Stable
	2	12	<1	−	−	−	−	−	Stable
		24	<1	<1	<1	+	−	−	Stable
		36	<1	<1	<1	+	−	−	Stable
	3	12	<1	<1	<1	+	−	−	Stable
		24	<1	<1	<1	+	+	+	Stable
		36	2	<1	<1	+	+	+	Stable
	7	12	<1	−	−	−	−	−	Stable
		24	<1	−	−	−	−	−	Stable
		36	<1	−	−	−	−	−	Stable
Distal femur	15	12	<1	−	−	−	−	−	Stable
		24	<1	−	−	+	−	−	Stable
		36	2	<1	<1	+	−	−	Stable
		48	4	<1	<1	+	−	−	Stable
	16	12	<1	<1	−	−	−	−	Stable
		24	<1	<1	−	−	−	−	Stable
	18	12	<1	−	<1	+	+	−	Stable
		24	<1	−	<1	+	+	−	Stable
Proximal tibia	20	12	<1	−	−	+	+	−	Stable
		24	<1	<1	<1	+	+	−	Stable
Proximal humerus	22	12	8	2	4	−	−	−	Instable
		24	12	2	4	−	−	+	Instable

[a] <1, less than 1 mm

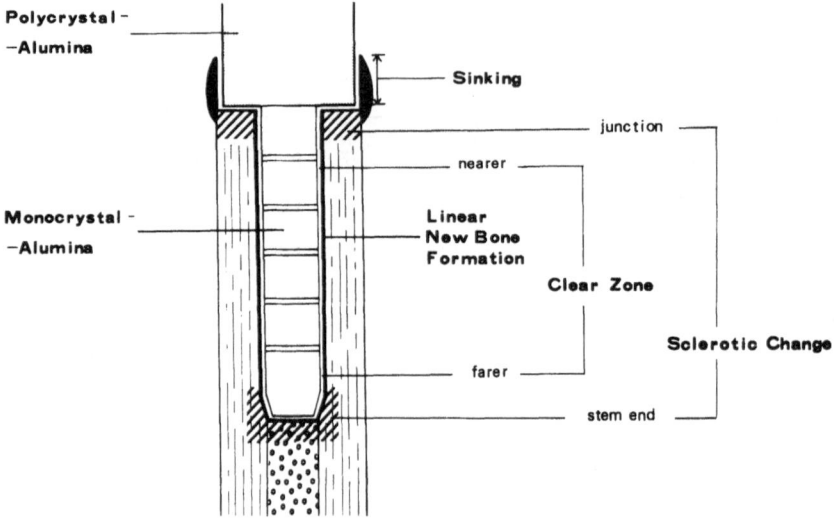

Fig. 2. Schema of radiographic analysis at the stem portion of the prosthesis

Discussion

The tissue compatibility of alumina ceramics has been clarified both in animal and clinical studies [3, 4]. But the compatibility is defeated at the portion where much more stress is concentrated as at the junction to the prosthesis. Sinking of the prosthesis and the appearance of a clear zone around the stem are found even in ceramic prostheses as in metal prostheses [5]. Although the facts that the clear zone does not progress over 1 mm and a linear new bone is formed around it are thought to be advantages for long-term fixation of the prosthesis. This fixation was obtained only when the ceramics correctly faced the cortical bone with as much area as possible to disperse the stress. Therefore, a careful method for the stem hole and antirotational channels as well as accurate choice in the size of the prosthesis is very important.

With regard to site, favorable results for replacement in the proximal femur and proximal humerus were obtained by use of the head-type prosthesis in a ball and socket joint and by satisfactory soft tissue reconstruction. In contrast, the results of replacement of the distal femur were unfavorable because of decreased supporting function after en bloc resection. Accordingly, the hinge-type prosthesis which can mechanically conpensate these defects is recommended for osteosarcoma in this region [6–10]. The ceramic-metal composite prosthesis, with the ceramics part in contact with the patient's bone and a metal hinge, will become available as it is now technically difficult to make an all-ceramics hinge prosthesis. In this concept, our specially made prosthesis for the proximal tibia in which tibial tuberosity is preserved is suitable because mechanical function is added to the morphological copy of the original bone.

References

1. Knahr K, Salzer M, Plenk H Jr, Grundschober F (1981) Experience with bioceramic implants in orthopaedic surgery. Biomaterials 2: 98–104
2. Salzer M, Knahr K, Locke H, Stärk N, Matejovsky Z, Plenk H Jr, Punzet G, Zweymüller K (1979) A bioceramic endoprosthesis for the replacement of the proximal humerus. Arch Orthop Traumat Surg 93: 169–184
3. Salzer M, Zweymüller K, Locke H, Stärk N, Plenk H Jr, Punzet G (1976) Further experimental and clinical experience with aluminum oxide endoprostheses. J Biomed Mater Res 10: 847–856
4. Akamatsu N, Hamada Y, Kozaki T (1983) Prosthetic replacement and other methods of treatment after massive bone resection. In: Chao EYS, Ivins JC (eds) Tumor prostheses for bone and joint reconstruction—The design and application. Thieme-Stratton, New York, pp 207–213
5. Harris WH, Schiller AL, Scholler JM, Freiberg RA, Richard S (1976) Extensive localised bone resorption in the femur following total hip replacement. J Bone Joint Surg 58-A: 612–618
6. Chao EyS, Sim FH (1983) Tumor prosthesis design—A system approach. In: Chao EYS, Ivins JC (eds) Tumor prostheses for bone and joint reconstruction—The design and application. Thieme-Stratton, New York, pp 335–359
7. Kotz RJ, Engel AE (1983) Cement-free design of a tumor prosthesis for osteosarcoma of the distal femur and proximal tibia with a new fixation technique for the ligamentum patellae. In: Chao EYS, Ivins JC (eds) Tumor prostheses for bone and joint reconstruction—The design and application. Thieme-Stratton, New York, pp 399–408
8. Malawer M (1985) Surgical technique and results of limb sparing surgery for high grade bone sarcoma of the knee and shoulder. Orthopedics 8-5: 597–607
9. Sim FH, Bowan WE Jr, Wilkins RM, Chao EYS (1985) Limb salvage in primary malignant bone tumors. Orthopedics 8-5: 574–581
10. Tomota K (1985) Ceramic prosthesis of cervical vertebra in metastatic tumor of the spine. Arch Jpn Chir 54-1: 16–22

Clinical Application of Ceramics in Bone Tumors

ATSUMASA UCHIDA, HIDEKI YOSHIKAWA, YASUAKI AOKI, HIDEKI HAMADA, EIJI KURISAKI, and KEIRO ONO[1]

Summary. Alumina ceramic was used in a tumor prosthesis in 26 patients who had resections of bone tumors. Hingeless ceramic total knee replacement and hemiarthroplasty showed unexpectedly satisfactory results. These results suggest that the development of alumina cermaic creates a more biocompatible and biomechanical condition. Calcium hydroxyapatite ceramics were used as a bone substitute after resection and curettage of benign bone tumors and were incorporated well into bony tissue. No toxic effect was found during the follow-up period.

Key words: Alumina ceramic—Bone tumors—Calcium hydroxyapatite ceramic

Introduction

In recent years, the use of ceramics in bone and joint surgery has received considerable attention, particulary as permanent implants for joint replacement. Ceramic materials can be grouped into bioinert and bioactive ceramics. The bioinert material most used is high-purity alumina. Alumina ceramics have been found to be biocompatible, provoking little reaction from tissues, and to have sufficient mechanical properties. Moreover, these ceramics have a low friction coefficient and a high wear resistance. Therefore, the use of alumina in a tumor prosthesis based on an optimal design is thought to be very convenient. In contrast, a representative bioactive ceramic is calcium hydroxyapatite. This ceramic has been considered for use in biodegradable bone replacement because of its mechanical and biological properties. The concept of biodegradability implies that the material is replaced by bone as it degrades. Therefore, this ceramic is thought to be useful for filling defects in bone after the resection and curettage of benign bone tumors. In this paper, the short-term results in clinical application of these bioinert and bioactive ceramics are reported.

[1] Department of Orthopaedic Surgery, Osaka University Medical School, Osaka, Japan

Materials and Methods

Twenty-six patients underwent reconstruction by alumina ceramic prosthesis after wide resection of bone tumors. The tumorous conditions consisted of 14 osteosarcomas, four metastatic tumors, two Ewing's sarcomas, two giant cell tumors, two malignant fibrous histiocytomas of bone, and others. The group undergoing prosthetic replacement of the knee joint consisted of ten patients, including five cases of hingeless total knee replacement and five cases of hemiarthroplasty as a spacer of the bone defect. Four of seven cases of upper humeral tumor underwent replacement by a new-type constrained total shoulder prosthesis; the remainder received replacement by ceramic head prosthesis. Three metastatic tumors of the upper femur and two primary bone tumors of the distal radius were replaced by hemiarthroplasty with a ceramic head prosthesis. Total ankle prosthesis with an artificial tibial was used for malignant fibrous histiocytoma of the middle tibia. Three patients with metastasis of the middle portion of the long bone underwent replacement by segmental prosthesis without joint structure. Porous calcium hydroxyapatite ceramic was used for the filling of bone defects produced by curettage and resection in 20 benign bone tumors and tumorous conditions of fibrous dysplasia, enchondroma, solitary bone cyst, osteoid osteoma, and aneurysmal bone cyst.

Results and Discussion

The total knee prosthesis used in this series is composed of a combination of alumina ceramic on high-density polyethylene for the articulating surface and an alumina single-crystal long stem. In general, fixation of the intramedullary long stem to the bone was attempted with no cementationprocedures. Five patients were treated with this prosthesis and their follow-up extended from 27 to 60 months. An excellent result from the functional evaluation system of Enneking was obtained in a 33-year-male with a giant cell tumor. In osteosarcoma, one patient had a good result, but three patients were fair. The functional rating mainly depended on preservation of the extensor apparatus of the knee (Table 1). Reconstruction of the collateral and cruciate ligaments was not performed. Although all patients had static instability of the knee joint, few troubles and symptoms were caused by this instability. One patient had an infection, which was treated with continuous irrigation without removal of the implant. There was no mechanical failure during the follow-up period. These results suggest that the hingeless design is also useful as a tumor knee prosthesis if it is possible to preserve sufficient muscle strength, particularly the extensor apparatus. Moreover, if reconstruction of the ligamentous stabilizer is performed, this design demonstrates many benefits for the tumor prosthesis. In young patients in whom a leg length discrepancy of 5 cm or more is expected following wide resection of bone, hemiarthroplasty with a ceramic prosthesis can be performed in anticipation of growth of the remaining opposite growth plate, and correction of the leg length discrepancy can be made at the time of revisional surgery. The functional results of hemiarthroplasty were unexpectedly satisfactory for the follow-up period ranging from 12 to 38 months. The functional ratings according to Ennek-

Table 1. Clinical assessment of ceramic total knee prosthesis

Case	Age (yrs)	Sex	Diagnosis	Follow-up (months)	Motion	Pain	Stability	Deformity	Strength	Functional activity	Emotional acceptance	Rating
1.	21	M	OS	60	P	E	F	F	F	G	G	F
2.	17	M	OS	59	E	E	G	E	G	E	E	G
3.	13	M	OS	47	F	P	G	E	P	P	P	P
4.	33	M	GCT	38	E	E	E	G	E	E	E	E
5.	13	M	OS	27	F	G	F	F	F	F	F	F

Case 3 had deep infection, which was treated with irrigation and drainage without removal of prosthesis

OS osteosarcoma, GCT giant cell tumor, E excellent, G good, F fair, P poor

Table 2. Functional results of hemiarthroplasty by knee ceramic prosthesis

Case	Age (yrs)	Sex	Diagnosis	Follow-up (months)	Motion	Pain	Stability	Deformity	Strength	Functional activity	Emotional acceptance	Rating
1.	13	F	OS	13	F	E	G	G	P	F	G	F
2.	12	M	OS	34	E	E	F	F	G	G	G	F
3.	13	M	OS	33	F	E	G	P	F	G	G	F
4.	13	F	OS	30	G	E	G	P	G	E	E	G
5.	12	F	OS	18	F	G	G	F	G	G	G	F

OS osteosarcoma, E excellent, G good, F fair, P poor
Case 1 had revisional surgery by hinged total knee prosthesis at 13 months after hemiarthroplasty

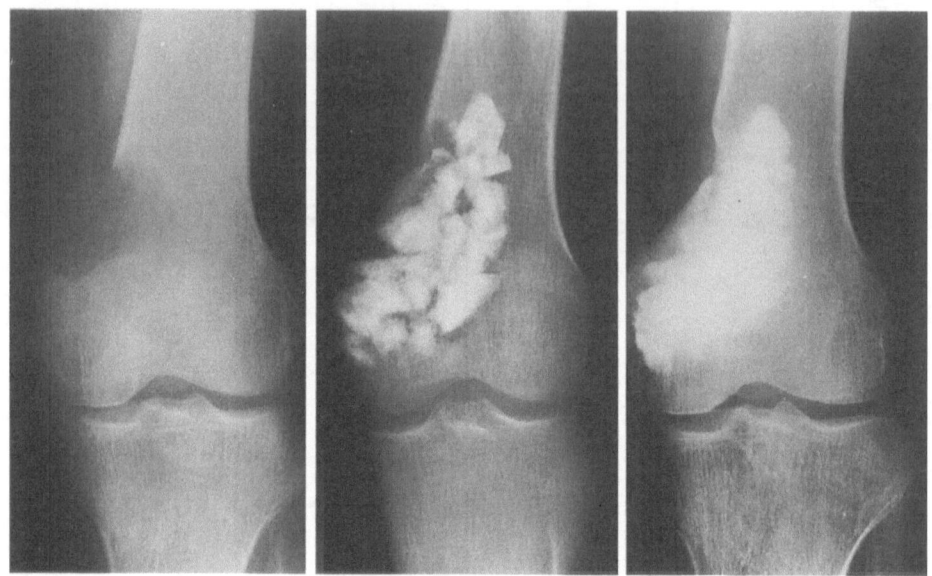

a   b, c

Fig. 1a–c. A 28-year-old female patient was treated by implantation of calcium hydroxy-apatite combined with autogenous iliac bone. The boundary between the bone and calcium hydroxyapatite ceramic materials is gradually becoming indistinct in post-operative X-ray. Giant cell tumor. **a** Preoperation, **b** 1 month postoperation, **c** 14 months postoperation

ing were one good and four fair, but their functional activity, emotional accep-tance, and pain showed good results (Table 2).

The articular cartilage opposite the ceramic implants was only slightly injured even after 2 years postoperation. These changes in the cartilage are thought to be caused by the structural incongruity rather than the adverse effect of alumina ceramic on articular cartilage. These results also suggest that temporary use as a hemiarthroplastic prosthesis after wide resection is useful in young patients.

Reconstruction of the shoulder joint after wide resection also has many dif-ficult problems, particulary the fixation of the scapular component. We made a new constrained ceramic total shoulder prosthesis, having a broad scapular attachment and reversed ball and socket design. Two osteosarcomas were recon-structed with this type of prosthesis after wide resection, and there was no loosening during the short-term follow-up period. Hemiarthroplasty of the hip and wrist joints with a ceramic head prosthesis and segmental prosthetic replace-ment without joint structure of the long bone were performed after resection and showed excellent results without adverse effects. There was one prosthetic fracture of the ceramic stem of the humeral head, but there was no symptomatic loosening in spite of the presence of a clear zone around the alumina ceramic. Moreover, it was observed that alumina ceramic is a better prosthetic material than metal regarding reactivity of the tissue around the implanted material. These results suggest that the development of alumina ceramics would create more favorable conditions for the tumor prosthesis.

For the use of calcium hydroxapatite ceramic, we have made general guidelines based on our animal experiemental results [1, 2]. Bone defects of 7 cm or more in diameter in metaphyseal regions and all sizes of bone defects in diaphyseal regions were filled with this ceramic combined with autogenous bone. Bone defects of 7 cm or less in metaphyseal regions were filled with ceramic only. These results demonstrated that these ceramics were incorporated very well into the bony tissue within several months after implantation (Fig. 1). There were no infections and toxic effects. Moreover, there were no mechanical problems after surgery. We believe that porous calcium hydroxyapatite ceramic is a useful material in bone replacement.

References

1. Uchida A, Nade S, McCartney E, Ching W (1984) The use of ceramics for bone replacement. J Bone Joint Surg 66-B: 269–275
2. Uchida A, Nade S, McCartney E, Ching W (1985) Bone ingrowth into three different porous ceramics implanted into the tibia of rats and rabbits. J Orthop Res 3: 65–77

Intraoperative Radiotherapy and Ceramic Prosthesis Replacement for Osteosarcoma

TAKAO YAMAMURO[1], YOSHIHIKO KOTOURA[1], KATSUYUKI KASAHARA[1], MASAJI TAKAHASHI[2], and MITSUYUKI ABE[2]

Summary. As our principal method for the treatment of osteosarcoma, we have adopted since 1978 a limb-saving procedure by a combination of chemotherapy and intraoperative radiotherapy (IOR); in addition, ceramic prosthesis replacement of the irradiated tumor has been carried out in some cases. We have performed IOR with a large dose of electron beams (50–60 Gray) in 21 patients with osteosarcoma between 1978 and 1984. No local recurrence was observed in the irradiated area. Serial histological examination of ten tumors removed 2–10 months after IOR demonstrated a consistent and marked cytocidal effect on the primary lesion, while IOR exhibited very little complications in the surrounding soft tissues. It was not indicated, however, in lesions of the spine and pelvic girdle, because serious radiation injuries to the spinal cord and internal organs could not be ruled out. The overall cumulative survival rate was 32%. Since 1982, when a new regimen of chemotherapy was adopted, the estimated culumative 5-year survival rate of ten patients increased to 60%. IOR did not prevent lung metastasis of the osteosarcoma, but it always allowed consistent local control of the tumor with little damage to the soft tissues in the extremities. A tumor prosthesis made of alumina ceramics can be used with satisfactory results for tumors developing in the distal femur, provided its design is based on a careful biomechanical analysis.

Key words: Irradiation—Ceramic prosthesis—Osteosarcoma

Introduction

Osteosarcoma was long regarded as the most radio-resistant malignant tumor. However, if it is carefully exposed away from the soft tissues and is covered with a layer of normal tissue, megavoltage radiation sufficient to kill all the tumor cells can be delivered with very little damage to the soft tissues. In 1964, Abe et al. [1] developed intraoperative radiotherapy (IOR) for advanced abdominal cancers with significantly better curative effects than other methods. Since 1978, we have used IOR in combination with chemotherapy and prosthetic replacement as our principal method for treating osteosarcoma in an attempt to preserve the affected limb. In 1983, we demonstrated, by serial histological examination of the removed tumors receiving IOR, that a large dose of electron

Departments of Orthopaedic Surgery[1] and Radiology[2], Faculty of Medicine, Kyoto University, Kyoto, Japan

beams was extremely effective in controling local lesions of osteosarcoma in the
extremities [2]. The present paper describes our IOR procedure, the ceramic
prosthesis design to replace the tumor if necessary, and the results of this combination therapy for osteosarcoma.

IOR Procedure

When a primary bone tumor is confirmed to have a malignant nature by biopsy
and has not expanded into the soft tissues according to computed tomographic
(CT) scanning, IOR is indicated. Prior to IOR, one routine course of chemotherapy is usually given. The area of IOR is determined primarily by the CT
findings, but also with reference to the results of bone scintigraphy and
angiography.

The irradiation area is exposed in the operating room. An extensive skin incision is made over the tumor, and the soft tissues are widely opened and retracted, leaving a layer of normal tissue directly covering the tumor. The skin,
muscles, vessels, and nerves are retracted away from the irradiation area as
much as possible so as to avoid damage by IOR. As a rule, the irradiation is
performed with 12- to 26-MeV electron beams from a betatron at a dose of
50–60 Gray. The dose distribution of electron beams in the focus is studied
preoperatively by CT number with a computer so that the focus is subjected to at
least 80% of the radiation dose. We found that the multifocal bilateral irradiation method is the best for minimizing complications of the soft tissues and increasing the dose distribution of electron beams in the focus. When the size of
the treatment cone is not large enough to cover the entire area of irradiation, the
cone is moved proximally or distally, overlapping by 1 cm with the adjacent area
to compensate for dose reduction in the margins. For example, three irradiation
fields with a 10×8-cm treatment cone with 1-cm overlap at the margins of each
irradiation field cover an area of 10×22 cm. After irradiation on the lateral side,
the treatment cone is rotated 180° and the corresponding medial side is similarly
irradiated. Formerly, when irradiation was only unilateral, skin and nerve damage and muscle contracture were observed on the contralateral side. These side
effects of radiation therapy have been almost completely eliminated since we
began irradiating from both sides.

The irradiation usually takes about 30–40 min. During irradiation, the patient
under general anesthesia is observed through a TV camera, and the electrocar-
diogram, pulse, and blood pressure are monitored in the control room. After the
irradiation, the wound is carefully washed and closed, and a drain is installed.

Materials

Twenty-one patients with osteosarcoma were treated by IOR between December 1978 and March 1984. These patients consisted of 15 males and six females
and were aged from 6 to 51 years at the time of IOR. The site of the lesion was
the distal femur in 12 cases, proximal tibia in seven, proximal humerus in one,
and iliac bone in one.

Eleven patients received only IOR, and eight underwent prosthetic replacement 3 months after IOR with ceramic prostheses. Two of seven patients with tibial osteosarcoma developed extensive skin necrosis and eventually underwent above-the-knee amputation.

Results and Discussion

Skin at the Site of IOR

Usually, the surgical wound heals primarily with no particular problems after IOR, and no irradiation injuries of the skin are noted. Among 21 patients who underwent IOR, two with tibial osteosarcoma developed skin necrosis due to extensive skin dissection and eventually required amputation. None of the patients underwent limb amputation due to irradiation injury of the skin. Thus, particularly in the case of tibial osteosarcoma, an extensive skin dissection for IOR sometimes results in ischemic skin necrosis, sine the microvessels in the underlying tissues soon become necrotic after IOR. To prevent such ischemic skin necrosis, a long skin incision on the medial surface of the tibia and unnecessary dissection between the skin and underlying muscles should be avoided.

Local Recurrence of the Tumor

Local recurrence of the tumor was examined in 19 patients, excluding the two who required limb amputation. No recurrence was observed in the irradiated area, suggesting that sufficient local control can be achieved by a dose of 50–60 Gray. Two patients showed recurrence in the nonirradiated area, one due to tumor implantation in the muscle by the biopsy procedure and the other due to insufficiency of the irradiated area. Therefore, particular caution is necessary for the biopsy technique and the irradiation method.

Bone Scintigraphy

Bone scintigraphy with Tc-MDP (methylene diphosphate) was performed preoperatively in all the patients with osteosarcoma, and the scintigrams invariably showed a high uptake in the primary lesions. The bone scintigraphy was again performed 3–6 months after IOR in 11 patients, excluding the two who underwent amputation and eight who underwent prosthetic replacement. The postoperative scintigrams invariably showed a marked decrease of uptake in the irradiated area as compared with those taken preoperatively (Fig. 1).

Serum Alkaline Phosphatase Level

The serum alkaline phosphatase level was examined at regular intervals in 13 patients, excluding the eight who underwent prosthetic replacement. The level, which was elevated, more less, before IOR, returned rapidly to normal 2–3 weeks after IOR in all patients (Fig. 2). This reduction was comparable with that observed in patients who underwent limb amputation without IOR. If the level remains high even after IOR, metastasis to other bones or the lung is suspected.

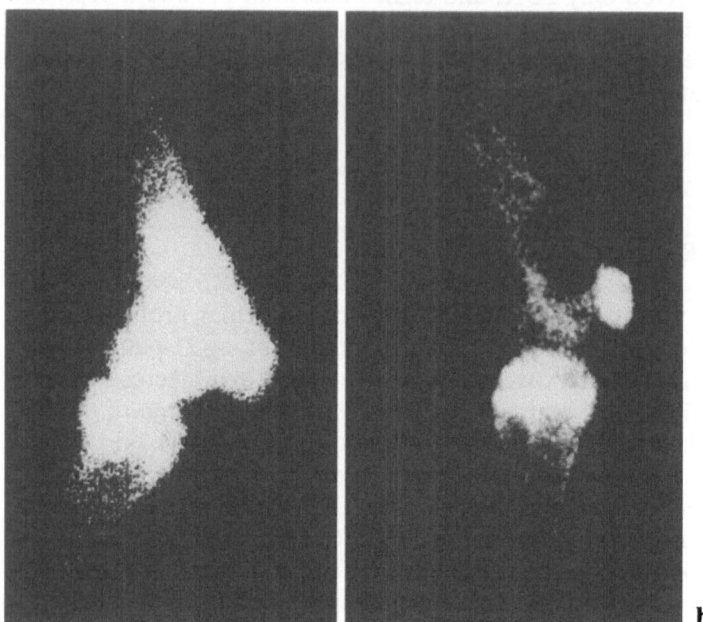

a   b

Fig. 1a, b. Bone scintigraphy with Tc-MDP in a 15-year-old male. **a** A preoperative scintigram shows marked uptake in the distal femur. **b** A scintigram taken 3 months after IOR shows little uptake in the distal femur, except for the patella which was eliminated from the irradiation field

Histological Findings

Histological examination of the resected primary lesions was carried out in ten patients who underwent limb amputation or prosthetic replacement 2–10 months (average 3 months) after IOR. In two patients who had received uni-directional irradiation, a few scattered tumor cells appeared viable in the super-ficial layers in spite of the presence of marked cellular changes and extensive destruction of the tumor. In the other ten patients who had received multifocal bilateral irradiation, complete necrosis of the tumor cells was observed through-out the specimen except for a few scattered, markedly altered, presumably nonviable tumor cells in small clusters (Fig. 3).

IOR consistently had a marked effect on the primary lesion in all patients as shown above by the various examinations. This absence of an individual varia-tion of the effect is characteristic of this treatment modality.

Cumulative Survival Rate

The overall cumulative 5-year survival rate was 32% in 18 patients, excluding the two patients who showed metastasis to other areas at IOR and one in whom the lesion originated in the iliac bone. The 5-year survival rate in eight of these patients who were treated primarily with adriamycin and methotrexate (MTX)

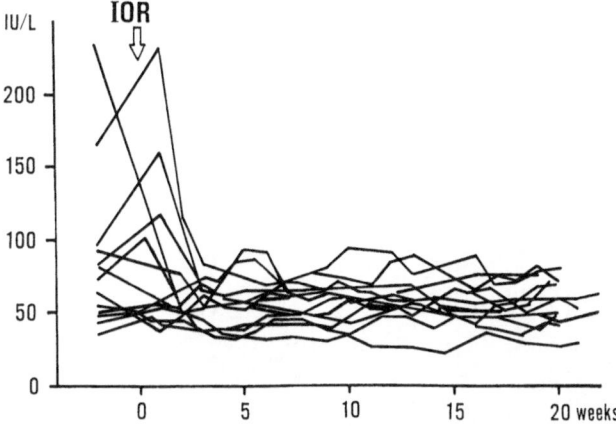

Fig. 2. Serum alkaline phosphatase level in 13 patients, excluding those who underwent prosthetic replacement. Note the rapid decrease of the level in all patients 2–3 weeks after IOR

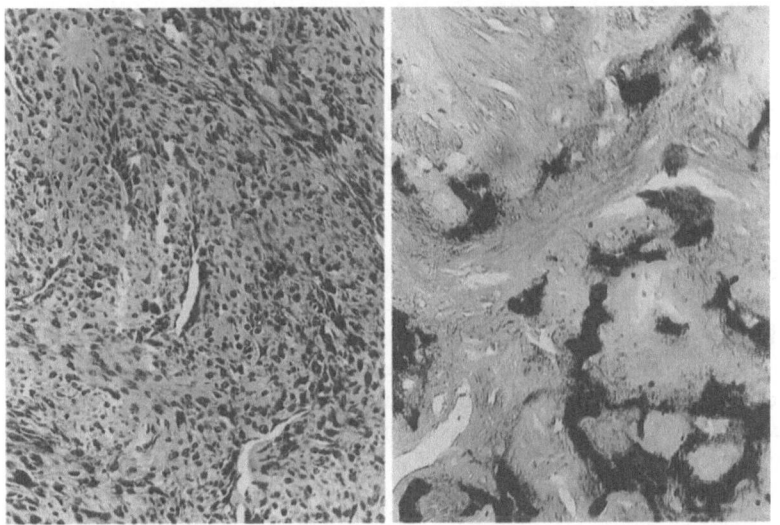

Fig. 3a, b. Histological findings of osteosarcoma developed in the proximal tibia of a 22-year-old male. **a** Microphotograph of the tumor tissue taken by biopsy before treatment shows a typical finding of osteosarcoma, × 20. **b** Microphotograph of the tumor removed 6 months after IOR shows complete necrosis of the tissue except for a few scattered, markedly altered, presumably nonviable tumor cells

was 17%; while more recently in ten patients treated primarily with adriamycin and cisplatin, the estimated cumultive 5-year survival rate was 60%. Thus, IOR has little benefit for the survival rate, although it is extremely effective for local control of osteosarcoma. IOR must, therefore, be performed in combination with adequate chemotherapy.

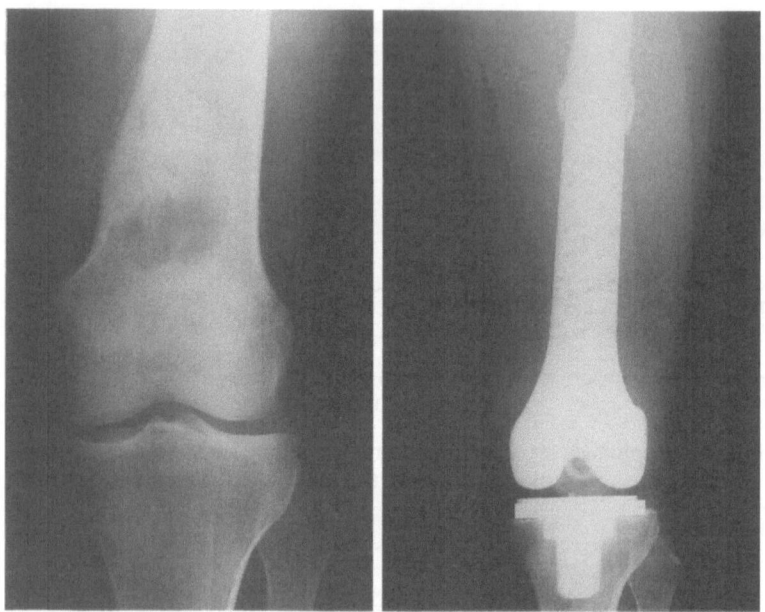

a   b

Fig. 4a, b. Osteosarcoma developed in the femur of a 44-year-old female. **a** Preoperative roentgenogram. **b** Roentgenogram taken 4 years after IOR and ceramic prosthesis replacement shows satisfactory alignment of the prosthesis. Note new bone formation over the junction with the femur ensuring firm connection

Design and Results of Ceramic Tumor Prostheses

The irradiated bone tended to break following a minor trauma after 3 months of IOR. Therefore, we routinely replaced the irradiated tumor in the distal femur with a ceramic prosthesis. In other locations such as the proximal humerus and proximal tibia, however, prosthetic replacement was not performed as a rule to preserve the insertion of large muscles, and a brace was applied or bone graft was performed in combination with intramedullary nailing when a fracture occurred.

As a material for fabricating a tumor prosthesis, alumina ceramic is more advantageous than metal alloys in terms of biocompatibility, mechanical strength, corrosiveness, fatigue, friction, and wear. Our tumor prosthesis is a nonconstrained two-compartmental artificial joint, in which the monocrystalline alumina stem (sapphire stem) is linked to the polycrystalline alumina bulk filling a major bone defect via a glass binder. The bearing surface of the tibial plateau is made of high-density polyethylene. Sapphire, while not inferior to other metal alloys in mechanical properties, is limited in availability for its proper length, the maximum being about 13 cm for the femur. Therefore, the tumor prosthesis must be carefully designed based on the results of biomechanical analysis, taking the tumor size and stem length into consideration. The replacement operation is carried out through the same incision as that made for IOR.

The irradiated bone segment, which is easily noticeable due to its color change, is excised with 2 cm of the nonirradiated bone segment proximally. The prosthesis stem is inserted securely into the marrow cavity without using bone cement. For the last 8 years, we have experienced no cleavage or loosening of the prosthesis. The patients can walk almost normally and bend the knee joint 60°–90°. Linkage between the prosthesis and bone becomes very firm usually 6 months postoperatively by newly formed bone covering the junction (Fig. 4).

References

1. Abe M, Takahashi M, Yabumoto E (1975) Techniques, indications, and results of intraoperative radiotherapy of advanced cancers. Radiology 16: 693–702
2. Nagashima T, Yamamuro T, Kotoura Y, Takahashi M, Abe M, Nakashima Y (1983) Histological studies on the effect of intraoperative irradiation of osteosarcoma. J Jpn Orthop Ass 57: 1681–1697
3. Yamamuro T (1985) Recent advances in orthopaedic ceramic implants. J Jpn Orthop Ass 59: 339–348

Moderator's Comment

TAKAO YAMAMURO[1]

Bioceramics is the name given to a group of ceramics which are used as biomaterials and in biotechnology science. They are classified into two groups according to their bioactivity. Bioinert ceramics are extremely stable in vivo and do not react with the surrounding tissues, while bioactive ceramics dissolve, to a greater or lesser extent, adsorb or crystallize minerals on their surface in vivo, and bind chemically with bone tissue.

Bioinert ceramics are highly biocompatible, antithrombogenic, noncarcinogenic, and nonteratogenic. Therefore, they appear to be usable as biomaterials, providing great biological safety. High stability in vivo is a characteristic of bioinert ceramics. They do not dissolve or corrode at all in the living body even after a long period of implantation, and they do not chemically react with any elements, molecules, cells, or tissues in vivo. Great mechanical strength is another characteristic of such bioinert ceramics as alumina, zirconia, and alumina-titanium carbonitride. For example, alumina ceramic is nearly ten times greater in compressive strength and its monocrystal in nearly two times greater in bending strength than Vitallium. The alumina ceramic exhibits much less deterioration even after a long period of implantation that such metal alloys as stainless steel and Vitallium.

If required, the surface of bioinert ceramics can be polished to a roughness (Ra) of less than 0.4 μm, which is about one-tenth that of the femoral head of the metal prostheses now on the market. If they are polished to such a condition and are used for the bearing surface of an artificial joint, a wear resistant and low frictional prosthesis can be fabricated. Recently, great advances in technology have made it possible to synthesize alumina ceramics with a high material quality, and this material has been used for tumor prostheses for the last 10 years in Europe and Japan.

Improvements not only in the quality of the ceramic material but also in the prosthetic design based on a precise biomechanical analysis are required to bring these ceramics to wide clinical use with long-term safety. One design of a ceramic tumor prosthesis presently used in Japan is illustrated in Fig. 1. This

[1]Department of Orthopaedic Surgery, Faculty of Medicine, Kyoto University, Kyoto, Japan

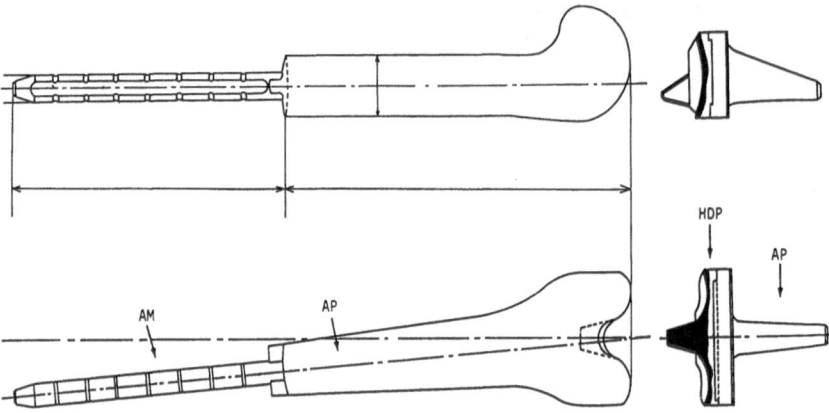

Fig. 1. A design of ceramic prosthesis for a bone tumor developing in the distal femur. *AM* alumina monocrystal, *AP* alumina polycrystal, *HDP* high-density polyethylene

prosthesis, which is used to replace a bone tumor developing in the distal femur, is a two-compartmental and nonconstrained artificial knee joint with a high degree of freedom. Alumina ceramic monocrystal is used for the stem as it is mechanically stronger than polycrystal, while the latter is used to replace the main bone defect since it is suitable for complicated molding. The tibial plateau on the concave side is made of high-density polyethylene. The shape of the articular surface is nearly identical to that of the total condylar type, but the intercondylar eminence is elevated to minimize medial-lateral instability as well as to prevent overextension and dislocation at maximum flexion. The prosthesis stems are securely inserted into the marrow cavity without using bone cement.

In this session, experience with ceramic tumor prostheses are presented, along with their availability, advantages, disadvantages, and various designs.

Chapter 7

Prosthesis vs. Osteochondral Graft, Alternative Substitute for Bone Tumor

A Comparison of Vascularized and Conventional Bone Grafts for Bridging Large Bone Defects

KENNETH L.B. BROWN and JEAN F. WELTER[1]

Summary. Clinical reports have shown that vascularized bone grafts heal faster, show more hypertrophy, and are more reliable in poorly vascularized beds than conventional, cortical grafts. Recent animal studies have failed to substantiate the advantages claimed in patients.

Twenty-six adult dogs were divided into two groups. In one forearm, a 7-cm segment of both the radius and ulna was removed. A 9-cm free vascularized fibular graft was harvested from one leg and a conventional 9-cm fibular graft was obtained from the opposite leg. In group I, the radial defect was bridged by the vascularized graft while the ulnar defect was bridged by the conventional graft. In group II, the positions were reversed. Grafts placed in the radius were subjected to considerably greater weight-bearing stresses than those placed in the ulna. An external fixator was used to stabilize the forearm. X-rays were taken every two weeks and hypertrophy of both grafts was measured on a Bioquant image analyzer. The dogs were killed 2, 3, 4, 6, and 12 months after receiving two doses of tetracycline. After killing the animals, arteriograms were performed and the transplants were torqued to failure with an Instron materials testing machine.

The vascularized grafts remained viable throughout and rapidly became encased in a peripheral callus. The conventional grafts underwent "creeping substitution" following revascularization, but the interstitial lamellae remained necrotic. Hypertrophy by peripheral callus was delayed in the conventional grafts, but by 6 months they approached the size of the vascularized fibular grafts. The mechanical strength of the grafts correlated well with their size. From 6 to 12 months, remodeling occurred in both grafts with lamellization of the peripheral bone and development of a medullary canal.

Key words: Hypertrophy—Vascularized bone

Introduction

There are many methods of reconstruction available for large bone defects created by tumor excisions. In many cases, biological reconstruction still offers the best long-term solution, especially in young patients. Autogenous cortical bone

---

[1] Department of Orthopaedic Surgery, The Montreal Children's Hospital, McGill University, Montreal, Canada

grafts are preferred by many surgeons because of their superior osteogenic capacity, ease of incorporation, and lack of immunological problems. Unfortunately, only a few surface osteocytes survive transplantation. The dense cortical bone acts as a diffusion barrier, so much of the graft becomes necrotic. The repair process is dependent upon revascularization from the surrounding bed through the existing necrotic osteons and the dead bone must be resorbed before new bone can be laid down. The resulting porosity substantially weakens the graft and often results in graft fracture, especially when the grafts are more than 12 cm long. Conventional cortical bone grafts do not appear to have much capacity for hypertrophy other than by callus formation following fracture repair. As a result, large medullary rods or plates are often necessary to add strength to the limb until the grafts are incorporated. Complete incorporation takes about 2 years in humans. The process may be increased considerably when there is a poorly vascularized soft tissue bed, as is often the case following tumor excisions.

There have been many clinical and experimental reports in the literature illustrating the problems associated with the repair of large cortical autografts. Most of these complications are related to the process of revascularization and resorption of the dead graft. If this "creeping substitution" could be eliminated or shortened, the use of cortical autografts would be much more reliable.

The implementation of microsurgical techniques has made it possible to reestablish the nutrient blood supply to bones following distant transfer. This has converted the problem from one of graft incorporation to essentially fracture healing, since the vascularized graft appeared to behave very much like a segmental fracture. The first clinical report was by Taylor et al. in 1975 [1]. Many others followed and all claimed faster union and rapid hypertrophy. There have been several experimental studies of vascularized bone grafts, but their conclusions are often contradictory and this has led to controversy. Weiland et al. [2] found earlier union, fewer complications, earlier hypertrophy, and greater mechanical strength. Doi et al. [3] also found earlier union in vascularized grafts, as did Haw et al. [4]. However, Dell et al. [5] found no difference in the union rate, nor did Adalaar et al. [6] Vascularized grafts were found to be much stronger than conventional grafts by Moore et al. [7], but Dell et al. [5] found that vascularized bone grafts were only transiently stronger and that there was very little hypertrophy.

One of the reasons for the conflicting results is the wide variation in animal models. Some grafts had only their periosteal blood supply preserved [2, 6, 7]. Other grafts were transplanted to areas of low stress [5] or were stress-shielded by large plates [2]. None of these models resembled the usual clinical situation, in which there is a large bone defect in a major weight-bearing bone. There is no perfect animal model which can exactly duplicate the clinical circumstances, but we developed one which closely resembles it. We had planned to create a defect in the tibia of a dog. On one side, we would insert a vascularized fibular graft, while on the other tibia a conventional fibula would be transplanted. This proposal did not meet the approval of our Animal Care Committee and we adopted our present model.

Materials and Methods

In one forelimb of an adult dog, a 7-cm segment of both the radius and ulna was removed. A 9-cm vascularized fibular graft was harvested from one hind limb. This was a modification of our previously published technique, which preserved the endosteal and periosteal blood supplies [8]. A conventional 9-cm fibular graft was obtained subperiosteally from the opposite leg. The forelimb was stabilized with an external fixator (which was worn for the duration of this study) and full weight-bearing was allowed. Twenty-six dogs were divided into two groups. In group I, the radial defect was bridged by the vascularized graft, while the ulnar defect was bridged by the conventional graft. In group II, the positions were reversed with the conventional fibula in the radius and the vascularized fibula in the ulna. The popliteal artery was anastomosed to the median artery and the popliteal vein was anastomosed to the antecubital vein. The average time of operation was $10\frac{1}{2}$ h. It is known that the radius in the dog is subjected to much greater weight-bearing stresses in vivo, but we did not really know what the differences between the radius and ulna would be in our model, especially with an external fixator applied. By having two groups of dogs with the grafts reversed, we hoped to decrease the influence of this unknown variable. In fact, our results showed that the grafts behaved differently depending on the bone segment replaced and further indicated the importance of stress in improving hypertrophy.

Radiographs were taken at two-week intervals to determine the union time and to measure hypertrophy. The hypertrophy of both grafts was measured from the X-ray films using a Bioquant System IV image analysis system. The dogs were killed at 2, 3, 4, 6, and 12 months. Prior to killing, two doses of tetracycline were given to label new bone formation. After killing the animals, arteriograms were made and the limbs were explored to find the anastomoses. The radius and ulna were then harvested. The fibular transplants and their proximal and distal graft-host junctions were included. The ends were potted in methylmethacrylate and mounted in a jig, which converted the linear pull of an Instron materials testing machine to a rotary force. The grafts were then rapidly torqued to failure at 550°/s and the resulting stress deformation curve was recorded with an X-Y plotter. The broken bones were reassembled and cut into four segments and embedded in methylmethacrylate. A Gillings-Hamco diamond saw was used to cut thin sections; they were mounted on plastic slides and milled to a 100-μm thickness with a Reichert Polycut E microtome with an Ultramiller attachment. Contact microradiographs were made and the unstained section was used to study tetracycline fluorescence. Alternate slices were further milled to a thickness of 5 μm and then stained with Goldner's trichrome stain. The cross sections were measured with the Bioquant System IV image analysis program to measure hypertrophy and porosity. The microradiographs and tetracycline-labeled specimens were studied to measure resorption and new bone formation.

Results

This report is based on our evaluation of 26 dogs. Thirty-eight were operated upon, but 12 dogs had to be deleted from the series due to severe infections, anastomosis failures, or three-legged gait.

All graft-host junctions were solidly united by 2 months following surgery. There was no difference in the union time between the vascularized and conventional grafts. There were seven graft fractures; two were in the ulna and five were in the radius. Four of the seven fractures were in the vascularized fibula, while three were in the conventional grafts. All fractures healed uneventfully without any changes in the dogs weight-bearing status.

Group I: Vascularized Fibula in Radius and Conventional Fibula in Ulna

At 2 months, all graft-host junctions were solidly united, but there was not much difference in the radiological appearance. There were marked differences at the microscopic level. The conventional fibula was very porous throughout its surface due to osteonal resorption. Revascularization was already widespread in the graft as shown by the tetracycline labels, but there was not much peripheral callus and the interstial lamellar bone was still very necrotic. The original vascularized fibula was intact and encased by an active peripheral callus. The original bone was viable throughout and the nutrient artery and vein were well visualized in the center of the graft (Fig. 1). The grafts continued to show hypertrophy during the next 2 months, but the increase was much greater in the vascularized grafts (Figs. 2, 3) where the peripheral callus more than doubled its initial size. At 6 months, the vascularized fibular graft reached its maximum size, and remodeling occurred at 6–12 months. The central part of the graft resorbed to form a medullary canal and the peripheral callus became lamellated to form a dense cortex. The rate of hypertrophy of the conventional graft was much slower than the vascularized fibular graft but it eventually became almost as large. At 1 year, the grafts were similar in size and shape. The vascularized grafts were significantly stronger at 4 and 6 months but not subsequently. There was a marked variability in the strength of paired bones in the same animal; there must therefore have been a very large difference between the tested bones for the difference to be significant. To help decrease the variability between animals, we paired the values for the vascularized fibula and conventional fibula taken from each animal and determined the differences in the individual values from the mean of the pair.

Group II: Conventional Fibula in Radius and Vascularized Fibula in Ulna

The repair process in the vascularized and conventional grafts was similar to group I but there was considerably less hypertrophy of the vascularized grafts. The forces in the vascularized graft were reduced when it was placed in the ulna and presumably this is the reason for the change. Hypertrophy was still greater than in the conventional grafts but the differences were not as marked. The conventional graft did not show much more hypertrophy than it did in group I, when it was in a less stressed bone. It seems that the repair process could not allow for adaptation to the increased forces until much later in the incorporation process. There was no significant difference in the strength of the conventional and vascularized fibulas in this group.

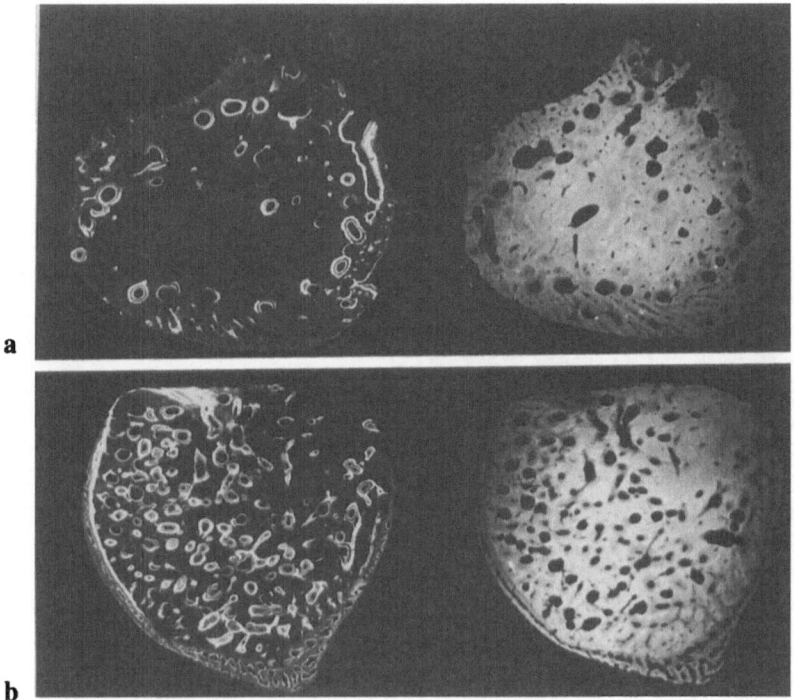

Fig. 1a, b. Group 1 dog at 2 months. **a** Tetracycline-labeled photomicrograph and microradiograph of the vascularized fibula. **b** Conventional fibular graft has markedly increased porosity

Discussion

Some authors have reported that the pattern of repair in vascularized transplants is similar to that in conventional grafts but merely accelerated. In our study, the patterns were quite different. Vascularized transplants showed marked peripheral new bone formation and little activity in the center of the graft, leaving the original transplant intact for about 6 months and then gradually remodeling. Conventional grafts, on the other hand, exhibited marked osteonal resorption, while peripheral new bone deposition was minimal at first and gradually increased.

The conventional grafts in this study fared better than we would have expected in patients. All of the conventional grafts were revascularized by 2 months after transplantation. This may have been due to the close proximity to the well-vascularized muscle of the other transplant and the thin flat shape of the dog fibula, which favored rapid revascularization.

In this study, vascularized fibular grafts increased in size by peripheral new bone formation. The response was better when it was subjected to the greater weight-bearing stresses in the radius. The grafts to the ulna did not respond as well; therefore, in this group, there was not a clear advantage of the vascularized

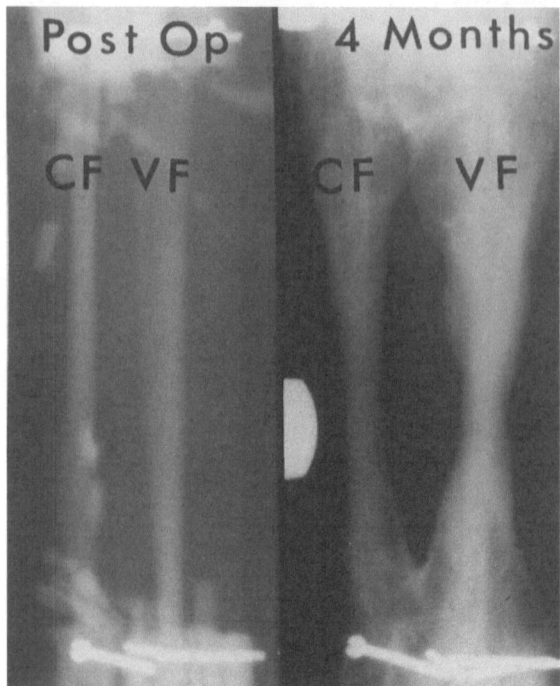

Fig. 2. Composite radiograph of a group 1 dog immediately postoperation and at 4 months. The vascularized fibula (*VF*) is in the radius; the conventional fibula (*CF*) is in the ulna

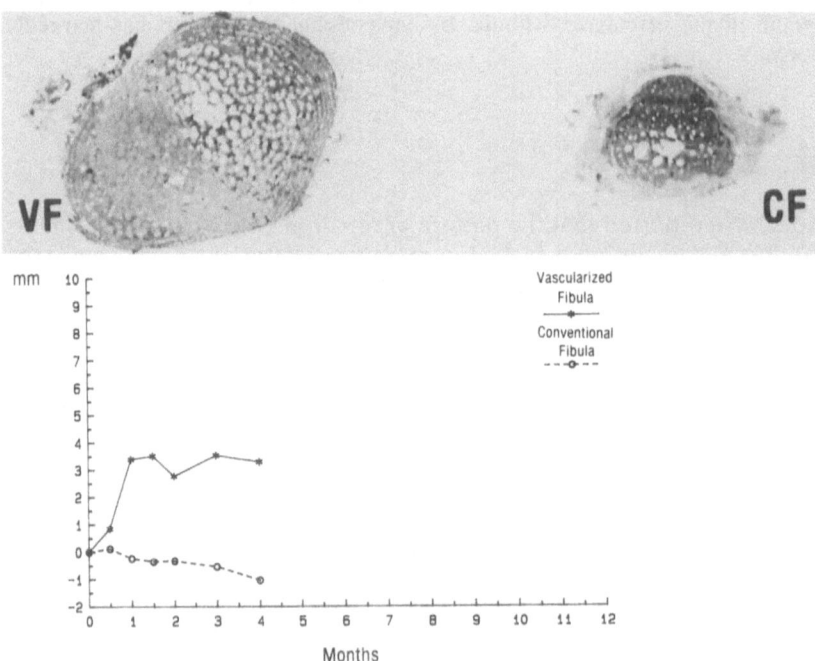

Fig. 3. Stained sections and growth curve from dog 7839. Group 1, 4 months *Graph* shows change from initial diameter as measured on the X-ray vs. time. The vascularized fibula is much larger. The outline of the original fibula is evident in the *lower left corner*

over the conventional fibular graft. This group correlates better with the model of Dell et al. [5], whose orthotopically transplanted fibulas bore little stress.

In clinical practice, vascularized fibular grafts should offer a distinct advantage when major bone defects must be bridged, especially when the surrounding bed is poorly vascularized. Utilization of an external fixator prevents the stress shielding, which can occur with large plates or intramedullary devices. The fixator can be modified as healing and hypertrophy occur so the graft can absorb more load. This should maximize the rate of graft hypertrophy and ultimately lessen the immobilization time for the patient.

Acknowledgment. This research was funded by the Medical Research Council of Canada.

References

1. Taylor GI, Miller GD, Ham FJ (1975) The free vascularized bone graft. Plast Reconstr Surg 55: 533–544
2. Weiland AJ, Phillips TW, Randolph MA (1984) Bone grafts. A radiologic, histologic and biomechanical model comparing autografts, allografts, and free vascularized bone grafts. Plast Reconstr Surg 54: 368–379
3. Doi K, Tominaga S, Shibata T (1977) Bone grafts with microvascular anastomoses of vascular pedicles. An experimental study in dogs. J Bone Joint Surg 59-A: 809–815
4. Haw CS, O'Brien BMcC, Kurata T (1978) The microsurgical revascularization of resected segments of the tibia in the dog. J Bone Joint Surg. 60B: 266–269
5. Dell PC, Burchardt H, Glowczewskie FP Jr (1985) A roentgenographic, biomechanical and histological evaluation of vascularized and non-vascularized segmental fibular canine autografts. J Bone Joint Surg 67-A: 105–112
6. Adalaar RS, Soucacos PN, Urbaniak JR (1974) Autologous cortical bone grafts with microsurgical anastomosis of periosteal vessels. Surgical Forum 25: 487–489
7. Moore JB, Mazur JM, Zehr D, Davis PK, Zook EG (1984) A biomechanical comparison of vascularized and conventional autogenous bone grafts. Plast Reconstr Surg 73: 382–386
8. Brown KL, Marie P, Lyszakowski T, Daniel RK, Cruess RL (1983) Epiphyseal growth after free fibular transfer with and without microvascular anastomoses. Experimental study in the dog. J Bone Joint Surg 65B: 493–501

Vascularized Bone Graft for Limb Salvage Surgery of Malignant Bone Tumor

Katsuro Tomita, Kazuo Ikeda, Hiroyuki Tsuchiya, and Susumu Nomura[1]

Summary. From the viewpoint of good biological replacement and permanent and active availability, we have preferred to utilize free vascularized fibular or iliac bone grafts as the first choice in reconstruction after wide resection of malignant bone tumor. From 1981 to 1987, in 13 of 36 cases of malignant bone tumor, a vascularized bone graft was employed. The cases included three osteosarcomas, three chondrosarcomas, two malignant fibrous histiocytomas, including four aggressive cases of giant cell tumor. The sites of lesion were the femoral shaft (two), distal femur (four), proximal tibia (three), proximal fibula (one), distal tibia (two), and proximal humerus (one). When the joint required removal, arthrodesis was necessary in four cases in the knee joints and two cases in the ankle joints. Fusion of the grafts was recognized after an average of 4 months and the patients could return to normal activity at 1.5 years. During the average 27 months follow-up, no patient showed local recurrence, but one died of metastases at 4 years, and one were obliged to perform amputation in one patient 1 year after operation. The functional evaluations of seven cases after 2 years were all excellent, including cases of arthrodesis. The advantages of vascularized bone graft are stressed.

Key words: Vascularized bone graft—Limb salvage surgery—Bone tumor

Introduction

Among the reconstruction techniques of the limb following radical resection of malignant bone tumor, artificial prosthesis has been used extensively with some success to replace the massive bone defect. The final goal of limb salvage, however, is permanent and active availability of the preseved limb for the rest of the patient's natural life; therefore, materials guaranteeing the permanence of the reconstructed limb are of the utmost importance. From the viewpoint of the best biological replacement, any kind of artificial material would be inferior to a bone autograft, which ensures ideal incorporation and allows the patient permanent activity of the salvaged limb for the rest of his life. Many investigators have reported that large nonvascular allografts and autografts ultimately fail because of incomplete and inadequate revascularization and mineralization [1]. On the other hand, free vascularized bone graft demands a meticulous micro-

[1] Department of Orthopaedic Surgery, Kanazawa University School of Medicine, Kanazawa, Japan

surgical technique; if successful, however, it offers the best living biological replacement in reconstruction.

For this reason, we have preferred to utilize a free vascularized fibular or iliac bone graft as the first choice in reconstruction after wide resection of a malignant bone tumor. This method was applied mainly on the knee joint area of active, younger patients under 40 years of age. However, we have also tried to extend the indication in location and age.

Materials and Methods

In 13 of 36 cases of malignant bone tumor during the past 6 years (1981–1987), we have employed vascularized bone graft (Table 1). The histological diagnosis was osteosarcoma (four cases), chondrosarcoma (three), malignant fibrous histiocytoma (two), including special aggressive cases of giant cell tumor (four). The operation age ranged from 14 to 55 years old, the average age being 27.8 years. Eight patients were male and five female. The sites of the lesion were: femoral shaft (two), distal femur (four), proximal tibia (three), proximal fibula (one), distal tibia (two), and proximal humerus (one). The length of defect after wide resection was 6–12 cm, with an average of 15.3 cm in malignant tumors.

To bridge large defects in bone, free (nine cases) or rotational (two) vascularized fibular grafts were applied in most cases, except in two where free vascularized iliac grafts were applied. One vascularized fibular graft was inserted as a main support and in many cases an additional bone with or without vascularization was placed parallel to give more stability, which was accomplished by an external fixation. In eight cases, an osteocutaneous flap was additionally employed to cover the large defect of soft tissue and skin following wide resection. When the joint required removal, arthrodesis was necessary in four cases in the knee joints and two cases in the ankle joints. Vessel grafts folllowing wide excision were necessary in three cases, all of which were in osteosarcoma.

Tibial and peroneal nerve grafts, 10 cm in length, were also tried in one case, which showed moderate sensory recovery in the course of a year.

Case Reports

Case 1. This was a 26-year-old man with osteosarcoma on the distal tibia; the distal third of the tibia, fibula, muscles, and skin were removed to obtain a safe oncological margin, leaving only the gastrocnemius, posterior tibial vessels, and nerve. Two vascularized fibular grafts were then bridged with pedicle skin and a soft tissue flap. At present (1.5 years postoperation), the grafts are thick enough to support weight, and the patient can carry out most daily activities without any problem.

Case 5. This was a case of chondrosarcoma on the lower femoral shaft in a 41-year-old man. Wide en bloc resection was carried out followed by insertion of one vascularized and one nonvascularized fibular graft. Full weight bearing was allowed 1.5 year later until hypertrophy of the grafted fibula was recognized.

Table 1. Vascularized bone graft for limb salvage of malignant bone tumor

Case	Age (yrs)	Sex	Diagnosis	Site	VBG + others	Complication	(R, M)	Course	Evaluation
1.	26	M	Osteosarcoma	D-tibia	2-fibula + AD		(−, −)	Alive (20 mos)	G
2.	36	F	Osteosarcoma	P-humerus	1-fibula + AP		(−, −)	Alive (10 mos)	F
3.	14	M	Osteosarcoma	D-femur	2-fibula + AD	Infection	(−, −)	Alive (8 mos)	
4.	21	M	Osteosarcoma	P-fibula	1-fibula		(−, −)	Alive (7 mos)	
5.	41	M	Chondrosarcoma	S-femur	1-fibula	Fx.	(−, −)	Alive (4 yrs)	E
6.	30	F	Chondrosarcoma	S-femur	2-fibula + nail		(−, −)	Alive (2 yrs)	E
7.	55	M	Chondrosarcoma	P-tibia	1-fibula		(−, −)	Alive (2 yrs)	E
8.	22	M	MFH	P-tibia	1-fibula	Fx.	(−, +)	Died (4 yrs)	E
9.	26	F	MFH	P-tibia	1-ilium + AD		(−, −)	Alive (2 yrs)	E
10.	21	M	GCT	D-femur	1-fibula + AD		(−, −)	Alive (6 yrs)	E
11.	31	F	GCT	D-tibia	1-fibula + AD		(−, −)	Alive (4 yrs)	E
12.	23	F	GCT	D-femur	2-fibula + AD	Non-U.	(−, −)	Amputation (1 yr)	P
13.	22	M	GCT	D-femur	1-ilium		(−, −)	Alive (6 mos)	

VBG vascularized bone graft, *R* local recurrence, *M* metastasis, *D* distal, *P* proximal, *S* shaft, *AD* arthrodesis, *AP* arthroplasty, *Fx* fracture, *Non-U* nonunion, *MFH* malignant fibrous histiocytoma, *GCT* giant cell tumor

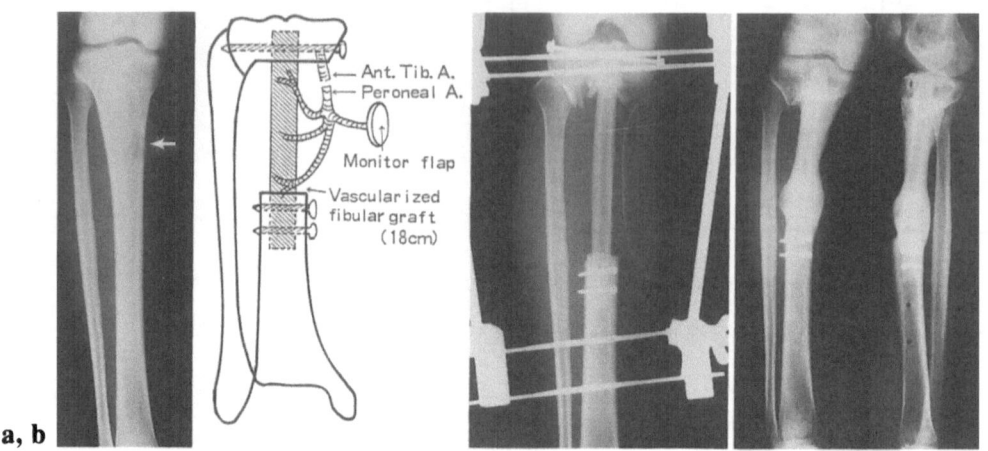

Fig. 1. a Malignant fibrous histiocytoma (MFH); surgical staging IIA. **b** Schema of free vascularized fibular graft. **c** X-p after operation. **d** One and a half years after operation

The patient returned to his job as a taxi driver 2 years after the operation. He has been quite well with no recurrence or metastasis of the tumor.

Case 8. This was a case of malignant fibrous histiocytoma on the tibia (surgical grading; IIA) in a 21-year-old male (Fig. 1). Wide en bloc resection was carried out. In this 14-cm defect, an 18-cm vascularized bone graft was inserted and external fixation was set; thus, the patient was allowed early mobilization. In the course of rehabilitation (4 months later), the graft cracked; however, this stimulated new bone formation, and the graft became thicker. The patient returned to his job 1 year later. He lived quite an active life, but because of liver metastases died 4 years later.

Results

Fusion of the grafts was indicated by X-ray after an average of 4 months and the patients could resume normal activity 1.5 years later (maximum 2 years). Fractures of the grafts were not an obstacle to bone union; on the contrary, they provided a good stimulation to induce bone hypertrophy. A case of infection could be managed well by curettage and closed irrigation with antibiotics, but fusion was delayed. One case of nonunion was due to postoperative thrombosis and we were obliged to amputate 1 year later. Chemotherapy was introduced in osteosarcoma and malignant fibrous histiocytoma pre- and postoperatively; however, in comparison with patients not receiving chemotherapy, there was no difference in bone union. During the average 27 months follow-up period, none of the patients showed local recurrence, but one died of metastases at 4 years. The functional evaluations of the seven cases after 2 years were all excellent, including cases of arthrodesis.

Discussion

Compared with other artificial prostheses for limb preservation, the advantages of bone autograft are as follows. It is an ideal material physically and bio-mechanically, resulting in ideal incorporation and biological replacement. It guarantees permanent stability and availability of the preserved limb and an active life-style with no fear of breakage. These advantages are intensified by applying a vascularized bone graft [2]. Of course, we realized that there are many disadvantages with a vascularized bone graft, such as demanding an advanced microsurgical technique, length of operating time (approximately 5–10 h), difficulty of procuring, limitation in size, arthrodesis admitted near the joint lesion, occasional failure of bone fusion, long period before becoming ambulatory, preserving vessels for anastomosis, preoperative arterial infusion of chemotherapy not recommended. Additionally, problems may occur with the vascularized fibular graft, such as accidental damage to the peroneal nerve, temporary weakness in extension of the hallux, instability of the ankle joint (these can be avoided by preservation of the peroneal muscle attachment and the distal quarter of the fibula).

However, among the many advantages of vascularized bone grafts are [3]: (a) More reliable and faster fusion of the graft can be expected; (b) once the graft is fused and incorporated, it becomes thicker and stronger with time (graft hypertrophy is usually accelerated in response to stress); (c) it can be applied on larger defects up to 20 cm; (d) additional application of an osteocutaneous flap is possible; (e) it is more resistant to infection than an artificial prosthesis.

In conclusion, we highly recommend a vascularized bone graft as the first consideration in limb salvage surgery.

References

1. Springfield DS (1978) Massive autogenous bone grafts. Orthop Clin North Am 18 (2), 249–256
2. Pho RWH (1983) Free vascularized bone and joint transplant in bone tumor resection. In: Chao EYS, Ivins JC (eds) Tumor prostheses for bone and joint reconstruction—the design and application. Thieme-Stratton, New York, pp 93–97
3. Tomita K (1983) Giant cell tumor of the lateral condyle of the femur treated by massive resection and rotational vascularized fibular graft. In: Chao EYS, Ivins JC (eds) Tumor prostheses for bone and joint reconstruction—the design and application. Thieme-Stratton, New York, pp 99–101

Limb Saving Surgery Without Endoprosthesis on Malignant Bone Tumors

Osamu Inoue, Kunio Ibaraki, Hiromichi Norimatsu, Munetoshi Kayo, Masanori Takeuchi, and Akira Arakaki[1]

Summary. Four cases of vascularized fibular graft and three cases of rotationplasty for reconstruction after wide resection in malignant bone tumors are presented. Since endoprosthetic reconstruction does not offer life-long durability and can cause limb discrepancy in growing patients dual vascularized fibular grafts should be considered for reconstruction of the diaphysis in the lower extremity. For reconstruction of the proximal humerus, the vascularized proximal fibula can be utilized, occasionally with the epiphyseal plate to minimize limb discrepancy in growing patients. Rotationplasty can be recommended because of good function even in lesions at the femoral diaphysis, neck, or proximal tibia.

Key words: Limb saving surgery—Vascularized fibular graft—Knee and hip rotationplasty

Introduction

Limb saving surgery with the endoprosthesis is not often indicated, especially in growing patients, because of its short durability and because it can lead to limb discrepancy. In cases of this kind, vascularized fibular graft or rotationplasty has been adopted in our department. In the past 3 years, four cases of vascularized fibular grafts and three cases of rotationplasty have been performed among 12 young candidates for malignant bone tumors in our department.

Case Presentation

Case 1. Teleangiectatic osteosarcoma (recurrent IIB) at the right lateral femoral condyle in a 28-year-old female was treated by marginal resection and arthrodesis by a vascularized fibular graft with intramedullary rod fixation. Bony union was observed at 4 months, and the patient was able to walk without support until local recurrence and distant metastasis 3 years after the first operation (Fig. 1a).

---

[1]Department of Orthopaedic Surgery, School of Medicine, University of the Ryukyus, Okinawa, Japan

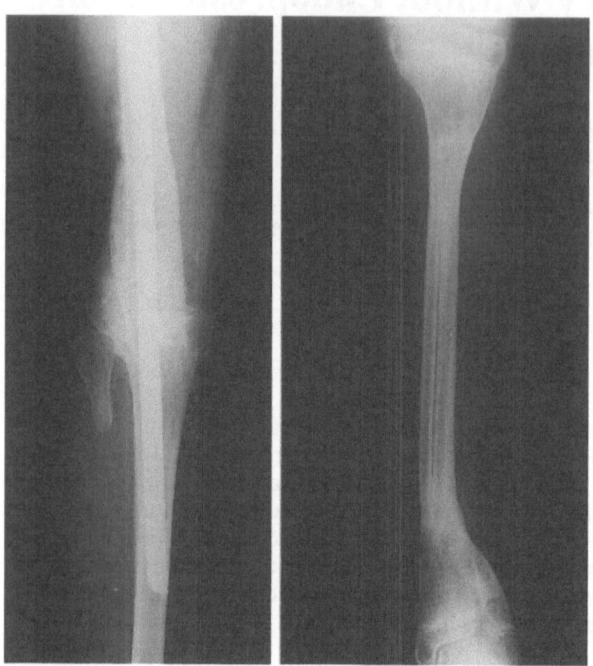

Fig. 1. Vascularized segmental fibular grafts for lower extremity. **a** Case 1, 28-year-old female. Osteosarcoma at right femoral condyle. Vascularized fibular graft with intramedullary rod. **b** Case 2, 10-year-old. Adamantinoma at left tibia. Reconstruction of the whole diaphysis by dual vascularized fibular grafts

Case 2. Adamantinoma at the left tibial diaphysis (IA) in a 10-year-old boy was treated by resection of the whole diaphysis of the tibia and reconstructed by fibular transposition with vascular pedicle. One year later, vascularized fibula from the opposite leg was grafted along with the previous fibula, which showed no sign of hypertrophy. Two years after the first operation, his left knee joint is supple (extension 0°, flexion 110°) and stable, but the ankle joint has a slight valgus deformity (Fig. 1b).

Case 3. Osteosarcoma at the right proximal humerus (IIB) in a 19-year-old boy was treated by wide resection and replacement with a ceramic endoprosthesis. The patient's right shoulder could not be used properly because of pain and anterior subluxation of the prosthesis. So, the ceramic implant was replaced by a vascularized proximal fibular graft. Ten months later, resorption and fragmentation at the grafted fibular head were observed. Exploration revealed no recurrence of the tumor. Although the range of motion is restricted, the shoulder is painless and stable (Fig. 2a, b).

Case 4. Ewing's sarcoma at the right humerus (IIA) in a 5-year-old boy was preoperatively treated by Rosen's T-9 chemotherapy followed by whole bone irradiation. The whole diaphysis of the humerus and surrounding soft tissues was

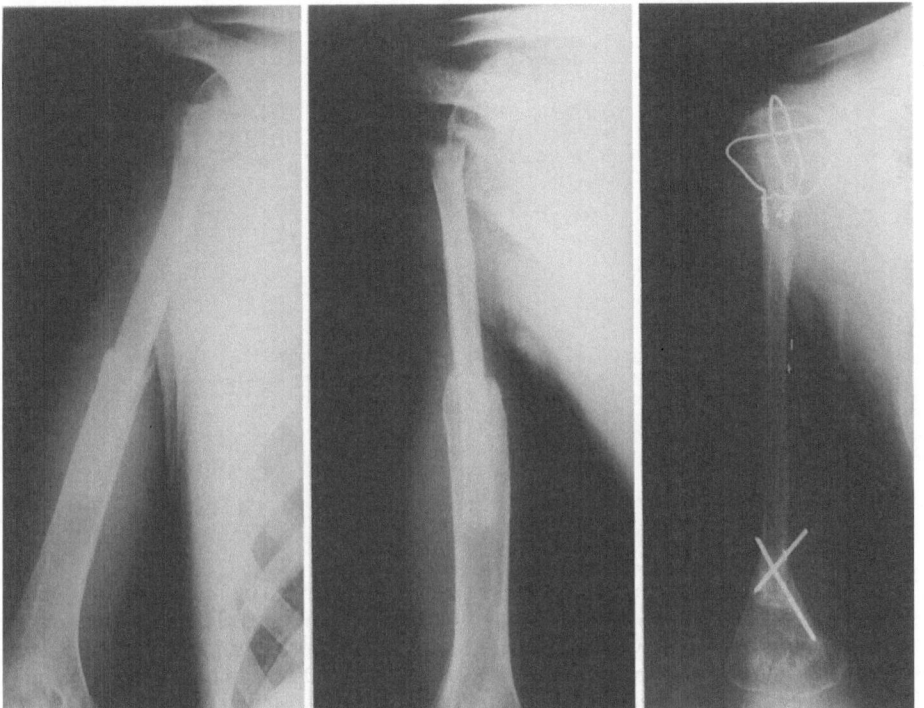

a, b   c

Fig. 2. Vascularized proximal fibular grafts for upper extremity. **a** Case 3 19-year-old boy. Osteosarcoma at right proximal humerus. 4 months after operation. **b** Same patient as in **a**. Resorption and fragmentation of the grafted fibular head were observed at 10 months after operation. **c** Case 4, 5-year-old boy. Ewing's sarcoma at right humeral diaphysis. Vascularized proximal fibula with epiphyseal plate was grafted 7 months after operation

replaced by vascularized proximal fibula with the epiphyseal plate, which was fixed by wires to the preserved humeral head with a rotator cuff. Seven months after the surgery, although bony resorption is observed around the wires, the growth plate still remains open (Fig. 2c).

Case 5. Ewing's sarcoma at the left femoral diaphysis (IIA) in a 10-year-old boy was preoperatively treated by Rosen's T-9 chemotherapy followed by irradiation. The femoral diaphysis was then replaced by an endoprosthesis designed at the Chiba Cancer Center. One year later, the loosened hip screw penetrated the skin, which resulted in a deep infection. The implant was removed and rotation-plasty was performed, preserving the femur above the subtrochanteric region. Although the rotated ankle joint is now 7 cm proximal to the opposite knee joint, the patient can walk with a slight limp without support (Fig. 3a).

Case 6. Osteosarcoma at the left proximal femur (IIB) in a 15-year-old boy was treated by periacetabular and proximal femoral wide resection and followed by

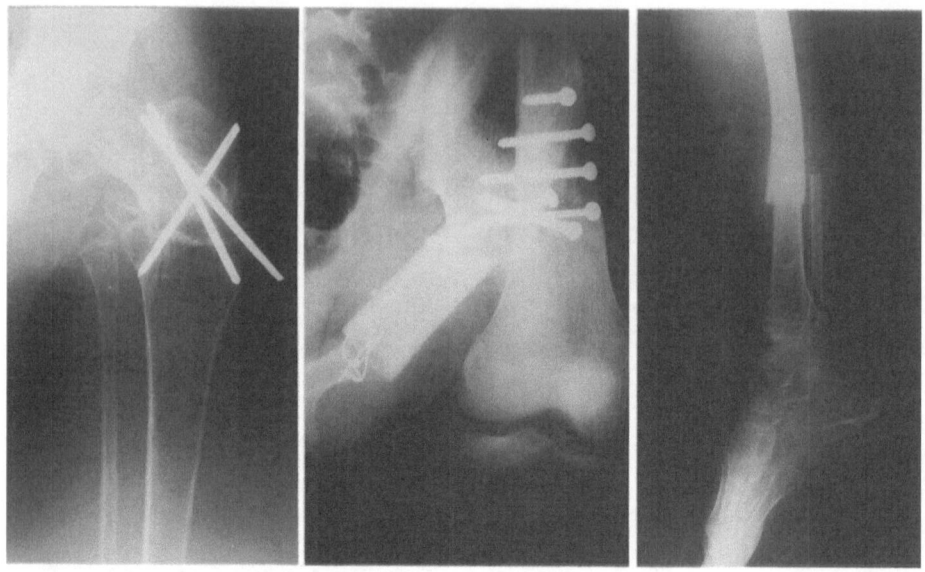

a   **b, c**

Fig. 3. Rotationplasty for lower extremity. **a** case 5, 10-year-old boy. Ewing's sarcoma at left femoral diaphysis. Salvage procedure 1 year after endoprosthetic reconstruction. **b** Case 6, 15-year-old boy. Osteosarcoma at left femoral neck. Primary procedure after periacetabular wide resection. **c** Case 7, 15-year-old boy. Osteosarcoma at left proximal tibia. Salvage procedure 5 years after endoprosthetic reconstruction

hip rotationplasty. The day after surgery, fasciotomy and resection of the avascular muscles were performed since the circulation was disturbed by expanded muscles. However, a large open wound and peroneal nerve palsy remained. One year after surgery, the open wound was closed successfully by a vascularized musculo-cutaneous (M-C) flap of the latissimus dorsi. Although the range of motion in the reconstructed hip is 0°–40° and that in the knee is −15°– 60°, the patient goes to school using a pelvic-supported long-leg brace and a crutch with sufficient weight bearing on the heel (Fig. 3b).

Case 7. Osteosarcoma at the left proximal tibia (IIB) in a 14-year-old boy was treated by wide resection and hemiendoprosthetic replacement. Five years after the first operation, the limb discrepancy became 10 cm and the knee joint was unstable. Since the flexor or extensor muscles of the ankle was well preserved, roationplasty was performed. During surgery, the peroneal was severed because the neurovascular bundles were not identified in the scar tissue. Five months after surgery, the ankle joint was stable and good enough to sustain the weight despite a decreased range of motion of −10°–50° (Fig. 3c).

Discussion

Arthrodesis of the knee joint in high-malignant bone tumors at the distal femur, such as in case 1, has a potential risk if the resectional margin is minimized in order to save the bone stock, as reported [1]. For reconstruction of the whole diaphysis in the lower extremity, such as in case 2, a dual vascularized fibular graft should be performed [2] because hypertrophy of the grafted bone may not be expected after the extensive resection, which is quite different from immediate hypertrophy of a grafted vascularized fibula usually observed in congenital pseudoarthrosis of the tibia [3]. For the reconstruction of the proximal humerus, such as in case 3 or 4, a vascularized fibular graft is perferable to an endoprosthetic implant because of the stability and minimal tissue reactions. The epiphysis of the grafted fibula in case 3 was resorbed although a case of simple fibular graft in the substitute of proximal humerus has been reported with no sign of resorption after 29 years [4]. In growing patients, a vascularized fibular graft with a growth plate, such as in case 4, may not disturb the bone growth and minimize the limb discrepancy. Experimentally, a vascularized fibula with a growth plate in puppies seems to be successful in 60%–80% of cases only if the metaphyseal nutrient artery is preserved J.R. Urbaniak, personal communication. In rotationplasty after resection of the femur below the subtrochanteric region, such as in case 5, the ankle joint is positioned several centimeters above the opposite knee. However, the function of the limb with a brace is as good as in rotationplasty in lesions of the distal femur. Hip rotationplasty, such as in case 6, has an advantage of stability in the reconstructed hip with less Trendelenburg limping when a long leg brace is applied. However, the range of motion in a reconstructed hip joint may be limited, as previously reported [5]. In rotationplasty of lesions of the proximal tibia, as reported in a few cases [6], at least the gastrocnemius and anterior tibial muscles have to be preserved to maintain the function of the ankle joint; moreover, a sufficiently wide margin at the proximal tibia is often difficult to preserve [1] because the neurovascular bundles are close to the tibia or fibula.

Once reconstruction in malignant bone tumors by vascularized fibular graft or rotationplasty has been performed successfully, life-long durability and function are almost certain. The problem of limb discrepancy can be solved by knee or hip rotationplasty for the lower extremities, or by a vascularized fibular graft with the epiphyseal plate for the upper extremities, although the latter is not well proven.

References

1. Enneking WF (1983) Musculoskeletal tumor surgery Churchill Livingstone, New York, pp 680–684
2. Okubo K, Murota K, Tomita Y (1985) Dual free vascularized fibula grafts for treatment of large bone defect of the femur. Seikeigeka 36: 917–926
3. Tamai S et al. (1980) Vascularized fibular transplantation. Int J Microsurg 2: 205–212
4. Clark K (1959) A case of replacement of the upper end of the humerus by a fibular graft reviewed after twenty-nine years. J Bone Joint Surg 41B: 365–368
5. Winkelmann WW (1986) Hip rotation-plasty for malignant tumors of the proximal part of the femur. J Bone Joint Surg 68A: 362–369
6. Ramach W, Kotz R, Salzer N, Knahr K, Sekera J (1983) The rotation-plasty for osteosarcoma of the knee region. Second workshop on the design and application of tumor prosthesis for bone and joint reconstruction. Vienna, pp 27–29

Chondrocyte Viability and Cryopreservation of Frozen Osteochondral Allografts

Michael G. Rock[1]

Summary. Osteochondral allograft transplantation has met with varied success due in large part to the lack of ongoing viability of articular cartilage. Methods have been developed to maximize the viability, the current cryopreservative of choice being dimethyl sulfoxide. However, no time frame has ever been defined in musculoskeletal transplantation during which the tissue should optimally be used, maximizing chondrocyte viability and cartilage function. Therefore, we embarked on a research project sacrificing patellae from multiorgan transplant donors and subjecting them to biomechanical and biochemical testing as well as chondrocyte viability as tested by scintography and culturing techniques. From our results, the matrix as assessed by biomechanical and biochemical testing does not alter during 3 months of being subjected to −80°C and subjected to the storage techniques recommended by the Musculoskeletal Branch of the American Association of Tissue Banks. Furthermore, dimethyl sulfoxide had no apparent influence on the matrix proper and when assessing chondrocyte viability did not seem to encourage more cellular viability than simple saline. Chondrocyte viability could be maintained for 2 weeks at −80°C, after which the viability dropped off precipitously.

We, therefore, have been capable of defining a time frame—within the first 2 weeks—in which chondrocyte viability persists after procurement from multiorgan transplant donors and being kept at −80°C. Thereafter the chondrocyte, being maintained within the matrix composite, no longer has the capacity to produce type II hyaline cartilage. We also shed doubt on the efficacy of dimethyl sulfoxide as a cryopreservative: There does not appear to be any statistical difference in the integrity of the matrix or capacity of the chondrocyte to maintain viability with the use of dimethyl sulfoxide. We, therefore, encourage orthopedic surgeons interested in *osteochondral* reconstruction to utilize the tissue within 2 weeks of procurement.

Key words: Allograft—Osteochondral—Chondrocyte—Viability of tumor cells—Biomechanical analysis—Biochemical examination

Introduction

The continued use of prosthetic implants in articulating segments after reconstruction for tumor has been fostered by the inconsistent and variably successful transplantation of osteochondral allografts [1]. The ultimate success of articular cartilage transplantation depends on several critical factors. The chondrocytes

---

[1] University of Western Ontario, London, Ontario, Canada

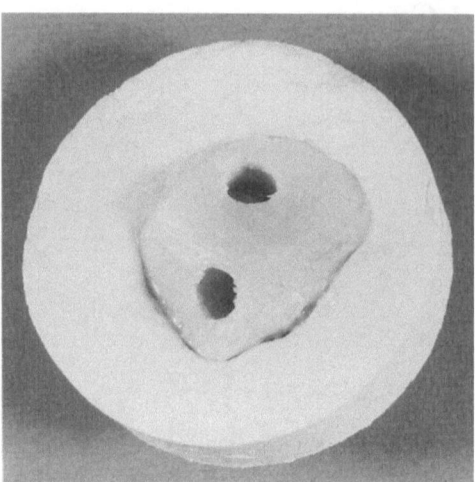

Fig. 1. Patella mounted in PMMA
allowing retrieval of osteochondral
plugs in a predetermined sequence

must survive the process of freezing and maintenance at −70°–80°C and survive
transplantation with the capacity to continue to produce type II collagen. The
matrix should also be biomechanically adequate to sustain normal joint function
and the host should have sufficient proprioception to minimize undetected
repetitive injury. Finally, the allograft should ideally anatomically replace the
resected articulating segment. The use of fresh osteochondral allografts may
address the chondrocyte and matrix viability, but in the vast majority of situations necessary for musculoskeletal reconstruction the use of fresh allografts is
not feasible, necessitating the use of forzen tissue. The need to preserve cartilage
and bone for subsequent use is therefore well recognized. Extensive research has
been conducted by Tomford [2] and Mankin et al. [1] in determining the opti-
mum means with which to maintain this tissue. Given that the majority of
osteochondral segments utilized for orthopedic surgeons would be subject to
such storage, we feel that it is important to define the cartilage integrity and
viability at various stages from procurement. At present, there are time frames
within which various body parts should be utilized for transplantation. No such
time frame exists for osteochondral tissue.

We thought it sufficiently important to address this issue and to assess present
cryopreservative means as to its efficacy and to define guidelines for practicing
orthopedic surgeons in the use of articulating allografts to maximize success
upon transplantation. This is particularly important in light of increasing tenden-
cies among orthopedic surgeons to prefer biological tissue over large metallic or
ceramic implants.

Materials and Methods

At University Hospital, we are fortunate in having a very prolific transplant
service, affording the opportunity of obtaining osteochondral tissue 12–15 times
a year. At the same time of procuring long bone and pelvis, we also obtained

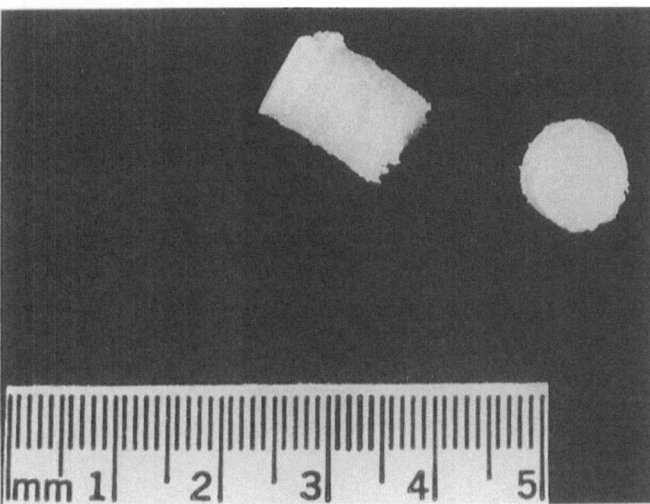

Fig. 2. Osteochondral plugs obtained with intact cartilage, subchondral and medullary bone

both patellae from the donor for research purposes. The donor patellae were acceptable only if the articular cartilage exhibited no evidence of degeneration or stage zero chondromalacia, as defined by Bentley [3]. The thrust of this research project was to look at matrix and chondrocyte integrity at varying stages of being subject to $-70°-80°$C as well as assessing the efficacy of dimethyl sulfoxide, the currently proposed cryopreservative of choice. One of the patellae was subjected to 10% dimethyl sulfoxide (DMSO) for 30 min, whereas the other was submersed in saline. The patellae were then removed, mounted in polymethyl methacrylate to allow for easy retrieval of osteochondral plugs, utilizing a trephine within a trephine instrument. This allowed us to obtain articulating cartilage, subchondral bone, and cancellous bone of the patellae all in continuity. At the same time, we also obtained full-thickness cartilage specimens from the periphery of the trephine defect for biochemical assay. Therefore, at the time of procurement, full-thickness osteochondral plugs were removed from the patellae, one subjected to DMSO and the other to saline, upon which immediate biochemical and biomechanical testing was conducted. The remainder of the patellae were wrapped appropriately in sterile bandages, kept at 4°C for 18 h and then transferred to a deep freezer, as recommended by the Musculoskeletal Branch of the American Association of Tissue Banks. At 2, 6, and 12 weeks, the patellae were removed and under sterile conditions, osteochondral plugs and full-thickness cartilage specimens were obtained in similar fashion from both patellae with subsequent repeating of the biochemical and biomechanical testing. Therefore, at the conclusion of the study, we could effectively compare matrix composition and function as well as chondrocyte function and viability at the time of procurement, 2 weeks, 6 weeks, and 12 weeks, assessing specifically the effect of deep-freeze conditions as well as assessing the efficacy of DMSO as a cryopreservative.

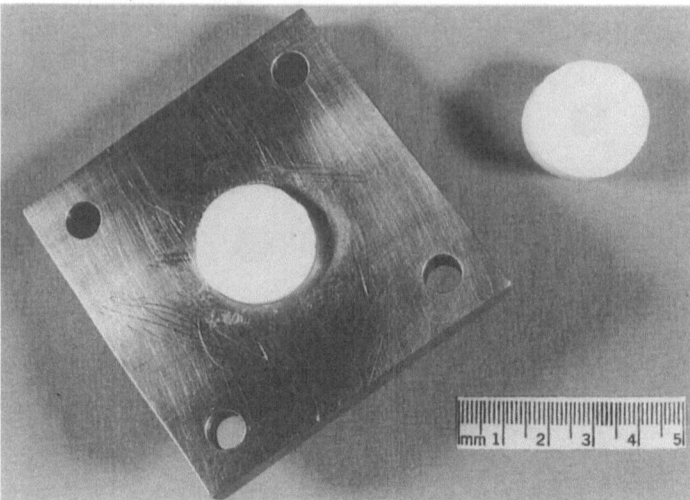

Fig. 3. Osteochondral plugs embedded in PMMA to allow the articular cartilage to be at perpendicular to the needle and plunger on the material testing system for calculation of cartilage depth and creep rate

Biomechanical Tests

The thickness of the cartilage was determined by deflection of a fine needle on the materials testing system (MTS). Three measurements of thickness were determined for each specimen to give an average cartilage thickness. The depth of the cartilage and its accurate calculation was instrumental in determining what we term the "creep rate," defined as the rate of change of percent indentation between 20% and 35%. We believe this more truly represents the viscoelastic response of cartilage to indentation, being smaller with normal cartilage and increasing with increasing cartilage softness or indentability. This creep rate was calculated with a specimen mounted in polymethyl methacrylate and subjected to uniaxial indentation tests on an MTS, using a 4-mm-diameter stainless steel indenter and a constant load of 50 N. The creep rate was, therefore, calculated for each of the ten pairs of patellae at times zero, 2, 6, and 12 weeks.

Biochemical Tests

The full-thickness cartilage specimens removed at the above-mentioned times were then prepared for quantitation of glycosaminoglycan hexosamine. Each specimen was finely chopped, allowed to dry thoroughly, and then weighed on a Mettler microgramatic balance. After the samples were dried, they were digested at 60°C for 18–24 h in a solution of 1% papain plus 0.05 M EDTA and 0.005 M cysteine. A 10% trichloracetic acid solution was then added to the digested cartilage and cooled at 4°C for 2 h, centrifuged at 2500 rpm for 45 min to precipitate out unwanted protein. A 95% ethanol and 5% potassium acetate solution was then added to the supernatant and cooled at −20°C for 8 h, then

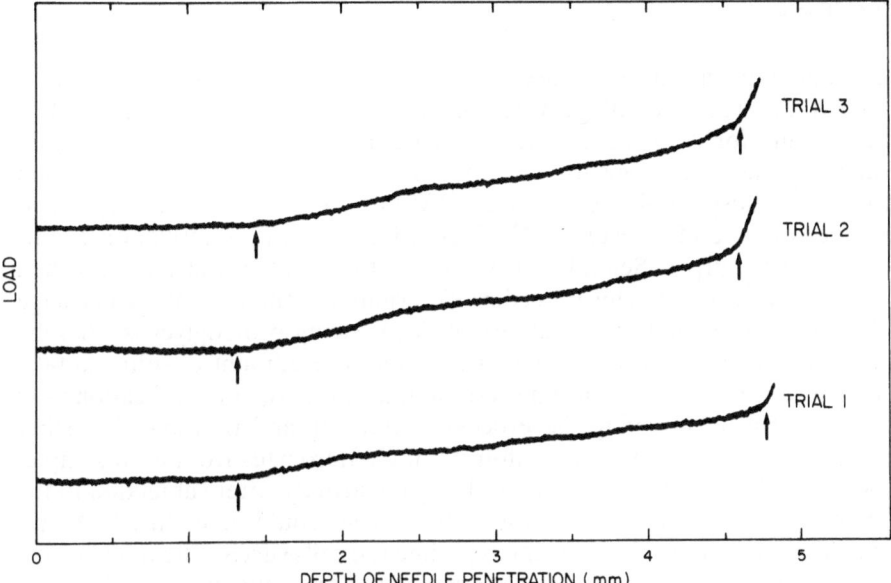

Fig. 4. Calculation of cartilage depth

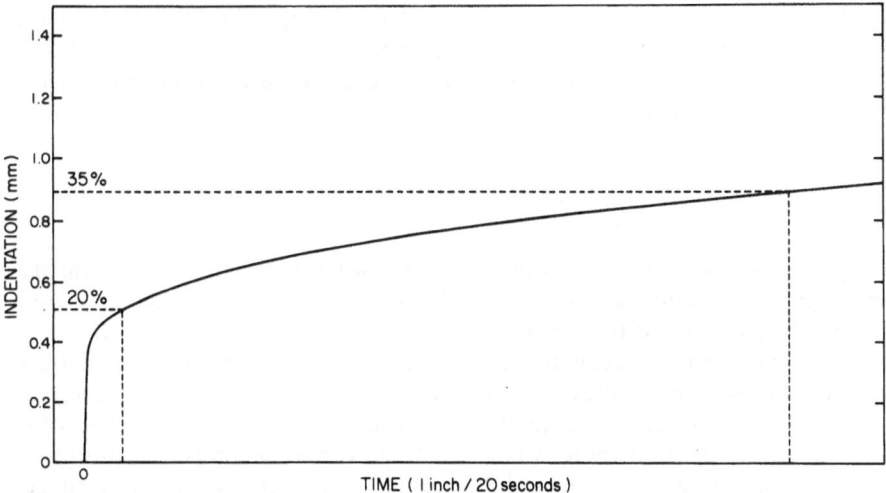

Fig. 5. Calculation of creep rate

centrifuged to obtain glycosaminoglycan samples. Quantitation of glycosamino-glycan hexosamine was performed according to the method described by Smith and Gilkerson [4].

By assessing both the biomechanical and biochemical properties as mentioned above, we feel we adequately assessed the matrix composition and function of the ten specimens in the DMSO-treated and -untreated group.

Viability Tests

At the same time as the sequences already mentioned, samples of DMSO-treated and -nontreated cartilage were obtained and placed in culture Hams F12 culture medium for 24 h. After this 24-h conditioning, 50 mCi sodium sulfate were added to these solutions for 4 h. The samples were then removed, washed three times in phosphate-buffered saline (PBS) to remove any nonincorporated radioactive sulfur, and digested in NCS (solution for liquid scintillation counting, Amersham Corp.). Scintillation fluid was then added and any absorbed radioactivity determined. This procedure determined if the cells of the cartilage stored in the freezer had the capability of synthesizing proteoglycans, thereby indicating at least some level of cellular survival. The amount of sulfur uptake was compared with the initial or time zero sample and gave us an indication as to the number of cells surviving the process of freezing and thawing. A further adjunct to the study involved the culturing of chondrocytes from each sample. This process helped to determine the viability of cartilage after subjection to the cryopreservation and freezing processes. If the cells could be cultured, the results would help to determine the length of time the cells survive the freezing and storage processes. The chondrocytes were isolated from the matrix only at the predetermined times, reflecting more accurately viability as a composite. Isolated chondrocytes subjected to freezing do not clarify the issue of their response in martix to those conditions. The type of collagen produced by the cultured cells was analyzed using the method of O'Driscoll et al. [5]. The main reason for culturing the chondrocytes was to determine their viability after storage with and without cryopreservative at $-70°-80°C$ and to determine the time frame over which this viability occurs.

Results

Tables 1–4 show the results of biomechanical testing of the intact osteocartilaginous plugs and biochemical testing on the same specimens in the same time frames. With reference to the creep rate, one can see that apart from the individual variations among specimens the average values are relatively unchanged from the time of procurement, i.e., time zero, through times 2, 6, and 12 weeks. This was subjected to statistical analysis and there was no significant variation noted. It is of interest that there was virtually no difference between the specimen treated with DMSO and those that were not. Similarly, when the results of the hexosamine concentration noted in Tables 3 and 4 are examined, there is no statistical difference between specimens at the time of procurement and those taken at various stages up to 3 months after subjection to $-80°C$. The presence or application of DMSO made absolutely no difference. This would argue in favor of no alteration in the matrix utilizing standard bone banking principles over a 3-month time frame of maintaining the tissue at $-80°C$. Furthermore, the lack of any beneficial effect of DMSO is not entirely unexpected. The benefit of the DMSO may rest in its capacity to maintain the chondrocyte viability and not necessarily the matrix itself.

Table 1. Creep rate in specimens treated without dimethyl sulfoxide

Specimen	Weeks			
	0	2	6	12
1	0.082	0.053	0.055	0.052
2	0.173	0.233	0.073	0.054
3	0.052	XXX	0.026	0.076
4	0.070	0.033	0.056	0.028
5	0.347	0.097	0.111	0.117
6	0.231	0.021	0.025	0.037
7	0.029	0.059	0.057	0.057
8	0.034	0.024	XXX	0.065
9	0.073	0.061	0.098	0.115
10	0.082	0.045	0.155	0.133
Average	0.117	0.070	0.073	0.073
SD	0.102	0.065	0.042	0.036

XXX specimen destroyed

Table 2. Creep rate in specimens treated with dimethyl sulfoxide

Specimen	Weeks			
	0	2	6	12
1	0.082	0.050	0.182	0.102
2	0.110	0.298	0.099	0.057
3	0.141	0.040	0.038	0.060
4	0.095	0.547	0.085	0.253
5	0.155	0.195	0.229	0.547
6	0.054	0.012	0.019	0.022
7	0.048	0.030	0.039	0.046
8	0.025	0.027	0.021	0.022
9	0.085	0.061	0.074	0.060
10	0.101	0.073	0.061	0.056
Average	0.090	0.133	0.085	0.123
SD	0.040	0.171	0.070	0.163

Viability Testing

We have been able to determine that chondrocyte viability maintained in the composite matrix environment can continue to show viability for up to 2 weeks of being subjected to −80°C. The specimens taken at 6 and 12 weeks do not show any acitivity nor can they be cultured. In the specimens tested to date, this has consistently been the case, indicating continued viability of the chondrocytes for 2 weeks after procurement at −80°C. We further compared the rate of viability among cells treated with DMSO and those that were not. There did not appear to be any statistical significance between the two subgroups. Compared

Table 3. Hexosamine concentration in specimens treated without dimethyl sulfoxide

Specimen	Weeks			
	0	2	6	12
1	41.0	46.5	47.4	60.6
2	39.3	38.2	42.9	54.5
3	49.9	60.9	66.5	40.3
4	53.2	58.0	51.7	47.4
5	39.5	54.3	51.7	33.5
6	35.0	38.0	41.0	51.3
7	42.2	59.2	60.9	60.5
8	57.1	61.4	XXX	48.5
9	53.1	49.1	50.3	58.2
10	38.6	57.6	68.0	70.2
Average	44.9	52.3	53.4	52.5
SD	7.68	8.92	9.72	10.7

XXX specimen destroyed

Table 4. Hexosamine concentration in specimens treated with dimethyl sulfoxide

Specimen	Weeks			
	0	2	6	12
1	40.3	49.8	48.1	41.6
2	43.0	27.8	50.1	XXX
3	39.4	45.9	59.0	48.9
4	41.7	58.0	65.9	39.1
5	36.1	57.9	38.8	33.5
6	41.3	52.3	41.5	59.1
7	39.7	35.1	40.5	71.9
8	63.8	65.1	73.5	30.7
9	57.4	58.0	61.5	61.3
10	58.2	64.7	58.3	58.4
Average	44.2	51.5	53.7	49.4
SD	12.4	12.2	11.7	14.1

XXX specimen destroyed

with the time zero sample, 80%–100% cellular activity was noted. We then proceeded to identify the cartilage that was being cultured within that first 2-weeks and confirmed that it was type II articulating cartilage.

Discussion

We have by this research endeavor attempted to answer and define some of the parameters that may allow osteochondral transplantation with anticipated success. We have addressed the issue of chondrocyte viability, concluding that the matrix biomechanically and biochemically do not alter significantly over at least the first 3 months from procurement while being subjected to $-80°C$. The viability of the articulating chondrocytes, however, drops off precipitously at 2 weeks which is commensurate with soft tissue transplantation (D. Jackson, S. Arnocksy, personal communication). It would appear, therefore, that the chondrocytes within the matrix will continue to be viable and continue to have the capacity of producing type II collagen from 2 weeks from the time of procurement, with this capacity dropping off precipitously at that time. This would certainly introduce another spectrum to osteochondral transplantation in allowing utilization of this tissue within the first 2 weeks, recognizing the distinct possibility of cartilage viability during that time. This would afford the orthopedic surgeon additional time for further investigation, staging, and more elective planning procedures for reconstruction than is presently possible with fresh osteochondral transplantation.

What is possibly disconcerting is the lack of effect from the DMSO. In none of the studies performed to date does there appear to be any benefit or detrimental effect with its use. However, we are at the point now of reevaluating its use in the routine storage of osteochondral tissue. Possible evaluation of other cryopreservative agents may be indicated.

What we have not addressed in this study are two additional parameters that may be as important as the viability question in allowing success upon transplantation. These are the congruity between host and allograft, particularly when it comes to articulating segments. We know from unipolar replacement of proximal femoral fractures that any alterations in size exceeding 1 mm markedly alters the biomechanical dynamics of the articulation. Therefore, efforts should be directed toward maximizing congruity between the allograft and recipient and the means with which to do this is to encourage computer-directed assisted digitalization of the implant to coordinate with the recipient. The other parameter is lack of proprioception in the transplanted tissue. If para-articular soft tissues can be preserved to some degree and if one of the articulations is that of the host then possible appreciation of proprioception and pain preservation can be maintained.

References

1. Mankin HJ, Doppeli SM, Sullivan RT, Tomford WM (1982) Osteoarticular and intercalary allograft transplantation in the management of malignant tumors of bone. Cancer 50: 156–164
2. Tomford WW (1983) Cryopreservation of articular cartilage. In: Friedlaender GE, Mankin HS, Sell KS (eds) Biology, banking and chemical applications. Little Brown, Boston
3. Bentley G (1970) Chondromalacia patella. J Bone Joint Surg 52A: 221–232
4. Smith RL, Gilkerson E (1979) Quantitation of glycosaminoglycan hexosamine using 3 methyl-2-benzothiazolone hydrazone hydrochloride. Anal Biochem 98: 478–480
5. O'Driscoll SW, Salter RB, Keeley FW (1985) A method for quantitative analysis of ratios of types I and II collagen in small samples of articular cartilage. Anal Biochem 145: 277–285

Limb Salvage and Massive Segmental Allograft Replacement for Malignant or Aggressive Bone Tumors After Wide Resection

Sachio Masuda, Yoichi Sugioka, Masahiro Ushijima, and Norio Shinohara[1]

Summary. Between September 1957 and January 1985, 20 patients with active, aggressive, or malignant bone tumors were treated in our clinic by radical resection of the tumor and massive segmental allograft replacement. There were 12 men and eight women and the ages ranged from 8–48 years (mean 27.7 years). Follow-up ranged from 28 months to 27 years (mean 13.2 years) for the 18 survivors. Eight of the twenty had giant cell tumors. Four patients had central osteosarcomas and two chondrosarcomas. In 16 of the 20 receiving the allografts (stored at $-20°$--$40°C$), the bones were trimmed as required and fixed in place using an intramedullary rod, screw, or by plating after resection. In four others, freeze-dried allografts were set up, using the same method. Results were graded as excellent, good, fair, or poor, according to Enneking's system for functional evaluation. Fourteen (77.8%) had successful transplants (graded excellent or good), four had tumor-related complications, and nine (45.0%) had complications unrelated to the tumor. In four (20%) there was a failure of union at the junction and allograft fracture occurred in three (15.0%) of the twenty. Thus, recurrence and rates of complications for high-grade lesions (stage IIB) were high.

Key words: Wide resection—Limb salvage—Massive allograft

Introduction

Wide en bloc resection is an acceptable alternative to amputation for the management of low-grade sarcomas of bone and giant cell tumor, which sometimes takes on the form of a local aggressive tumor [1]. This technique is now considered to be an alternative to amputation for osteosarcoma, as the tumor-free margin is enhanced by preoperative chemotherapy [2]. The margin for resection can be determined preoperatively in all cases by correlating the extent of the tumor demonstrated by roentgenography, angiography, bone scanning, and computerized tomography. Wide resection for limb salvage is not a new concept. Phemister [3] advocated local resection followed by bone graft reconstruction and this has been followed by more advanced techniques for treating a tumor in the extremities, and reconstruction by autologous transplants, allografts, or prosthetic replacement. Although autogenous grafts seem to be the treatment of

---

[1] Department of Orthopedic Surgery, Faculty of Medicine, Kyushu University, Fukuoka, Japan

choice for complete restitution of a small defect, the resulting large segments of bone require for stability a combination of long cortical grafts and cancellous grafts to stimulate osteogenesis.

Materials and Methods

Between September 1957 and January 1985, 20 patients with active, aggressive, or malignant bone tumors were treated in our clinic by radical resection of the tumor and massive segmental allograft replacement. There were 12 men and eight women and the ages ranged from 8 to 48 years (mean 27.7 years). Follow-up ranged from 28 months to 27 years (mean 13.2 years) for the 18 survivors. Prior to surgery, roentgenography, tomography, angiography, bone scanning, and/or computerized tomography were used. Eight of the twenty had giant cell tumors, two of the eight were recurrences following ineffective surgical treatment, and the other six had an expansile lytic lesion with a pathological fracture. Four patients had central osteosarcomas and one parosteal osteosarcoma. Two patients had chondrosarcomas, all with cortical destruction and soft tissue extension. In two patients, a fibrous dysplasia was evident. The one malignant fibrous histiocytoma was located in the proximal humerus and the one benign osteoblastoma was located in the iliac bone. There were numerous spotty calcific areas in the radiolucent lesion. One patient had a mono-ostotic metastasis of follicular carcinoma of the thyroid gland in the proximal humerus. According to the system for staging benign and malignant musculoskeletal lesions, fibrous dysplasia, osteoblastoma, or giant cell tumor with an active or aggressive behavior were in stage II–III. Malignant fibrous histiocytoma was stage IIA, chondrosarcomas and osteosarcomas were stage IIB, and the parosteal osteosarcoma was stage IB. In 16 of the 20 patients, the allograft bones (stored at $-20°--40°C$) were trimmed as required and fixed in place, using an intramedullary rod, screw, or by plating after resecting the lesion. Included in this group were four distal femora, four distal radii, four proximal humeri, two proximal tibiae, one femoral shaft, and one pelvic bone. In four other patients, freeze-dried allografts were set up using the same method and included two proximal tibiae, one tibial shaft, and one pelvic bone.

Results and Discussion

Of the 20 patients receiving an allograft replacement, 18 were followed and a comprehensive end result analysis was made (Table 1). In one of these eighteen, a distant metastasis occurred 15 months after surgery and the patient died 42 months postoperatively. The results were graded as excellent, good, fair, or poor, according to Enneking's system for functional evaluation. Fourteen (77.8%) had successful transplants (graded excellent or good) and were able to live a normal life (Fig. 1). In four patients, three malignant bone tumors and one giant cell tumor led to tumor-related complications, and in three there was a local recurrence of the tumor. In one, a distant metastasis became evident. Nine patients (45.0%) had complications unrelated to tumor recurrence or dissemina-

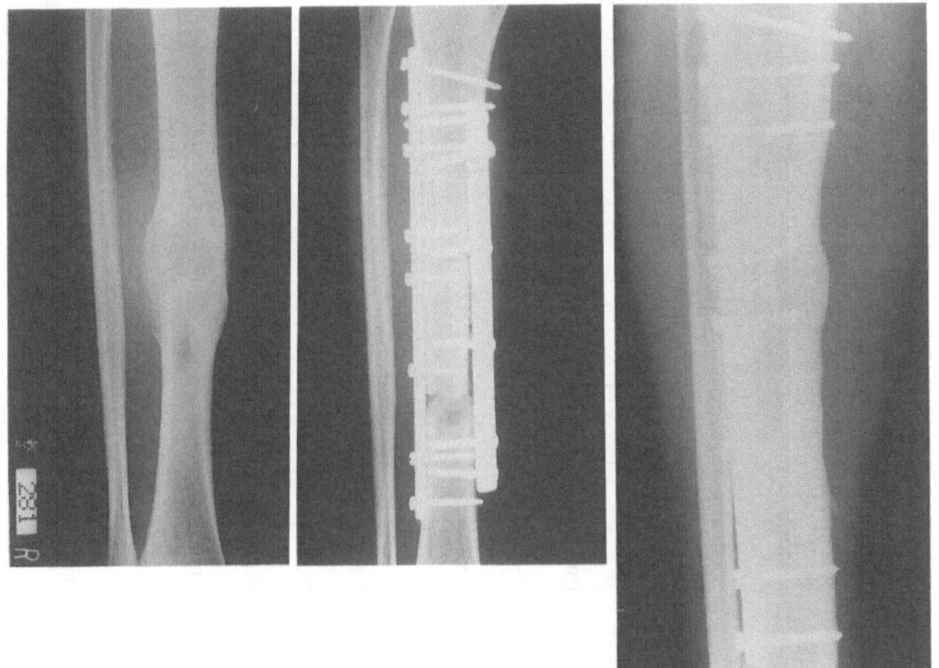

Fig. 1a–c. A 36-year old man **a** with a fibrous dysplasia of the tibial shaft was treated with **b** segmental resection and freeze-dried allograft replacement (b). **c** Fourteen years after surgery there is firm incorporation of the graft

tion; four had to undergo reoperation, including two for whom secondary autogenic grafting procedures had to be done for a nonunion and marked resorption of the grafts. In four (20%), there was a failure of union at the graft-host junction (Fig. 2). One was revised to a custom prosthesis due to a local recurrence and no others required a second graft or plating of the nonunion site. Fracture of the allograft occurred in three (15.0%) of the twenty, only after union of both graft junctions (Fig. 3). One patient underwent additional surgery with reinsertion of the autograft.

The range in time of development of fractures was 4–31 months. Allograft fracture seemed to occur frequently in cases of a rapid heeling. These cases of nonunion or fracture were always accompanied by extensive resorption of the graft. One infection occurred 5 months later in a patient who underwent a freeze-dried allografting. Partial removal of the allograft and autografting led to good results. According to the staging system advocated by Enneking [4], 11 cases in our series were stage II–III (stages of benign musculoskeletal lesions). Seven (excluding solitary metastatic bone carcinoma) were considered to be stage IIA or IIB (high-grade lesions). Thus, the recurrence and complication rates for stage IIB lesions (six cases) were high. Massive segmental allografting offers an effective alternative to reconstruction after tumor resection [1, 2, 5]. However, the number of complications and the necessity of reoperation after

Table 1. Massive segmental allografting

Case	Age (yrs)	Sex	Diagnosis	Stage[a]	Site and type of graft	Complications, disposition	End result[b]	Length of follow-up
1	45	M	Giant cell tumor	3	Dist. femur, frozen bone	Recurrence, amputation		27 yrs
2	31	M	Giant cell tumor	3	Dist. radius, frozen bone arthrodesis	(−)	Good	21 yrs
3	19	M	Parosteal osteo-sarcoma	IB	Dist. femur, frozen bone	(−)	Excellent	19 yrs
4	40	M	Giant cell tumor	2	Dist. radius	Nonunion, autograft	Good	19 yrs
5	29	M	Giant cell tumor	3	Prox. tibia, frozen bone	Instability	Good	17 yrs
6	16	M	Fibrous dysplasia	2	Tibial shaft, freeze-dried	Infection, autograft	Excellent	15 yrs
7	36	M	Fibrous dysplasia	2	Tibial shaft, freeze-dried	(−)	Excellent	15 yrs
8	37	F	Giant cell tumor	2	Prox. tibia, freeze-dried	(−)	Good	14 yrs
9	48	M	Benign osteo-blastoma	3	Iliac bone, freeze-dried arthrodesis	(−)	Good	13 yrs
10	15	M	Chondrosarcoma	IIB	Pubic bone, frozen bone	Recurrence, autograft	Excellent	13 yrs
11	36	F	Giant cell tumor	2	Dist. radius, frozen bone	Nonunion	Good	13 yrs
12	13	F	Osteosarcoma	IIB	Dist. radius	Fracture, resorption, autograft	Good	11 yrs
13	8	F	Osteosarcoma	IIB	Dist. femur, frozen bone arthrodesis	Fracture	Fair	3 yrs 6 mos
14	23	M	Chondrosarcoma	IIB	Femoral shaft, frozen bone	Nonunion, recurrence, prosthesis	Poor	4 yrs 4 mos Died of tumor

(Table continued on the following page)

Table 1. (*continued*)

Case	Age (yrs)	Sex	Diagnosis	Stage[a]	Site and type of graft	Complications, disposition	End result[b]	Length of follow-up
15	34	F	Malignant fibrous histiocytoma	IIA	Prox. humerus, frozen bone prosthesis	Nonunion, resorption	Fair	3 yrs 8 mos
16	46	M	Giant cell tumor	3	Dist. femur, frozen bone arthrodesis	(−)	Good	3 yrs 5 mos
17	11	F	Osteosarcoma	IIB	Prox. humerus, frozen bone arthrodesis	Fracture, resorption	Poor	2 yrs 7 mos
18	19	F	Osteosarcoma	IIB	Prox. humerus, frozen bone prosthesis	Recurrence		9 mos Died of tumor
19	19	M	Giant cell tumor	2	Prox. tibia, frozen bone	(−)	Excellent	2 yrs 4 mos
20	54	F	Metastasis of carcinoma		Prox. humerus, frozen bone prosthesis	(−)	Good	2 yrs 6 mos

[a] After Enneking's staging of musculoskeletal tumors
[b] After Enneking's system for functional evaluation

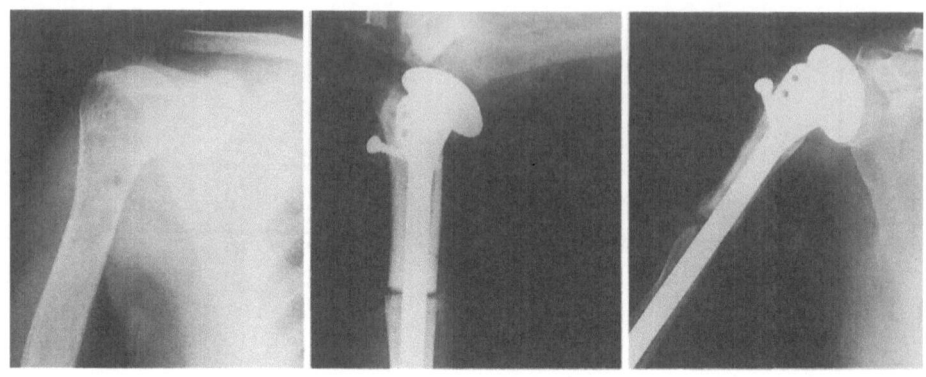

a   b, c

Fig. 2a–c. A 34-year-old woman with **a** a stage IIA malignant fibrous histiocytoma of the proximal humerus was treated with **b** segmental resection, allografting, and prosthesis. **c** Even 2 years later, there was no union of the allograft to the host bone

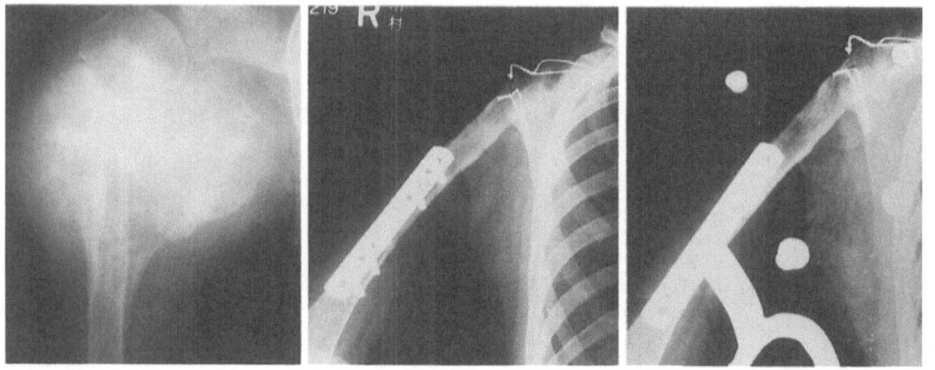

a   b, c

Fig. 3a–c. An 11-year-old girl with stage IIB osteosarcoma of the proximal humerus. **a** Radiogram showing a sclerotic change in the tumor due to the preoperative high-dose methotrexate therapy. **b** Tikhoff-Linberg resection, allografting, and arthrodesis were performed. **c** Fourteen weeks later, there was union of the proximal junction, but fracture, nonunion, and resorption of the graft occurred

initial surgery indicate that the techniques can be improved. In the case of high-grade lesions that require extensive resection and adjuvant chemotherapy, the results can probably be improved by using allograft replacement together with other techniques such as vascularized autografting.

Acknowledgment. This work was supported by a Grant for Cancer Research from The Ministry of Health and Welfare, Japan.

References

1. Alho A, Karraharju EO, Korkala O, Laasonen E (1987) Hemijoint allografts in the treatment of low grade malignant and aggressive bone tumours about the knee. Int

Orthop 11: 35–41
2. Mankin HJ, Doppelt SH, Sullivan TR, Tomford WW (1982) Osteoarticular and intercalary allograft transplantation in the management of malignant tumors of bone. Cancer 50: 613–630
3. Phemister DB (1945) Rapid repair of defect of femur by massive bone graft after resection for tumors. Surg Gynec Obstet 80: 120–127
4. Enneking WF (1986) A system of staging musculoskeletal neoplasms. Clin Orthop 204: 9–24
5. Parrish FF (1973) Allograft replacement of all or part of the end of a long bone following excision of a tumor. J Bone Joint Surg 55-A: 1–22

Megaprosthesis—Massive Osteochondral Allograft

DOMINIQUE POITOUT[1]

Summary. Autologous grafts, unlike allogenic grafts, have an important osteogenic potential. But, in as much as the procurement volume is limited, they do not permit bone or joint reconstruction where there has been partial or total resection as a result of either a bone tumor or a posttraumatic lack of substance. For this reason, we have elected since 1976 to use fresh allogenic bone grafts and since 1981 deep-frozen allogenic grafts to rebuild the skeleton (191 cases, 1976–1986). Deep-freezing alone allows the preservation of voluminous bone pieces in satisfactory conditions of sterilization. This type of preservation keeps the bone architecture in an optimal biological and biomechanical state.

With the bone cells destroyed and the bone being recolonized by the host's own cells, there is no immunological risk of inadequate blood and leukocyte compatibility between donor and recipient. If the bone is to be totally integrated by the skeleton within a few years following the graft, the functional value of the cartilaginous surfaces has to be altered after a massive osteocartilaginous graft.

Ligament grafting and a reconstructive prosthesis surrounded by deep-forzen preserved bone are currently the object of experimental study and the results thus far are encouraging.

When great precautions are taken during the surgical procurement as well as during the grafting intervention (sterility, stability, and appropriate muscular surrounding), the long-term results are excellent in 80%–85% of cases.

Key words: Megaprosthesis—Massive osteochondral allograft—Deep-frozenbone—Bone tumor—Bone reconstruction

The use of preserved bone is not a recent technique and sources even cite Cosme and Damien, who, according to legend, accomplished the transplantation of a leg 1800 years ago on a sacristan of their basilica in Rome. Scientifically speaking, the first published case of bone grafting occurred in Amsterdam in 1810 and was performed by Van Mechren. Although autologous grafts have for some time proven effective, allografts have often been used since 1879 when MacEwen treated a humeral pseudoarthrosis with a fresh graft from an amputated member. Since then, authors have published numerous accounts of long-term positive results.

[1] Service of Orthopedic and Traumatologic Surgery, C.H.U. Nord, Chemin des Bourrely, Marseille, France

Table 1. Fresh and frozen allografts used since 1976

Type	Number
Spongious allografts used for osteotomy	118
Spongious allografts used to Papineau or socket filling	12
Corticospongious allografts used for acetabulum reconstruction	42
Massive osteochondral allografts	6
Massive diaphyseal allografts	2
Massive metaphyso-diaphyseal allografts with prothesis	6
Massive pelvic bone	5

Table 2. Massive allografts used since 1981

Type	Number
Femur	6
Total femoral replacement with two prosthesis	1
Massive diaphyseal allograft	1
Metaphyso-diaphyseal femoral upper part with megaprosthesis	2
External condyle	1
Condyle and trochlea	1
Tibia	7
Massive diaphyseal allograft	1
Tibial articular plate	1
Metaphyso-diaphyseal tibial upper part with megaprosthesis	3
Massive osteochondral grafts of upper part of tibia	2
Humerus	
Massive osteochondral graft of upper part	1
Pelvic bone	5
Pelvic bone with hip prosthesis	2
Iliac bone + half sacrum + vertebra	1
Cotyle with hip prosthesis	1
Pubic bone and half cotyle	1

In Marseille, we have used fresh allografts since 1976; our use of deep-frozen grafts to rebuild the human skeleton dates back to 1981. In the 191 operations of both types performed over the last 10 years, the results have been excellent. The grafts comprising that total are listed in Tables 1 and 2.

The advantages of banking bone are readily apparent. Simplifying the surgeon's task and patient convenience are the most obvious, since a bank offers a surgeon bone material, in varying dimensions and quality, permitting immediate interventions that could not be performed otherwise.

Allograft Biology

Allografts are well incorporated by the skeleton. If osteoid or blood cells (mostly leukocytes) as well as blood vessels and nerves have an inner antigenic potential leading to immunoreaction, the proteinic matrix and the minerals fixed on it become either nonantigenic or less antigenic. Clinically speaking, the reactions are almost nonexistent with the use of massive allografts. In any case, the immunological response is mostly due to blood transfusions, which produce different HLA groups.

When the evolution [1, 5, 6, 8] of autologous and allogenic grafts are compared, no significant differences are noted other than the integration of heavy allografts, which lasts 12–18 months more.

However, the two types of graft become revascularized, the dead bone being replaced by new bone due to creeping apposition. The late times of the sintigraphy are very demonstrative (24 h).

Preservation of Large Osteocartilaginous Pieces

Many methods of preservation have been described since the use of allografting was introduced to orthopedic surgery, but deep-freezing preservation alone seems to be the most effective and problem free. Since 1981, we have worked on *deep-freezing massive cartilaginous swabs in liquid nitrogen* at a temperature of $-196°C$. This method permits indefinite preservation of the entire bone and also maintains the preservation vitality of the osteocartilaginous cells [5, 7–10].

Biomechanical Properties

Because of bone revascularization, the mechanical resistance of cortical allografts attains only 50%–60% that of a normal bone for a period of 8–18 months after grafting. A period of 2–3 years is necessary before the bone returns to its normal biomechanical density and resistance.

The biomechanical properties of allografts can be impaired by the preservation or storage process. Deep-freezing seems to ameliorate allograft mechanical resistance, which reaches 110%–120% of fresh bone resistance. On the other hand, lyophilization and massive irradiation (greater than 3 Mrad) leads to less mechanical resistance of the grafts (55% for lyophilization and 60%–70% for massive irradiation) [6, 7, 9, 11].

Results and Indications

Four types of intervention use allografting, as described below.

Spongious Grafts

In 1982, we published a comparative study of 219 fresh autologous grafts and 71 allografts, showing that the histological, immunological, and clinical development were very similar. Among the autologous grafts, 76% maintained correction of the axle of 4° (range 2°–8°); among homologous grafts, this figure was 69% (range 3°–9°; Table 3).

The time required for consolidation was the same for the two groups and the subsequent radiological examination did not disclose any differences in incorporation.

After this study, we decided to use allografts systematically each time the indication was determined (osteotomy, Papineau, filling up sockets or cysts).

Table 3. Delay of renewal of load

	Autologous grafts before 1979 (%)	Homologous grafts and autologous grafts since 1979 (%)
Partial load		
Week 6	8	15
Week 8	22	52
Week 12	70	95
Total load		
Month 3	5	19
Month 4	25	64
Month 6	75	93

Corticospongious Grafts

This method is employed primarily to rebuild the acetabulum. Between 1981 and 1986, we rebuilt 42 hips with femoral head and neck pieces. To this allografting is added a total hip prosthesis in almost every case. We used an adhesive filling material (cemented) prosthesis rather than the screw type, although we did use the latter in two cases.

The results were excellent, there was no infection, and only one graft crushing after 12 months. The latter occurred in the case of a patient who had undergone 77 surgical interventions in different places and who needed a total acetabulum graft.

Massive Diaphyseal and Epiphysio-Metaphyseal Grafts

Massive diaphyseal or epiphysio-metaphyseal replacement can be achieved with no particular difficulty (centromedullar pinning being one of the most common methods as it leaves the muscular masses close to the graft).

We believe there is a midpoint between massive metal prostheses, sometimes responsible for long-term mechanical problems, and massive osteocartilaginous grafts.

We usually perform both techniques: Massive prostheses surrounded by an allograft. Joint prosthesis has the advantage of avoiding problems like ligamentary laxity (Figs. 1–3).

On the other hand, because of the possibilities it offers in long-term recolonization and quick muscular reinsertion, allografting leads to less hazardous results.

In some particular cases, we chose a massive articular prosthesis surrounded by allografts (one total femoral replacement, six massive prosthesis surrounded by allografts, five massive pelvic bones) [3, 4, 7, 8] of the femur and the tibia.

Osteocartilaginous Grafts

If possible, it is preferable to graft only a thin layer of subchondral tissue and spongy tissue so that chondrocyte nutrition can be given by the synovial fluid as well as epiphyseal neovascularization (Figs. 4–6). If the entire capsule, or the

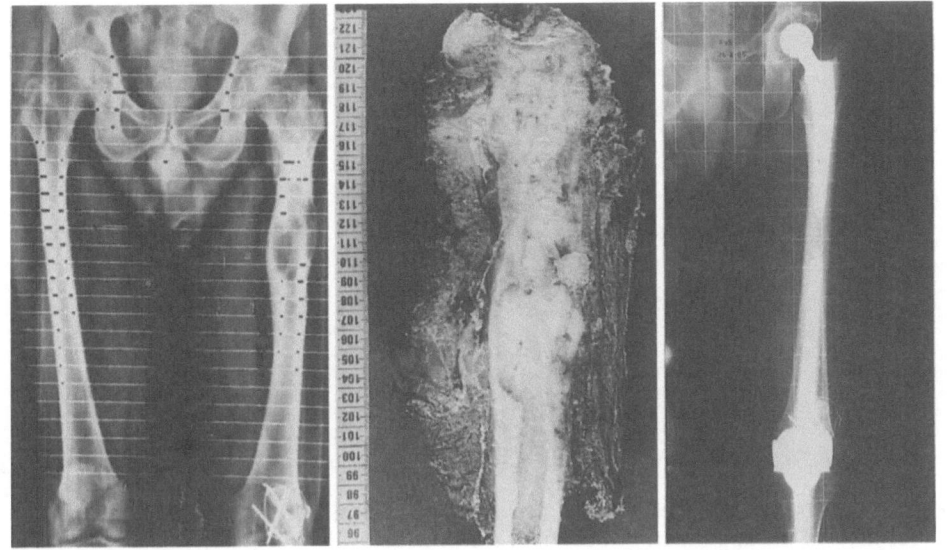

Fig. 1. a Chondrosarcoma of the upper two-thirds of the femur. **b** Total femoral resection. **c** Reconstruction of the whole femur with diaphyso-metaphyseal allograft surrounding upper and lower prosthesis

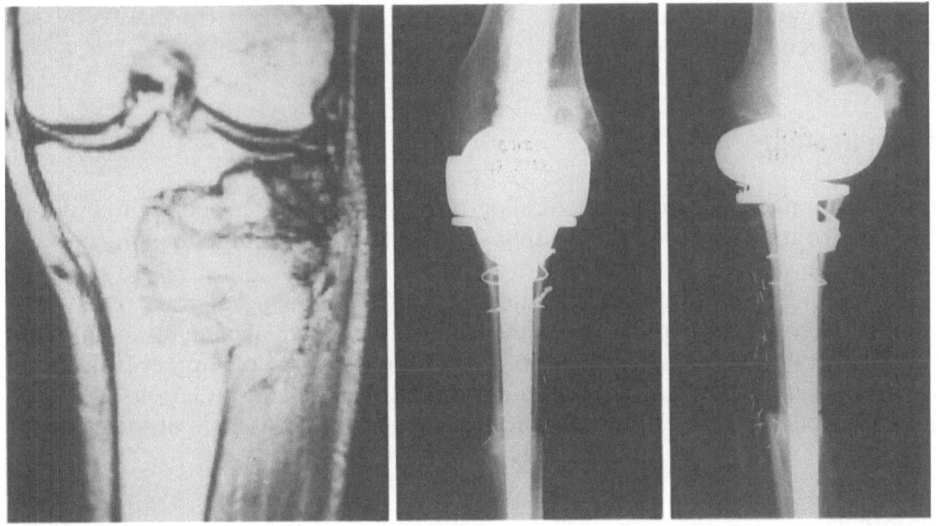

Fig. 2. a Giant cell tumor of the upper end of the tibia with ligamentary and articular obstruction. **b, c** Reconstruction by prosthesis surrounded by massive allograft

majority of it as well as the host's ligaments, can be reinserted on the graft the joint stability is very acceptable (Fig. 7, 8) [2, 3, 5, 6, 12].

If an articular necrosis develops it is painless and may require only a partial replacement of the articular surface by a small prothesis a few years later.

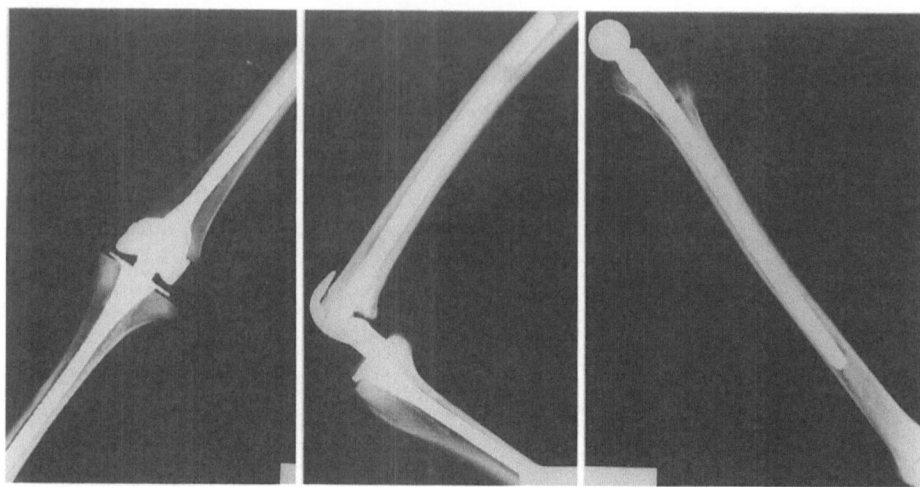

a   b, c

Fig. 3. a, b Massive prosthesis of the knee surrounded by allogenic articospongious graft.
c Prosthesis of the upper part of the femur surrounded by the allograft

There may also be an articular laxity which could justify, in the long term, the use of either a prosthetic ligament or a deep-frozen ligamentary graft. In instances when it is evident that the muscles and ligaments have to be removed, as is often the case in tumors near a joint, it is preferable to use an articular prosthesis surrounded by an allograft. Since 1981, we have performed only six massive osteochondral allografts.

Complications

Complications linked to the use of allografts have been described in great detail by several authors. In fact, the complications actually determine the limits of this surgery.

With the exception of complications due to local tumoral recurrency (the tumoral exeresis having to present the same carcinological value as an amputation), several other complications are inherent to this type of surgery (infection, fracture, joint instability, necrosis and arthrosis, lack of consolidation). According to various statistics, these complications represent 10%–15% of the cases [4, 6, 11].

Infections

By far the most frequent and serious of known complications, infections often lead to amputation or removal of the graft; in cases where the graft can be preserved, the functional results are often less than satisfactory. So far, we have had four cases of sepsis in all our grafting interventions. In 191 cases, this represents 2%. For operations of this nature we normally use betadin as well as local and general antibiotherapy.

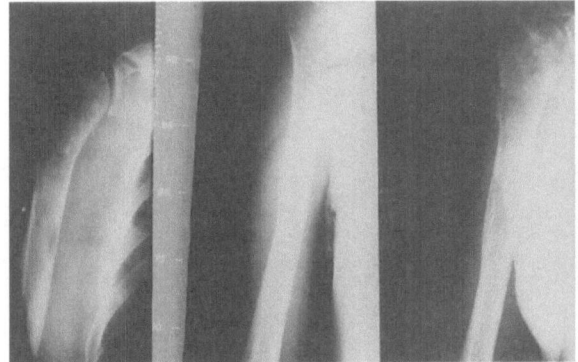

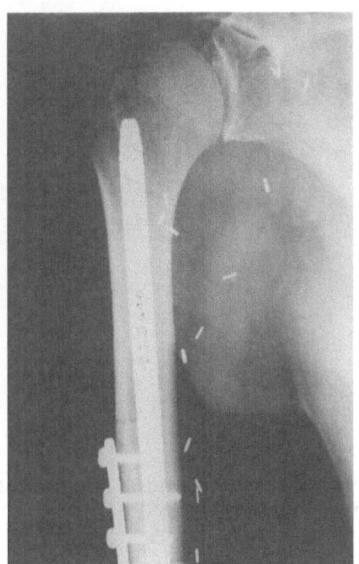

a

Fig. 4. a Chondrosarcoma of the upper end of the
humerus. **b** Allograft of two-thirds of the humerus

b

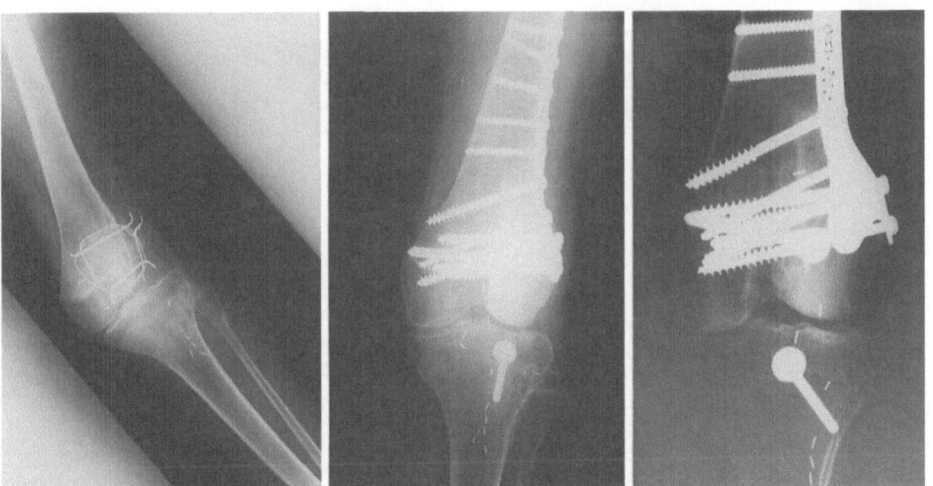

a, b   c

Fig. 5. a Traumatic destruction of the external condylum of the femur. **b** Osteochondral
allograft of the external condylum of the femur. **c** Two years later the graft had been
recolonized and integrated

Fractures

When fractures are observed during the period of graft fragility, the explanation
is frequently found in inadequate osteosynthesis. If fractures occur, they must be
treated like any other normal fracture by being osteosynthetized and surrounded
with autologous grafts. In this manner, they usually consolidate satisfactorily.

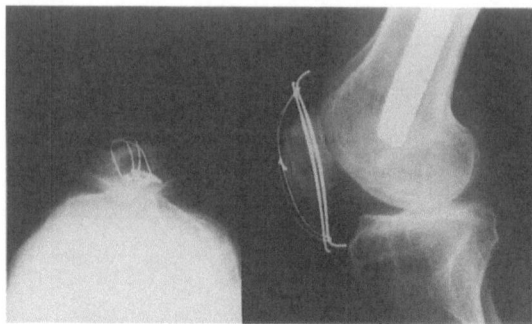
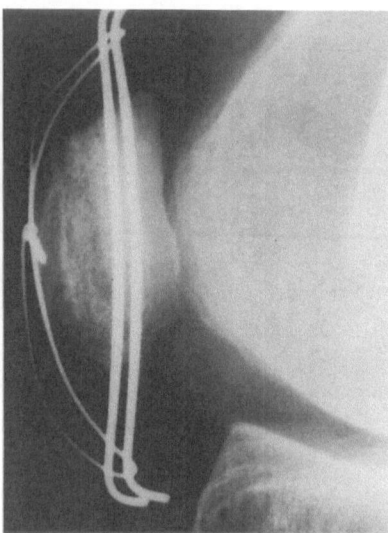

Fig. 6. a Osteochondral allograft of the patella.
b Eight months later

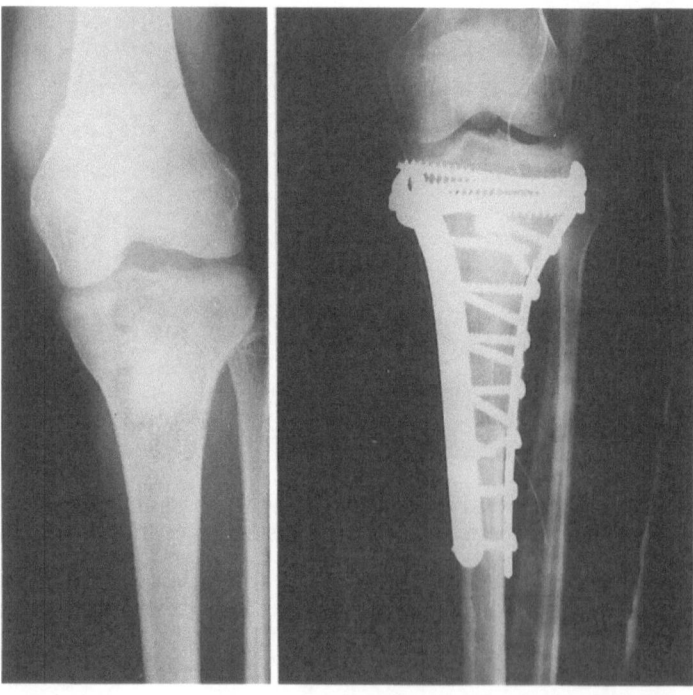

Fig. 7. a Osteogenic sarcoma of the upper end of the tibia. **b** Osteochondral allograft of
the upper end of the tibia

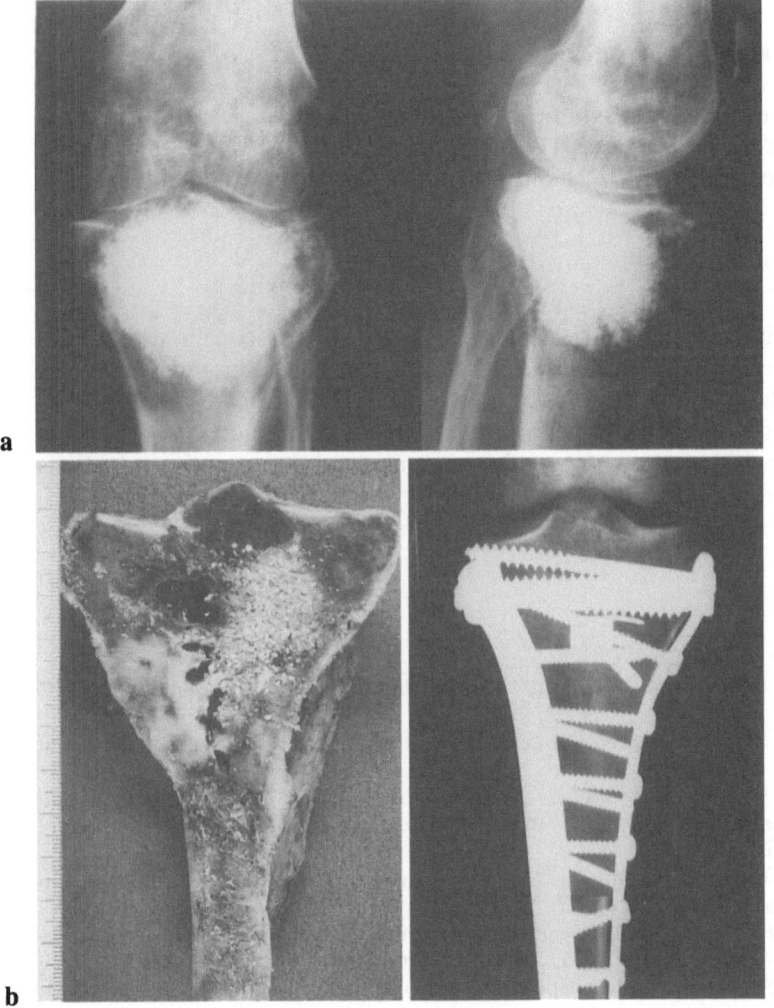

Fig. 8. a Giant cell tumor of the upper end of the tibia. **b** Piece of resection. **c** Reconstruction with osteocartilaginous allograft

Joint Instability

In spite of the problems linked to the fixation of the ligament and capsule of osteocartilaginous grafts, joint instability is exceptional and occurs in less than 5% of the cases. We have had no problems in our cases.

Necrosis and Arthrosis

In almost 80% of the cases, if the histological aspect of the grafted gristle is abnormal, the series having the greatest long-term results do not show surface arthrosis or any other important changes in joint surface morphology until after more than 10 years.

Lack of Consolidation

Lack of consolidation of grafted bone extremities is quite rare. Usually, an average of 8 months' delay is necessary for complete fusion. If after that period consolidation does not occur, fresh autologous tissue has to be added locally.

Conclusion

As a result of this study, based on 191 cases since 1976, we conclude that allografts used to replace a lack of bone substance are well tolerated and incorporated by the skeleton satisfactorily.

The ultimate aim of the orthopedic surgeon and traumatologist is to rebuild the locomotor system partly destroyed by traumatic and degenerative infections and congenital or neoplasic diseases.

The use of osteocartilaginous allogenic grafts assists us in this endeavor.

References

1. Friedlander G (1983) Immune response to osteochondral allografts. Clin Orthop 174: 58–67
2. Gross A, McKee N, Pritzker K, Langer F (1983) Reconstruction of skeletal deficits at the knee. Clin Orthop 174: 96–106
3. Mankin HJ, Doppelt SH, Sullivan TR, Tomford WW (1982) Osteo-articular and intervalary allograft transplantation in the management of malignant tumors of bone. Cancer 50: 613
4. Mankin HJ, Doppelt S, Tomford W (1983) Clinical experience with allograft implantation. Clin Orthop 174: 69–86
5. Poitout D (1985) Conservation et utilisation de l'os de banque. Cahier d'enseignement de la S.O.F.C.O.T. no. 23. Expansion Scientifique, Paris, pp 157–177
6. Poitout D (1986) Greffes utilisées pour reconstruire l'appareil locomoteur. Masson, Paris
7. Poitout D, Novakovitch G (1986) Allogreffes et banque d'os. Encyclopédie médico-chirurgicale. Appareil Locomoteur 14015 AIO-5, Paris, p 6
8. Poitout D, Novakovitch G (1987) Utilisation des allogreffes en oncologie et en traumatologie. Int Orthop 11: 169–178
9. Roy-Camille R, Laugier A, Ruyssen S, Chenal C, Bisserie M, Pene F, Saillant G (1981) Evolution des greffes osseuses cortico-spongieuses et radiothérapie. Revue Chir Orthop 67: 599–608
10. Tomford WW, Fredericks GR, Mankin HJ (1982) Cryopreservation of intact articular cartilage. Trans Orthop Res Soc 7: 176
11. Tomford WW, Doppelt S, Mankin HJ (1983) 1983 Bone bank procedures. Clin Orthop 174: 15–21
12. Tomford WW, Mankin HJ (1983) Investigational approaches to articular cartilage preservation Clin Orthop 174: 22–27

The Use of Proximal Femoral Allografts in the Treatment of Bone Tumors

Michael H. Jofe, Mark C. Gebhardt, and Henry J. Mankin[1]

Summary. One of the most challenging problems in orthopedic oncology is the reconstruction following resection of tumors of the proximal femur. Various techniques have been proposed, one of which is the use of frozen cadaveric allografts, either as an osteoarticular implant or coupled with a standard proximal femoral replacement prosthesis (Austin Moore, bipolar or total hip replacement). Since 1971, 44 of these proximal femoral allografts have been performed by members of the Orthopaedic Oncology Service of the Massachusetts General Hospital. Of these, 28 met the dual criteria of being performed for malignant tumours and having at least a 2-year follow-up. Fifteen of the patients underwent osteoarticular allografts and 13 had allograft segments coupled with metallic hip prostheses (nine Austin Moore, two bipolars, and two long-stem THRs). The average period of follow-up was 57.6 months. The mean age at the time of operation was 49 years, with a range of 20–77 years. The average length of the femoral segments implanted (as measured from greater trochanter to host-donor junction sites) was 18.4 cm and the longest was 31 cm. The patients were graded according to function, degree of pain, and tumor-related complications. Twenty patients (71%) were rated as acceptable, having no to minimal pain and being ambulatory without support. When the tumor-related failures were deleted (to evaluate the allograft procedure in isolation), successful results rose to 80%. The osteoarticular series fared less well than the combination allograft prosthesis group, but the series were not directly comparable. The late complications included six fractures, two nonunions, and five infections. It was possible to treat most of these allograft-related complications and no patients required amputation. If the final results are evaluated to include the results of patients initially deemed failures (excluding tumor-related failures), but subsequently salvaged by a second reconstructive procedure, the final functional score was 96% satisfactory. Tumor-related complications included nine metastases, two local recurrences, and five deaths. Allograft transplants with or without prosthetic implants should be considered as a means of reconstruction when major tumor resections require sacrifice of a segment of the upper end of the femur.

Key words: Bone tumor—Proximal femur—Allograft

Introduction

The surgical management of aggressive and malignant bone tumors of the proximal femur frequently includes wide local resection of the tumor and adjacent

---

[1] Orthopaedic Oncology Service, Massachusetts General Hospital, Boston, MA, USA

soft tissues. Once successfully achieved, reconstruction is sometimes difficult because of the amount of bone resected, the magnitude of the soft tissue loss, and the number of muscles remaining with which the patient can be expected to control and move the hip. Although many methods have been reported for the reconstruction of the resultant skeletal defect [1–6], the use of allograft bone may offer some distinct advantages, principally in terms of availability, retention of cartilage surfaces, and, if accepted by the body, conversion of the implant to living tissue. In previous reports, we have described the use of fresh frozen cadaveric allografts in a number of anatomical sites [7, 8], but because the biomechanical factors and functional issues at the hip are considerably different it seemed appropriate to study the proximal femoral segment replacements separately. Twenty-eight patients who had been treated for malignant tumors of the proximal femur by resection and allograft replacement and followed for at least 2 years (with a mean follow-up of almost 5 years) serve as the basis for this report.

Materials and Methods

Since November 1971, the Orthopaedic Oncology Unit at the Massachusetts General Hospital has performed 410 allograft transplantations, mostly following resection of bone tumors. Of the 266 sequential cases followed for more than 2 years, 44 cases involved the upper end of the femur. Of these, 28 cases met the criteria for inclusion in this current series, i.e., a diagnosis of aggressive or malignant neoplasm treated by resection and replacement of the proximal femur and femoral head by either an allograft alone or an allograft and a prosthesis (Austin Moore, bipolar or total hip replacement). Sixteen patients with benign disease or failed total hip replacements were excluded. All patients in our series underwent routine evaluations including plain radiographs, CT or MR images, bone scintography, and angiograms and were staged according to the Musculoskeletal Tumor Society Staging System [9]. The allografts were procured and stored as previously described [10, 11].

The operative technique was individualized, although some general principles were followed. In every case, the biopsy tract was excised in continuity with the specimen and the marginal or wide resection included a segment of normal bone and surrounding soft tissue [9]. The sciatic nerve was routinely identified and protected. The allograft bone was rapidlly thawed, cut to match the bony defect, and held in place with either two DC plates or the medullary portion of a long-stem endoprosthesis (a small plate was often used at the host-donor junction site to control rotation). The host tendons were firmly sutured to the gluteus medius and iliopsoas insertion sites of the allograft. All wounds were closed over suction drainage. Patients were kept at bedrest for 2–3 weeks to allow for repair of the soft tissues. Intravenous antibiotics were used for approximately 2 weeks, following which the patients were maintained on oral antibiotics for 3 or more months. Anticoagulation usually using Coumadin was routinely carried out for 4 months unless a specific contraindication exsited. Following the period of bedrest, partial weight bearing was begun using crutches and continued until radiological evidence of healing was seen. For the patients who should healing at the host-donor junction site, the period of assisted weight bearing averaged 5.6 months. Physical therapy protocols were individualized according to the specific operation and proved to be very valuable in restoration of function.

There were two types of proximal femoral reconstruction used. In younger patients in whom the tumor did not extend into the hip joint and in whom an excellent proximal femur-acetabulum fit could be obtained, an osteoarticular allograft was performed (15 patients). In older patients in whom a portion of the acetabulum had to be resected or a suitable fit could not be made, a composite allograft prosthesis was inserted (13 patients). In these cases, a long-stem Austin-Moore (nine cases) bipolar prosthesis (two), or total hip replacement (two) was inserted in standard fashion into the proximal femoral allograft in a press-fit manner.

All of the patients have been closely followed and none have been lost to follow-up. Patients were evaluated according to the functional grading system developed previously reported [7]. Results were classified as *excellent* in those patients who had no evident disease, had normal function of the grafted part, and were able to return to normal activities with minimal limitations. A result was considered to be *good* in an individual who had no evidence of disease but had reduced function of the graft part. Neither a brace nor support were necessary to return to most daily activities. A *fair* result was recorded in a patient who had no evidence of recurrence of the tumor but a significant functional deficit which required a brace or support. A *failure* was noted in any patient who required resection of the graft or amputation of the limb because of local or systemic effect of the tumor, fracture, or infection.

Results

Table 1 presents the demographic data for the 28 patients in the series and compares them with those for 239 patients who have had allograft implants in other than the proximal femur and have been followed for the requisite 2 years. As is evident, the mean age for the patients was considerably greater than the rest of the series ($P < 0.001$) and the number of males exceeded females. Analysis of the diagnostic pattern shows that a greater percentage of virulent tumors were included in the proximal femoral group than in the remaining patients. The percentage of cases in stages IIA, IIB, and III for the proximal femoral series was 68%, distinctly different from the value of 23.5% for the overall group ($P < 0.0001$). Eleven of the patients received chemotherapy and three chemotherapy and radiation. Fourteen patients were treated by surgery alone.

Eleven of the grafts were implanted in the left side and 17 on the right. The average length of the femoral segment implanted (as measured from greater trochanter to host-donor junction site) was 18.4 cm and the longest was 31 cm. Fifteen of the patients had no osteoarticular replacement and 13 had an allograft in combination with a prosthesis (long-stem Austin Moore endoprosthesis in nine, a bipolar device in two, or a long-stem total hip replacement in two). Cement was used in only one of two total joint replacements and was implanted into only the distal fragment of two of the Austin Moore prostheses to improve fixation and prevent rotation.

Table 1. Demographic data for proximal femoral allograft replacement

	Proximal femoral grafts (28)	Total series excluding proximal femora (239)
Mean age	49.0 years	30.9 years
Sex		
Males	17 (60.7%)	99 (41.4%)
Females	11 (39.3%)	140 (58.6%)
Follow-up	57.6 months	70.6 months
Diagnosis		
Chondrosarcoma	12 (42.9%)	40 (16.7%)
Osteosarcoma	6 (21.4%)	26 (10.9%)
Giant cell tumor	4 (14.3%)	81 (33.9%)
Metastatic carcinoma	2 (7.1%)	5 (2.1%)
Lymphoma	2 (7.1%)	0 (0.0%)
Ewing's sarcoma	1 (3.6%)	5 (2.1%)
Myeloma	1 (3.6%)	1 (0.4%)
Stage		
0	0 (0.0%)	31 (13.0%)
I	9 (32.1%)	152 (63.6%)
II	14 (50.0%)	47 (19.7%)
III	5 (17.9%)	9 (3.8%)

Table 2 shows the details for the tumor and allograft complications. Nine of the twenty-eight (32.1%) of the patients developed metastases (two of these also had local recurrences) and (18%) died of the disease. In addition, there were six fractures, five infections, two nonunions and one unstable joint in the series (since several of the patients had more than one complication, the figures are not additive). When the complication data are compared with the remaining 239 patients, it is evident that the proximal femoral allograft patients are at higher risk for metastasis or death and their infection and fracture rates are greater. Union, on the other hand, appears to be more predictable.

The patients who died of disease included two with metastatic carcinoma, one of whom had widespread metastatic carcinoma from the prostate and the other, who died of a self-administered overdose of narcotics, with medullary carcinoma of the thyroid. The remaining three deaths occurred in patients with osteosarcoma, two of whom presented with pulmonary metastases (stage III disease). Four additional patients remain alive with metastatic disease; two with chondrosarcoma, one with lymphoma under treatment with chemotherapy, and one who has had two pulmonary resections for osteosarcoma.

The five infected patients included two who developed late infections following open reduction and internal fixation for fractures. The remaining three showed no specific predisposing cause. One of these five patients died of widespread metastatic prostatic carcinoma, but the other four were salvaged by surgical debridement and insertion of a new device and remain free of infection at 2–5 years following the salvage surgery. All are classified as *good* on the functional evaluation system.

Six of the 28 patients sustained a fracture of the allograft, one of which healed

Table 2. Complications for proximal femoral allograft replacements

	Proximal femoral grafts (28)	Total series excluding proximal femora (239)
Tumor complications[a]		
Local recurrence	2 (7.1%)	20 (8.4%)
Metastasis	9 (32.1%)	27 (11.3%)
Died of disease	5 (17.9%)	18 (7.5%)
Allograft complications[a]		
Infection	5 (17.9%)	28 (11.7%)
Fracture	6 (21.4%)	41 (17.2%)
Nonunion	2 (7.1%)	30 (12.6%)
Unstable joint	1 (3.6%)	14 (5.9%)
No tumor failures	19 (67.9%)	199 (83.3%)
No allograft complications	16 (57.1%)	142 (59.4%)
No tumor or allograft complications (successful)	12 (42.9%)	114 (47.7%)

[a] It should be noted that the complication rates shown are not additive, since many of the patients had more than one complication. In fact, the "true" values as far as the patient groups are concerned are as indicated in the "No tumor failures" row and below

spontaneously and four of which were treated with open reduction and internal fixation (two were successful and two became infected—see above). In the remaining case, the graft was resected and successfully replaced. The two cases in which nonunion occurred were noted to have a significant gap at the host-donor junction site. After failure of the hardware at 8 months and 1 year respectively, both were successfully treated with replacement of the hardware and addition of iliac crest autograft. The patient with an unstable hip developed a local recurrence of her osteosarcoma and died of disease at 2.5 years following initial treatment.

In summary, 19/28 (68%) of the patients remain tumor free (a rather extraordinary figure, considering the nature of the tumors with which we are dealing), and 16/28 (57%) had no allograft complications, a value which approximates that for the entire series. Of the 28 patients, 12 (43% were considered successful, in that they had neither allograft nor tumor complications and did not require additional surgery to achieve their excellent or good results.

The *initial results* include only evaluation of the first procedure. Analysis shows that 9/28 (32.1%) were designated as excellent and 10/28 (35.7%) as good. There was one patient who was fair and 8/28 (28.6%) were considered to be failures—two as a result of tumor recurrences, four for infection, and two for fracture. The *current results* report the patient's condition at the time of writing, independent of the number of procedures. In relation to the tumor, 19 (68%) have no evident disease, four (14%) are alive with disease, and five (18%) have died from disseminated tumor. Analysis of the functional results shows that 8 of the 23 survivors are currently scored as excellent (35%), 14 as good (61%), one as fair (4%), and none as *failure* for an overall success rate of 96%.

The differences between the numbers shown in the initial results and current results reflect not only the deletion of the five tumor deaths but also evaluation

Table 3. Comparison of osteoarticular allografts and allograft plus prosthesis for 28 proximal femoral alloimplants

	Osteoarticular (15)	Allografts plus prostheses (13)
Age	48.2	50.4
Sex		
Males	13 (87%)	4 (31%)
Females	2 (13%)	9 (69%)
Follow-up	50.6 months	65.8 months
Stage		
0	0	0
I	4	5
II	7	7
III	4	1
Tumor		
Recurrence	2	0
Metastasis	5	4
Died of tumor	4	1
Allograft complications		
Infection	4	1
Fracture	4	2
Nonunion	2	0
Unstable joint	1	0
Initial results		
Excellent	3	6
Good	6	4
Fair	0	1
Failure	6	2
Current status		
Excellent	3	5
Good	8	8
Fair	0	1
Failure	0	0
Died of disease	4	1

of the patients after they underwent reoperation for the complications. In all, there was a total total of 22 reoperations performed in 13 of 28 patients and only one of these was necessitated by tumor recurrence. The remainder were performed to treat complications of the allograft procedure and consisted of the following: six total hip replacements (one for osteoarthritis of the hip at 4.5 years, two for painful Austin Moore prostheses at 7.5 and 8 years, respectively, and three for restoration after resection of the graft for infection), seven open reduction and internal fixations for either allograft fracture or nonunion, and three cases with resection of the graft, maintaining skeletal length with a tobramycin-impregnated polymethyl methacrylate spacer and reinsertion of a new allograft after a prolonged course of antibiotics.

Table 3 compares the 15 members of the osteoarticular (OA) and 13 patients in the allograft plus prosthesis (AP) groups. As can be noted, the mean age for the OA group is slightly greater and the sex distribution markedly skewed in favor of males (this distribution is almost certainly related to the fact that more of our donors are male and hence the likelihood of our bank providing a donor femoral head which fits in the host acetabulum is much greater for males than for females). The OA group has a slightly more virulent group of tumors in that 11/15 are stage II or III, compared with 8/13 for the AP group, and this is reflected in the tumor results. Infection and allograft fracture occurred in eight instances among the 15 patients in the OA cohort, while they occurred in only 2/13 in the AP group; both of the nonunions and the single unstable joint occurred in OAs.

The initial results for the two groups show that 9/15 (66%) of the OA group were excellent or good while 10/13 (76.9%) of the allograft prosthesis group were similarly successful. When the current results are compared 11/15 of the OA group are excellent or good and four have died. The AP group is almost the same with 11/13 successful, one labeled as fair, and one patient dead.

Discussion

Reconstruction of the proximal femur following major tumor resection presents many technical problems. Autografts, while shown by Enneking et al. [2] and Wilson and Lance [1] to be successful in other anatomical areas, are unlikely to provide the structural support required in the proximal femur and also cannot offer either an articular surface or a shaft in which to introduce a prosthetic implant. Custom prostheses have been advocated by a number of surgeons and are currently in vogue [4-6], but most of these reports have a short follow-up and the complications of loosening and fracture of the device are likely to present significant problems in the future.

Allograft transplantation, although still in a developmental stage, would seem to offer several advantages for tumor reconstruction. The parts are readily available in different sizes and shapes, include articular surfaces, and if intact are likely to be able to withstand the biomechanical stresses acting on the proximal femur. The allogenic bony implants, although still not ideal in terms of such complications as allograft fracture, infection, and slow and occasionally unpredictable rate of healing of the host-donor junction site (particularly in patients who are receiving chemotherapy), are still an attractive system particularly for the upper end of the femur [7, 8].

This present study demonstrates that allografts are a reasonable option in reconstruction of the proximal femur following major tumor resections. The initial success rate is approximately 70% (77% with tumor failures deleted) and, more importantly, studies for the current status of these patients show that 95% of the survivors have successful implants and are functionally restored over an average 57-month period of follow-up. Of interest is the superior performance of the AP patient group as compared with those who underwent OA grafts. Although it is tempting on this basis to consider performing all these cases with the AP system (without cement), the evidence is not conclusive because of differences in the composition of the series.

It seems apparent to us on the basis of these data and a review of other series that the overall success rate achieved in these patients is not only acceptable but equivalent or better to those by other management systems. The percentage of excellent and good results is sufficiently high to encourage us to continue to refine and improve the methods, and it further suggests that with some control over complications the method may have a much broader application in orthopedic oncology.

References

1. Wilson PD Jr, Lance EM (1975) Surgical reconstruction of the skeleton following segmental resection for bone tumors. J Bone Joint Surg 47A: 1629–1656
2. Enneking WF, Eady JL, Burchardt H (1980) Autogenous cortical bone grafts in the reconstruction of segmental skeletal defects. J Bone Joint Surg 62A: 1039–1058
3. Winkelmann WW (1986) Hip rotationplasty for malignant tumors of the proximal part of the femur. J Bone Joint Surg 68A: 362–369
4. Burrows HJ, Wilson JN, Scales JT (1975) Excision of tumors of the humerus and femur with restoration by internal prosthesis. J Bone Joint Surg 57B: 148–159
5. Scales JT (1975) Massive bone and joint replacement involving the upper femur, acetabulum and iliac bone. In: The hip. Proceedings of 3rd open scientific meeting of the Hip Society. Mosby, St Louis, pp 245–275
6. Kotz R, Ritschl P, Trachtenbrodt J (1986) A modular femur-tibia reconstruction system. Orthopedics 9: 1639–1652
7. Mankin HJ, Doppelt SH, Sullivan TR, Tomford WW (1982) Cancer 50: 613–630
8. Mankin HJ, Doppelt SH, Tomford WW (1983) Clinical experience with allograft implantation. The first ten years. Clin Orthop 174: 69–86
9. Enneking WF, Spanier SS, Goodman MA (1980) Current concepts review: the surgical staging of musculoskeletal sarcoma. J Bone Joint Surg 62A: 1027–1030
10. Doppelt SH, Tomford WW, Lucas A, Mankin HJ (1981) J Bone Joint Surg 63A: 1472–1479
11. Tomford WW, Doppelt SH, Mankin HJ, Friedlaender GE (1983) 1983 bone bank procedures. Clin Orthop 174: 15–21

Titanium Long-Stem Prosthesis Combined with Bone Allografts in Reconstructive Surgery of High-Grade Bone Sarcomas

Gérard Delepine[1] and Nicole Delepine[2]

Summary. From 1984 to 1987, 70 long-stem titanium prostheses coated with massive bank allografts were used to reconstruct bone defects secondary to in bloc resection for high-grade bone sarcomas (average length of bone defect 22 cm). Such a combination permits immediate weight bearing and avoids articular and mechanical problems of massive allografts.

With an average follow-up of 20 months, the functional result, rated excellent or good in 57 patients (63%), was better than expected after implantation of a large prosthesis. Good muscle reattachment, as evident in reoperated cases, improves hip stability after resection of the upper femur, limits extension lag after resection of the upper tibia, and permits active lateral rotation after proximal humerus resection. Radiological follow-up shows progressive peripheral ossification, bone calus after 6 months, and cortical healing after 18–24 months.

No bone resorption of the diaphysis or graft and no radiological sign of pseudarthrosis have been observed except in cases of infection or local recurrence. No endo- or exocortical resorption of the diaphysis, cement fracture, sign of loosening, or implant failure (stem fracture or polyethylene failure) have been found.

By providing mechanical stability of the prosthesis and better functional results of the allografts, without major infections or immunological problems, such a combination seems to us to be indicated in high-grade bone sarcoma when the patient's chances for survival appear long enough.

Key words: Titanium prosthesis—Massive allograft—Limb salvage surgery

Introduction

After conservative surgery for bone sarcomas, reconstructive procedures involves massive prostheses or bone allografts. Both have their advantages and drawbacks. Bank allografts permit muscle reattachment, usually give better functional results and better long-term tolerance but require a long period without weight bearing and are threatened by infection, nonunion, and secondary stress fractures, especially in the lower limbs if chemotherapy and radiotherapy have to be performed. For these reasons, large stainless steel prostheses are

[1] Unite d'Oncologie Orthopedique du Pre Gentil, Rosny Sous Bois, France
[2] Oncologic Pediatric Unit, Hospital Robert Debre, Paris, France

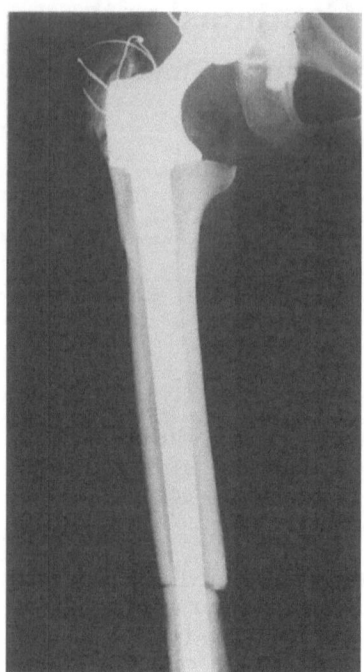

Fig. 1. Massive allograft coating long stem upper femoral prosthesis after en bloc resection for Ewing's sarcoma. Patient's trochanter was knotted on the allograft with titanium wires

actually preferred by most surgeons in spite of their high rate of mechanical problems—stem fractures, progressive bone resorption, loosening. Two main reasons explain these failures—the excessively long lever arm of the massive prosthesis and the excessively high rigidity of stainless steel. Both can be avoided by using long-stem titanium prostheses coated with a massive bank allograft. Titanium is almost twice as light and twice as elastic as stainless steel. Massive bank allografts can change the lever arm of the large prosthesis to a short one of a common prosthesis as soon as bone healing occurs.

Materials and Methods

From 1984 to 1987, we used 70 long-stem titanium prosthesis coated with massive bank allografts to reconstruct bone defects secondary to in bloc resection for limb sarcomas. The histological investigations revealed 34 cases of osteosarcoma, ten cases of Ewing's sarcoma, eight cases of chondrosarcoma, seven cases of fibrosarcoma or malignant histiocytofibroma, and 11 others. According to Enneking's classification, the grade was IA in two, IB in three, IIA in one, IIB in 52, and IIIB in 12 cases.

The tumor location was the distal femur in 34 cases, proximal or upper diaphyseal femur in 15 cases, upper humerus in 11 cases, and proximal tibia in ten cases. Average length of the bone defect after resection was 22 cm (minimum 15, maximum 37). Average age of the patients was 27 years (minium 6, maximum 87).

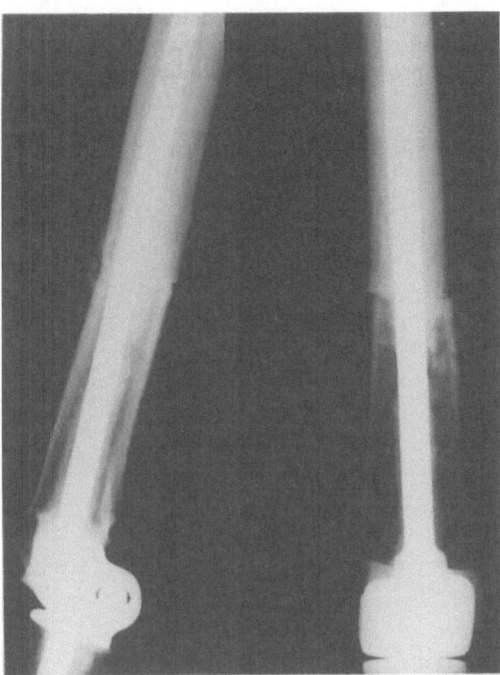

Fig. 2. Long stem titanium prosthesis coated with allograft. Peripheric bone callus 3 months after operation. (No chemotherapy was necessary in that core of low grade chondrosarcoma)

Prosthesis

All implants were long-stem custom-made titanium prostheses with individualized sizes according to the authors' designs. Forged titanium alloy was chosen for its better mechanical properties (twice as elastic, twice as light as stainless steel). The average fabrication duration was 10 days.

The *upper femoral prosthesis* had a metaphyseal part similar to the Merle d'Aubigne model C prosthesis, with modular heads allowing the choice of head material and size. In adults, we chose a 32-mm head associated with a cemented high-density polyethylene cup. The stem was straight; the length and diameter were individualized to each patient (Fig. 1).

The *knee prosthesis* was a hinge prosthesis with a titanium axis and polyethylene bearings. The size of the epiphyseal part of the prosthesis was small enough to be inserted from the age of 5 years and its smooth edges avoided any soft tissue trauma. No trochlea was necessary. A patellar prosthesis was used only after extra-articular resection. The femoral stem had a 5° valgus angle (Fig. 2).

The *proximal humeral prosthesis* had a metaphyseal antirotation part and an individualized epiphyseal part and stem, permitting a good fit with the scapula and lower humeral diaphysis. Holes permit rotatory cuff reattachment (Fig. 3).

Special Needs

In five young patients, we used a special growing prosthesis, and in three total femoral replacements a combination of upper and lower prostheses coated with

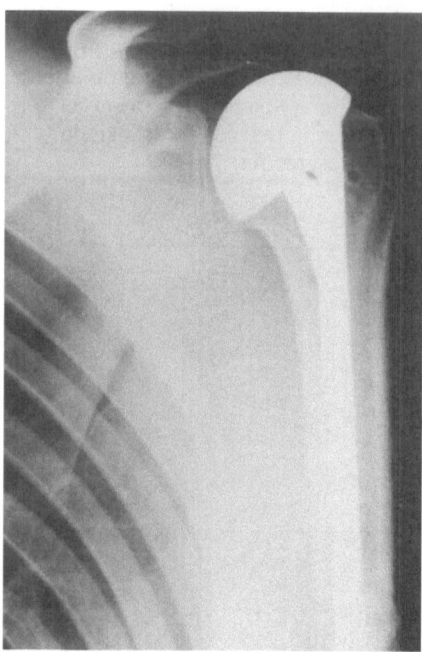

Fig. 3. Upper humeral resection for osteosarcoma. Reconstruction with custom made prostheses coated with bone graft

a diaphyseal allograft was employed.

The allografts were all provided by the bone bank of Hopital Henri Mondor in Creteil (Prof. D. Goutallier). They were removed under sterile conditions in the operating room and immediately freezed to −30°C. They were stored at −30°C for a period not exceeding 6 months and preoperatively sterilized by beta irradiation (2.5–3.5 Mrad). The graft was removed from the fridge 3 h before operation, cut with an oscillating saw, and then smoothly reamed. The allograft was cemented onto the prosthetic stem and the prosthesis was then cemented into the residual diaphysis. In 30 cases, en bloc resection could preserve the periarticulated tendons that were reattached to the graft either directly through the graft, with their bony insertion, or with the tendon of the allograft. Titanium wires passing through the prosthesis seem to be more reliable than other procedures. A fresh autogenous graft harvested from the opposite epiphysis was placed around the allograft-diaphysis junction.

Postoperative Cases

Weight bearing was immediate (except in one case), but active motion was restricted for 45 days in the upper tibia and proximal humerus to help muscle reattachment. Fifty-six patients underwent postoperative chemotherapy (average duration 10 months), and 38 local radiotherapy (35–55 Gy).

Follow-up

All patients were clinically followed up by the same physician and underwent X-ray examination, HLA antibody tests, quantified bone scan, computed tomography (local and chest) every 3 months, and, usually, magnetic resonance imaging. The average follow-up was 20 months (minimum 5, maximum 39 months).

Results

Oncological Results

To date, 12 follow-up patients (six initially metastatic patients) have died, and two others have had pulmonary metastasis. For patients with localized disease, the nonmetastatic survival rate was 91% after 12 months and 86% after 30 months. Three local recurrences and two deep infections occurred, necessitating amputation (one case) of ablation of the prosthesis (two cases).

Functional Result

Following two early deaths, the functional results could only be evaluated in 68 operative cases. According to Enneking's rating system, the final functional results were excellent in 20 cases (29%), good in 37 cases (54%), fair in seven cases (10%), and not satisfactory in four cases (6%). The functional result depends mostly on the tumor size and location and on postoperative radiotherapy. The result is nearly always improved by good reattachment of the preserved muscles and tendons on the allograft, as evident from clinical examination and macroscopic and microscopic findings of reoperated patients. In the proximal femur, the main advantage is hip stability. In spite of immediate weight bearing, we have not observed early dislocation. In one case with trochanteric pseudarthrosis that became evident 18 months after surgery; hip instability appeared subjectively before hip dislocation and was cured by trochanteric reinsertion. In the upper tibia, the advantage of patellar tendon reinsertion was evident to limit extensor lag. To provide benefit more quickly and easily, we prefer to transplant both the allograft and patellar tendon, which gives better closure, no need for cast immobilization, and improved final mobility. After lower femur reconstruction, the functional result was quite similar to that with a massive prosthesis. After upper humeral resection, a prosthesis with a titanium allograft coating gives the best hanging strength, better active abduction, and some active lateral rotation, which no current prosthesis allows. HLA antibodies against the graft were detected in only three cases with no evidence of clinical or radiological implications. Quantified bone scintigraphy showed slow but progressive revascularization of the graft from the surrounding muscles.

Radiological Following

The allograft-diaphysis junction showed progressive peripheral ossification. The bone calus appeared mostly within 6 months (quicker in young children or when no chemotherapy was used). Cortical healing came later (18–24 months). No bone resorption of the diaphysis or graft and no radiological signs of pseudarthrosis have been observed except in two cases (one infection, one local recurrence).

Clinical examination and macroscopic findings of reoperated cases showed that muscle reinsertion always occurred (1–2 months) and that tendon reattachment could be obtained. However, we observed three clinically evident secondary tendon ruptures and four secondary radiological fractures of patellar tendon bony insertions, rotator cuffs, or gluteus tendons. Titanium wires knotted through the prosthesis seemed to provide the most reliable reattachment.

Seven fractures of allograft-coated long-stem prostheses were observed in plain radiographs without any clinical complications. They all healed spontaneously. These secondary fractures indicate the poor mechanical condition of the graft compared with normal cortical bone and the associated mechanical stress.

This more physiological transfer of mechanical stresses both through long-stem titanium prostheses and massive allografts indicates that bony modification of the diaphysis is very poor: Non-endo- or exocortical bone resorption was observed and distal periostis appeared in only four cases. No cement fracture, loosening, or implant failure (stem fracture or polyethylene failure) were found.

Conclusion

Sterilized allograft-coated long-stem titanium prostheses give, without major infections or immunological problems, better functional results and mechanical transfer of stresses to bone than stainless steel massive prostheses. Such a combination avoids mechanical and articular problems of massive allografts. It is indicated in high-grade sarcoma when the patient's life expectancy appears to be greater than 1 year.

Chapter 8

Reconstruction After Resection of Large Bone Tumors About the Hip and Pelvis

Long-Term Performance of Custom Prosthetic Replacement for Neoplastic Disease of the Proximal Femur

Kok-Sun Khong, Edmund Y.S. Chao, and Franklin H. Sim[1]

Summary. We analyzed 84 hips in 82 patients with proximal femur prosthetic replacement as a reconstructive procedure after tumor resection. Forty-nine patients had primary disease while 37 patients had metastases. The mean follow-up time was 30.4 months in all patients; the median survival was 79 months for primary cases and 9 months for metastatic cases. The most common surgical indication was tumor size and position in primary cases and pathological fractures in metastatic cases. Nine cases had primary tumor recurrence. Overall functional scores were good and excellent in 54.7%, while only one patient required revision for femoral loosening. There were radiographic lucencies around 10 of 22 acetabular components at 5 years. Implant-related osteopenia was seen in 31 of 72 assessable femurs. There is a definite role for bipolar implants in both primary and metastatic disease.

Key words: Proximal femur prosthesis—Primary tumor—Metastatic disease

Introduction

Orthopedic oncology centers have reported improving results in limb salvage surgery in almost all anatomical areas [8, 9]. This improvement may be attributed to earlier diagnosis, more accurate staging methods, advances in neo-adjuvant therapy, aggressive ablative surgery, varied choices in reconstructive procedures, and patient preference. The advancement of limb salvage techniques has been greatest in the treatment of proximal lesions of long bones, particularly the proximal femur since functional results for hip disarticulation or hemipelvectomy have been dismal. State-of-the-art reconstructive procedures utilized for primary lesions involving the proximal femur include hip arthrodeses by vascularized and nonvascularized fibular grafts, massive allograft replacement, and custom-designed proximal femoral replacement arthroplasty [8].

The question of limb salvage in patients with metastatic disease has not been resolved. Many of these patients have failed palliative radiotherapy, and the majority present with problematic pathological fractures. Reasonable treatment goals include alleviation of pain and reacquisition of ambulatory status. The

[1] Orthopedic Biomechanics Laboratory, Department of Orthopedics, Mayo Clinic/Mayo Foundation, Rochester, MN, USA

most common site of metastatic involvement is the proximal femur. Lesions above the lesser trochanter are not well managed by internal fixation devices. For these lesions, especially in the elderly, prosthetic replacement of the proximal femur provides a viable option [6]. This paper presents our experience in proximal femur replacement for the purpose of identifying the common indications and to review patients' functional and clinical results so that the proper role of such surgery can be defined. Such results may also suggest future implant modifications.

Materials and Methods

Between January 1971 and December 1984, 140 patients underwent proximal femur replacement at our institution. In 82 patients, 84 hips involved neoplastic disease. Forty-nine patients (50 hips) had primary disease, while 33 patients (34 hips) had metastases. All patients were followed up for a minimum of 2 years, until death, or when limb or implant was removed or revised. All hips were staged by the system adopted by the Musculoskeletal Tumor Society [4]. When evaluating radiographs, lucencies around the femoral component and zones I, II, and III for acetabular cups were measured [3]. They were graded by the 2-mm limit or when they were complete. The Kaplan-Meier method was used to analyze survivorship.

The functional results were studied using the clinical examination parameters rated according to a grading system recommended by the Musculoskeletal Tumor Society [5]. In this system, various parameters partinent to proximal femur and hip joint reconstruction are incorporated. There are seven parameters (joint active motion, pain, stability, deformity, strength, emotional acceptance, and function), which were rated "excellent," "good," "fair," or "poor," according to preset criteria. An overall rating was achieved by combining an individual rating on each parameter. The prosthetic device used was also evaluated using a scoring system similar to that used in functional evaluation [5].

Results

The mean follow-up time was 45.4 months for primary cases but only 8.9 months for patients with metastases. In the primary tumor group, 27 of 49 patients (55.1%) were still alive at last review, with 25 disease-free and two with disease. Two died of unrelated causes and one of surgical complications. In the metastatic cases, all but three have died and all have disease remaining, one in the same limb and two elsewhere. With regard to prostheses, 75 hips (89.4%) retained their original implants. Four prostheses were revised to a second custom device, two hips were disarticulated for infection, and three required hemipelvectomy for control of disease. The median age at surgery was 50.5 years for primary (range, 14–81 years) and 60 years for metastatic cases (range, 40–80 years; Table 1).

Half of all primary tumors were chondrosarcomas. There were three dedifferentiated chondrosarcomas. Osteogenic sarcoma accounted for ten and fibro-

Table 1. Demographic, pathological, and operative data of patients with proximal femur and hip joint replacement

	Patient group	
	Primary	Metastatic
Demographic data		
Total patients	49	33
Males	30	14
Females	19	19
Hips	50	34
Median age	50	60
Pathological data		
Surgical staging		
Benign 3	2	—
Malignant IA	5	—
Malignant IB	5	—
Malignant IIA	16	—
Malignant IIB	21	—
Malignant III	1	34
Surgical margins		
Intralesional	4	11
Marginal	9	9
Wide	37	13
Unknown	—	1
Surgical indications		
Tumor size/location	30	11
Pathological fracture	8	22
Inadequate margins	8	—
Tumor recurrence	4	—
Nonpathological fracture	—	1
Operative data		
Resection length (mm)	144[a] (30–220)	105[a] (45–175)
Replacement length (mm)	150[a] (52–250)	110[a] (49–200)
Operating time (min)	175[a] (100–390)	150[a] (90–290)
Estimated blood loss (ml)	1740	1650
Time to ambulation (days)	9 (5–20)	7 (4–32)
Hospital stay (days)	16[a] (10–79)	22[a] (11–48)

[a] Significantly different between primary and metastatic groups ($P < 0.05$)

sarcoma for five hips. Two cases of recurrent benign giant cell tumor were also included. In metastatic malignancies, the most common primary was breast adenocarcinoma in 13 hips. The two hips with gian cell tumor were staged "benign aggressive." There were five stage IA, five IB, 16 IIA, and 21 IIB lesions. There was one patient with a stage III primary tumor, and all 30 metastatic cases were classified as stage III for purposes of statistical analysis. The indication for resection was tumor size and position in 60% of primary but only in 32.4% of metastatic lesions. Pathological fracture was the main indication in 52.9% of metastatic hips.

Resection margins were graded as wide in 74% of primary tumors, but only in 38.2% of metastatic lesions. This is statistically significant ($P < 0.01$). There were nine marginal resections in each group. Four primary tumors had intra-lesional margins (8%), while 11 metastatic tumors had intralesional margins (32.4%). Of the primary hips with lesional margins, two had disease in the distal femur, one had resection at the fracture site, and one patient with osteogenic sarcoma of the femoral neck had involvement of the hip joint. Of primary lesions that had prior surgical intervention, 75% were performed at another in-stitution. There was no significant difference in the survival of these patients when compared with those who did not have prior intervention. The mean resec-tion length was significantly longer (141.5 mm versus 111.6 mm) in those with previous surgery ($P < 0.001$).

The median duration of operation was significantly lower ($P < 0.05$) in the metastatic group than in the primary group. Median resection length was signif-icantly less in metastatic lesions than in primary lesions. This is explained by the fact that more intralesional and marginal margins were obtained in femurs with metastases. The postoperative hospital stay was shorter in patients with primary lesions than in those with metastases ($P < 0.05$). There was no correlation be-tween resection length and other parameters related to function, surgical results, morbidity, and complications.

There was a total of 63 total joint proximal femur replacement prostheses (72.6%), 20 bipolar-type components, and one custom Leinbach endoprosthe-sis. All femoral and acetabular components were cemented by the technique prevalent at the time. There was a comparable distribution between primary and metastatic cases, and the age-groups were equally matched. The mean resection length was significantly more in joint-replacing components (135 versus 113 mm; $P < 0.01$), as was replacement length (151 versus 132 mm; $P < 0.05$). In addi-tion, the estimated blood loss (1518 versus 2205 mm; $P < 0.02$), blood trans-fusions (4 versus 5.7 units; $P < 0.01$) and postsurgical hospital stay (17.7 versus 22.6 days; $P < 0.05$) were significantly less in the bipolar group.

In the primary group, 12% of the patients had preoperative adjuvant therapy and 33% required postoperative adjuvant therapy. In the group with metastases, the majority had some form of adjuvant therapy. Only ten (30%) patients had no preoperative therapy. Thirteen received no postoperative therapy (40%), but six with primary breast tumor had already received maximum irradiation to the femur.

There was no statistical correlation between patient survival and tumor stage in this series. In primary lesions, wide and marginal margins resulted in better patient survival than did intralesional margins (Fig. 1a). However, resection margins made no difference in survival of patients with metastatic tumors (Fig. 1b). Four of the 84 initial femoral components and one acetabular com-ponent were revised and five limbs were amputated. Two revisions were for im-plant fracture at $2\frac{1}{2}$ and 12 years, respectively.

Forty-four patients (53.7%) did not have any complications (Table 2). The most common intraoperative " complication" was oversized implants in 11 hips (13.1%). Instability occurred in ten hips (11.9%) and, with one exception, all were total joint replacment implants; they were symptomatic within 3 months of implantation, with six having their first episode within 1 month. Five were treated by closed reduction and spica cast immobilization for 6 weeks and two required open reduction. Deep infection occurred in four hips (4.8%).

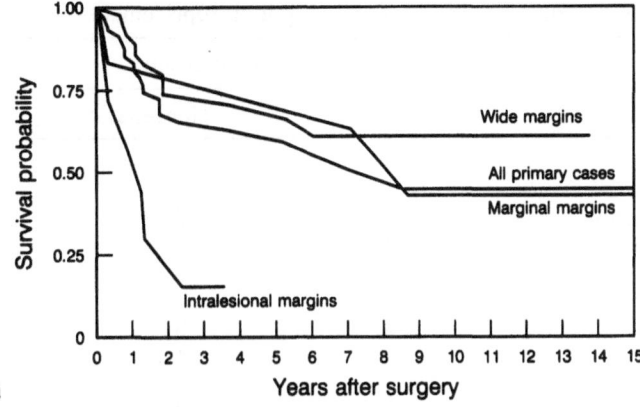

a

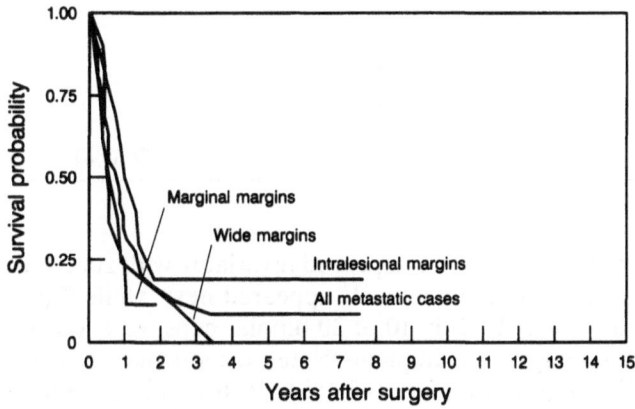

b

Fig. 1a, b. Kaplan-Meier survivorship of proximal femur replacement patient as a function of margin of tumor resection. **a** Survival probability in primary group; **b** Survival probability in metastatic group

There were nine primary tumor recurrences (18%).

Results of functional evaluation were available for 64 hips (76.2%; Table 3). While five of the seven categories had a majority of excellent and good scores, the overall score was lowered because of the lower grades in "stability" and "strength" categories. As a result, only 48.5% of assessable hips were graded as "good" and "excellent." There was no difference between "primary" and "excellent." There was no statistical difference between primary and metastatic groups, and also none between total-joint replacement-type and bipolar-type implants. Implant performance was much better with 80% of 65 assessable prostheses rated "good" and "excellent." Again, the majority of categories were graded as "excellent" (Table 4).

Only two femoral components could be graded radiographically loose at 1 and 11 months, respectively. None of the 25 prostheses with longer than a 2-year follow-up could be determined loose. At final follow-up, 10 of 22 acetabular components (45.5%) were considered loose radiographically. None, however, have been revised for loosening, and symptomatically only three of the eleven

Table 2. Complications in patients with proximal femur and hip joint replacement

Type of Complication	Patient group	
	Primary	Metastatic
Preoperative medical	5	13
Intraoperative		
Inadequate prosthetic dimension	9	2
Stem protruding through femur	2	—
Sciatic nerve palsy	4	—
Postoperative		
Medical	4	3
Hematoma	1	1
Residual foreign body	—	2
Instability	6	4
Deep infection	1	3
Operative mortality	—	1
Late complications		
Implant failure	2	—
Clinical loosening	1	—
Rumor recurrence	9	—
Reoperative rate	17 (34.0%)	7 (20.6%)

patients complained of any pain. Lucent lines appeared invariably with zone I at the bone-cement interface. Lucent lines in zone III appeared next, while these lines occurred the least within zone II. Only 10 of 20 bipolar cups were assessable, with two showing medial migration. Implant-related osteopenia was considered present in 32 of 72 assessable femurs (43.1%). In 6 of 72 assessable radiographs, significant ectopic bone formation was observed around the femoral component.

Discussion

While arthrodesis for minimal bone loss after tumor resection, such as in internal hemipelvectomy, is highly successful, the bridging of a wide intercalary defect in proximal femur resection requires both vascularized and large amounts of non-vascularized grafts and, possibly, allografts to ensure fusion. Double vascularized fibular grafts can be used, but donor site morbidity and the risk of graft fracture should be contemplated. Furthermore, the patient is immobilized for many months and full weight bearing is seldom possible for up to 1 year. In patients with uncertain prognosis, this long period of recovery may prove inferior to amputation. When massive allografts have been used to improve initial structural integrity, the problems relevant to large allografts must also be contended with. Certainly, in patients with metastatic disease, rapid relief of pain and the ability to mobilize and remain independent are quite important in allowing good quality of their short remaining lives.

The "alloimplant" has a distinct advantage since a revision long-stem femoral component can be cemented into the allograft segment and serve as the joint-

Table 3. Functional evaluation results of the patients (n = 64) with proximal femur and hip joint replacement to following the parameters and rating scale recommended by the Musculoskeletal Tumor Society

Rating	Motion	Pain	Stability	Deformity	Strength	Acceptance	Function	Overall[a] Rating
Excellent	36 (56.3%)	37 (57.8%)	9 (14.1%)	40 (62.4%)	13 (20.3%)	11 (17.2%)	37 (57.8%)	3 (4.7%)
Good	22 (34.4%)	15 (23.4%)	14 (21.9%)	20 (31.2%)	21 (32.8%)	39 (60.9%)	15 (23.4%)	28 (43.8%)
Fair	6 (9.4%)	10 (15.6%)	35 (54.7%)	4 (6.3%)	25 (39.1%)	8 (12.5%)	4 (6.3%)	25 (39.1%)
Poor	0 (0%)	2 (3.1%)	6 (9.4%)	0 (0%)	5 (7.8%)	6 (9.4%)	8 (12.5%)	8 (12.5%)

Figures are numbers of patients and percentage distribution in *parentheses*
[a] For the "excellent" category, six out of seven parameters must be rated "excellent"; for the "good" category, six out of seven parameters must be rated "good" or better; the remaining categories for the overall rating are determined in a similar manner

Table 4. Implant device evaluation results in proximal femur and hip replacement patients (n = 65) following the parameters and rating scale recommended by the Musculoskeletal Tumor Society

Rating	Anatomical restoration	Availability	Morbidity	Tissue reaction	Loosening	Failure	Overall[a] rating
Excellent	59 (90.7%)	41 (63.1%)	61 (93.9%)	1 (1.5%)	47 (72.3%)	52 (80.0%)	26 (40.0%)
Good	2 (3.1%)	19 (29.2%)	2 (3.1%)	32 (49.3%)	11 (16.9%)	4 (6.2%)	26 (40.0%)
Fair	4 (6.2%)	5 (7.7%)	0 (0.0%)	32 (49.3%)	4 (6.2%)	5 (7.7%)	10 (15.4%)
Poor	0 (0.0%)	0 (0.0%)	2 (3.1%)	0 (0.0%)	3 (4.6%)	4 (6.2%)	3 (4.6%)

Figures are number of patients and percentage distribution in *parentheses*
[a] As in Table 3

replacing portion, as well as having an intramedullary stem in the remaining distal femur for stability. The other major advantage is in the attachment of the remaining hip musculature to the biological material for optimal line of muscle action, rather than to a smooth metal surface or to surrounding scar tissue or adjacent muscle. However, the major problems with massive allografts are still unsolved. Bony incorporation is slow and may never be complete. The incidence of infection even in centers dealing with allografts routinely is still in the region of 10%–20% [7]. Should infection occur in an alloimplant, limb removal is probably mandatory. On the other hand, early aggressive debridement of infected custom metallic implants saved two of four patients from losing their limbs. Furthermore, the question of the immune-compromised host adapting to massive allogenic material remains unanswered, especially when the patient is receiving chemotherapy or radiation therapy.

Preoperative sizing for the femoral component is usually based on measurements from preoperative full-length radiographs in two planes with the planned line of resection determined by current imaging evaluation of tumor margins. It is, however, only at the time of surgery that resection margins are truly determined. Unexpected tumor extension or the presence of previously undetected microskip lesions will mean nought to prior sizing. To wait weeks or months for implant design and fabrication when a tumor requires immediate resection is also impractical. Should the implant be too short, the loss of tension may cause hip dislocation. A modular prosthetic system for use not only in the proximal femur-hip region, but also in other anatomical areas, is being developed as well [1]. Interchangeable parts will assure compatibility with varying resection lengths and bone dimensions. Soft tissue attachment to implants through porous pads is also under investigation. Such an option, if successfully developed, may improve hip joint function by alleviating the Trendelenburg phenomenon. By restoring the normal line of action of the hip abductors, the problem of abductor weakness giving rise to both an abnormal gait and being a possible etiological factor for acetabular component loosening could be eliminated.

Finally, the question of implant-related osteopenia of the femoral shaft must be addressed. The design of the femoral stems has changed from an I-beam configuration with a large diameter to the current more slender fluted or splined cross section. Initial stability can be accomplished using bone cement and long-term prosthetic fixation and can rely on the new concept of extracortical bone bridging and ingrowth over the porous-coated segmental portion of the implant [2]. When bone crosses the shoulder region of the prosthesis and is incorporated into the porous layer, the joint load will bypass the stem and be transmitted directly to the femoral cortex, thereby minimizing the effect of stress-shielding osteopenia. Should the stem fail through fracture or loosening at a future date, this bone collar may continue to maintain the skeletal integrity.

Acknowledgment. This study was supported by grant number CA 23751, awarded by the National Cancer Institute, DHHS.

References

1. Chao EY, Sim FH (1985) Modular prosthetic system for segmental bone and joint replacement after tumor resection. Orthopedics 8: 641–651
2. Chao EY, Okada Y, Hein T, Sim FH, Pritchard DJ, Shives TC (1987) Extracortical bone bridging: A new concept for implant fixation. In: Transactions of 33rd annual meeting of the orthopedic research society, Jan. 19–22, San Francisco. p 435
3. DeLee JG, Charnley J. (1986) Radiological demarcation of cemented sockets in total hip replacement. Clin Orthop 121: 20–32
4. Enneking WF (1984) Staging of musculoskeletal neoplasms. In: Uhthoff HK, Stahl E (eds) Current concepts of diagnosis and treatment of bone and soft tissue tumors. Springer, Berlin Heidelberg, pp 5–21
5. Enneking WF (1987) A system for the functional evaluation of the surgical management of musculoskeletal tumors. In: Enneking WF (ed) Limb salvage in musculo-skeletal oncology. Churchill Livingstone, New York, pp 5–16
6. Lane JM, Sculco TP, Zolan S (1980) Treatment of pathological fractures of the hip by endoprosthetic replacement. J Bone Joint Surg 62-A: 954–959
7. Mankin HJ (1983) Complications of allograft surgery. In: Friedlaender GE, Mankin HJ, Sell KW (eds) Osteochondral allografts. Biology, banking and clinical applications. Little Brown, Boston, pp 259–274
8. Sim FH, Bowman WE Jr, Wilkins RM, Chao EYS (1985) Limb salvage in primary malignant bone tumors. Orthopedics 8: 574–581
9. Simon MA, Aschliman MA, Thomas N, Mankin HJ (1986) Limb-salvage treatment versus amputation of the distal end of femur. J Bone Joint Surg 68-A: 1331–1337

References

Total Massive Hip Prosthesis for Tumors of Upper Femur

Analysis of Twenty Cases

J.P. Courpied and B. Tomeno[1]

Summary. Twenty cases of total massive hip replacement are analyzed. Of the 20 tumors, 15 had primary malignant bone disease and the site of occurrence was always the upper end of the femur. The mean length of femoral resection was 16 cm. The prosthesis used was mainly the Cochin type with a 32-mm head and a short lever arm. After resection, the range of follow-up was 1–10 years with an average of 4.5 years. Twelve patients remain free from disease and two have been lost to follow-up. According to Enneking's classification, the functional results are as follows: four are excellent, 11 are good, four are fair, and one is poor. The best stability of the hip was obtained when it was possible to conserve the lateral part of the trochanter with the attachment of muscles. After the procedure, hip immobilization with a plaster cast seems to reduce the risk of dislocation. The behavior of the prosthesis is discussed according to the bone resorption around the stem of the prosthesis and X-ray signs on the acetabular component.

Key words: Upper femur tumors—Resection for tumor—Total massive hip replacement

Twenty-four cases of massive hip prosthesis were performed between 1973 and 1986 at Cochin Hospital. For four patients, the follow-up was only 6 months (two recent cases, one patient died, and one was lost to follow-up) and, therefore, they are not included in the study.

Materials and Methods

Among the 20 patients, 11 were males and nine females. The average age was 40 years (range, 20–67). Fifteen tumors had primary malignant bone disease. Of these, six were classic chondrosarcomas, four were clear cell chondrosarcoma, and one was a mesenchymal chondrosarcoma. There were also two cases of metastases and three benign bone tumors. According to Enneking's classification, three of the primary malignant tumors were of type IIA and 12 were of type IIB.

After resection, the range of follow-up was 1–10 years with an average of 4.5 years.

---

[1]Service de Chirurgie Orthopedique, Hopital Cochin, Paris, France

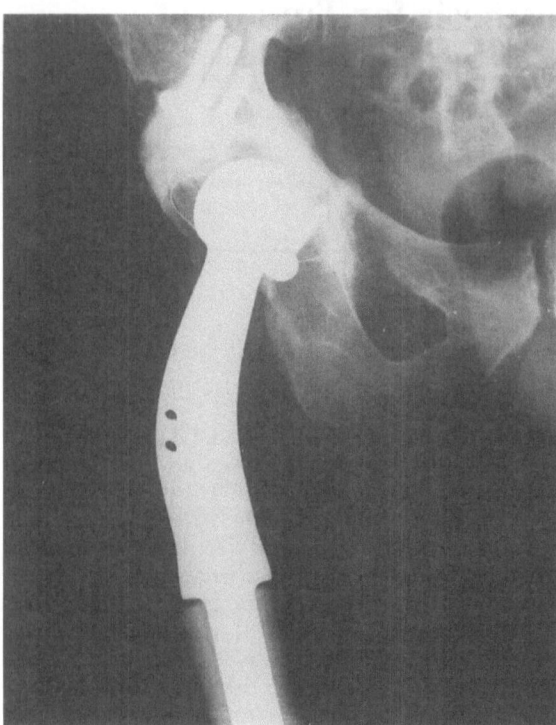

Fig. 1. En bloc arthrectomy after chondrosarcoma. Reconstruction with acetabular allograft and Cochin prosthesis

Resection of Tumor

Resection of the primary malignant tumors was wide in 11 cases and wide but contained in the four other cases. Resection of the two metastases was marginal.

The site of occurrence was always the upper end of the femur. However, in two cases of chondrosarcoma, en bloc arthrectomy was necessary because of articular extension of the tumor. The average length of femoral resection was 16 cm (range 10–25 cm). The muscular resection depended on the extent of the disease. It was possible in four cases to conserve the lateral part of the greater trochanter together with the attachment of the gluteus medius and vastus lateralis and then to fix this bone shell onto the prosthesis. When this procedure was not possible, we attempted to suture the remains of vastus lateralis and the fascia lata to the remaining gluteus maximus tendon and then to attach them onto the prosthesis in order to restore an abductor and flexor mechanism.

The prostheses used were one Muller, 17 Cochin [1], and two metal-on-metal prostheses. These two last prostheses became loose and revisions were performed with Cochin prostheses; so here we pay particular attention to the Cochin prosthesis.

The Cochin prosthesis is a metal-on-polyethylene cemented prosthesis with a chrome-cobalt femoral component, a 32-mm head and a short lateral level arm (Fig. 1).

After the operation, 15 patients were kept in traction for 3 weeks and among these seven were immobilized with a simple hip cast for an additional 4 weeks.

Oncological Results

There were three local recurrences after resection for one metastasis, one osteosarcoma, and one chondrosarcoma. In the two latter cases, the resection was wide. Metastases occurred rapidly and the three patients have died. There were three metastases after two chondrosarcomas and one after Ewing's sarcoma. All these complications occurred during the first 2 years after the initial surgical procedure.

Today, the oncological status of our patients is as follows: 12 are continuously disease free, one is alive with disease, five have died of the disease, and two have been lost to follow-up.

Functional Results

According to the Musculo skeletal Oncology Society classification, there were four excellent, 11 good, four fair results, and one poor result. Fifteen patients are free of pain, and in the five other cases the pain is modest. Active mobility is excellent in three, good in seven, and fair in nine cases; it is poor in one case after removal of the prosthesis for an early infection. The active range of flexion depends on the continuity of the abductor and flexor muscles; the average is 55°, but it is usually between 70° and 90° degrees if a shell bone or good muscle attachment—as described above—have been preserved. In the same way, active abduction is often about 20° in these good cases.

Stability of the hip is excellent in five cases, good in ten, fair in four, and poor in one (the case with removal of the prosthesis after infection). The length of femoral resection is not directly related to the stability of the hip. However, conservation of a trochanteric shell bone (four cases) always results in excellent stability.

All the patients but four use one stick out of doors and half of them can discard the stick at home. Success in achieving a stable hip depends on muscle preservation and a prosthesis having a femoral component with a short lateral lever arm.

Extra Oncological Complications

There were two early infections. In one case, exploration of the hip and cleaning gave a good result but in the other, the prosthesis had to be removed. There were three cases of dislocation. In one case, the dislocation occurred only once. In the two other cases, dislocations were recurrent and reoperation was performed. Modification of the orientation of the cup was successful in one case. In the other case, several procedures were carried out, involving reconstruction of the soft tissues posteriorly followed by hip immobilization. This hip has not dislocated in the 2 years of follow-up. In all the cases where dislocation occurred, there had been no hip immobilization after the initial procedure. We therefore think that the application of a plaster cast for 3–6 weeks postoperatively is advisable to reduce the risk of dislocation.

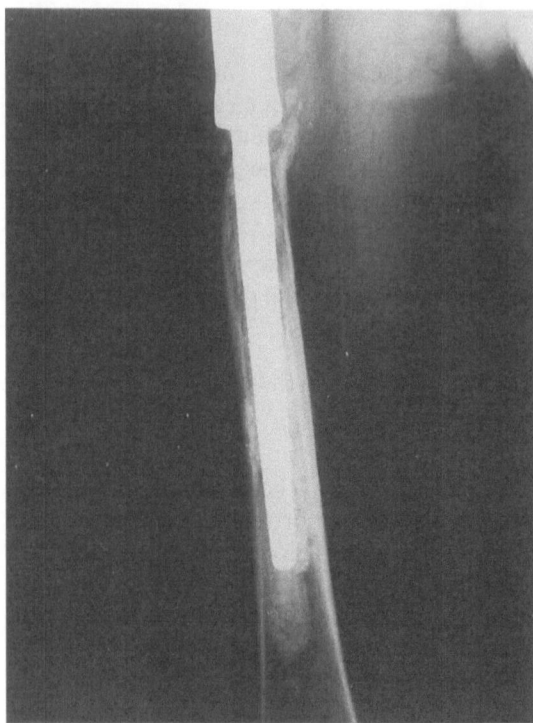

Fig. 2. After 5 years of follow-up there is seating resorption and endosteal cavitation. Functional result is still very good

Behavior of Prosthesis

On Femoral Side

None of the femoral components have broken. There was often bone resorption; this occurred where the femoral component rested on the shaft (five cases), at the periphery of the shaft with cortical resorption (four cases), or at the bone-cement junction with endosteal cavitation (three cases; Fig. 2). Among these three last cases, one loosening occurred and revision was performed 6 years after the initial procedure. Reconstuction was carried out with a massive allograft (upper half of a femur) and a long-stem prosthesis.

These various types of resorption appeared early and were the result of stress shielding. They seemed to occur most frequently when adjuvant therapy was administered before surgery.

In five cases, we observed extensive ossification along the big part of the stem, which appeared soon after resection. Usually, the functional result was good, perhpas because of good muscle reinsertion onto this new bone.

On Acetabular Side

In two cases there was slight wear (or creep) of the acetabular cup. In three other cases, we observed the following asymptomatic abnormalities: a radiolucent line, disruption of the metal marker ring, and fracture of a screw placed adjacent to the cup. These features may possibly indicate an aseptic loosening. Finally, loosening occurred in one case with recurrent dislocation. Reoperation was performed with an acetabular graft. All these acetabular problems occurred after 4 or 5 years of follow-up.

Discussion

In tumors of the upper end of the femur, resection-reconstruction gives creditable results. If possible, conservation of a small part of the greater trochanter with the attachment of muscles is a very good procedure: It leads to good active mobility and good stability of the hip.

We think that postoperative care must include immobilization of the lower limb: traction for 2 weeks after the initial procedure and then a plaster cast for 3 or 4 weeks. This immobilization allows good healing of the muscles around the hip and a slight stiffness of the joint. This is a better procedure against dislocation.

Results with the Cochin prosthesis design are favorable. None of the femoral components have broken and the short lever arm ("humerus-like") reduces the limp when the muscles are not sufficient. Osteolysis of the shaft may be a consequence of chrome-cobalt stem high rigidity [2], and it seems to us that a titanium alloy stem would be better than the current one. Another possibility would be to use a long-stem prosthesis with a massive allograft of the upper femur. Then, if union between the graft and shaft occurs, the stresses will be better tolerated.

The most disquieting problem is the cup fixation; after 5 years of follow-up, a lucent line or loosening appears. The head size is perhaps implicated in these mechanical features but it would seem dangerous to use a small head size because of dislocation. The use of a ceramic head to decrease joint friction would perhaps be a good solution.

References

1. Postel M, Langlais F (1977) Prothese de reconstruction aprés resection épiphyso-diaphysaire supérieure du femur pour tumeur. Rev Chir Orthop 63: 285–301
2. Dobbs HS, Scales JT, Wilson JN, Kemp HBS, Burrows HJ, Sneath RJ (1981) Endoprosthetic replacement of the proximal femur and acetabulum. J Bone Joint Surg (Br) 63-B: 219–224

Resection of Tumors of the Pelvis and Proximal Femur

Evaluation of Survival, Local Recurrence and Function

René P.H. Veth[1], Hans K.L. Nielsen[1], Jan Oldhoff[2],
Heimen Schraffordt Koops[2], Dinesh Mehta[3], Liedeke Postma[6],
Ludwig N.H. Göeken[4], J. Wolter Oosterhuis[5], and Bart Verkerke[7]

Summary. Nineteen patients with bone tumors of the pelvis and proximal femur were treated surgically by resection and reconstruction. Histological types included five primary bone tumors, 11 metastatic lesions, and three benign tumors. At review, four primary bone tumor patients were still alive without evidence of disease. The length of the observation period varied from 2 to 8 years. Seven of the eleven patients with metastatic bone disease had died. Their average postsurgical survival time was 17.2 months. All patients were able to walk with or without a cane. Failure of an endoprosthesis occurred in one case. According to the Enneking Evaluation System, the functional results in proximal femur replacement were one good and one fair in primary malignancies and nine good in metastatic disease. Both pelvic replacements and the three total femur replacements scored fair. There were two good and one excellent scores among the benign lesions (two pelvic, one proximal femur).

Key words: Bone tumor—Resection—Reconstruction

Introduction

Advances in cancer chemotherapy, radiotherapy, and surgery have led to an increase of reconstructive procedures in patients with primary malignant or metastatic tumors of the skeleton [1, 3, 6]. In high-grade tumors, the surgical procedure may consist of the eradication of the tumor and a reconstructive procedure [8]. In the region of the hip, one may consider prosthetic replacement; in the region of the pelvis, an internal hemipelvectomy may be chosen, followed by either an arthrodesis or a pseudarthrosis.

In primary bone tumors, such as osteosarcoma, the combined treatment with pre- and postoperative chemotherapy and extensive surgery including prosthetic replacement proved to be a reliable method in selected patients.

In patients with metastatic disease of the skeleton, a quick recovery should be the first aim of the treatment protocol. Impending and actual pathological fractures can be treated by resection of the lesion and implantation of a

Departments of Orthopaedic Surgery[1], Surgical Oncology[2], Radiotherapy[3], Rehabilitation[4], athology[5], and Division of Paediatric Oncology[6], University Hospital Groningen, Groningen, The Netherlands
Twente University of Technology[7], Enschede, The Netherlands

mega-endoprosthesis [2, 5, 8]. In our view, this type of treatment should also be performed in cases where chemo- and/or radiotherapy have proved to be inadequate.

In other metastatic lesions, one might consider a combination of osteosynthesis and implantation of methyl methacrylate. Following the functional grading system of Enneking, we report on 19 patients who were treated for tumors of the pelvis and proximal femur.

Materials and Methods

This paper concerns the results in 19 patients, who were treated by adjuvant therapy, resection, and reconstruction. Five had a primary malignant and 11 a metastatic bone tumor. In addition, three patients suffering from benign tumors are presented. Histological types included: osteoblastic osteosarcoma (patient 1), teleangiectatic osteosarcoma concomitant with an aneurysmal bone cyst (patient 3), and chondrosarcoma grade 2 in three cases. In all patients, the lesion proved to be stage IIB according to Enneking [1]. In one chondrosarcoma case (patient 2), the lesion was confined to the left iliac bone and superior ischium [4]. Eleven patients suffered from metastatic disease. Histological types included breast cancer (six patients), prostate cancer (two), multiple myeloma (two), and adenocarcinoma of unknown origin (one). Histological types in the benign cases were: giant cell tumor (one), aneurysmal bone cyst (one), and synovitis villonodularis (one; Table 1).

This study included 11 female and eight male patients with an average age of 53.2 years (range 14–76 years).

Neither impending nor pathological fractures were encountered in the primary malignant tumor cases. Four patients with metastatic bone disease showed an impending fracture, and seven patients a pathological fracture. Of these 16 lesions, three were localized in the femoral neck, five in the intertrochanteric, four in the subtrochanteric, two in the femoral diaphyseal, and two in the paracetabular region. Primary bone tumors were evaluated preoperatively according to the Enneking staging system [1]. In osteosarcoma cases, multidrug chemotherapy according to the protocol of Rosen et al. [7] was administered pre- and postoperatively. In chondrosarcoma patients, no adjuvant therapy was described.

The criteria for reconstruction in primary bone tumors of the femur were described previously [10]. Briefly, they are as follows: adequate resection of the tumor; moderate soft tissue extension without involvement of the neurovascular bundle; absence of metastases, or metastases which responded well to treatment; optimal local and general conditions; expected good cooperation of the patient.

The decision to treat the metastatic lesion was based on the following criteria: inadequate reaction to adjuvant therapy; life expectancy beyond 6 weeks; potential facilitation of the care of the patient with good mobility and less pain; a lytic lesion more than 2.5 cm in diameter; destruction of the cortex of more than 50%; potential greater benefit from surgery than from closed treatment.

In primary malignant tumors, only resections classified as "wide" according

Table 1. Patients with tumors of the hip region

Patient no.	Sex	Age (years)	Histology	Resection length	Follow-up (months)	Survival time (months)	Enneking results
1	F	47	Osteosarc.	240 mm	104	+104	Good
2	M	30	Chondrosarc.	Para-acetabular + total hip	71	+71	Fair
3	F	14	Osteosarc.	210 mm	53	+53	Fair
4	M	59	Chondrosarc.	Total femur	42	+42	Fair
5	F	61	Chondrosarc.	Total femur	26	26	Good
6	F	65	Mult. myeloma	180 mm	28	30	Good
7	M	66	Prost. cancer	120 mm	43	+47	Good
8	F	57	Breast cancer	120 mm	24	+24	Good
9	F	63	Breast cancer	Saddle	5	7	Fair
10	F	76	Breast cancer	30 mm	9	11	Good
11	F	55	Breast cancer	120 mm	8	11	Good
12	F	37	Breast cancer	Total femur	12	15	Fair
13	F	65	Breast cancer	60 mm	12	+16	Good
14	M	65	Prost. cancer	180 mm	12	+12	Good
15	F	45	Adeno. cancer	60 mm	3	4	Good
16	F	50	Mult. myeloma	120 mm	2	3	Fair
17	M	56	Giant cell	Cryosurg.	22	+22	Good
18	M	16	A B C	Curettage	35	+35	Good
19	M	35	Synovitis villo nodularis	120 mm	10	+10	Good

+ Patient still alive

to Enneking [1] were acceptable. Resection in metastatic disease should be classified as "marginal." In 14 patients, fixation of the prosthesis (Interplanta Anatomical Replacement-Link, Hamburg, Federal Republic of Germany was achieved with the aid of cement. In two patients, an uncemented intramedullary stem and two paracortical plates with screws were used. Bone resection varied from 60 mm to total excision of the femur (Table 1).

For acetabular fitting, a Bicentric (Howmedica, Limerick, Republic of Ireland) cup was used. Two patients had a total femur replacement (Howmedica).

In two patients, a para-acetabular resection [4] was performed in combination with a cemented pelvic and total hip replacement (Stanmore, England) and a saddle prosthesis (Link, Hamburg, FRG), respectively. In all patients, mobilization was started 2 days postoperatively. Ambulation with crutches was allowed 2 weeks postoperatively. Full weight bearing was permitted after 12 weeks.

Results and Discussion

The length of the follow-up period is presented in Table 1. At the time of this review, four of five primary malignant bone tumor patients were alive without any evidence of disease (Table 1).

The postsurgery survival times of the two osteosarcoma patients were 4.0 and 8.0 years; those of the chondrosarcoma cases were 3.0 and 5.0 years. One chondrosarcoma patient died 2 years after surgery. Seven patients with metastatic disease died and four are still alive. The average survival of the group of seven patients was 11 months (range 3–33 months); that of the remaining four patients was 24 months (range 8–47 months).

The combined active flexion, abduction, and rotation of the hip joints was 140° or more in four primary bone tumor patients and 110° in one. In the patients who suffered from metastatic disease, active motion of the hip joint was 160° or more in all cases. Flexion of the knee joint was limited in two primary malignant bone tumor cases (patients 3 and 4)—a range 0°–30° and 0°–45°, respectively. In none of the metastatic or benign cases was limitation of knee function observed.

According to the Enneking Evaluation System [1], strength could be rated "good" in all cases. Complete relief of pain was accomplished in 17 patients. Two patients suffering from metastatic disease needed nonnarcotic analgetics.

In the primary bone tumor cases, the emotional acceptance rating was good in three and fair in two patients. The results in the metastatic group were good in nine and fair in two cases.

According to the Enneking Evaluation System, the end results should be classified as good in 13 and fair in six cases.

Complications

Failure of the prosthesis was observed in one case (patient 4). In this patient, a Bicentric (Howmedica, Limerick, Republic of Ireland) cup had been dislocated. Because of additional damage to the acetabular cartilage, a Müller (Protek, Bern, Switzerland) cup was cemented in. Peroneal palsy was found in one patient (patient 4); this could be attributed to dislocation problems of the prosthesis. Infection, deep venous thrombosis, loosening, and fracture of the prosthesis were not observed in any of the patients. No perioperative deaths occurred and no evidence was found of local tumor seeding due to surgery.

In primary malignant bone tumors, the biopsy should preferably be performed by the same surgical team who will plan and perform the resection and reconstruction. In patients 3 and 4, the initial biopsy was carried out in another hospital. The abnormal localization and size of the biopsy urged us to perform a total femur replacement in patient 4 and a large muscle resection in patient 3. After resection, all chondrosarcoma specimens showed vital tumor cells on histological examination. In osteosarcoma patients, the Huvos qualification after chemotherapy was grade IV in patient 1 and grade III in patient 3.

We concur with Scales and Wright that the contour of the femur should be transposed on the stem of the prosthesis as much as possible [8]. We reject the use of fixation techniques of muscles to the prosthesis. In our opinion, the attached muscles will become necrotic and make this device useless. It also seems to be important to test the mobility of the adjacent joints when closing the wound. One should never attach remnants of fascia to one another if this compromises good mobility of the joints [10].

In our opinion, noncemented fixation techniques are preferable in primary malignant bone lesions [9, 10]. As the risk of loosening increases with the prolonged survival of these patients, one should aim at a fixation technique which enables revision of the prosthesis without a major risk of bony fractures. According to Oda and Schuman, the failure of pathological fractures to unite, the short life expectancy of the patient, and the compromise of stability of fixation due to weakened bone surrounding the metastatic lesion warrant the use of megaprostheses in fractures that would normally be treated by closed treatment, traction, or internal fixation [5].

Finally, good aftercare, especially optimal nutrition, prophylactic administration of antibiotics, antithrombotic measures, early mobilization, and well-trained physiotherapists are essential in the treatment of this group of patients.

References

1. Enneking WF (1983) Muscoloskeletal tumor surgery. Churchill Livingstone, New York
2. Johnsson R, Carlsson A, Kisch K, Mortiz U, Zetterström R, Persson MB (1985) Function following mega total hip arthroplasty compared with conventional total hip arthroplasty. Clin Orthop 192: 158
3. Mnaymneh W, Malinin THI, Mackley JT, Dick HM (1985) Massive osteoarticular allograft in the reconstruction of extremities following resection of tumors, not requiring chemotherapy and radiation. Clin Orthop 197: 76
4. Nielsen HKL, Veth RPH, Olfdhoff J, Schraffordt Koops H, Scales JT (1985) Resection of a periacetabular chondrosarcoma and reconstruction of the pelvis. J Bone Joint Surg 67-B: 413
5. Oda MAS, Schuman DJ (1983) Monitoring of pathological fracture. In: Stoll BA, Pabhoo S (eds) Bone metastasis. Raven, New York, p 271
6. Oldhoff J, Schraffordt Koops H, Nielsen HKL, de Vries JA (1983) Femurosteosarcoma treated by high dose methotrexate, resection and reconstruction with a custom

made endoprosthesis. In: Chao EYS, Ivins JC (eds) Tumor prosthesis for bone and joint reconstruction—The design and application. Thieme-Stratton, New York, pp 141–149

7. Rosen G, Caparros B, Huvos AC, Keshoff G, Nirenberg A, Cacavia A, Marcove RC, Lane JM, Mehta B, Urban C (1982) Preoperative chemotherapy for osteogenic sarcoma. Cancer 49: 1221

8. Scales JT, Wright KWJ (1983) Major bone and joint replacement using custom implants. In: Chao EYS, Ivins JC (eds) Tumor prosthesis for bone and joint reconstruction—The design and application. Thieme-Stratton, New York, pp 149–168

9. Veth RPH, Nielsen HKL, Oldhoff J, Schraffordt Koops H, den Heeten GJ, van Krieken F, Kamps W (1983) Reconstructive procedures in patients with a malignancy of the femur. In: Kotz R (ed) Proceedings of 2nd international workshop on the design and application of tumor prostheses for bone and joint reconstruction. Egermann, Vienna, p 180

10. Veth RPH, Nielsen HKL, Oldhoff J, Schraffordt Koops H, Postma A, Kamps W, den Heeten GJ, Hartel RM, van Krieken F, Göeken LNH, Göeken LNH, Oosterhuis JW (1985) The treatment of primary tumors of the femur with chemotherapy (if indicated) resection and reconstruction with an endoprosthesis. J Surg Oncol 30: 252

Reconstruction After Resection of Bone Tumors About the Hip

GEORGI ZAFIROSKI, BLAGOJ MIŠEV, PETAR GEORGIEV, IVANKA STEFANOSKA, and
GEORGI ZOGRAFSKI[1]

Summary. Thirty-two patients with aggressive bone tumors, low-grade malignant bone tumors, and bone metastases involving the hip region were treated by wide resection and reconstruction. Indications for resection and reconstruction of bone defects have definitely broadened with improved adjuvant chemotherapy, better surgical techniques, and replacement possibilities.

The choice of procedure was dependent on surgical staging according to Enneking, localization of the defect, extent of postresection defect, and general stage of disease. For replacing bone and joint defects after tumor resection, we used prosthetic replacement and biological material. Length of the resection extended from 18 to 24 cm (average 20 cm). A review was made after an average follow-up of 3.5 years, which is too short a time to assess the oncological value of this type of treatment but sufficiently long to assess the functional results and surgical technique. The functional results varied depending on whether the procedure was performed for palliation or for care. In 12 patients custom femoral components were used, in 17 standard total hip prostheses with a long stem were inserted, and in three patients after resection and cryosurgery bone grafts were used. Results for the group of patients with custom-made hip prostheses were as follow: seven patients may be classed as "good," two as "fair," and three as "poor." Of the 17 patients with standard implants, 13 were rating as "good," two as "fair," and two as "poor." The five (15.62%) bad functional results were due to one cardiac arrest, two local recurrences, one infection, and one sciatic nerve palsy. The clinical and biomechanical analysis indicates that these procedures are effective in carefully selected patients.

Key words: Bone tumors—Reconstruction—Bone resection

Introduction

Limb preserving surgery for so-called potentially malignant or low-grade malignant bone tumors and bone metastases has received increasing attention during the last 10 years. Giant cell tumor, peripheral chondrosarcoma, fibrosarcoma, parosteal osteosarcoma, aggressive tumors that tend to recur locally, and a solitary focus of bone metastasis are included in this group. The recent evidence that chemotherapeutic agents may have significant antisarcoma activity and technical

---

[1]Clinic for Orthopaedic Surgery, Faculty of Medicine, University of Skopje, Skopje, Yugoslavia

Table 1. Distribution of pathological findings and surgical reconstruction

Pathological findings	Surgical reconstruction			
	Number	Custom-made	Standard implants	Bone grafts + cryosurgery
Giant cell tumor	3	—	—	3
Chondrosarcoma	7	6	1	
Fibrosarcoma	1	1		
Bone Metastases	21	5	16	
Total	32	12	17	3

advances in reconstructive surgery and radiation therapy have fostered an enthusiastic era of protocols for saving extremities [2–4]. Thus interinstitutional cooperation and a surgical staging system for lesions of bone and soft tissue have become necessary [1]. The choice of procedure is dependent on: surgical staging by Enneking, localization of the defect, extent of postresection defect, and general stage of disease [1]. Careful preoperative assessment is necessary to determine whether the lesion is suitable for nonablative surgical treatment or for resection and reconstruction of the defect [2–4, 6–8]. Limb preserving surgery for such aggressive lesions has been supported by the relatively good preliminary results obtained by bone resection and various methods of reconstruction [3, 4, 6–8]. In considering the surgical management of locally aggressive or low-grade malignant bone tumors, the recent attitude has stressed the use of wide resection limb salvage surgery rather than amputation [4, 8].

From 1974 through 1986, 32 patients underwent reconstruction after resection of bone tumors and bone metastasis about the hip. After resection of the bone tumor, patients did not have servere functional deficits or cosmetic deformities. We hope that limb salvage surgery will be acceptable alternative to disarticulation or hemipelvectomy for the management of bone tumors around the hip.

Materials and Methods

Between 1974 and 1986, 32 patients with aggressive or malignant bone tumors and bone metastases were treated by radical resection of the tumor about the hip and reconstruction. Of these patients, 18 were women and 14 men, their ages ranging from 24 to 71 years (mean 52 years). The follow-up period in the group was from 6 months to 10 years (mean 3.5 years). No patients were lost to follow-up. Reconstruction as a limb saving surgical procedure was indicated in benign-aggressive bone tumors (G_0), low-grade malignant bone tumors (G_1), and a solitary focus of bone metastasis. The diagnoses for which the reconstruction after resection of bone tumor about the hip were performed are shown in Table 1. Of the 32 patients, seven had chondrosarcoma, two of these were recurrent following one to two unsuccessful prior surgical treatments and two had a pathological fracture. Three of the patients had giant cell tumor; one of these was

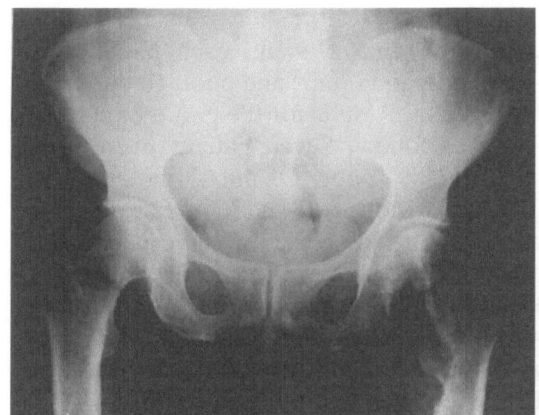
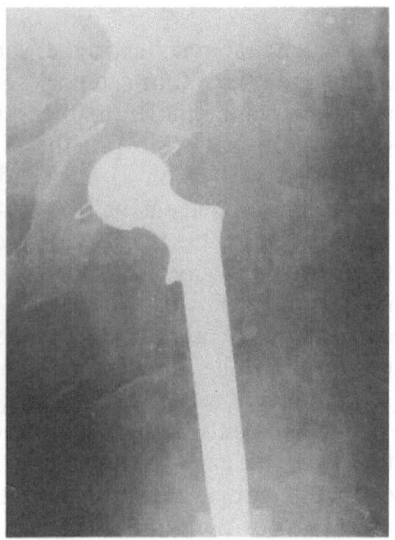

Fig. 1. a Preoperative roentgenogram of a metastatically affected proximal left femur and pathological fracture in a 58-year-old female with breast cancer. Eleven years after mastectomy, the patient was without evident disease. **b** Resection of the proximal femur and implantation of a tumor prosthesis. The patient had good function of the hip and was working using considerable physical strain. Two years later she developed lung metastasis but is still alive

recurrent. One of the patients had fibrosarcoma with a pathological fracture in the subtrochanteric region after open biopsy. All of these 11 patients were benign-aggressive bone tumors or with low-grade malignancy. One of the eleven patients had localization of the tumor in the caput femoris, four in the colum femoris, and six in the trochanteric and subtrochanteric region. Of the 21 patients with metastatic bone focus, eight were metastatic carcinoma of the breast, four were metastatic carcinoma of the kidney, three were metastatic carcinoma of the lung, two were metastatic carcinoma of the stomach and colon, one was metastatic carcinoma of the thyroidea, and one metastatic carcinoma of unknown origin. The most common localization of the metastases was the colum femoris and trochanteric or subtrochanteric region.

In 29 of the 32 patients, the resection involved a hip joint and endoprosthetic replacement was performed. In seven patients with primary malignant bone tumors and in five patients with bone metastasis, custom femoral components were used. The length of resection extended from 18 to 24 cm (average 20 cm; Fig. 1). In 16 patients with bone metastasis and one patient with primary malignant bone tumor, standard total hip prostheses with a long stem were employed. In two patients with giant cell tumor and one patient with bone metastasis, after en bloc resection of the proximal part of the femur and cryosurgery we carried out bone grafts in two patients and used mythyl methacrylate in one.

Results and Discussion

The functional results of the surgery were analyzed and each patient was assigned to one of four categories—excellent, good, fair, and poor. In our series of 32 patients, no patient had excellent results. Results for the group of patients with custom-made hip prostheses were as follow: Seven patients were good (58.33%), two (16.66%) fair, and three (25%) poor. Of the 17 patients with standard hip replacement, 13 (76.47%) were good, two (11.76%) fair, and two (11.76%) poor. Of the three patients with en bloc resection, cryosurgery and reconstruction were performed in two with bone grafts and in one with methyl methacrylate cement; two (66.66%) were rated good and one (33.33%) fair. The end result evaluation of 32 patients with reconstruction after resection of bone tumors about the hip were as follow: 22 (68.7%) patients were rated good, five (15.62%) were rated fair, and six (18.75%) were rated poor.

All 32 patients generally tolerated the procedure well, although, as can be noted by the early complications, the surgery was difficult. One patient developed a cardiac arrest during surgery. He was resuscitated but died 3 weeks later. Two of the patients had hemorrhages during the surgery and postoperatively; the hemorrhages in both cases subsided spontaneously after massive blood transfusion. Two of eleven patients with primary bone tumors had a local recurrence (18.18%)—one 6 months after surgery and one after 4 years. Two of them required disarticulation of the hip and died 1 year later of metastatic disease. Three patients with primary malignant bone tumors have died of metastatic disease 42.5 and 56 months after surgery. Of the 32 patients, two (6.25%) developed transient nerve palsy and both of them recovered within 4 months. Infection occurred in two patients (6.25%)—one deep and one superficial. In our experience, a serious problem was dislocation of the prosthesis. Of 29 patients, two (6.89%) developed early dislocation of the prosthesis. In one of them, this was solved with closed reduction and in the other open reduction of the prosthesis occurred. To prevent the tendency of these prostheses to dislocate, we applied the acetabular component horizontally in marked anteversion, the femoral component was 1 cm longer than the resected bone segment, and there was 1 month postoperative total immobilization. One patient had more than one complication.

The two patients with metastatic carcinoma are of interest. One, a 62-year-old man with hypernephroma underwent custom-made total hip reconstruction and radical resection of bone metastasis and died 28 months after surgery, but he did not have a local recurrence. The other, a 58-year-old woman with breast carcinoma 11 years after mastectomy developed bone metastasis in the proximal part of the femur and after custom-made total hip reconstruction 2 years later developed lung metastasis and is still alive. Fourteen patients with bone metastasis and surgical resection and reconstruction died between 6 and 20 months later.

A variety of methods have been used to reconstruct the hip joint and to restore hip function. Extensive cryosurgery can control low-grade and medium-grade chondrosarcomas following curettage or en bloc resection and bone replacement [5]. In recent years, interest has increased in en bloc resection not only for aggressive benign and low-grade tumors but also for limb salvage procedures involving high-grade lesions [4]. In the last decade with limb saving resection, more patients are undergoing reconstruction of the hip with custom-made prostheses, and with improved cancer treatment more patients are expected to survive the disease [6–8].

There have been two trends in the design of special prostheses for use following massive resection. The first involves modular prostheses, and the second noncemented prostheses of the madreporic type [3]. After resection and reconstruction of the bone defect of malignant bone tumors and bone metastasis, patients were without severe functional deficits and cosmetic deformities. There appeared to be little difference whether these patients were treated by amputation or en bloc resection in terms of their ultimate survival. Careful preoperative assessment is necessary to determine whether the lesion is suitable for nonablative surgical treatment or resection and reconstruction of the bone tumor about the hip. We hope that in future the material and the design of prosthetic implants will improve, and with improved cancer treatment more patients are expected to live linger with a better quality of life.

References

1. Enneking WF, Spanier SS, Goodman MA (1980) A system for the surgical staging of musculoskeletal sarcoma. Clin Orthop 153: 106–120
2. Enneking WF, Eady JL, Burchardt H (1980) Autogenous cortical bone grafts in the reconstruction of the segmental skeletal defects. J Bone Joint Surg 62A: 1039–1058
3. Kotz R (1983) Modular femur and tibia reconstruction system. In: Kotz R (ed) Proceedings of 2nd international workshop on the design and application of tumor prostheses for bone and joint reconstruction. Egermann, Vienna, pp 64–66
4. Marcove RC, Rosen G (1980) En bloc resection for osteogenic sarcoma. Cancer 45: 3040
5. Marcove RC (1982) A 17-year review of cryosurgery in the treatment of bone tumors. Clin Orthop 163: 231
6. Scales JT (1975) Massive bone and joint replacement involving the upper femur, acetabulum, and iliac bone. In: The hip. Proceedings of 3rd open scientific meeting of the Hip Society. Mosby, St Louis, pp 245–275
7. Sim FH, Chao EY, Peterson LFA (1975) Reconstruction following segmental resection of primary bone tumors of the hip. In: The hip. Proceedings of 3rd open scientific meeting of the Hip Society. Mosby, St Louis, pp 302–324
8. Sim FH, Hartz CR, Chao EY (1976) Total hip arthroplasty for tumors of the hip. In: The hip. Proceedings of 4th open scientific meeting of the Hip Society. Mosby, St Louis, pp 246–259

Bone Reconstruction Using Vascularised Bone Grafts

A 7-Year Review

PING-CHUNG LEUNG[1]

Summary. Tumor resection in the pelvic bone and proximal femur often leaves the difficult problem of reconstruction. Vascularized bone grafting has advantages over conventional grafts. In the past 7 years, 15 cases of locally aggressive lesion in the proximal femur and five similar cases in the pelvic bone were treated by the method of thorough excision and vascularized bone grafting. The femoral gaps were filled with vascular pedicled bone grafts based on the deep circumflex iliac vessels. In the pelvic cases, integrity between the spinal column and pelvic ring was lost in all cases and restoration was achieved through the use of a number of vascularized grafts, which included the vascular pedicled anterior iliac crest, muscle pedicled posterior iliac crest, free vascularized iliac crest, and fibular grafts. The results of healing were on the whole optimal for both regions. The vascular pedicled iliac creast graft used to bridge the pubic bones fractured but the patient was able to walk well. Two other cases of proximal femoral tumor suffered from fracture of the neck of the femur and were treated by screwing. The good results experienced give good support to the use of this technique.

Key words: Vascularized bone graft

Introduction

Large tumors around the hip and pelvis present difficult problems of treatment. Not only is tumour removal difficult because of the deep-seated nature of the lesions, but reconstruction for the large bone defects using the conventional means of bone replacement [1, 2] does not give good results. Since the pelvis and the hips transmit the body weight from the central spinal region to the lower limbs, their integrity is of vital importance to the normal ambulatory function of the human body. After the excision of large tumours in the hip or pelvic region, adequate and sound rebuilding of the defects must be established immediately so that early and efficient restoration of the strength may be re-established to allow the weight transmission from the trunk to the lower limbs. When extensive bone grafting is performed in the conventional way, i.e. non-vascularized, graft incorporation follows the rules of creeping substitution and the whole process needs

---

[1]Department of Orthopaedics and Traumatology, Chinese University of Hong Kong, Prince of Wales Hospital, Shatin, Hong Kong

Table 1. Tumours around the hip (proximal femur)

Type of tumour	Number
Giant cell tumour	6
Aneurysmal bone cyst	2
Fibrous dysplasia	3
Enchondroma	1
Chondrosarcoma (low grade)	1
Giant cyst	1
Osteoid osteoma	1
Total	15

Table 2. Tumours around the pelvis

Type	Site	Radiological size (cm)
Giant cell tumour	Rt. ala of ilium and sacrum	12 × 7
Giant cell tumour	Lt. ala of ilium	6 × 4
Aneurysmal bone cyst	Lt. ala of ilium	6 × 5
Chondrosarcoma	Pelvic bones	10 × 6
Chondroma	Sacrum and rt. ilium	11 × 8

months to be accomplished. During this period, the patient needs to restrain carefully from weight bearing, which might mean several months of bed-rest followed by crutch walking to remove the weight-bearing strain. Using a special vascularized bone graft, however, will significantly reduce the graft incorporation time and, hence, the whole rehabilitation process is hastened. Large vascularized bone grafts become united to the adjacent bone by a callus-forming process resembling fracture healing followed by re-modelling. Unlike conventional block grafts, the final bony resorption would be minimal; hence, the functional results are expected to be better.

Materials and Methods

Large vascularized bone graft reconstructions around the hip and pelvis after tumour resection were done mainly for benign or locally recurrent lesions when the life expectancy was expected to be long and adjuvant chemo- or radiotherapy did not have to be given. Such tumours included giant cell tumour, enchondroma, chondrosarcoma, aneurysmal bone cyst, fibrous dysplasia, and huge bone cysts.

Tables 1 and 2 list the tumours treated in the past 7 years.

Although most of the lesions were benign, a good marginal excision was thought advisable. Intralesional excisions should not be done because the chance of recurrence is high and recurrences tend to be problematic because of the deep-seated locations. In fact, for aneurysmal bone cysts, giant cell tumours and chondrosarcoma, a wide excision with a definite margin of healthy bone was removed.

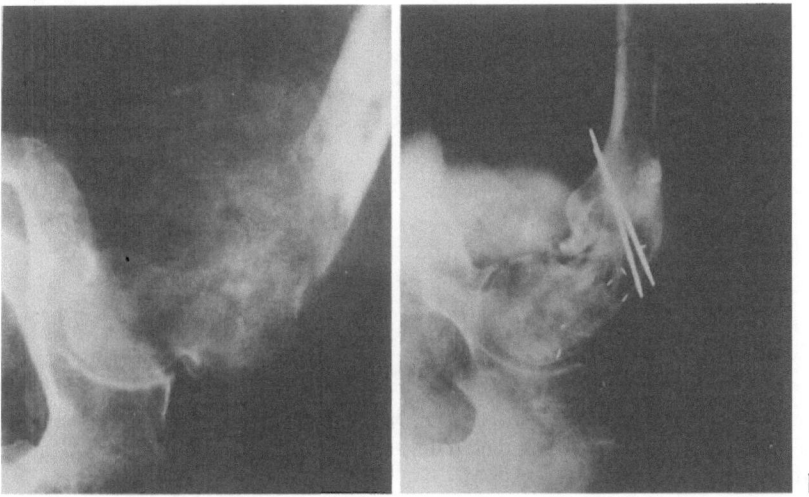

a   b

Fig. 1. a Pre- and **b** postoperative X-ray (4 months) of recurrent giant cell tumour of the proximal femur showing vascular pedicled iliac crest bone graft filling the large bone gap resulting after tumour resection

Hip Region

Since the lesions occurred at varying sites of the proximal femur, tumour resection left empty bone gaps in the intertrochanteric and proximal femoral region (11 cases), in the greater trochanter (three cases), and in the femoral head and neck (one case). The lengths of these defects varied from 8 to 13 cm and more than 50% of the circumference of the proximal femur was involved. The extensive involvement affected the strength of the bone to such a degree that if it had been left unsupported, fracture would have been inevitable.

A large piece of the iliac crest graft matching the bone gap to be filled, pedicled on the deep circumflex iliac vessels, was raised from the ipsilateral side in a fashion previously described by the author [3, 4]. The vessels gave off a number of branches before reaching the anterior superior iliac spine and then running close to the inner lip of the crest, where they became well protected. Extra care ought to be given around the anterior superior iliac spine region to make sure that no damage has been done to the vascular pedicle. The vascular pedicle was tunnelled below the psoas tendon. This soft tissue tunnel must be wide so that no compression occurs around the vascular pedicle. Fixation of the graft may not be necessary because it can always be securely latched in. Wiring or screwing may further strengthen the fixation. Remaining bone gaps were filled by cancellous chip grafts (Fig. 1).

Pelvic Region

Wide excision with ample free margins was the policy of resection so that recurrence could be avoided [5]. The resulting bone gaps varied from 8 to 15 cm

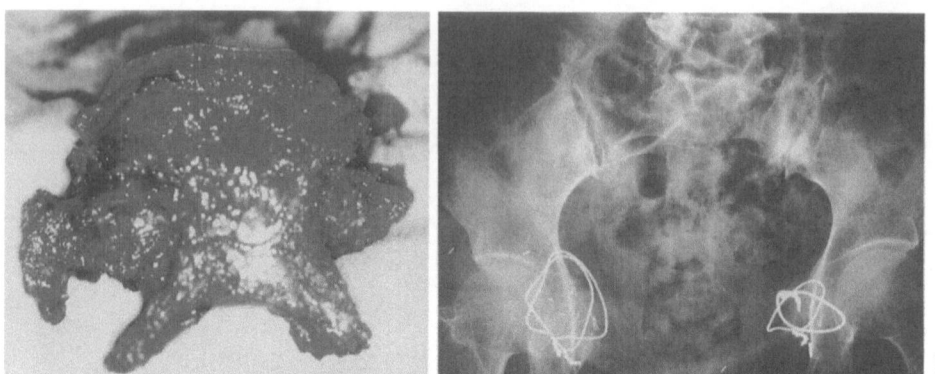

Fig. 2. a Operative specimen and **b** postoperative X-ray of recurrent chondrosarcoma of the pubic symphysis. A large vascular pedicled iliac crest graft bridged the wide bone gap resulting from tumour resection

and the pelvic ring was disrupted on all occasions. In the cases of chondroma, subtotal removal of the sacrum plus the posterior iliac crest on one side left a skeletally detached pelvis, which needed to be slung back to the lumbar spine. The wide gaps and diverging situations required a variety of vascularized bone to restore the skeletal integrity. In the case of pubic bone defects, an extra large (15 cm) vascular pedicled iliac crest bone was raised and rotated medially to bridge the remaining pubic rami. Fixation was achieved by wiring (Fig. 2). The same graft had been used as a free vascularized graft to fill up a large gap in the posterior iliac crest. The deep circumflex iliac vessels were anastomosed to the superior gluteal vessels. After sacrum resection, the lumbal vertebral laminae were wired to Luque rods, which were bent at their local ends to allow entry into the iliac bone at right angles. Two marginal pieces of posterior iliac crest, 3 cm wide and 12 cm long, were detached from the main iliac crest to glide medially towards the mid-line to give additional support to the hanging lumbar spine. The back muscles were left attached to these gliding bone grafts so that their blood supply was maintained. The grafts were wired at their medial ends to complete the rebuilding of the pelvic ring (Fig. 3).

The last case of aneurysmal bone cyst arising from the posterior iliac crest was excised and a free vascularized fibular graft folded onto itself in a double-barrel fashion was used to bridge the sacral ala and the acetabular region of the ilium (Fig. 4). Vascular anastomoses were performed between the inferior gluteal and peroneal vessels.

Results

In the hip cases, bed rest varied from 4 to 16 weeks, averaging 7 weeks in the uncomplicated cases. Healing occurred as with fractures, and postoperative evidence of viable grafts were proven by angiographic and isotope studies [6]. Complications included two cases of fracture of the neck of the femur in spite of

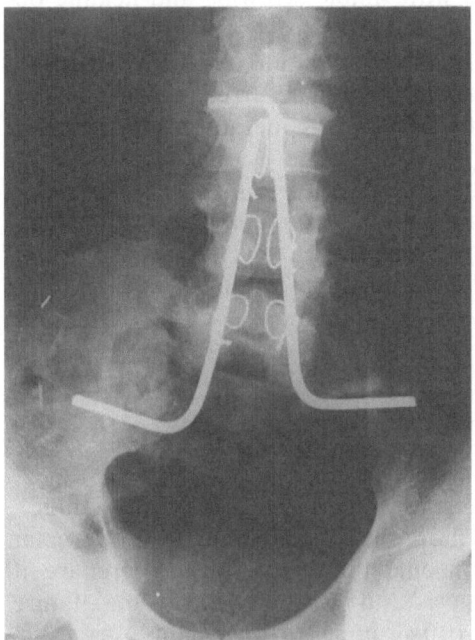

Fig. 3. Medial advancing muscle pedicled posterior iliac crest bone blocks were approximated at the mid-line to give more support to the vertebral column

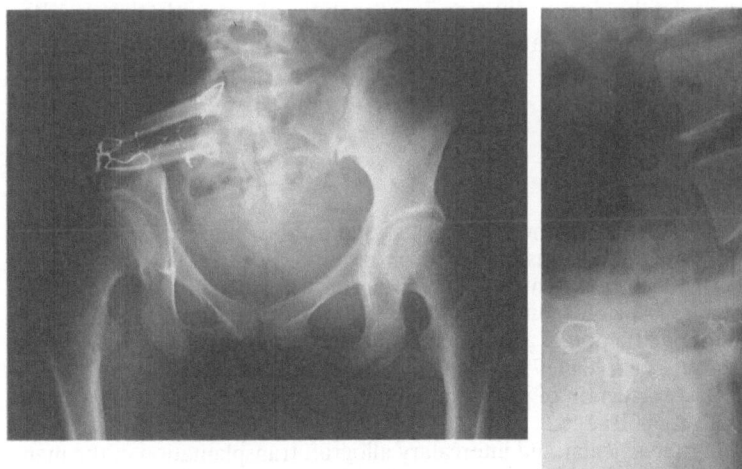
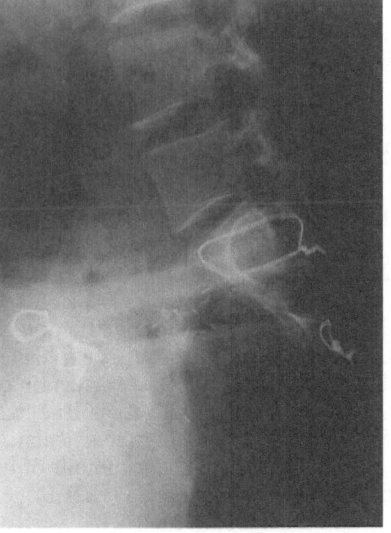

a

b

Fig. 4a, b. Double-barrelled free vascularized fibular graft bridging between the sacrum and iliac bone after tumour excision. **a** A-P view; **b** lateral view

intact viable grafts. These were treated with simple screwing and healing occurred rapidly in 3–4 weeks.

There was no case of recurrence with a follow-up period of 7–10 years (average $4\frac{1}{4}$ years). Limitations in hip flexion and abduction occurred in all cases. This was mild (10°–20° short of full range) in ten cases and moderate (20°–50° short of full range) in five.

In the pelvic cases, bed rest had to be prolonged for 3 months, after which assisted walking was started. Bone healing was evident radiologicaly and in technetium scanning after 2–3 months. Delayed graft fracture occurred in the case of long graft replacement for recurrent chondrosarcoma in the pubic rami. This occurred 6 months after the surgery, but the patient walked well with the pseudarthrosis that never healed.

Conclusion

Vascularized grafts give more reliable results of replacement: better viability, earlier incorporation, more strength and more rapid rehabilitation. The vascular pedicled iliac crest graft is particularly convenient in that it is easy to prepare, it does not involve microsurgical anastomosis and its cortico-cancellous nature gives it better quality of viability than cortical bones. Its proximity to the hip region has made it a valuable graft to replace bone defects lying within the radius of deep circumflex iliac vessels. When the deep circumflex iliac bundle cannot be used, the muscle pedicled posterior portion of the iliac crest may be mobilized, basing on the spinal and abodmoinal muscles, to be approximated towards the mid-line to complete the pelvic ring of bone.

When vascular pedicled bone flaps cannot be used, large bone gaps may be bridged with free vascularized bone grafts using microsurgical techniques. Although more technically demanding and more hazardous with the results, such grafts would be advisable because of the greater certainty with viability and shorter rehabilitation.

References

1. Parrish FF (1966) Treatment of bone tumours by total excision and replacement with massive autologous and homologous grafts. J Bone Joint Surg 48A: 968
2. Parrish FF (1973) Allograft replacement of all or part of the end of a long bone following excision of a tumour. J Bone Joint Surg 55A: 15
3. Leung PC (1983) Reconstruction of a large femoral defect using a vascular pedicle iliac graft. J Bone Joint Surg 65A: 8, 1179
4. Leung PC (1984) Reconstruction of proximal femoral defects with a vascular pedicled graft. J Bone Joint Surg 66B: 1, 32
5. Mankin HJ (1982) Osteoarticular and intercalary allograft transplantation in the management of malignant tumour of bone. Cancer 50: 613
6. Lau RSF, Leung PC (1982) Bone graft viability in vascularised bone graft transfer. Br J Radiol 55: 325

The Use of Bateman Bipolar Proximal Femoral Replacement in the Management of Proximal Femoral Metastatic Disease

Michael G. Rock[1]

Summary. Six patients, all metastatic in the proximal femur, who received Bateman bipolar proximal femoral replacement are reported here. These patients were uniformly subjected to the Musculoskeletal Tumor Society functional analysis, as was the prosthesis itself. The patients were afforded immediate pain relief and allowed early and vigorous ambulation with no morbidity to date attributable to the implant itself. The advantages of increased inherent stability, decreased tendency to protrude, ease of application, and ready accessibility are distinct advantages with the Bateman system. Four of the six patients died as a result of their disease but were, like the two remaining live patients, independent and free of pain at the time of follow-up or death. Most patients used a quad cane and could flex and abduct against gravity. Generally, the patients functioned at a good level and the prosthesis was good to excellent.

Key words: Bipolar hip prosthesis—Bone matestasis—Proximal femur

Introduction

The proximal femur is a common site for both primary sarcomas and metastatic disease. With the advent of limb sparing surgery in the management of bone sarcomas, many reconstructive procedures have been conceived and attempted, the results of which are now becoming evident (Figs. 1, 2). The use of femoral megaprosthesis in the management of primary and metastatic bone tumors was analyzed in 49 patients by Capanna et al. [1]. It became obvious that the use of this large implant was not without morbidity contributing to a difficult postoperative course and rehabilitation. In critically assessing the clinical and radiographic outcome of these patients, it became apparent that 20% of patients experienced at least one dislocation and radiographic loosening in 28% of femoral and 14% of acetabular components within several years of implantation. There was also 70% absorption of the host medial calcar at the implant host junction. The recommendations of Capanna et al. were to reconstruct the proximal femur with an implant that would exceed the length of the resected specimen by 1 cm; that the acetabular cup should be more horizontal proximating 20° and anteverted 30°; the femoral stem should be 16 cm long with press-fit characteristics.

[1]The University of Western Ontario, London, Ontario, Canada

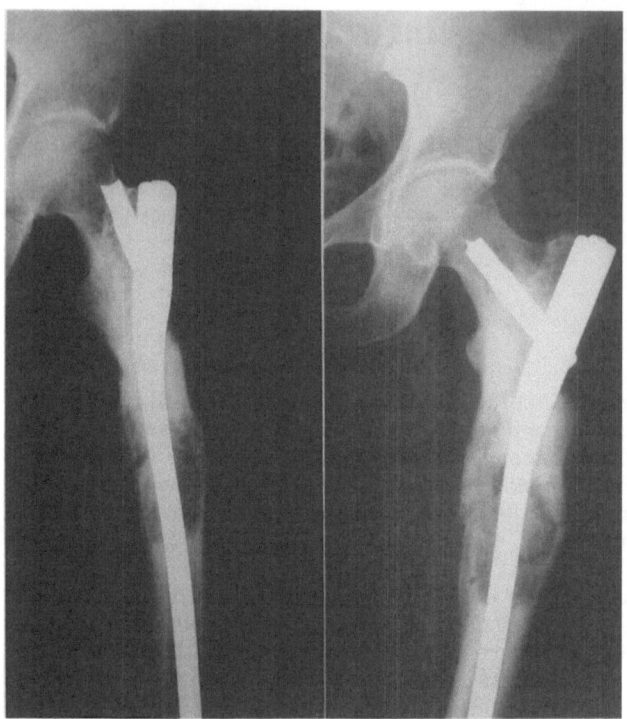

Fig. 1. Metastatic breast carcinoma in a 63-year-old female treated with a zickel nail.

The long-term survival of custom prosthetic devices is not accurately known. Sim et al. [2] note that at 5 years 83% of custom hip implants used in the management of primary bone tumors are still functional. Given the young age of most primary sarcoma patients, their inevitably activity level and demands, it is not unexpected that the implant will fail and will inevitable require additional reconstruction or possibly even ablative surgery. Therefore, in the management of primary bone tumors of the proximal femur, I have preferred a more biological substitute in the form of intercalary allograft and long-stem noncemented porous-coated implant with a bipolar acetabular articulation.

However, for patients with metastatic disease, the proximal megaprosthesis continues to represent an expedient means of regaining ambulation. In an effort to minimize the complications noted by Capanna et al., I used the Bateman bipolar femoral prosthetic replacement (Fig. 3) in six patients with metastatic disease. The inherent advantages of this system are that availability, ease of insertion, and the press-fit characteristics obviate cementing the femoral component. Absorption at the implant host junction is reduced due to the greater surface contact and serrated shaft stem junction. Possibly the greatest advantage of utilizing a bipolar articulation is the inherent greater stability and considerable less risk of protrusion that with unipolar articulation.

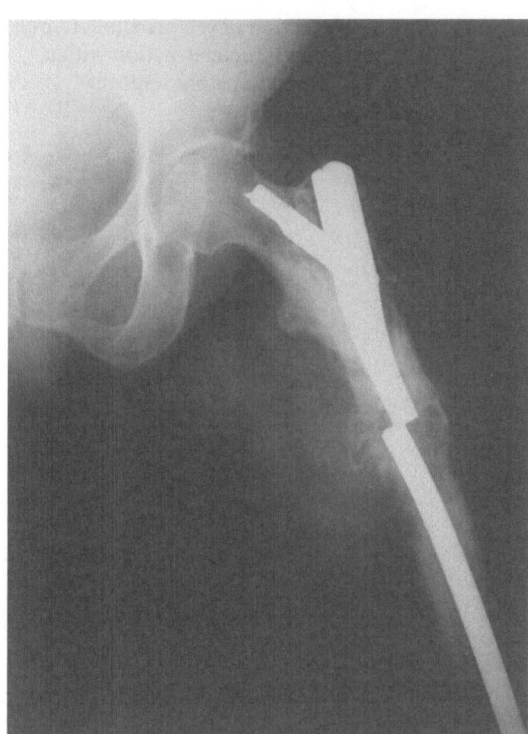

Fig. 2. Same patient in Fig. 1. One year later, the implant failed

Methods

Six patients with known metastatic proximal femoral involvement were treated with en bloc resection of the metastatic focus and reconstruction with a proximal femoral Bateman bipolar prosthesis. All of these patients had primary tumors diagnosed for which appropriate management had been initiated 6 months to 4 years previously. None of these patients were treated with anticipated cure in mind. All of them had other foci of metastases rendering their prognosis poor. The primaries were the breast in three cases, the prostate in one, the lung in one, and the colon in one.

Prior to surgery, the proximal femoral templates were used from the Bateman system to calculate the length of necessary resection, attempting to select a prosthesis that was at least 5 mm longer than the resected bone. Calculation of the acetabular size could also be conducted prior to surgery, although a wide selection of components was readily available at the time of surgery to articulate with the 22-mm femoral head. The shaft lengths available are 80–150 mm with a consistent stem length of 19 cm. The shaft lengths used in the six patients were 100 mm in one, 120 mm in three, and 150 mm in one. The approach was that of a standard lateral incision and, given that none of these patients were potentially curative, excision of tumor was performed without sacrificing a wide cuff of normal tissue. Therefore, the para-articular soft tissues, including the abductors,

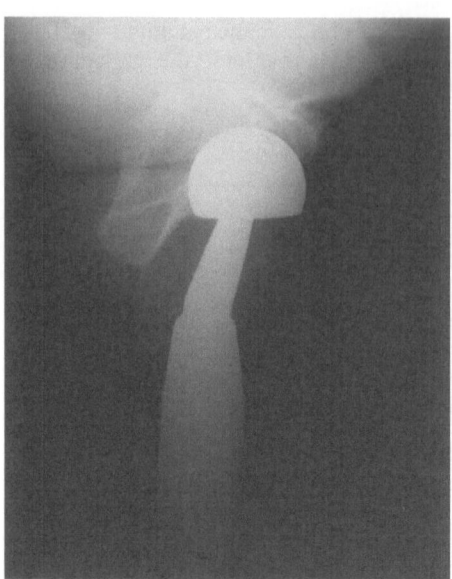

Fig. 3. Resection of the proximal femur was performed; reconstruction with a Bateman bipolar custom femoral prosthesis

vastus lateralis, and external rotators of the hip, were sacrificed close to respective bony contact to allow for a more appropriate soft tissue reconstruction. If the hip joint or capsule was not contaminated by tumor, the capsule was reflected off the proximal femur, tagged, and subsequently reconstituted around the bipolar acetabular component.

After excision of the specimen, it was measured for accurate determination of the resected length. If, as was usually the case, the femoral component was longer than the resected specimen, minimal alteration could be made to the host to accommodate the implant, recognizing that it should be at least 5 mm longer than the resected specimen. The femoral shaft was reamed with a flexible AO reamer to accommodate the large quadrilateral stem. Press-fit fixation of the stem was thus assured.

If the femoral head was still intact, it was measured, and from this measurement an appropriate acetabular component was selected. If not, trial acetabular components were used to gauge the most appropriate component. The femoral component was inserted first, and then the biarticulation was applied to the femoral head, after which the composite system was reduced into the acetabulum. Stability was checked by various flexion and rotation maneuvers. If the capsule still remained, it was brought over the acetabular component for additional support.

By placing the leg in maximal abduction, the tendinous portions of the abductors and vastus lateralis were approximated. If this was not possible, the abductors were advanced distally into the iliotibial band. The rest of the closure was standard.

Postoperatively, the patient was maintained in abduction due to the soft tissue advancement with the use of a Thomas splint. Recognizing the need to gain ambulation quickly in these patients within several days of surgery, they were

Table 1. Functional assessment

Patient	Motion	Pain	Stability	Strength	Acceptance	Complications
H.O.	Excellent	Excellent	Fair	Fair	Excellent	Excellent
C.A.	Excellent	Good	Fair	Fair	Good	Excellent
B.S.	Excellent	Excellent	Good	Fair	Excellent	Excellent
G.A.	Excellent	Excellent	Good	Fair	Good	Good
M.S.	Excellent	Excellent	Fair	Fair	Good	Excellent
D.C.	Excellent	Good	Fair	Fair	Excellent	Excellent

Table 2. Prosthetic evaluation

Patient	Anatomic restoration	Availability	Morbidity	Tissue reaction	Migration	Failure
H.O.	Excellent	Excellent	Good	Good	Excellent	Excellent
C.A.	Good	Excellent	Fair	Good	Good	Excellent
B.S.	Excellent	Excellent	Good	Good	Excellent	Excellent
G.A.	Excellent	Excellent	Good	Good	Excellent	Excellent
M.S.	Good	Excellent	Fair	Good	Good	Excellent
D.C.	Good	Excellent	Good	Good	Excellent	Excellent

taken out of the Thomas splint to be placed in an abduction pillow when in bed and recumbent. When ambulatory, a special brace that had been prepared by occupational therapists was utilized to maintain the leg in approximately 20° of abduction. The patients could then ambulate with the use of walkers and progress to canes at the discretion of the therapist. At 6 weeks postsurgery, the abduction splint was removed and active flexion and abduction exercises initiated.

Ten to fourteen days after the surgery and with the anticipation that primary wound healing was to occur, adjuvant radiation therapy was given to control local residual disease. Approximately 2000 rads was given over a 2-week period.

Results

All patients were ambulatory within the 1st week after surgery. All patients showed primary wound healing. The abduction splint was well tolerated by all patients. Four of the six patients died of their disease an average of 8 months after resection, whereas two patients were still alive at 2 and $2\frac{1}{2}$ years after surgery.

Four patients progressed to use only a quad cane for ambulation. The two remaining patients needed to use a walker due to their general frailty and other metastatic deposits. All patients developed antegravity forward flexion and abduction but could not overcome minimal resistance. All patients were subjected to the functional assessment as recommended by the Musculoskeletal Tumor Society for the hip, and the prosthesis was evaluated in similar terms

(Tables 1, 2). Even in the presence of fair designations in strength and stability, the overall functional assessment was "good." The assessment of prosthetic function was "good," posssibly even "excellent." The immediate resolution of pain in their patient population was dramatic, rapidly decreasing the need for analgesic administration and allowing their activities to increase toward self-sufficiency. The survival data reflect the serious implications of metastatic disease to bone.

Conclusions

The use of the Bateman bipolar proximal femoral replacement is advocated in the management of proximal femoral metastatic disease with impending or actual pathological fracture. The deficiencies of custom femoral replacements have been addressed in previous reports contributed to by the author [1], prompting the utilization of a bipolar acetabular. The results of the data have been very encouraging with no postoperative morbidity, rapid return to function, and restoration of quality of life. The advantages of the bipolar system are those of inherent stability, accessibility, and ease of insertion.

References

1. Capanna R, Rock M, Giunti A, Picci P, Campanacci M (1986) Femoral megaprosthesis in the management of bone tumours. a study of 49 cases. J West Pacif Orthop Ass 22: 1
2. Sim F, Pritchard D, Ivans SC, Shives TC (1979) Total joint arthroplasty applications in the management of bone tumors. Mayo Clinic Proceedings 54: 583–589

Resection and Reconstruction of Periacetabular Malignant and Aggressive Tumors

JOHN H. HEALEY, JOSEPH M. LANE, RALPH C. MARCOVE, KAREN DUANE, and JAMES C. OTIS[1]

Summary. We studied 34 patients who were treated for malignant and highly aggressive bone tumors of the pelvis and periacetabular region. Each was treated by limb sparing local excision of the tumor to evaluate the local tumor control and functional results. There were 20 males and 14 females (mean age 33.5 years). Diagnoses were of chondrosarcoma (12 cases), osteogenic sarcoma (eight), Ewing's sarcoma (six), malignant fibrocystiocytoma (two), and six other tumors. Radiation and/or chemotherapy were given both pre- and postoperatively in 24 of the patients. Staging was IA (two), IB (five), IIB (24), III (one), and 3 (two). Surgical margins were wide (27), wide with contamination (one), marginal (three), and intralesional (three). Resections were classified by Enneking's types: I (eight), IIA (four), IIB (five), IIC (13), and other (four). Reconstructions were as follows: girdlestone (ten), pseudoarthrosis (two), acetabular/sacral fusion with fibular graft (five), allograft pelvis/hip replacement (four), arthroplasty (four), femoral/pelvic fusions (seven), and local bone grafting (two). Twenty-two (65%) patients sustained major complications. After a mean follow-up of 45 months, 25 patients were NED, three were alive with disease, and six had died of disease. Local recurrence developed in five cases (15%). Functional results were excellent (one), good (five), fair (ten), and poor (three). Gait analysis was done on 12 patients. Asymmetry between the duration of stance phase correlated best with the functional results. Oxygen consumption and gait velocity had no correlation. In conclusion, local excision of periacetabular lesions can provide local tumor control and acceptable functional results.

Key words: Sarcoma—Hip—Function—Reconstruction—Limb salvage

Introduction

Decisions regarding the indications for and advisability of limb sparing surgery require careful documentation of oncological and functional results. The need is particularly acute in malignant pelvic lesions, which are infrequently treated by limb sparing surgery. The number of variables encountered have precluded statistical analysis of results. Significant progress has been made in unifying international standards for these complex resections and reconstructions. The Musculoskeletal Tumor Society System allows for clear preoperative staging.

[1]Memorial Sloan-Kettering Cancer Center, Hospital for Special Surgery, New York, NY, USA

Procedures have been clearly defined based upon their margin and containment by adjacent normal tissue. While these systems have worked for the extremities, substantial confusion apparently remains when referring to pelvic tumors. In the absence of sufficient tumors of a given histogenesis, widely understood definitions of margin, and uniformity of treatment, there is as yet no appropriate way to evaluate local excision of pelvic lesions for their oncological adequacy. Enneking's functional analysis, updated for their meeting, imparts a sense of objectivity to the functional evaluation. Though it remains unvalidated, it is the best measure currently available. The instruments are now in place to begin quantifying the oncological and functional adequacy of the mushrooming number of local excisions, and "limb sparing" operations now being performed for sarcomas. This report supplies information on one of the largest series of pelvic and periacetabular tumors treated by local excision. In conjunction with other series, some rational choices regarding limb sparing verus ablative surgery can be made. Furthermore, gait analysis is employed as a tool to measure more objectively the functional results.

Materials and Methods

Thirty-four patients with malignant and highly aggressive benign pelvic tumors underwent periacetabular excision at the Memorial Sloan-Kettering Hospital between 1977 and 1986. Twenty male and fourteen female patients were treated; the mean age was 33.5 years (range 8–75 years). Primary diagnoses were chondrosarcoma (12 patients), osteogenic sarcoma (eight), Ewing's sarcoma (six), malignant fibrocystiocytoma (two), and six other tumors. All told, there were 32 malignant tumors. The other two lesions were a grade II, stage 3 giant cell tumor that had failed radiation therapy, having replaced the entire ischium and medial acetabulum with a large soft tissue component, and desmoplastic fibroma with aneurysmal bone cyst degeneration, a large soft tissue mass, and destruction of the central acetabulum. Surgery was the principal treatment in all patients. Various combinations of adjuvant therapy were used: preoperative radiation (RT) and pre- and postoperative chemotherapy (CT) in four patients; pre- and postoperative CT in ten patients; pre- and postoperative CT and RT in four patients; preoperative RT in one patient; postoperative CT in four patients; postoperative RT in one patient; no adjuvant therapy in ten patients. Tumors were staged as follows: stage 3 (two cases), IA (two), IB (five), IIB (24), and III (one).

Preoperatively, staging was done by plain radiographs, bone and/or gallium scans, and computed tomography scan or arteriography. Local excision was performed for 33 patients with localized disease and one patient with resectable metastatic disease and severe local morbidity. Local excision was chosen for patients who were thought to have no involvement of the femoral vessels, sciatic or femoral nerves, or viscera.

An extended ilioinguinal incision was used, often in conjunction with a posterior "southern" approach to the hip, or occasionally with the utilitarian incision of Enneking. Extracapsular excisions were employed due to the propensity for extracompartmental malignant tumors to extend along the ligamentous structures of the hip joint. Special care was taken to achieve adequate margins in areas such as the iliopsoas and the hip adductor musculature, where tumor extension is commonly found. The following excisional procedures were done: hip socket and proximal femur (one case), inferior hemipelvis including the acetabulum (three), inferior hemipelvis including part of the acetabulum (seven), a portion of the hemipelvis including the entire hip joint and proximal femur (12), and the entire hemipelvis lateral sacrum, hip joint, and proximal femur (11). Using the Enneking system to classify pelvic resections, there were eight type I, four type IIA, five type IIB, and 13 type IIC lesions. An additional four patients had variations of type IIC resections referred to as type IID resections.

Wide margins were obtained in 27 cases. One additional patient had a wide excision with intraoperative contamination. There were three marginal and three intralesional excisions, one of which was a curettage and cryosurgery procedure and another a palliative marginal excision of the stage 3 chondrosarcoma.

Reconstructions were varied. Ten patients were left with a girdlestone-type reconstruction. These patients were generally mobilized 1–3 weeks postoperatively. Traction was rarely used. Two patients had intentional pseudarthroses established. Five patients had acetabular-sacral fusion with a nonvascularized fibula extending from the posterior-lateral acetabulum to the sacrum. Pubic symphyseal fusion was added in young patients who had mobile joints. Four patients had allograft replacements with the hemipelvis and proximal femur including the entire hip joint. Four patients had modified total hip replacements. This included one patient who had also received a Chiari-type osteotomy and acetabular shelf procedure to reconstruct the acetabular roof and one patient who had a socket implanted in the sacrum. Seven patients had fusions (five iliofemoral and two ilioischial fusions). These included three iliofemoral fusions with an average intercalary musculoosseous graft of 6 cm harvested from the iliac crest. Internal fixation was achieved by a cobra plate in most cases, using bolts or bone bolts within the pelvic wing to secure cortical screws. Two patients had bone grafting restoring the contour of the socket and prolonged non-weight bearing.

Functional results were graded by the Enneking classification for hip and pelvic lesions. Pain, motion, stability/deformity, strength, and function/patient acceptance were graded. Both descriptive and numerical scores were employed.

In an attempt to quantify objectively the differences between these diverse patients, we functionally evaluated 12 patients in the pathokinesiology laboratory. This included nine patients in the current series and three with similar resections or amputations not performed during the time covered in this review. The functional analyses were of two types: (a) measurement of energy consumption, and (b) stride analysis. Energy consumption was measured when the patient ambulated around the perimeter of the laboratory at a self-selected speed of ambulation. The rate chosen by a patient was used to adjust the monitoring-pacing lights, which were placed at regular intervals around the room. After walking at this chosen rate for 3 min, achieving the steady state of oxygen consumption, the patient's expired air was collected in a meteorological balloon (Douglas Bag Technique) during the next 3 min of walking. The pacing lights were then adjusted to flash at a rate 20% faster than the chosen rate. The patient adjusted the speed of ambulation for another 3 min and the expired air was again collected. Prior to ambulation, a resting sample of expired air was collected over

4 min. The expired air was analyzed for O_2 and CO_2 content, and the total volume was measured. These values along with patient's age, weight, walking rate, and air sample collection time were used to calculate the walking rate in meters per minute, net anergy cost in milliliters of O_2 per kilogram of body weight, and the relative energy cost in milliliters of oxygen as a percentage of the maximum aerobic capacity for both the chosen and accelerated walking rates.

Stride analysis requires that the patient ambulate along the 10-m walkway wearing insoles that are equipped with foot switches under the heel, first metatarsal, fifth metatarsal, and toes. These switches monitor the footfall pattern via wire connections to a waistpack recorder. Using a given distance of 6 m, the calculating unit derives and prints the gait velocity, cadence, stride length cycle time, and single-limb support time for each limb. The absolute and percentage normal values are printed for each parameter. Six trials were conducted, two at the chosen rate, two at the fast rate, and two at the slow rate. These rates were self-selective following verbal instructions by the examiner.

Results

Oncological Outcome

Local tumor control is a measure of any surgical procedure. Our local excisions were quite successful in this regard. Five patients (15%) developed local recurrence after 36, 34, 12, 6, and 4 months following IIA, IIC, IIA, IID, and IIB excisions, respectively, for two osteogenic sarcomas, two chondrosarcomas, and one Ewing's sarcoma. Thus, two of four (50%) IIA, one of five (20%) IIB, one of thirteen (8%) IIC, and one of four (25%) IID resection patients suffered recurrences. There was a trend for greater local recurrence in cases extending toward the sacrum. Disease in the periphery of the pelvis such as type I lesions had the lowest recurrence with none of eight cases.

After follow-up of 12–108 months (median 45 months), 25 patients were NED including 24 who were continuously disease-free. Three patients were alive without disease and six had died of disease. Removing the two patients with benign aggressive disease from the analysis, 23 of 32 patients are NED (72%). Deaths occurred at 36 months (osteogenic sarcoma), 15 months (Ewing's sarcoma), 12 months (chondrosarcoma), 9 months (chondrosarcoma), 1 month (chondrosarcoma), and 7 months (melanoma) postoperatively. Osteogenic sarcomas were well controlled with this aggressive surgical management and adjuvant chemotherapy. Six of eight patients are NED, one is alive with disease, and one patient died of disease. The standard T-10 regimen of high-dose methotrexate has enjoyed similar success treating pelvic lesions as has been reported for extremity lesions.

Operative Results

There were 22 patients (65%) who sustained 27 major complications (12 early, 15 late). Early complications included wound slough (five), neurological loss (three), major hematoma (one), dislocating hip replacement (one), the vascular rupture (two). The first vascular rupture was of the internal iliac artery following an extended type I iliac/sacral excision for a Ewing's sarcoma through irradiated skin. The wound broke down, infection developed, and arterial rupture occurred. The vessel was repaired and the sinus tract of the patient has slowly closed over the last 6 years. The second rupture occurred after an extended type IIC excision of a chondrosarcoma. Three weeks later, a delayed reconstruction with an allograft pelvis was performed. The pelvic graft was malrotated, leaving excessive pressure of the pubic ramus under the tented external iliac artery. Rupture ensued requiring vascular repair, which was complicated by infection, DIC, and death.

Late complications included delayed union (three cases) or nonunion (one) of iliopelvic fusions, allograft fracture (two), 70° structural scoliosis due to pelvic obliquity and limb length inequality (one), prosthetic dislocation (three), allograft infection (one), symptomatic incisional hernia (one), and painful instability requiring late fusion (four). Twenty-nine additional operative procedures were needed to address these problems such as wound debridement/skin grafting (three cases), prosthetic relocation (two), vascular repair (two), Chiari osteotomy (one), prosthetic arthroplasty (three), amputation (one), repair pseudarthrosis (one), bone grafting (seven), fusion (six), epiphyseodesis (one), girdlestone (one), and hernia repair (one). Due to the number of complications, no specific resection could be correlated with an increased complication rate. Specific reconstructive procedures suffered similar complications however. Iliofemoral fusions in the face of postoperative chemotherapy never healed primarily. Two allografts suffered late failure requiring revision. Prosthetic replacements were frequently unstable and complicated by dislocation. Disruption of the pelvic ring and skeletally immature patients produced severe structural changes, requiring surgery to reestablish pelvic ring continuity.

Attempts were made to go as widely around the tumor as possible during initial resection. This contributed to better local tumor control than reported elsewhere [1], but this improvement was at the sacrifice of some function and risk of local complication. It should be noted that the majority (13 of 22 patients) showed resolution of their problems without sequellae. The results were affected in nine patients, mildly in affected in three, moderately in two, and severely in four.

Functional Results

Enneking functional grades were given to 18 patients as seen in recent follow-up at a mean of 47.3 months after surgery. There were one excellent, five good, ten fair, and three poor results. When analyzed by reconstructive procedure (Table 1), there were deteriorating results as the articular surface was sacrificed, hip motion was diminished, or sacral/femoral stability was lost. No differences were seen when numerical values were substituted for qualitative descriptions of function.

Unavailable were five patients who had died of disease, four patients from overseas who had no orthopedic follow-up, two patients who had not completed treatment and for whom the postoperative period was too short to be evaluated, and five patients who had no recent follow-up. Of the nine living patients, off

Table 1. Functional results for reconstructive procedures

	Excellent	Good	Fair	Poor	Total
Girdlestone	0	0	5	3	8
Pseudarthrosis	0	1	1	0	2
Fusion	0	2	2	0	4
Allograft	0	1	1	0	2
Arthroplasty	0	1	1	0	2
Intact/cryosurgery	1	0	0	0	1

treatment estimates of function made from old records would be one good, four fair, and four poor results. In general, these patients had less remaining muscle and stability than the evaluated patients and for clinical reasons had undergone less extensive reconstructions. It should be noted that virtually without exception in both evaluated and nonevaluated groups, the patients apparently functioned better than they would have with a hemipelvectomy, with or without a prosthesis. Only patients with ongoing complications were limited to a greater extent than they would have been by hemipelvectomy.

Gait Analysis

Statistical analysis of results is not yet possible due to the multiplicity of resection, disparate adjuvant therapies, variations of reconstructions, and small numbers of patients thus far analyzed. Interesting trends are seen however. Nine patients were analyzed at a mean of 37.5 months after surgery. There were three type I (+), four type IIC, and two type IID resection patients studied. Preservation of an adequate weight-bearing socket was important in each of the parameters measured, namely free walking velocity, oxygen consumption, percentage maximum aerobic capacity, and stance phase symmetry. It did not, however, matter how this femoral/pelvic relation was reestablished. Good and bad results were found with each reconstructive procedure depending on the surgical success of that procedure.

The type of resection did strongly influence the gait parameters. Oxygen consumption averaged 0.198 l/min in type I, 0.195 l/min in type IID, and 0.245 l/min in type IIC resection patients (normal average = 0.160 l/min). This parameter best distinguished between resection types but varied considerably. It correlated directly to the magnitude of the muscle/bone excision around the hip joint and the intensity of adjuvant chemotherapy. There was no relation to the Enneking functional evaluation.

The percentage maximal aerobic capacity (PMAC) varied widely (14%–41%) but in all cases was well below the 50% cut-off limit, above which uninterrupted, sustained ambulation is not possible. Again, the magnitude of acetabular resection was the best indicator of results. Mean PMAC was 30.3% for type I (+) and 34.3% for type IIC resections. No relation was found between the type of reconstruction or Enneking's functional evaluation and the PMAC results.

Stance phase asymmetry between affected and unaffected limbs best reflected the functional results as assessed by Enneking evaluations. The relation is pres-

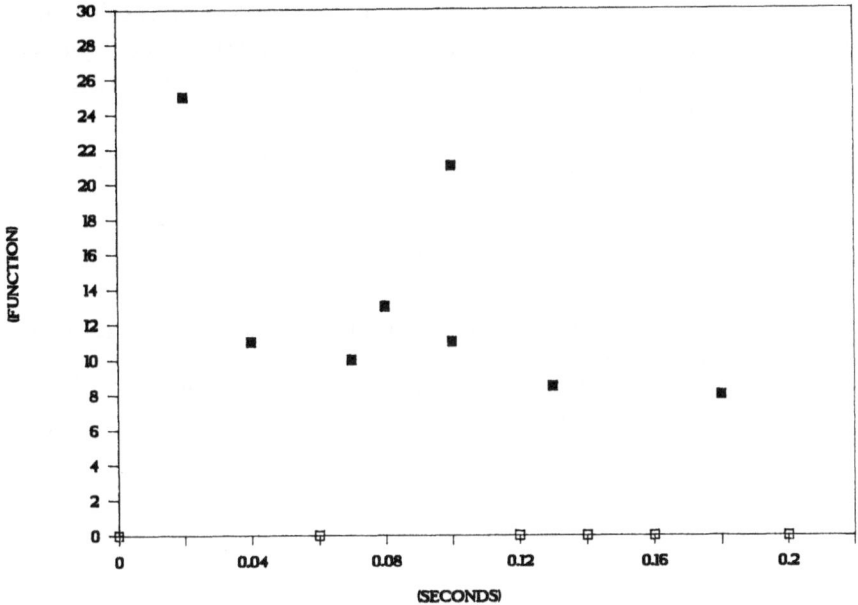

Fig. 1. Asymmetry versus function. The time difference between affected and unaffected limb single stance phase correlated best with functional score

ent whether qualitative or semiquantitative (5 points excellent, 3 points good, 1 point fair, 0 points poor) systems are used (Fig. 1). Stance phase asymmetry was unable to distinguish between the types of resections performed. Furthermore, the results varied markedly and did not necessarily reflect the success of the reconstruction.

Discussion

Periacetabular excision has acceptable oncological results with low recurrence rates in experienced surgical hands. Every effort must be made, however, to maximize surgical margins. Resection size correlates inversely with reconstructive difficulty and functional results. Early and late complications are common, and 9 of 34 patients were ultimately limited by complications.

Enneking's functional analysis correlated satisfactorily with resection size, and asymmetry of stance phase during ambulation. No correlation was present between functional score and the gait velocity, oxygen consumption, or PMAC.

Reconstruction should attempt to establish sacral/femoral stability. Functional score and gait parameters were best when this relation and limb length were optimized. No clear benefits were seen between reconstructive procedures that achieved these goals. Operative complications were at least as significant a determinate of function as the procedure. Hip fusion is theoretically appealing, but the results are discouraging because of limb shortening and nonunion (especially in the face of postoperative chemotherapy).

Current systems to evaluate function fail to assess: (a) functionally significant complications; (b) temporal alterations (deterioration?) of results; and (c) objective parameters such as limb length and gait analysis. These systems require validation with objective measures before they should be used to assess results of periacetabular excisions.

Acknowledgment. This study was supported by the Greenwall Foundation.

Reference

1. Campanacci M, Capanna R (1987) Closing remarks: Functional results of reconstruction for periacetabular resections requiring sacrifice of the hip joint. In: Enneking WF (ed) Limb salvage in musculoskeletal oncology. Churchill Livingston, New York, pp 187–192

Surgical Treatment of Bone Tumors Arising from Pelvic Ring

ATSUMASA UCHIDA, HIDEKI HAMADA, HIDEKI YOSHIKAWA, YASUAKI AOKI, SOHEI EBARA, and KEIRO ONO[1]

Summary. Six patients with periacetabular pelvic tumors were treated with a new type of constrained total hip replacement without reconstruction of pelvic continuity later wide resection. Five of six patients were able to walk with the supporting aids without pain after a follow-up of 6 months to 3 years. There was one local recurrence and one metastasis. No prosthetic failure and symptomatic loosening were found. Pelvic tumors away from the acetabulum were resected with wide margins and had no local recurrence. They had almost normal function. In sacral tumors (11 cases), there were two local recurrences and two deep infections. The preservation of the S_2 nerve root appears to be adequate for normal control bladder and bowel functions. Moreover, stability of the spinal column can be obtained with complete preservation of the body of the S_1 vertebra.

Key words: Pelvic tumors—Constrained total hip—Reconstruction

Introduction

Hemipelvectomy is the standard surgical procedure for primary malignant tumors involving the pelvic bone. However, pelvic tumors are potentially curable by an adequate resection with adjuvant chemotherapy and radiotherapy. Moreover, the development of diagnostic imaging such as computed tomography and nuclear magnetic resonance imaging has greatly enhanced the accuracy of the anatomical location of tumors, and makes it easy to select the patients who have adequate resection. With regard to resection and reconstruction, the pelvic ring is divided into three parts—periacetabular regions, sacral regions, and pelvic bone away from the acetabulum. This paper describes the method of wide resection and reconstruction employed, the functional results in patients who had resections, and the incidence of local recurrence, metastasis, and complications after these procedures.

[1] Department of Orthopaedic Surgery, Osaka University Medical School, Osaka, Japan

Table 1. Tumorous conditions of pelvic tumors

Tumor type	No. of patients
Periacetabular	
Chondrosarcoma	3
Osteosarcoma	2
Malignant fibrous	1
Histiocytoma	1
Pelvic away from acetabulum	
Giant cell tumors	3
Ewing's sarcoma	3
Malignant lymphoma	1
Chondroblastoma	1
Sacral	
Chordoma	5
Giant cell tumors	5
Chondrosarcoma	1

Patients

All patients who were thought to have malignant bone tumors and locally aggressive benign lesions were considered for resection and reconstruction under the following circumstances: (a) when there was no evidence of metastasis; (b) when the anatomical location of the lesion would permit and adequate margin. There were six cases of periacetabular tumors: two osteosarcomas, three chondrosarcomas, and one malignant fibrous histiocytoma of bone. Eleven sacral tumors consisted of five chordomas, five giant cell tumors, and one chondrosarcoma. On the other hand, there were eight cases of pelvic tumors away from the acetabulum: three giant cell tumors, three Ewing's sarcoma, one malignant lymphoma of the ilium, and one large chondroblastoma of the iliac wing. These pelvic tumors were located in ilium in seven cases and in the pubis in one case (Table 1). In malignant tumors, all patients received pre- and/or postoperative adjuvant chemotherapy, and the patients who had an inadequate margin received postoperative radiotherapy. The functional results were assessed by Enneking's evaluation system.

Surgical Procedures

In periacetabular lesions, the whole acetabulum and adjacent portion of the ilium, ischium, and pubis were resected by including the hip joint. Lesions that showed intrapelvic extension required the removal of the iliacus and psoas muscles to achieve adequate margins. In contrast, gluteal muscles were removed for the lesions extending in the buttocks. Although there are several types of reconstruction after this wide resection, e.g., resection arthroplasty, arthrodesis, we selected the method of reconstruction using constrained total hip prosthesis without the restoration of pelvic continuity for reasons of stability of the hip joint, easy fixation of the prosthesis to the residual bone, and early rehabilita-

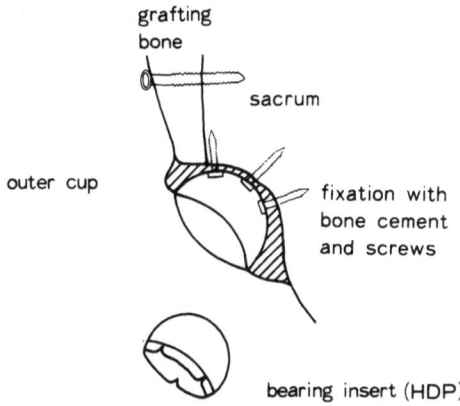

grafting
bone

sacrum

outer cup

fixation with
bone cement
and screws

bearing insert (HDP)

Fig. 1. Schema of constrained total hip replacement. Bone grafting was performed at the anterior and lateral sacrum for the rigid fixation of acetabular cup

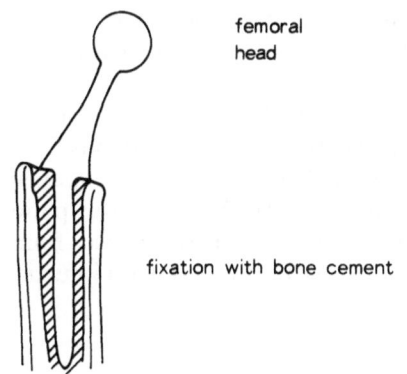

femoral
head

fixation with bone cement

tion. This constrained total hip is composed of three components. The metallic outer head is fixed firmly with screws, bone cement, and bone grafting to the remaining ilium and sacrum, and then the inner head with the long neck and stem is cemented into the femoral shaft. These two components are connected by a high-density polyethylene-bearing insert, and the constrained total hip replacement is accomplished (Fig. 1).

In sacral tumors, a combined abdominal sacral incision that provides access to both the intrapelvic and extrapelvic aspects was used. At the onset, the internal iliac artery and vein were exposed and ligated to reduced bleeding. The nerve roots that were to be removed for wide resection were identified and divided at their exit from the dura. With the remaining dura and intact nerve roots protected, osteotomy of the sacrum was performed and then connected with the sciatic notch on each side. In cases of complete preservation of the body of the S_1 vertebra, spinal stabilization was never required. In contrast, various types of stabilization of the vertebral column were performed in cases of impairment of the sacroilac joints. Bone grafting and spinal instrumentation were used for the stabilization.

Wide resection of the iliac wing was performed with the combined resection of the buttock and iliac muscles if required. Disruption of the sacroiliac joint after wide resection required reconstruction of this joint by bone grafting and approximation of the remaining part of the pelvic bone.

Results

Reconstruction with Constrained Total Hip Prosthesis

The functional results of six patients with this type of reconstruction were assessed by Enneking's evaluation system. Follow-up ranged from 6 months to 3 years. The functional ratings were two good, two fair, and two poor. However, five of six patients had no pain and all patients were able to walk with supporting aids. Moreover, two patients in the fair group had good results for the rating of emotional acceptance and functional activity. It was necessary to preserve either the psoas or gluteal muscle for rotational control of the hip joint. Enneking's functional results were correlated with the function of the preserved muscles after wide resection rather than the method of reconstruction of the hip joint (Table 2).

There was one local recurrence in the case of inadequate marginal resection. Local recurrence in case 2 (chondrosarcoma) was found in subcutaneous tissues around the incisional scar at 1 year after operation. There was one lung metastasis in the case of malignant fibrous histiocytoma (case 4). Although this patient died of pulmonary metastasis at 15 months, no local recurrence was found. There were no prosthetic failures, symptomatic loosenings, and deep infections (Fig. 2).

Sacral Tumors

The results in sacral tumors are shown in Table 3. Two patients underwent bilateral resection of the sacral nerve roots S_2 through S_5 in the course of the sacral resection, and two had bilateral resection of S_3 through S_5. Preservation of the S_2 nerve appears to be adequate for normal control of bladder and bowel functions. The two patients who had resection of the S_2 nerve did not have bladder incontinence, although they required intra-abdominal pressure to control the bladder. It was possible to control bowel function with preservation of the S_1 nerve root. Three patients had bilateral resection of S_1 through S_5, sacral roots. Two patients required intermittent catheterization to control the bladder, whereas the other patient could void spontaneously by increasing intra-abdominal pressure. There were two patients with unilateral resection of sacral nerve roots S_1 through S_5. they experienced to bowel incontinence and could void spontaneously by increasing intra-abdominal pressure. These results suggest that even in patients with unilateral resection of the S_1 nerve root, tolerable control of bowel and bladder function can be obtained. Although unilateral resection of the S_1 root caused weakness of plantar flexion in the ankle joint, it was possible for the patients to walk without the assistance of a brace. Various types of stabilization of the vertebral column were required in six patients with an impaired sacroiliac joint. Unilateral or bilateral sacroiliac fusions were performed in five cases and lumboiliac fusion with bone grafting and instrumental fixation in one

Table 2. Functional results of constrained total hip replacement

Case no.	Age (years)	Sex	Diagnosis	Follow-up	Motion	Pain	Stability	Deformity	Strength	Functional activity	Emotional acceptance	Rating
1	73	F	OS	36	P	P	P	P	P	P	F	P
2	67	M	OS	17	G	E	F	G	P	F	G	F
3	64	M	CS	15	G	E	G	E	F	G	G	G
4	51	F	MFH	15	P	E	P	G	P	P	F	P
5	36	M	CS	12	G	E	G	E	F	G	G	G
6	25	M	CS	6	G	E	F	E	F	F	G	F

Functional assessment was made by Enneking's Evaluation system
OS osteosarcoma, CS chondrosarcoma, MFH malignant fibrous histiocytoma of bone, E excellent, G good, F fair, P poor

Table 3. Functional results after resection of sacral nerve root

Functional results	Level of resection			
	S_3–S_5 ($n=2$)	S_2–S_5 ($n=2$)	Unilateral S_1–S_5 ($n=2$)	Bilateral S_1–S_5 ($n=3$)
Bladder				
Continent	2	0	0	0
Void by intra-abdominal pressure	0	2	2	1
Catheterization	0	0	0	2
Bowel				
Continent	2	2	2	1
Incontinent	0	0	0	2

S_3–S_5 indicates resection of S_3 through S_5 sacral nerve roots

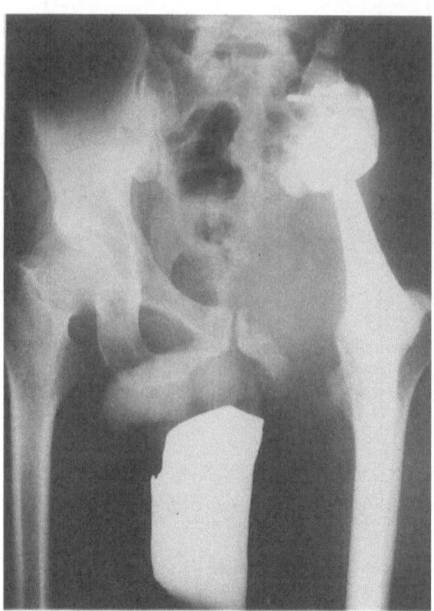

Fig. 2. Postoperative X-ray in case 5 (chondrosarcoma). No mechanical loosening and local recurrence were found 12 months after the operation. This patient was able to walk without a cane and returned to work

case. Stability of the spinal column can be obtained with complete preservation of the body of the S_1 vertebra. Local recurrence developed in two of these patients. One of the patients with a chordoma showed evidence of recurrence at 1 year postoperatively and was treated with radiation. The other patient with a giant cell tumor had recurrence at 6 months after operation and was reoperated. These two cases had inadequate resection of the tumors. There were two deep wound infections, requiring multiple debridement and drainage.

Pelvic Tumors away from the Acetabulum

In pelvic tumors away from the acetabulum, all patients had excellent results. Becuase all cases were operated with wide excision, they had no local recurrence for follow-up periods ranging from 1 to 20 years. Four of seven iliac wing tumors had disruption of pelvic continuity at the site of the sacroiliac joint after wide resection of tumors. The pelvic ring continuity was reconstructed by sacroiliac fusion with bone grafting and approximation of the remaining part of the pelvic bone. There was no pseudoarthrosis. On the other hand, although no reconstruction of pelvic continuity was performed after pubic resection, the function was normal.

Discussion

There are many problems regarding the reconstruction after wide resection that requires sacrifice of the acetabulum. Enneking and Dunham [1], Steel [2] and Nilsonne et al. [3] describe femoral-iliac arthrodesis without restoration of pelvic continuity as the best type of reconstruction and the functional results after pseudoarthrosis as upredictable. The disadvantage of arthrodesis, however, is the inevitable discrepancy in leg length. Therefore, Johnson [4] and Nielsen et al. [5] reported the reconstruction method of the pelvic defect after periacetabular resection by combining total hip athroplasty and restoration of the pelvic ring by prosthesis or cementation to prevent leg length discrepancy. This type of procedure also has the difficulty of rigid fixation of prosthesis and the risk of dislocation of the hip joint because of the removal of the extensive soft tissues to obtain a wide margin of tumor resection. Our constrained total hip atrthroplasty appears to provide a stable joint and easy fixation of the prosthesis. Although fixation of the acetabular component appears to be insufficient compared with conventional total hip replacement, there have been no signs of mechanical loosening during the follow-up period. Moreover, to obtain greater rigid fixation of the acetabular cup to the sacrum, we are now improving the design of the outer cup.

With regard to repair of the continuity of the pelvic ring, a good cosmetic and functional results might be best achieved by reconstruction of the normal anatomy. In contrast, there are some reports that it is not essential to repair the pelvic continuity for a good functional result. In our reconstruction method, there is no repair of the pelvic continuity, but no patients were disabled as a result of this disruption. The present results demonstrate that excellent postoperative assessment will be achieved if adequate margins can be obtained and stable joint reconstruction with preservation of sufficient muscle strength is performed.

Patients with resection of the iliac wing had almost normal function when the neck of the ilium was fused to the sacrum by bone grafting. Moreover, even in two patients who had no reconstruction of pelvic continuity after resection of the iliac wing, there was no impairment of the stability and motion of the hip joint at 2 or 3 years follow-up. Some patients had a slight limp because of the weakness of the hip abductor muscles.

In sacral tumors, there are many problems in surgical management [6]. Two local recurrence (2/11) and two deep wound infections (2/11) were found in this series. For the prevention of local recurrence, accurate preoperative diagnosis of the intrapelvic location of tumors must be achieved using various imaging methods, and surgical planning which provides an opportunity to obtain a wide margin of resection must be made. Moreover, chemotherapy and radiotherapy should be also used.

The preservation of the S_1 vertebra did not cause instability of the vertebral column, but we must consider the management for a large defect after sacral resection because a hematoma in the defect can cause a deep wound infection. Neurologically, preservation of the S_1 nerve root enables control of bowel and bladder functions after adequate training.

References

1. Enneking WF, Dunham WK (1978) Resection and reconstruction for primary neoplasms invoving the innominate bone. J Bone Joint Surg 60-A: 731–746

2. Steel HH (1978) Partial or complete resection of the hemipelvis: an alternative to hidquater amputation for periacetabular chondrosarcoma of the pelvis. J Bone Joint Surg 60-A: 719–730
3. Nilsonne V, Kreicberg A, Olsson E, Stark A (1982) Function after pelvic tumor resection involving the acetabular ring. Int Orthop 6: 27–33
4. Johnson JTH (1978) Reconstruction of the pelvic ring following tumor resection. (1978) J Bone Joint Surg 6-A: 747–751
5. Nielsen HKL, Veth RPH, Oldhoff J, Schraffordt Koops H, Sales JT (1985) Resection of a peri-acetabular chondrosarcoma and reconstruction of the pelvis—a case report. J Bone Joint Surg 67-B: 413–415
6. Huth JF, Bawson EG, Eilber FR (1984) Abdominal resection for malignant tumors of the sacrum. Am J Surg 148: 157–161

Innominate Bone Resection for Tumors with Limb Preservation

A Report of 36 Cases

BERNARD TOMENO and ANNE LANGUEPIN[1]

Summary. Thrity-six innominate bone resections for malignant tumors with limb conservation are analyzed. The functional results were almost always satisfactory for resections concerning only the ilium (12 cases) or only the pubic ring (eight cases) and, here, reconstruction was usually unnecessary of very easy. Reconstructions for resections concerning the acetabulum, either isolated (one case) associated with an ilium resection (six cases), a pubic resection (seven cases), or both (two cases), are more difficult; complications are frequent and functional results are seldom perfect, even using massive bone grafts or massive prosthetic components. Arthrodesis between the upper femur and pubic ring remains a reliable procedure; excluding the problem of mobility, the results are quite good.

Key words: Innominate bone tumors—Bone resections—Hemipelvectomy

Between 1954 and 1987, almost 2000 bone tumors were treated in our orthopedic department. About half of them were benign and half malignant. Sixty-six malignant tumors required innominate bone resection: 30 were treated by hemiquarter amputation and 36 by conservative techniques, using various reconstructive procedures.

General Data on 36 Cases

There were 16 males and 20 females, and the age ranged from 20 to 64 years (average 40.5 years). The tumors concerned were: 31 chondrosarcomas (nine secondary to an exostosis), two osteosarcomas, one fibrosarcoma, one malignant hemangioendothelioma, and one metastasis. The follow-up ranged from a few months to 20 years, with an average of greater than 4 years (52.6 months). Functional results, however, are only available for 28 of the 36 cases: One patient never returned, five soon died (three metastases and two major postoperative complications), and two were operated upon recently.

The site of the resection was: zone I isolated (ilium) in 12 cases, zone II isolated (acetabulum) in one case, zone III isolated (pubic ring) in eight cases,

---

[1] Pavillon Ollier, Hôpital Cochin, Paris, France

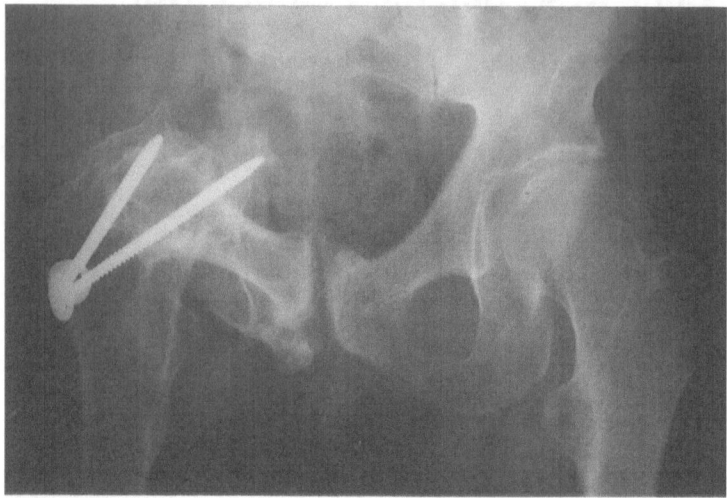

Fig. 1. Resection of acetabulum and ilium for a chondrosarcoma. Reconstruction with an arthrodesis between femur and ischium. Good functional result after 6 years in spite of a little shortening and an asymptomatic dislocation into the pubic symphysis

zones I and II in six cases, zones II and III in seven cases, and zones I, II, and III (hemipelvis) in two cases [2, 3].

Tumor Control

Seven local recurrences occurred: six after insufficient resection (intralesional or contaminated) and one in spite of good surgical margins. One can seldom achieve wide margins in these kind of resections; most often it is necessary to be marginal in one or several zones of the dissection. Six patients had metastasis (four associated with local recurrences). Five of these six patients died.

Functional Results

Complications were due to the topography of the tumor and the bone resection, the extent of muscular, nervous, and vascular sacrifice, and, of course, depended on the type of reconstruction. Surgical complications were frequent; they occurred in 18 of the 36 patients. We noted 14 minor complications. Of these, there were seven cases of small skin necrosis and superficial sepsis requiring only minor treatment, two venous thromboses without sequelae, three peroneal nerve palsies (only one complete and definite), and two prosthetic luxations treated by closed reduction. There were six major complications, including two cases of failure of reconstruction (reoperated) and four cases of major wound necrosis with deep infection (leading to two postoperative deaths). We also observed one patient with crural nerve palsy and one with major genitourinary sequelae as a result of the resection.

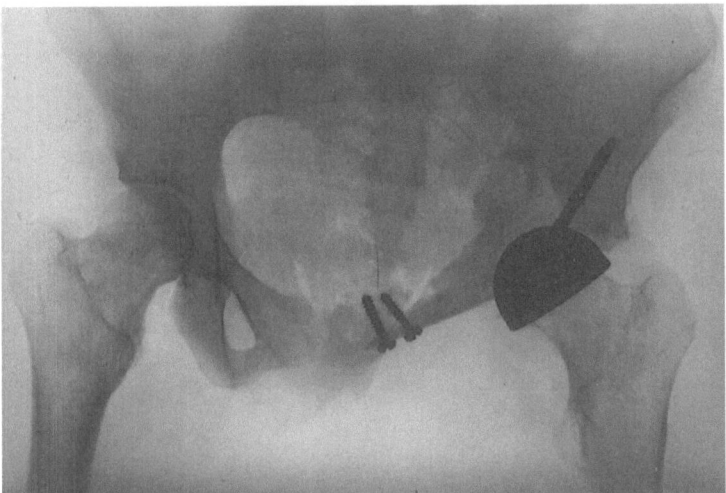

Fig. 2. Resection of acetabulum and pubis for chondrosarcoma. Reconstruction with a cup and an allograft. After 12 years, partial resorption of the allograft, leading to a total hip prosthesis

The global functional result in 28 cases were excellent in nine cases (four zone I, five zone III), good in 12 cases (six zone I, one zone II, two zone III, two zones I + II, one zones II + III), fair in four cases (one zone I, two zones II + III, one zones I + II + III), and poor in three cases (one zones I + II, two zones II + III).

Results according to the reconstructive procedures in the 28 cases were as follows. Thirteen patients did not require reconstruction. There were five resections of part I, with two excellent results, two good, and one fair, and eight resections of part III (five excellent, three good). Five patients were treated with an arthrodesis between the remaining acetabulum and sacrum after resection of zone I. Two of the patients are excellent and three are good. Three fixations of the upper femur under the remaining ilium were performed after resection of parts II + III. Two of the patients are poor and one is fair (all have instability, use crutches, and have shortening and pain). There were three arthrodeses between the femoral head (or great trochanter) and pubis (Fig. 1). After resection of parts I + II, who had a good result with minor or no shortening and a pseudo-mobility into the pubic symphysis. After 3–5 years, this joint showed some radiological changes (arthritis, dislocation) but with a good clinical result. The third case had a poor result because of crural palsy (nerve resected with the tumor).

There were four reconstructions using a prosthesis or a massive bone graft after resection of part II (isolated or associated with parts I or III). Two had a good result, and two a fair result. One good result was after reconstruction of an isolated part II with conventional hip prosthesis and autografts. The other good result was after cup arthroplasty and massive allograft bridging of the defect (zones II + III). This latter patient underwent reoperation 12 years later, receiving a total hip arthroplasty (Fig. 2). There was one fair result after resection of

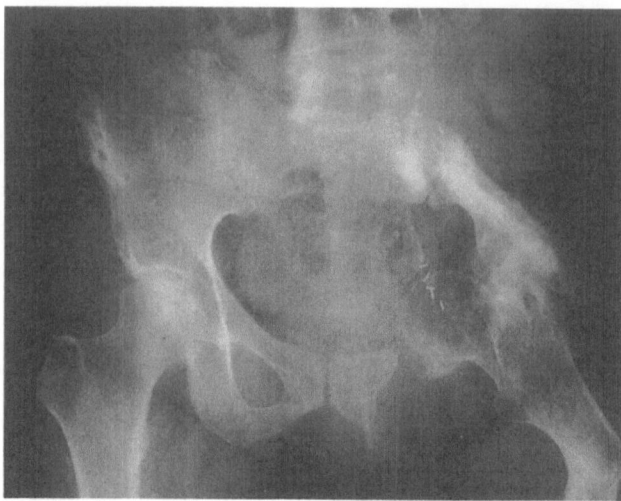

Fig. 3. An alternative to reconstruction of a complete innominate bone. Arthrodesis between sacrum and great trochanter using a bone graft and complementary directional osteotomy of the femur

the three zones. An arthrodesis with authografts was attempted here between the trochanter and sacrum (Fig. 3).

Unfortunately, some interesting reconstructions are not available for this study because the follow-up period is too short. In particular, there were three subtotal replacements of the hemipelvis with a massive allograft (two patients died of metastasis after some weeks, the other case is too recent).

Conclusions

Conservative surgery for pelvic bone tumors remains difficult with a high rate of complications [1, 4–9]. Oncological results are usually good. Functional results when the soft tissue sacrifices are not too great are as follows. Usually, they were satisfactory after isolated resections of part I or III, and here reconstruction was not necessary except in some cases with a large defect between the acetabulum and sacrum. The results were bad for upper femur fixations under the iliac wing after resection of zones II + III. They were acceptable after a successful arthrodesis between the upper femur and pubic ring for resections of parts I + II. The results were either good or poor after ambitious reconstructions (massive hemipelvic allograft, sophisticated osteosynthesis, or major prosthetic replacement). Here, they depend especially on the possible (and rather frequent) complications.

References

1. Burri C, Claes L, Gerngross H, Mathys R (1979) Total internal hemipelvectomy. Arch Orthop Traumt Surg 94: 219–226

2. Enneking WF (1966) Local resection of malignant lesions of the hip and pelvis. J Bone Joint Surg 48A: 996–1007
3. Enneking WF, Dunham WK (1978) Resection and reconstruction for primary neoplasms involving the innominate bone. J Bone Joint Surg 60A: 731–746
4. Erikson U, Hjelmstedt A (1976) Limb saving radical resection of chondrosarcoma of the pelvis. J Bone Joint Surg 58A: 568–570
5. Johnson JTH (1978) Reconstruction of the pelvic ring following tumor resection. J Bone Joint surg 60A: 747–751
6. McLaughlin RE, Sweet DE, Webster TH, Merrit WM (1975) Chondroblastoma of the pelvis suggestive of malignancy. Report of an unusual case treated by wide pelvic excision. J Bone Joint Surg 57A: 549–551
7. Merle d'Aubigne R, Meary R (1963) Resection ou amputation dans les tumeurs cartilagineuses malignes du squelette. Mem Acad Chir 89: 755–769
8. Schollner D, Ruck W (1974) Die Beckenendoprothese. Eine Alternative zur Hemipelvectomie. Z Orthop 112: 968
9. Steel HH (1978) Partial or complete resection of the hemipelvis. J Bone Joint Surg 60A: 719–730

Results of Treatment After Resection of Large Bone Tumors of the Pelvic Girdle

W. Winkelmann and K.P. Schulitz[1]

Summary. Since 1978, we have done 23 resections of large bone tumors of the pelvic girdle. Four patients had a giant cell tumor, three patients a chondrosarcoma, eight patients Ewing's sarcoma, five patients an osteosarcoma, two patients a chordoma, and one patient a fibrosarcoma. Of special interest are the results of eight patients who had a tumor arising from the wing of the ilium, extending into the sacrum. The follow-up time was more than 5 years in five patients, more than 4 years in four patients, and more than 2 years in seven patients. After tumor resection, we performed a reconstruction of the pelvic girdle in four patients only. The functional results were comparable with those without reconstruction.

Three patients developed a local recurrence and died of their malignant disease. One of these patients died after only one intralesional resection of Ewing's sarcoma and postoperative irradiation; the other two patients died after wide resections of osteosarcoma and fibrosarcoma, respectively.

Key words: Bone tumor—Pelvic girdle—Functional results

Introduction

Excluding the sacrum, we divided pelvic tumors into four main types, according to their localization (Fig. 1). Tumors of the cranial part of the ilium are localized sufficiently distant from the hip joint to allow preservation of the joint. For tumors of the ilium which have grown close to the hip joint, particularly in growing patients, we have developed a new surgical procedure (Fig. 2).

The growth plate forms a barrier to tumor invasion. It is possible to remove the ilium at the triradiate cartilage, leaving more than two-thirds of the acetabulum, which due to the failing support results in a hip joint which cannot be stressed. Following osteotomy of the pubic bone and ischium, the rest of the acetabulum is pulled over the femoral head, the limb is pushed up cranially, and the acetabulum is fixed to the sacrum (Fig. 2). In this way, the extensive and deep defect following resection of the complete ilium is covered, resulting in

[1]Department of Orthopaedic Surgery, University of Düsseldorf, Düsseldorf, Federal Repubic of Germany

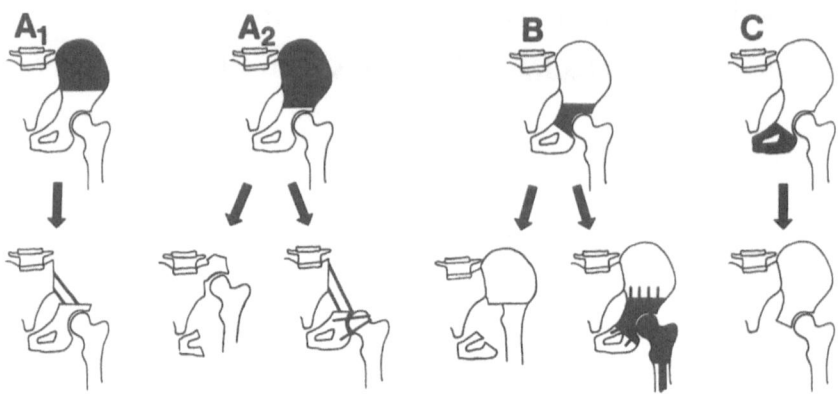

Fig. 1. The four main localizations of pelvic tumors and types of pelvic tumor resections

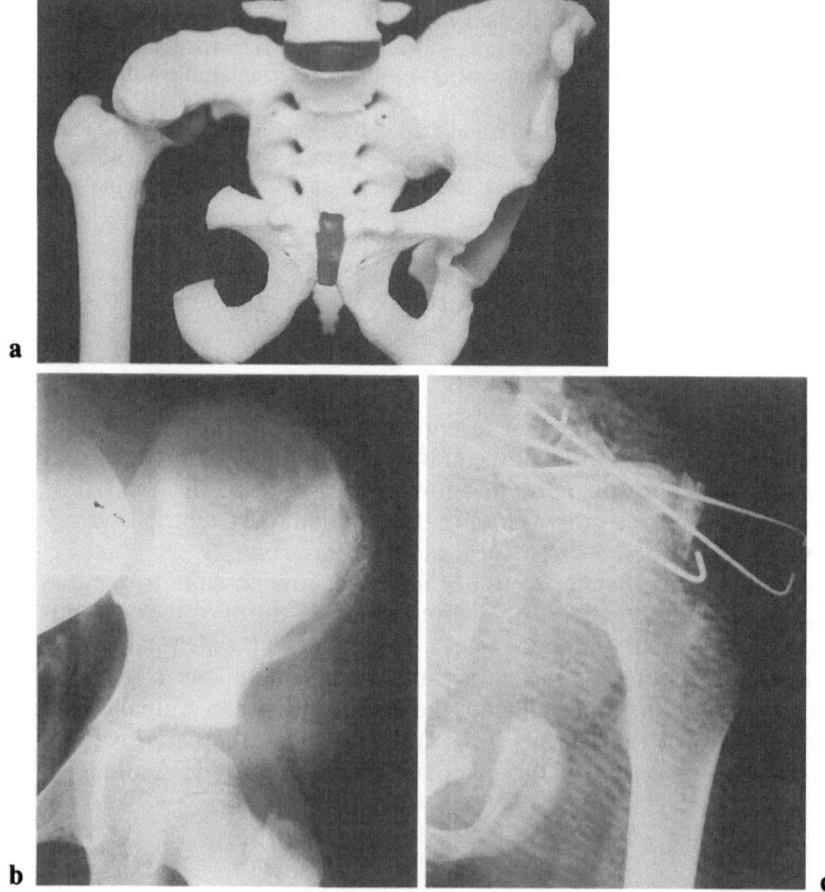

Fig. 2a–c. Hip joint transposition after complete excision of the ilium demonstrated in **a** a model and **b**, **c** in a 9-year-old girl with Ewing's sarcoma

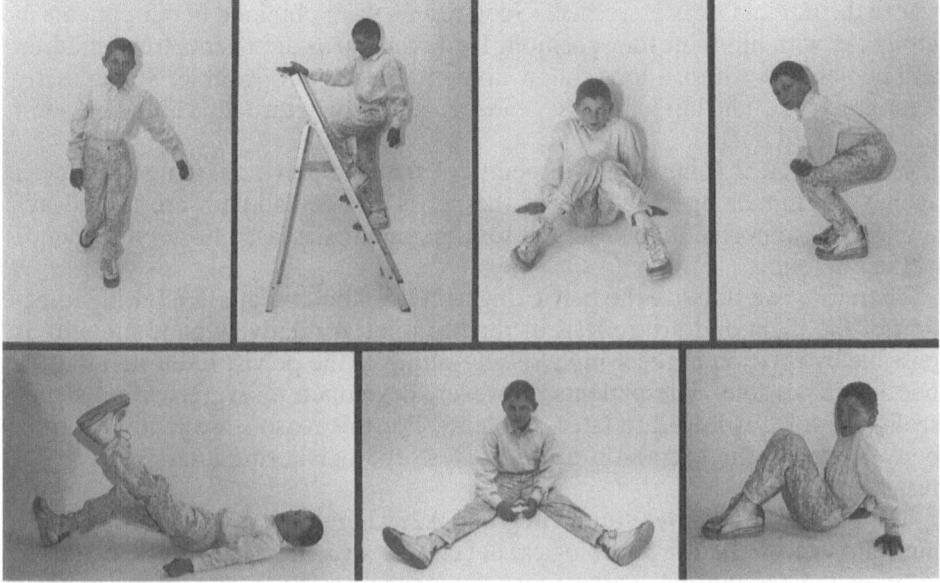

Fig. 3. Clinical pictures of an 11-year-old girl with a hip joint transposition after complete excision of the ilium 2 years after surgery

good cosmetic results. Of particular importance is the resulting practically un-limited movement and function of the joint (Fig. 3). The only disadvantage is that the leg is 4 cm shorter.

Another alternative following complete resection of the ilium is the arthro-desis with the remaining part of the acetabulum. Following resection of a peri-acetabular tumor, either an iliac-femoral fusion or implantation of a custom-made pelvic and proximal femur endoprosthesis can be carried out. Finally, there is the localization in the pubic bone and/or ischium. Here again, it is almost always possible to preserve the hip joint.

Material

Taking into consideration the four localization types and a follow-up of at least 2 years, 21 patients were assessed. Eight patients had Ewing's sarcoma, five pa-tients osteosarcoma, four patients giant cell tumor, three patients chondrosarco-ma, and one patient fibrosarcoma.

Results

The results were dependent on the localization of the tumor and the type of surgical procedure.

Of the 21 patients, four had excellent, nine good, six fair, and two poor results. The best results were seen in patients in the localization group A1 and C, where the hip joint was preserved. Good results were obtained in our patients in group A2 with hip joint transposition. However, these are results from children and adolescents where a long follow-up period is not yet possible. Should early wear and tear of the hip joint arise, endoprosthesis or arthrodesis of the hip joint can be carried out.

In group A1, it is important to point out that the pelvic ring must be closed again. The remaining distal part of the pelvis and acetabulum are not always sufficiently supported at the sacrum, resulting in an increased luxation tendency of the hip joint.

Therefore, we stabilize the pelvic ring with two fibular grafts. Following resection of the ilium and arthrodesis of the hip joint, a relatively good mobility is possible by rotation in the symphysis and tilting of the pelvis. Even standing on one leg is possible. The patients, however, developed a severe compensatory scoliosis, which will lead to later problems. For this reason, we tend to form a bony bridge to the sacrum in order to close the pelvic ring after that type of resection.

The poorest results were found in group A2, where not only a stiffening of the hip joint occurred but a neurological deficit followed the necessary resection of parts of the sacrum and nerve roots. Following resection of a periacetabular tumor and iliac-femoral fusion, a stable leg results. The spinal column remains perpendicular when the, partly severe, leg shortening is compensated. Due to the high rate of primary and secondary complications using a custom-made pelvic endoprosthesis, we are very cautious in its recommendation and have up until now used it only in patients with primary metastases.

Complications

Three patients developed local recurrence and died. Two of them (one with osteosarcoma, the other with fibrosarcoma) have had a resection with tumor-free margins. The third patients has had an intralesional resection of a large Ewing's sarcoma and postoperative radiotherapy with 60 Gy. This corresponds with the results of the German CESS-study in which ten of twelve patients with intralesional resection of pelvic Ewing's sarcomas and postoperative radiotherapy developed a local recurrence.

Reconstruction After Resection of Pelvic Bone Tumors

Takeshi Sawaguchi, Katsuro Tomita, Setsuji Akagawa, and Susumu Nomura[1]

Summary. We have classified pelvic tumor resections into five types according to the disruption of the structural continuity of the pelvic ring, sacrifice of the hip joint, and the necessity for reconstruction. Type IA is a resection of the iliac wing; type IB is a resection of the ischium; type II is a resection of the anterior part of the pelvic ring; type III is a resection of the periacetabular area. In type IIIA, only the acetabulum is resected; in type IIIB, both the acetabulum and the femoral head are reseted. Type IVA is a partial resection of the unilateral sacroiliac joint. Type IVB is a total resection of the unilateral sacroiliac joint. Type VA is a partial resection of the sacrum. Type VB is total sacral resection.

Reconstruction was not necessary in types I and II. Restoration of the hip function by arthrodesis or prosthetic replacement was always necessary in type III. Reconstruction of the pelvic continuity was indispensable in types IVB and VB. The necessity of restoring pelvic stability was dependent on the amount of sacroiliac joint resection in types IVA and VA.

Key words: Pelvis—Reconstruction

Introduction

Resection of malignant bone tumors of the pelvis involves formidable problems [1, 2]. Although obtaining a wide tumor-free surgical margin is essential as in other tumors of the extremities, it is often impossible to do so because of poor compartmentalization of the pelvis and technical difficulties in surgical resection due to the complicated anatomy. Therefore, adjunct chemotherapy and radiation therapy are necessary. Even if local control of tumors is obtained with these measures, there are still difficult problems caused by sacrifice of the pelvic structural continuity and the hip joint.

[1]Department of Orthopaedic Surgery, Kanazawa University, Kanazawa, Japan

Materials and Methods

Since 1975, 20 pelvic tumor resections (except four cases of hemipelvectomy) were performed at our institution. There were twelve males and eight females. The age ranged from 16 to 70 years with an average of 40. Histological study revealed three chondrosarcomas, two Ewing's sarcomas, two malignant fibrous histiocytomas, one osteosarcoma, three chordomas, three giant cell tumors, and six metastases.

We classified pelvic resections into five types according to the disruption of the continuity of the pelvic ring, sacrifice of the hip joint, and the necessity for reconstruction. Except for type II, each type has subtypes of A and B (Fig. 1).

Type I is a resection of the iliac wing (IA) or the ischium (IB). This type of resection does not jeopardize the pelvic ring and no reconstruction is necessary. There were two cases of IA resection, one was chondrosarcoma and the other was a metastatic tumor from the thyroid. In both cases, the iliac wing was resected and the abdominal muscles were sutured to the gluteus muscles. There was no functional deficit after this type of resection. There was one case of IB resection for a metastatic adenocarcinoma of the left ischium. The only functional deficit after this type of resection was pelvic obliquity when the patient sat down.

Type II resection involves sacrificing the anterior part of the pelvic ring. Stability of the pelvic ring is given by the posterior structures [3]. These are the sacroiliac joint and its surrounding ligaments, i.e., iliolumbar, anterior and posterior sacroiliac, sacrotuberous, and sacrospinous ligaments. As type II resection preserves these structures, the pelvic ring is stable and no reconstruction is necessary. There were two cases of type II resection: One was a chondrosarcoma of the left pubis and the other was a metastatic tumor of the right pubis. Type II resection was performed without reconstruction.

Type III is a resection of the periacetabular area. The hip joint is sacrificed. If no reconstruction is attempted, a flail hip is inevitable and the functional prognosis is poor. Reconstruction is always necessary for this type of resection to transmit the load from the trunk to the lower extermity [4]. In type IIIA, only the acetabulum is resected. The femoral head can be utilized for iliofemoral arthrodesis. In type IIIB, both the acetabulum and femoral head are resected. The options for this type of resection are prosthetic replacement and ischiofemoral arthrodesis. There was one case of type IIIA resection in a malignant fibrous histiocytoma of the right pubis in a 43-year-old male. After wide resection, iliofemoral arthrodesis was done with a cobra plate. There were two cases of type IIIB resection, one was a giant cell tumor of the left ilium in a 54-year-old female and the other was a giant cell tumor of the right acetabulum in a 29-year-old female. Both of them were replaced by a prosthetic pelvis made of alumina ceramics with a total hip component.

Type IV is a resection of the unilateral sacroiliac joint. In type IVA, there is sacrifice of a part of the sacroiliac joint but the pelvic continuity is preserved. If only a small portion of the sacroiliac joint is resected, no reconstruction is necessary [5]. When a large portion of the sacroiliac joint is resected, augmentation of the structure by internal fixation and bone graft is sometimes necessary. Type IVB is a total resection of the sacroiliac joint. Continuity and stability of the pelvic ring are lost. Reconstruction is always necessary to transmit the load and

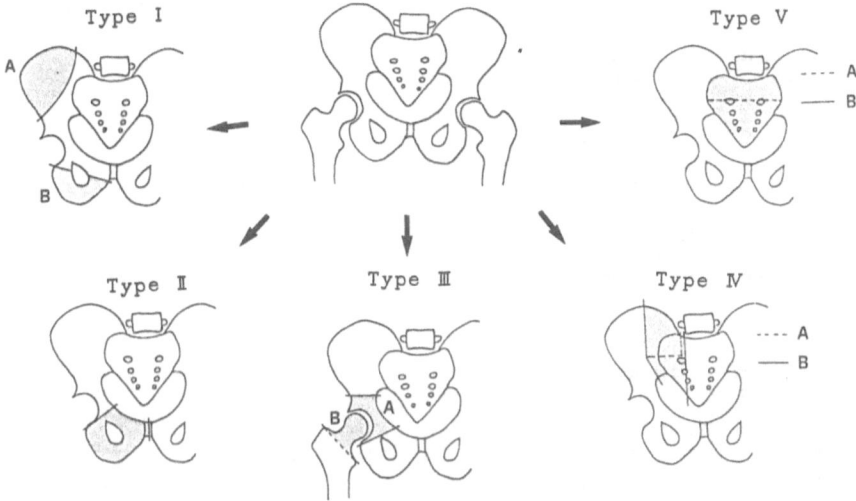

Fig. 1. *Type I* is a resection of the iliac wing (*IA*) or the ischium (*IB*). *Type II* is a resection of the anterior part of the pelvic ring. *Type III* is a resection of the periacetabular area. In *type IIIA*, only the acetabulum is resected. In *type IIIB*, both the acetabulum and femoral head are resected. *Type IV* is a resection of the unilateral sacroiliac joint. *Type IVA* is a partial resection of the sacroiliac joint. *Type IVB* is a total resection of the sacroiliac joint. *Type V* is a resection of the sacrum. *Type VA* is a partial resection of the sacrum. Type VB is a total sacral resection

gain stability of the pelvic ring. There were three cases of type IVA resection: one Ewing's sarcoma, one chondrosarcoma, and one metastatic tumor from renal cancer. In the latter two cases, the tumors were resected through a transiliac approach [6, 7]. The anterior part of the iliac wing was detached temporarily with abdominal muscular attachment; it was reattached or used as a vascularized bone graft after tumor resection for sacroiliac arthrodesis. There were three cases of type IVB resection: one osteosarcoma, one Ewing's sarcoma, and one metastatic tumor from a malignant teratoma. After resection of the tumor through the transiliac approach, the iliac wing was utilized to bridge between the sacrum and the acetabulum in all three cases.

Type V is a resection of the sacrum. The functional prospect is very much dependent on the level of the sacrified nerve [8, 9]. Type VA is a partial resection of the sacrum. The necessity for reconstruction depends on the amount of sacroiliac joint resection. Type VB is total resection of the sacrum. Total sacral resection was performed through a combined anterior and posterior approach [10]. Reconstruction should be done in order to support the spine. There were four cases of type VA resection: three chordomas and one metastatic tumor from meningioma. In two cases, no reconstruction was performed: There was one case of posterolateral fusion and one of augmentation of the sacroiliac joint by sacral bars. There were two cases of type VB resection: one of malignant giant cell tumor and one of malignant fibrous histiocytoma. In these cases, the structural continuity of the lumbar spine and the bilateral ilium was reconstructed by a massive bone graft obtained from the ilium and bilateral fibulas with the use of sacral bars and Harrington rods.

Table 1. Results of reconstruction

Type	Age (years)	Sex	Diagnosis	Reconstruction	Follow-up	Results	Status
IIIA	43	M	MFH	Iliofemoral arthrodesis	1 y 5 m	Good	CDF
IIIB	54	F	Giant cell tumor	Pelvic prosthesis	3 y 6 m	Fair	CDF
IVA	53	M	Metastasis	Bone graft + internal fixation	1 y 9 m	Excellent	CDF
IVB	40	M	Osteosarcoma	Bone graft + internal fixation	Expired		AWD
	17	M	Ewing's sarcoma	Bone graft + internal fixation	1 y 6 m	Poor	CDF
VA	64	M	Metastasis	Internal fixation	4 y 5 m	Excellent	CDF
	57	F	Chordoma	Posterolateral fusion	1 y 9 m	Excellent	CDF
VB	32	F	Giant cell tumor	Bone graft + internal fixation	2 y 5 m	Fair	CDF

MFH malignant fibrous histiocytoma, *CDF* continuously disease free, *AWD* alive with disease

Results and Discussion

Our 20 cases could be classified according to this system. Reconstruction of some kind was attempted in 11 cases: One iliofemoral arthrodesis, two ceramic pelvic prostheses, one sacroiliac arthrodesis, three iliosacral bridging bone grafts, one augmentation of the sacroiliac joint by sacral bars, one posterolateral fusion, and two sacral reconstructions after total sacral resection were performed. In only five cases could a wide margin be obtained; all of these patients are currently without local recurrence or metastasis. Four cases had complications: One was a fracture of the graft, and three were necrosis of the skin and deep infection.

Eight cases were followed for more than 1 year (average 2.5 years). One patient (type IVB resection, osteosarcoma) died due to local recurrence and metastasis. Six cases are currently disease-free.

The functional results were assessed according to the evaluation system. Three were rated "excellent," one "good," two "fair," and one "poor" (Table 1).

It is important to try to obtain wide resection of the tumors, even about the pelvis and hip, but this is often impossible. Effective adjunct chemotherapy and radiation are imperative. Although these methods may succeed in controlling local recurrence and distant metastasis, it is not enough to obtain satisfactory functional results. Reconstruction of pelvic stability and preservation of the hip function should be attempted in selected cases. Any kind of pelvic resection can be classified into one of the types or combinations of this classification system. We propose this classification system for pelvic resection as a means of determining the necessity of reconstruction.

References

1. Enneking WF, Dunham WK (1978) Resection and reconstruction for primary neoplasms involving the innominate bone. J Bone Joint Surg 60-A: 731–746
2. Enneking WF (1983) Pelvis. In: Enneking WF (ed) Musculoskeletal tumor surgery. Churchill Livingstone, New York, pp 483–529
3. White AA, Panjabi MM (1978) Clinical biomechanics of the spine. Lippincott, Philadelphia, pp 264–265
4. Johnson TH (1978) Reconstruction of the pelvic ring following tumor resection. J Bone Joint Surg 60-A: 747–751
5. Gunterberg B, Romanus B, Stener B (1976) Pelvic strength after major amputation of the sacrum. Acta Orthop Scand 47: 635–642
6. Sawaguchi T, Tomita K (1987) Transiliac approach for the sacroiliac joint tumor. Rinsho Seikei (in Japanese) 22: 751–760
7. Wilson PD (1972) A clinical study of the biomechanical behavior of massive bone transplants used to reconstruct large bone defects. Clin Orthop 87: 81–109
8. Stener B, Gunterberg B (1978) High amputation of the sacrum for extirpation of tumors. Spine 3: 351–366
9. Gunterberg B, Norlen B, Sundin T (1975) Neurourologic evaluation after resection of the sacrum. Invest Urology 13: 183–188
10. Huth JF, Dawson EG, Eilber FR (1984) Abdominosacral resection for malignant tumors of the sacrum. Am J Surg 148: 157–161

A Custom-Made Adaptable Pelvic Prosthesis

Reiner Gradinger and Erwin Hipp[1]

Summary. In the last 10 years, we have implanted 15 custom-made pelvic prostheses after internal hemipelvectomy. Although we have used computerized tomography in the last 5 years, we have been unable to obtain a proper fit allowing implantation without technical problems. Thus, we changed our method. The basis of the new method is: (a) Anatomical replacement of the acetabular socket; (b) intramedullary fixation with a spongy metal shaft into the ileum or sacrum; (c) intramedullary fixation into the os pubis; (d) these three parts of the prosthesis (a–c) are linked together with a screw (to the os pubis) and a conical connection (between the acetabular socket and the ileum-or sacrum-prosthesis).

During the last 6 months, we have treated six patients with malignant tumors in the pelvis with this type of prosthesis. There were three children (two cases of Ewing's sarcoma, one of osteosarcoma) and three adults (two chondrosarcoma, one metastasis of a thyroid carcinoma).

The operative technique is much easier with a partially custom-made adaptable prosthesis than with the total custom-made prosthesis, because we can adapt the different parts to the anatomical and pathological situation. The intramedullary shaft to the pelvis or sacrum is custom-made and ensures a proper fit with primary stabile anchorage, which is assured through transpelvic or transsacral screws, and secondary bone ingrowth to the spongy metal shaft. Initial results show that this could be the way to an individually adaptable, partially custom-made pelvic prosthesis.

Key words: Malignant bone tumours—Pelvis—Adaptable cementless pelvic prosthesis

Introduction

Since 1970, Nilsonne [6] has used internal hemipelvectomy to preserve the leg but without reconstruction of the resected part of the pelvis. The function of the leg after this kind of treatment is not satisfactory. It was for this reason that we and others [1–6, 7] tried to reconstruct pelvic defects by the use of prostheses. Different kinds of prosthesis were implanted. We used a custom-made metal prosthesis and a computerized custom-made polyacetal prosthesis. With both systems, we had difficulties intraoperatively in fitting the prosthesis into the pel-

[1] Department of Orthopaedics, Technical University of Munich, Klinikum Rechts der Isar, Munich, Fedeal Republic of Germany

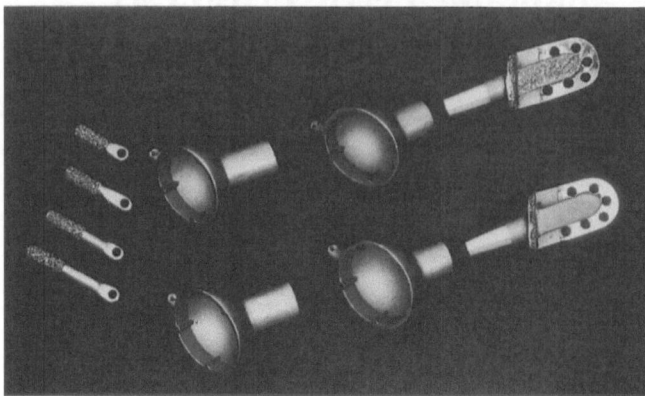

Fig. 1. Custom-made adaptable pelvic prosthesis with different lengths and sizes of acetabular sockets and support rods to the os pubis

vic defect. Either we had to resect bone and bend the prosthesis in the hospital workshop (metal) or we had to cut the prosthesis (polyacetal).

A second problem is how to fix the prosthesis. A durable loadable fixation by screws alone is impossible.

These were the reasons for developing a cementless implantable partially custom-made prosthesis.

Materials and Methods

During the last year, we have implanted six pelvic endoprotheses without bone cement. The patients were three children, two with osteosarcoma, and three adults, two with chondrosarcomata and one with metastasis of a thyroid carcinoma. In all six cases, the indications for internal hemipelvectomy and reconstruction with endoprostheses were for palliative treatment. In four cases, the tumors were so big that only a hemicorporectomy would have had a "curative" effect. In two cases (a 12-year-old female with osteosarcoma and a 17-year-old male with Ewing's sarcoma), the parents refused to consent to hemipelvectomy.

In four cases, we had to resect the os ileum subtotally, in two cases totally.

Our new prosthesis is composed of five parts (Fig. 1–3). The custom-made (computerized) shaft is covered with spongy metal and a lateral plate. The shaft can be placed in an intramedullary position in the remains of the os ileum and fixed additionally through the lateral plate into the os sacrum. When total resection of the os ileum is necessary, we can fix the prosthesis with a small spongy metal plate into the os sacrum from the front and fix it additionally through the lateral plate into the os sacrum. There are acetabular sockets of different sizes with conical connections of varying lengths. For this reason, we are able to choose the correct size and length intraoperatively. The polyethylene inlays we use are from the usual cementless endoprosthetic system with two different angles—one in the plane of the metal socket and one with a 10° angle overhang

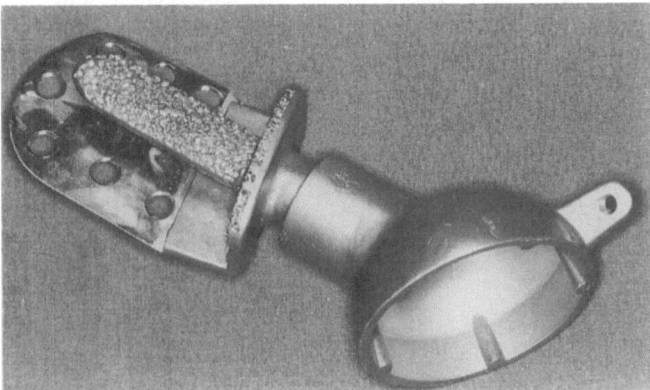

Fig. 2. Pelvic prosthesis for subtotal hemipelvectomy. Note the spongy metal shaft for positioning in the remains of the os ileum

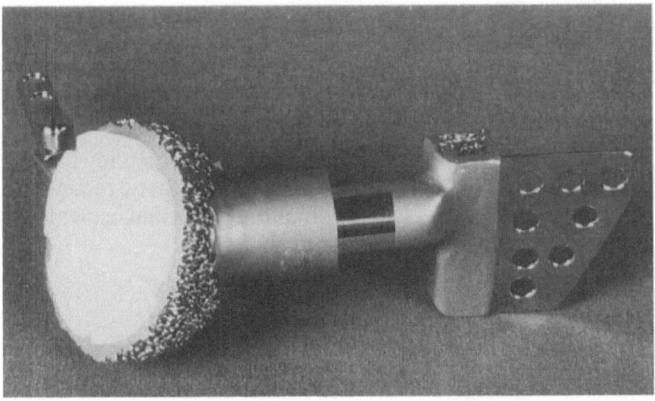

Fig. 3. Pelvic prosthesis for total hemipelvectomy

if there is a tendency to luxate. The connection from the metal socket to the os pubis is made by a supporting rod (also available in different lengths).

Results and Discussion

After an internal hemipelvectomy, we performed prosthetic replacement with a partially custom-made adaptable prosthesis (Figs. 4, 5). The operative technique is much easier, because we can adapt the different parts to the anatomical situation. At the moment, we still consider this prosthesis to be a prototype.

In four cases, the indications were for palliative treatment and twice were due to refusal of conventional hemipelvetomy. In the Enneking hip score, the results were fair, which is good for internal hemipelvectomy. This is the same result as

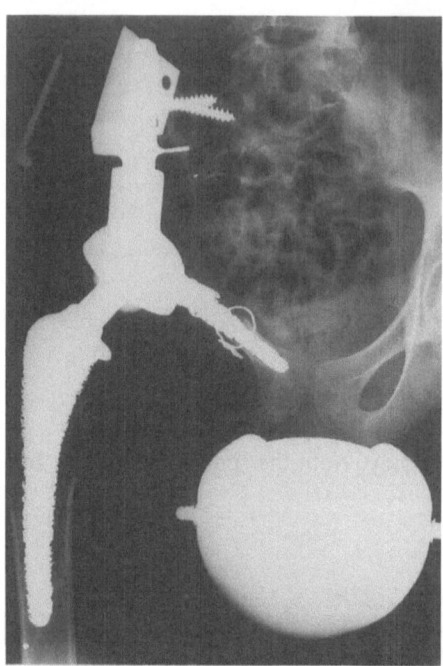

Fig. 4. Subtotal hemipelvectomy and cementless implantation of a pelvic prosthesis

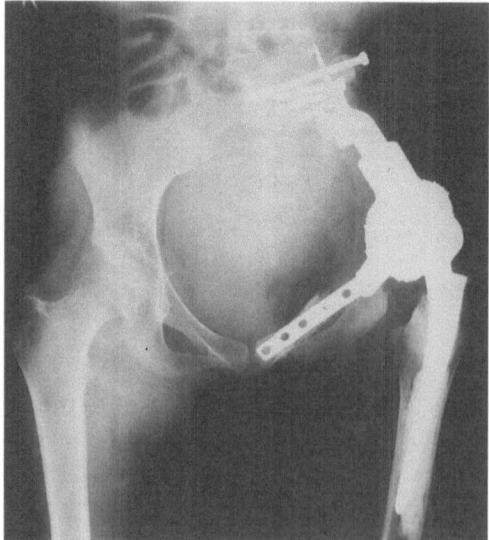

Fig. 5. Total hemipelvectomy and cementless endoprosthetic reconstruction of the pelvis and cementless femur shaft

we have achieved with other prostheses. One patient died 1 year after the operation because of multiple metastases. In this case, we had to remove the pelvic prosthesis because of infection and loosening. In the other five cases, we have seen a bony ingrowth in the spongy metal shaft. In one case, we were able to prove this histologically. It is our opinion that this is a first step toward achieving a durable cementless anchorage of pelvic prostheses.

References

1. Burri C, Claes L, Gerngross H, Mathys R (1979) Total "internal" hemipelvectomy. Arch Orthop Trauma 94: 219–226
2. Burri C, Schulte J (1980) Operationsindikation und chirurgische Technik bei Beckentumoren. Langenbecks Arch Chir 352: 465–469
3. Hipp E, Biehl T, Gradinger R (1986) Diagnostik und Therapie der primären malignen Knochentumoren. Demeter, Munich
4. Immenkamp M (1983) Surgical techniques in the treatment of tumors in the hip region. In: Chao YS, Ivins JC (eds) Tumor prosthesis for bone and joint reconstruction. Thieme-Stratton, New York, pp 235–238
5. Karpf PM, Mang (1978) Das Reticulum-Zellsarkom des Backens. Fortschr Med 96: 1559
6. Nilsonne U (1983) Use of internal hemipelvectomy to preserve the leg. In: Chao YS, Ivins JC (eds) Tumor prosthesis for bone and joint reconstruction. Thieme-Stratton, New York, pp 35–37
7. Russe W, Bauer, R (1983) Custom prosthetic replacement for internal hemipelvectomy. In: Chao YS, Ivins JC (eds) Tumor prosthesis for bone and joint reconstruction. Thieme-Stratton, New York, pp 231–234

The Saddle Prosthesis Mark II, Endo-Modell®

ELMAR NIEDER[1] and ARNOLD KELLER[2]

Summary. The Saddle Prosthesis was designed to treat patients with extensive loss of acetabular bone from any cause and was inserted in 76 cases of failed, aseptic, and infected total hip arthroplasties between 1979 and 1985 and recently also in some cases of acetabular tumors. Following analysis in 1987, the design has been changed. Freedom of rotation of the saddle has been integrated with respect to motion, muscle function, comfort, longevity, and modular use.

Key words: Saddle prosthesis—Total femoral replacement—Resection or loss of acetabular bone stock

The Earlier Model

To treat patients who have had resections for tumor or after extensive loss of acetabular bone from any cause, the saddle prosthesis was designed as a simple alternative to other methods of hip reconstructions (Fig. 1) [1–8].

Using the original model (manufactured by W. Link, Hamburg, FRG), 76 operations were performed in aseptic and septic revision cases between 1979 and 1985; 72 were followed (Figs. 2, 3; Table 1) [9]. At the time of operation, 33 cases were infected, 11 had a past history of infection and 28 cases, had never been infected.

In addition, some patients with acetabular tumors were also treated with the device.

Conclusion

Fifteen cases had a suboptimal outcome for reasons which were obvious (two primary, thirteen continued infections). Evaluation of the remaining 57 aseptic cases revealed five occasional design-related features which marred the quality of the result. These were: (a) A poor range of motion; (b) poor abductor

[1]Endo-Klinik, Hamburg, Federal Republic of Germany
[2]Fa. W. Link, Hamburg, Federal Republic of Germany

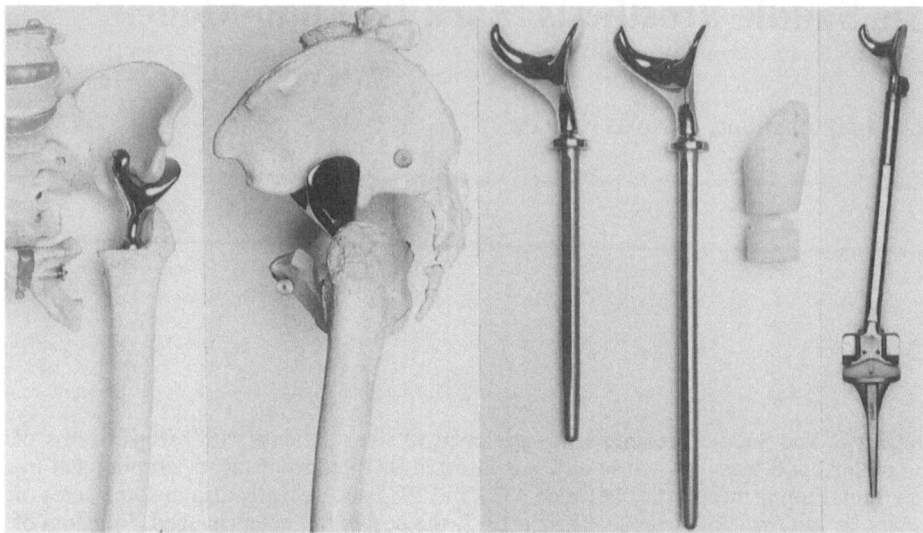

Fig. 1. Saddle articulation to iliac bone. Implanted models: 55 simple saddles, six saddles proximal femur, 11 saddles total femur

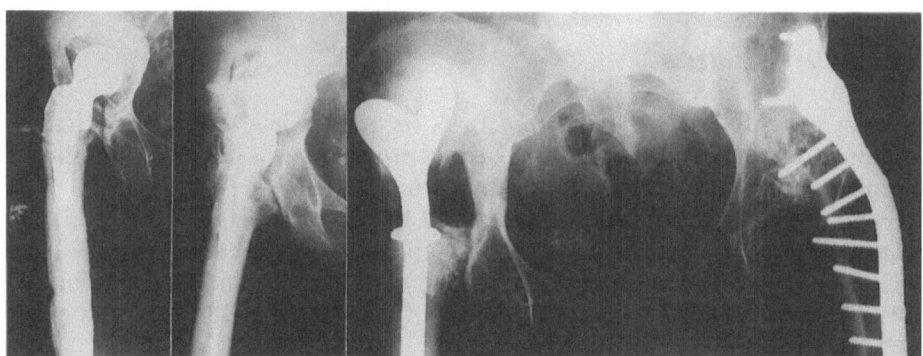

Fig. 2. Bilateral hip dysplasia, arthrodesis left hip—excessively high implantation of acetabular cup right hip, two septic revision arthroplasties, recurrence of infection, implantation of saddle, using ALAC. Four years postoperatively, no signs of infection, final rating 4→3

strength; (c) unacceptable discomfort in the hip region; (d) loosening and fracture of femoral stem; (e) progressive upward migration of prosthesis and fracture of iliac wing (Fig. 4).

Despite significant problems in certain patients, we remain convinced that the saddle is a useful addition to our armamentarium and believe that recent changes in the design will improve the quality of results.

Five modifications have been integrated. How successful these will prove to be is open to conjecture. The design changes and their theroetical benefits are as follows.

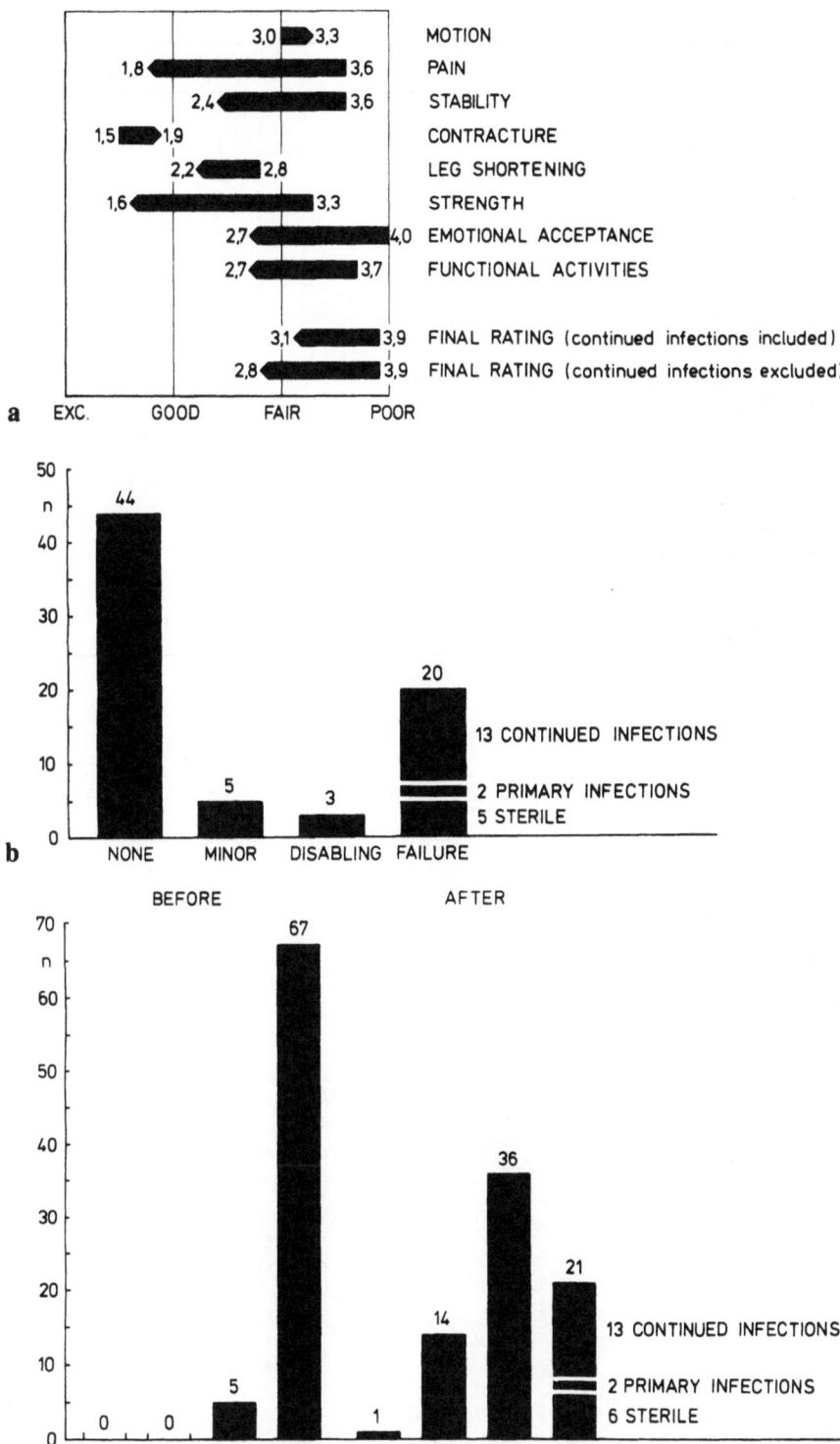

Fig. 3. a Primary factors. Average pre- to postoperative change in functional status using saddle prosthesis in revision total hip arthroplasty; **b** complications ($n = 72$); **c** final rating ($n = 72$)

Table 1. Complications

	No. of patients
Minor (good)	
Early postoperative dislocation	1
Infraprosthetic spiral femoral fracture	1
Painful nearthrosis	1
Early radiological signs of loosening	2
Disabling (fair)	
Malposition of prosthesis	1
Rotatory instability, locking mechanism of total femur engaged incorrectly	1
Significant (but asymptomatic) radiological evidence of stem loosening	1
Failures (poor)	
Continued infections	13
Primary infections	2
Noninfection-related failures	
Fracture of supporting iliac wing	2
Aseptic Loosening of stem and fracture	1
Recurrent dislocation of saddle	1
Excessive soft tissue tension	1

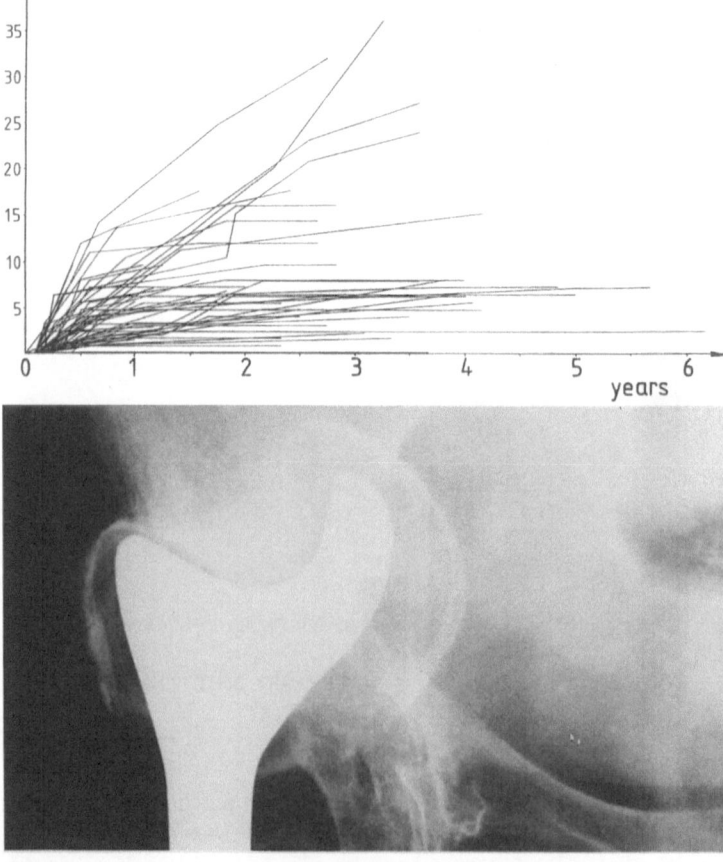

Fig. 4. Cranial migration related to time in aseptic cases. In the presence of sclerotic reactions, initial cranial migration decreased

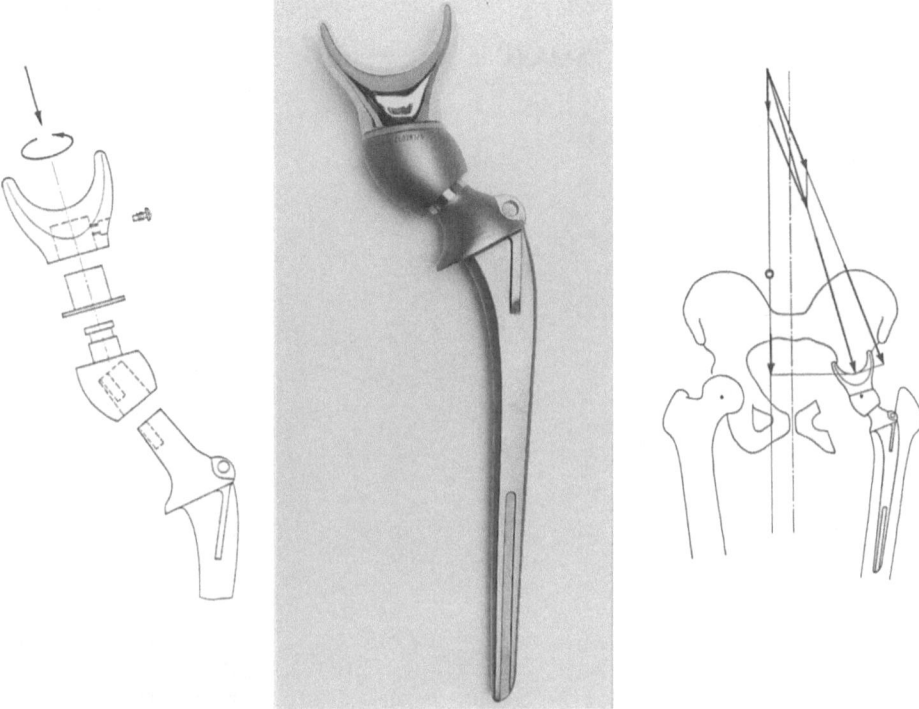

Fig. 5. New design. Polyethylene bearing for free rotation of saddle, perpendicular to the load-bearing axis

1. Freedom of Rotation

In the initial design, the prosthesis-bone articulation was a pure saddle arrangement, allowing only 2° of unconstrained freedom of motion. A small degree of rotation in the long axis of the femur was possible, but its range depended on an unscrewing action at the saddle. Restriction of rotation may have been the cause of disordered stress and load on perhaps the weakened pelvic bone and the femoral fixation, and may have also been the reason for discomfort and reduced flexion and abduction. For comfort in daily activity, a rotatory movement is absolutely essential.

Clearly, the saddle would function best if allwed to follow its own trajectories of motion. A bearing was therefore introduced inserted at right angles to the load-bearing axis to compensate for any required rotation (Fig. 5).

2. Increased Offset

The increased offset results in an increased abductor lever arm and improves the load-bearing characteristics of the saddle joint (Fig. 6). The position of the femur in a physiological alignment improves the function of all muscle groups around the hip if present and avoids impingement.

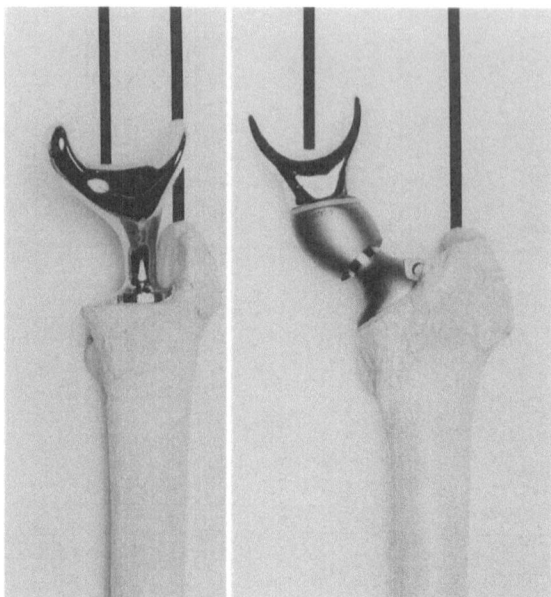

Fig. 6. The increased offset results in an increased abductor lever arm

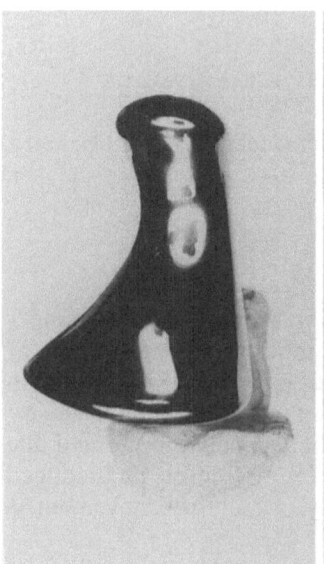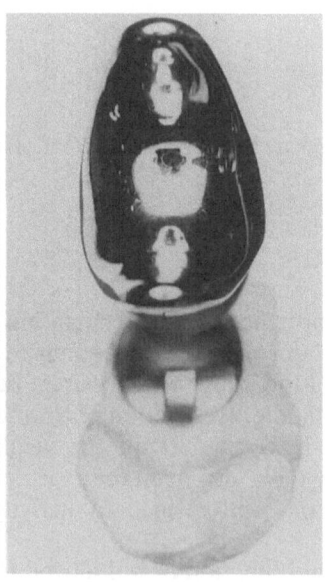

Fig. 7. The broader saddle results in load distribution over a larger area

3. Broader Saddle

The narrow load-bearing surface of the earlier saddle was thought to be necessary so as to allow some degree of axial rotation. With the inclusion of rotation in the prosthesis, a broader saddle can be allowed, thereby distributing load over a larger area with consequent reduction in pressure and perhaps a reduced tendency to upward migration due to bone resorption (Fig. 7).

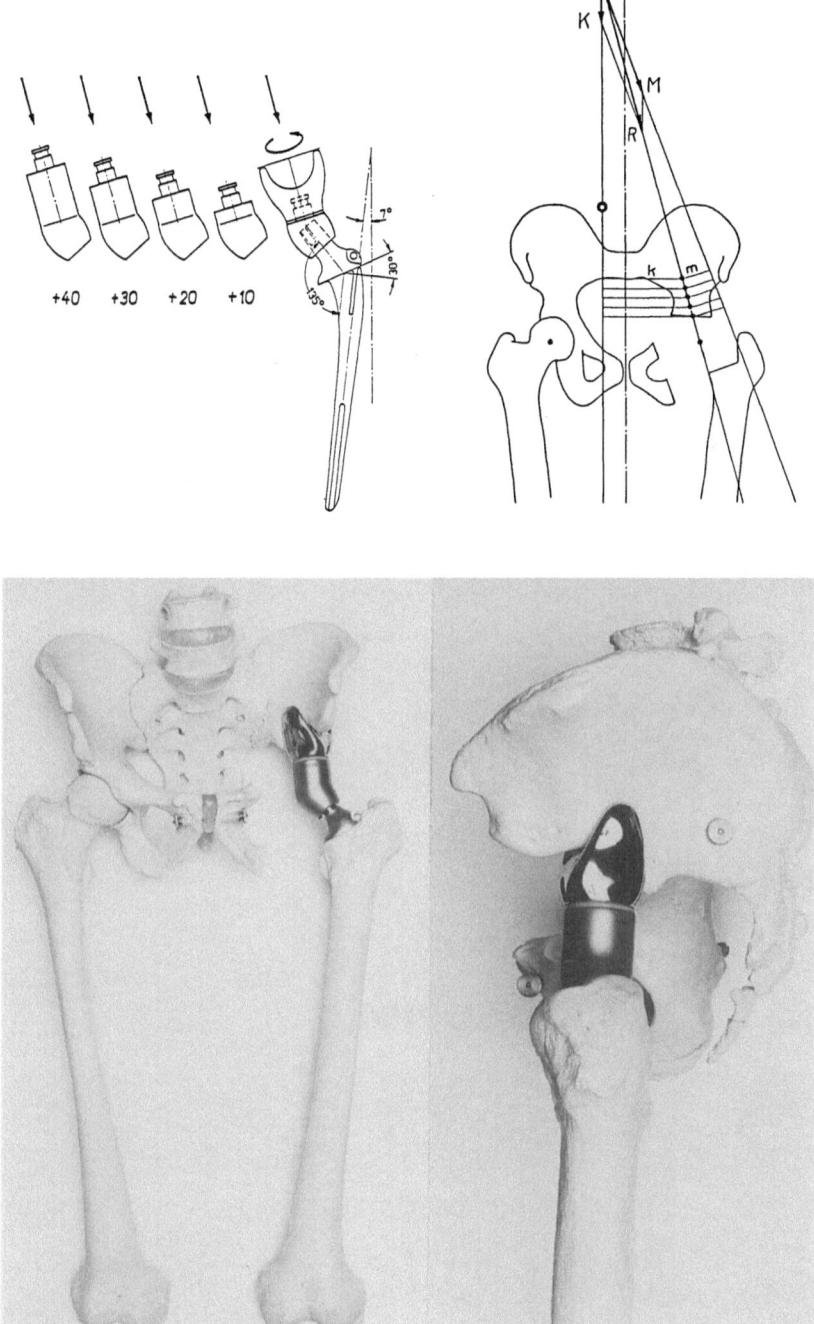

Fig. 8. Elongation of the system following the line of action of the hip force. In higher articulations, balance between moments from muscle force and body weight is maintained if muscles are present

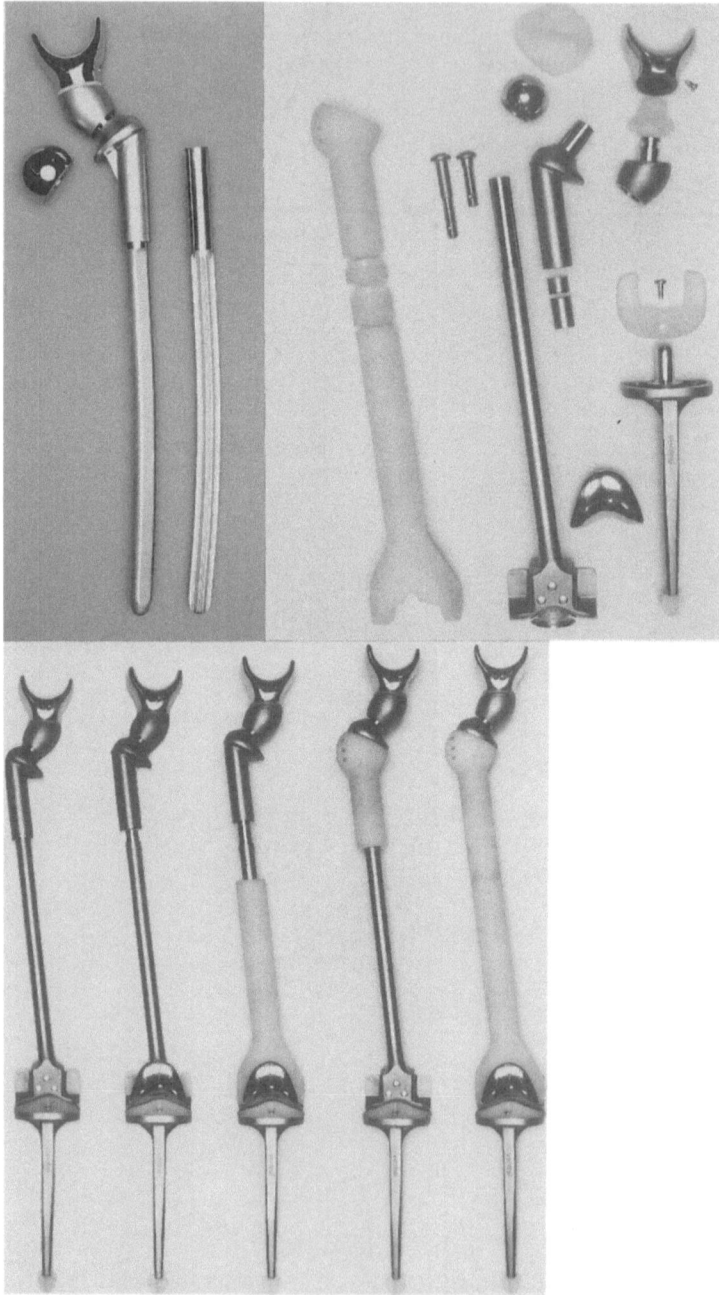

Fig. 9. Cemented revision and cementless reconstruction prosthesis; modular system of total femoral replacement; examples comprising a saddle. Preserved bone can be attached to the stem; lost or resected bone is replaced by polyethylene sleeves or ALAC for infected cases

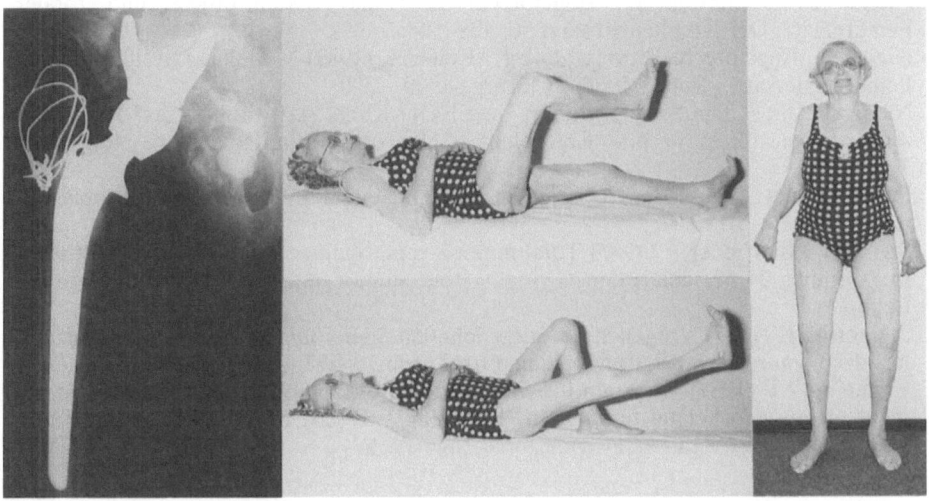

Fig. 10. Rheumatoid arthritis. Central migration of acetabular cup; unable to withstand partial weight bearing. Eight weeks postoperatively final rating 4→2

4. Correction of Length in Physiological Axis of Hip Loading

By means of a modular series of interpositional components, correction can be achieved in those cases which require articulation higher up the pelvic bone while the relative offset is preserved (Fig. 8). By following the line of action of the hip force, the site of loading follows the solid bone of the sciatic buttress.

5. Conical Mounting Allowing Modular Use

The conical mounting permits easy attachment to the full range of prostheses available in our unit, allowing conversion to conventional hip replacement in the event of subsequent pelvic reconstruction (Fig. 9).

The modifications to the initial design of the saddle are interrelated. It is hoped that they will improve the function and longevity for patients who require these advanced techniques of salvage (Fig. 10). Seven new-type prostheses have been inserted since April 1987 (26 at time of printing). We are encouraged by the early results.

References

1. Nieder E, Engelbrecht E (1982) Die Sattelprothese, eine Alternative in Grenz-situationen des alloplastischen Hüftgelenksersatzes. In: Wolter D (ed) Osteolysen—pathologische Frakturen 1. Paul-Sudeck-Symposium 1981. Thieme, Stuttgart
2. Steinbrink K, Engelbrecht E, Fenelon GCC (1982) The total femoral prosthesis—A preliminary report. J Bone Joint Surg (Br) 64: 305–312

3. Nieder E, Steinbrink K, Engelbrecht E (1983) Sattelprothese und totaler Femurersatz. Der Krankenhausarzt 56: 498–504
4. Nieder E, Engelbrecht E, Steinbrink K, Keller A (1983) Modulares System für den Femurtotalersatz—Endo-Modell. Chirurg 54: 391–399
5. Nieder E (1987) Die Sattelprothese. In: ENDO-Klinik (ed) Primär- und Revisions-Alloarthroplastik Hüft- und Kniegelenk. Springer, Berlin Heidelberg New York Tokyo
6. Otto K, Baars GW, Nieder E, (1987) Beckenknochendefekte in der Alloarthroplastik. Orthopäde 16: 261–276
7. Steinbrink K, Nieder E (1987) Total femoral replacement and the saddle prosthesis. In: Coombs R, Friedlaender G (eds) Bone tumor management. Butterworths, London
8. Steinbrink K (1987) Vorgehen bei ausgedehntem oder völligem Knochensubstanzverlust des Femurs nach Schaftlockerung. Orthopäde 16: 277–286
9. Enneking WF (1987) A system for the functional evaluation of the surgical management of musculoskeletal tumors. In: Enneking WF (ed) Limb salvage in musculoskeletal oncology. Churchill Livingstone, New York, pp 5–16

Pelvic and Sacrum Resections

Surgical Procedure and Outcome

PETER RITSCHL, WOLFGANG KICKINGER, HERBERT FELDNER-BUSZTIN,
REINHARD WINDHAGER, and RAINER KOTZ[1]

Summary. From 1970 to February 1987, 48 patients with major malignant tumors in the pelvic or sacrum region were treated surgically at the Orthopaedic Clinic of the University of Vienna.

Of 37 resections, 22 involved only the ilium, while in nine cases the ischium and/or the pubis were the bones resected. In six cases, we had to remove more than one of the pelvic bones as well as the hip joint. In those cases where we had to resect the hip joint, we used saddle prostheses four times for stabilization, once a pelvic-hip-endoprosthesis, and once an internal wire fixation. Of the resections involving the ilium, seven had to be stabilized with tibial grafts and one with a bone-cement-plasty.

The tumor involved the sacrum in 11 cases. Two tibial grafts, one internal wire fixation with subpositioning of the ilium, and one cement interposition were required in the cases of partial or hemisacrectomies.

Surgical planning, preoperative diagnostic measures, surgical approaches, and possibilities of internal stabilization are described in detail. Results are judged according to radicality and with a critical eye to the life quality of the patients after surgery.

Key words: Bone Tumor—Pelvis—Sacrum—Surgical procedure

Introduction

Tumor reduction through neoadjuvant polychemotherapy for malignant bone tumors increasingly allows limb salvage surgery at the pelvis as well [5]. If the resections are adequately wide, these operations are a possible alternative to hemipelvectomy. Functional results following such operations have gained more and more ground in recent years. The criteria set up by Enneking have made standardization of the functional assessment possible [3]. This is of considerable advantage, especially in tumors involving the pelvis. Firstly, even large tumor centers often perform only a small number of extensive pelvic resections; secondly, size and location of the tumor as well as methods of reconstruction vary widely. Therefore, a large number of operations and their standardized evaluation will contribute to the definition of the best surgical methods for each individual patient.

---

[1] Department of Orthopaedics, University of Vienna, Vienna, Austria

Table 1. Diagnoses made at Department of Orthopaedics of University of Vienna

	No. of patients
Metastases	13
Hypernephroma	6
Rectum carcinoma	2
Thyroidea	2
Adenocarcinoma	2
Cervix	1
Osteosarcoma	10
Ewing's sarcoma	7
Chondrosarcoma	6
Giant-cell tumor	4
Chordoma	2
Spindel-cell sarcoma	2
Others	4
Total	48

Methods

At the Department of Orthopaedics of the University of Vienna, 48 large resections involving the pelvis and sacrum were performed between 1970 and 1987. The diagnoses are listed in Table 1.

According to the three basic patterns of pelvic resection described by Enneking in 1978 [2], the findings were as follows.

Type-IA resections (22). Four of these were IP (type-I partial) resections with only partial removal of the ilium. Another four type-I resections were performed, removing the adjacent sacrum as far as the sacral foramina as well (Fig. 1).

Type-IIA resections (six). Here the femoral head was also resected. In three cases, an additional type-III resection had to be performed; in two cases large parts of the ilium and in one case the ischium and ilium also had to be resected (Figs. 2–4).

Type-IIIA resections (nine). These were made of the pubis and/or ischium (Fig. 5).

Of the 35 primary tumors, the resection was wide in 11 cases, marginal in seven and intralesional in 17. Of the 13 metastatic cases, the resection was wide in four, marginal in one, and intralesional in eight.

The planned surgical procedure was a wide en bloc excision for 26 primary tumors. In nine cases, the surgical intention was intralesional curettage. Intralesional surgery was often performed in patients with tumors in the region of

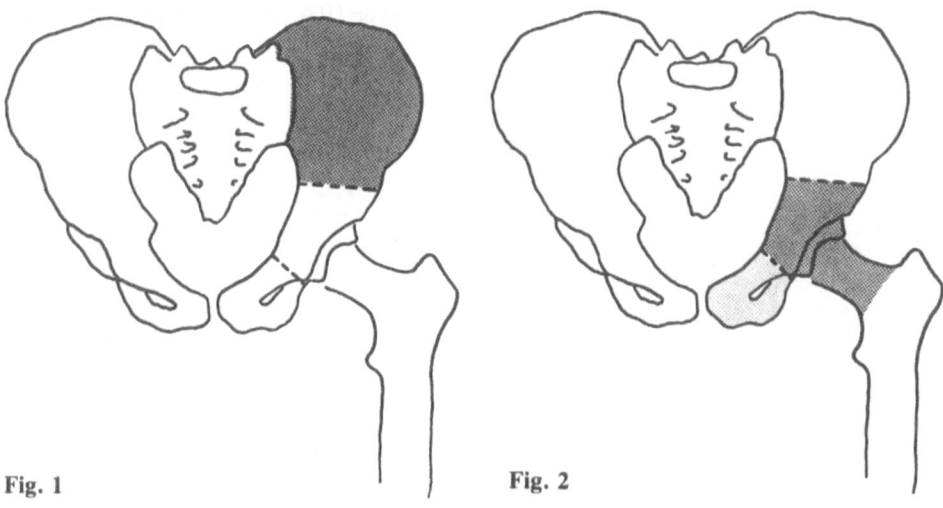

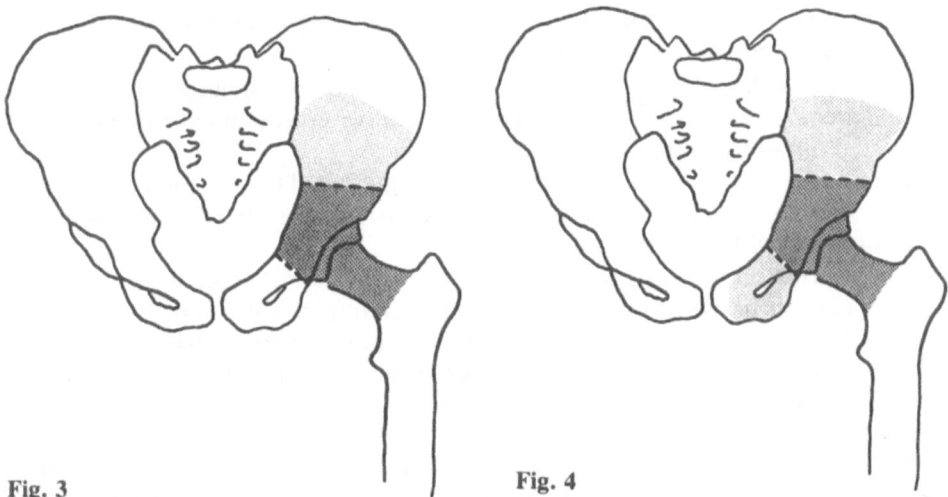

Fig. 1. Type IA ($n = 22$). Partial in four cases, with part of sacrum in four. Reconstruction was done in seven cases

Fig. 2. Type IIA + III ($n = 3$). Reconstruction was done with a saddle prosthesis

Fig. 3. Type IIA + I ($n = 2$). Reconstruction was done with saddle prosthesis and custom-made pelvis prosthesis

Fig. 4. Type IIA + III + I ($n = 1$). Reconstruction by saddle prosthesis. In one case after infection reconstruction with arthrodesis

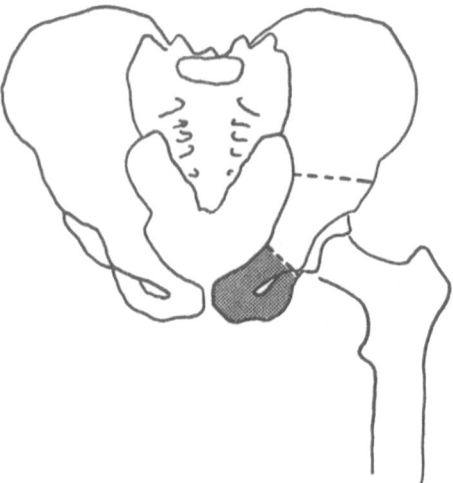

Fig. 5. Type IIIA ($n = 9$). No reconstruction

the sacrum and Ewing's sarcomas, who were given postoperative radiation treatment. Of the 26 intended wide resections, the tumor was entered at one point in eight patients (32%). Of the 13 metastasectomies, nine were planned as en bloc resections and the tumor was entered in four of these (44%).

A survey of the sacral tumors with regard to diagnosis, staging, surgical margin, and complications is shown in Table 2. Follow-up treatment of chordomas consisted of radiation therapy.

In one case with a recurrence of a malignant giant-cell tumor, total extirpation of the sacrum was performed after previous irradiation and stabilization was accomplished with two AO plates [7].

Reconstruction methods for the pelvis fall into the following five main categories: (a) soft-tissue reconstruction alone, resulting in a flail hip; (b) pseudarthrosis between the femur and the remaining parts of the pelvis, such as the ilium, ischium, pubis, or sacrum; (c) arthrodesis—iliofemoral, ischiofemoral, or sacrofemoral; (d) prosthetic replacement; (e) reconstruction with an osteochondral allograft.

In the resections of type IA and IA with parts of the sacrum, reconstruction with a tibial graft was performed in seven cases (Fig. 6). In one case, extensive skin grafting was necessary.

Reconstruction in the type-IIA resections was achieved with a saddle prosthesis [6] in four cases and in one with a custom pelvic prosthesis (Fig. 7). One of the saddle prostheses had to be removed due to infection. In a second procedure, 6 months later, arthrodesis with a tibial graft between the femur and remaining iliac crest was performed.

In none of the type-IIIA resections was reconstruction necessary (Fig. 8).

In the case of two patients with osteosarcoma, extensive occult spread had occurred to the common iliac vein and the vena cava, respectively. In one case, the iliac vein was bridged by a prosthetic graft (Gortex).

Postoperative complications encountered in the type-I and type-III resections

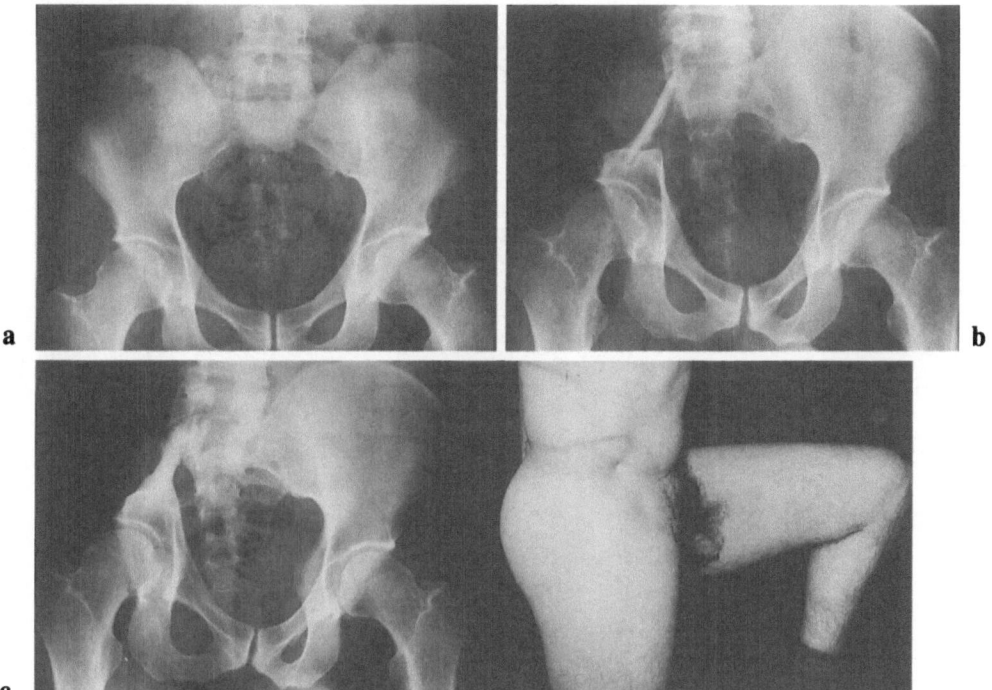

Fig. 6a–c. Subject H.S., 32 years old, male. **a** Osteosarcoma of the right ilium penetrating the adjacent sacrum. **b** Type-IA en bloc resection with wide margins and reconstruction with a tibia bone graft. **c** Five years after surgery. The tibia bone graft has clearly consolidated. Excellent result according to Enneking

were excessive bleeding in one case each and a wound-healing with infection in a type-III resection. The type-II resections including the adjacent ilium or ischium showed wound-healing complications in two and infections in two patients. In both cases, a saddle prosthesis had been used for reconstruction. One of them had to be removed. A large percentage of wound-healing complications and infections appeared in the sacrum resections (Table 2). Other material-related complications were two graft fractures in a total of nine tibial graft interpositions.

Comparison of the local recurrence rate with the wide, marginal, and intralesional procedures shows eight local recurrences in 25 intralesional resections and one local recurrence in eight marginal resections. In the 15 wide resections, no local recurrence was detected.

Of the 48 patients operated on at the Department of Orthopaedics of the University of Vienna, 22 have died, 20 of them from their primary disease. Two patients live with their disease. The other 24 have no evidence of disease.

Eighteen patients were available for follow-up. Five patients were not assessed because the follow-up period was less than 6 months. One patient was abroad, and two patients did not appear for examination.

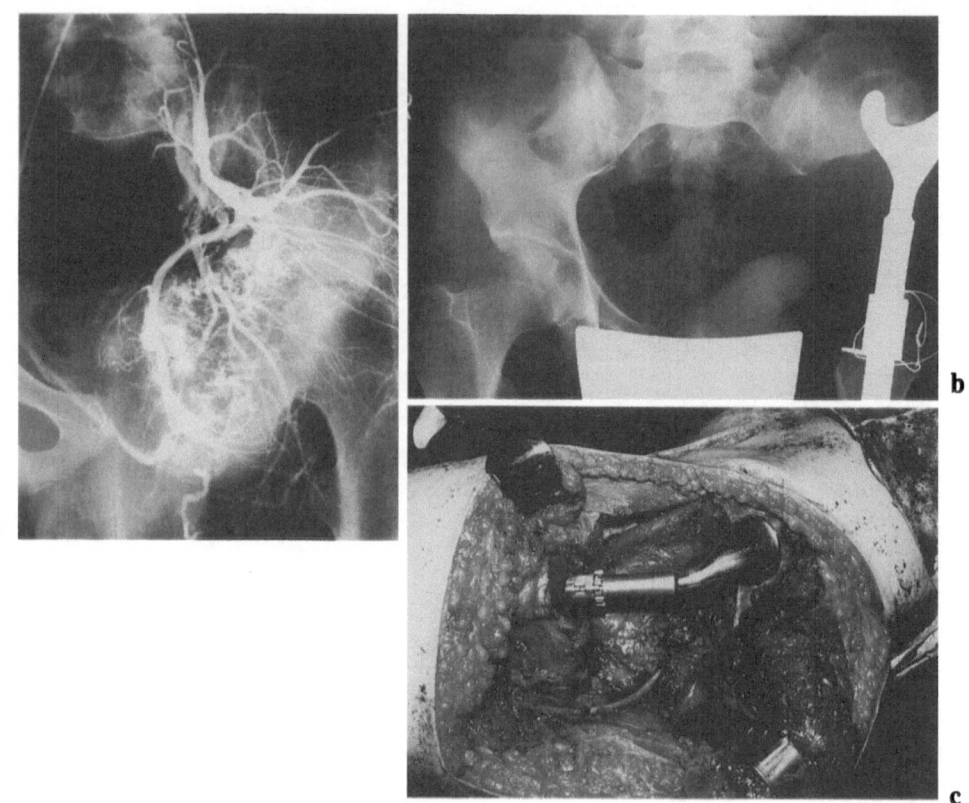

Fig. 7a–c. Subject N.T., 17 years old, male. **a** The angiogram shows the big soft-tissue extent of a periacetabular Ewing's sarcoma. **b** Resection type IIA + III + partial I with wide margins. Reconstruction with a saddle prosthesis. Overall rating according to Enneking was fair. Lack of motion and muscular strength. **c** Intraoperative situs with the implanted saddle prosthesis

Functional Results

Of the 18 evaluated patients, 11 had had type-IA resections. In three patients only, partial removal of the ilium had been performed. In six patients, stabilization had been achieved with a tibial graft. The individual functional results and the patient rating are compiled in Figs. 9–16.

The patient with the bad overall result had had no tibial graft after resection of a huge chondrosarcoma together with several nerve roots.

One patient with a type-IIA resection and concomitant removal of the ischium and pubis had an overall rating of fair. A saddle prosthesis had been used for reconstruction. In this patient, mainly muscle strength and motion were reduced. The three patients with resections in the area of the ischium-ilium and ischium-pubis had an overall rating of excellent in one case and good in two. Four patients with resection of the sacrum had an excellent rating in two cases and a good and a fair result in one case each.

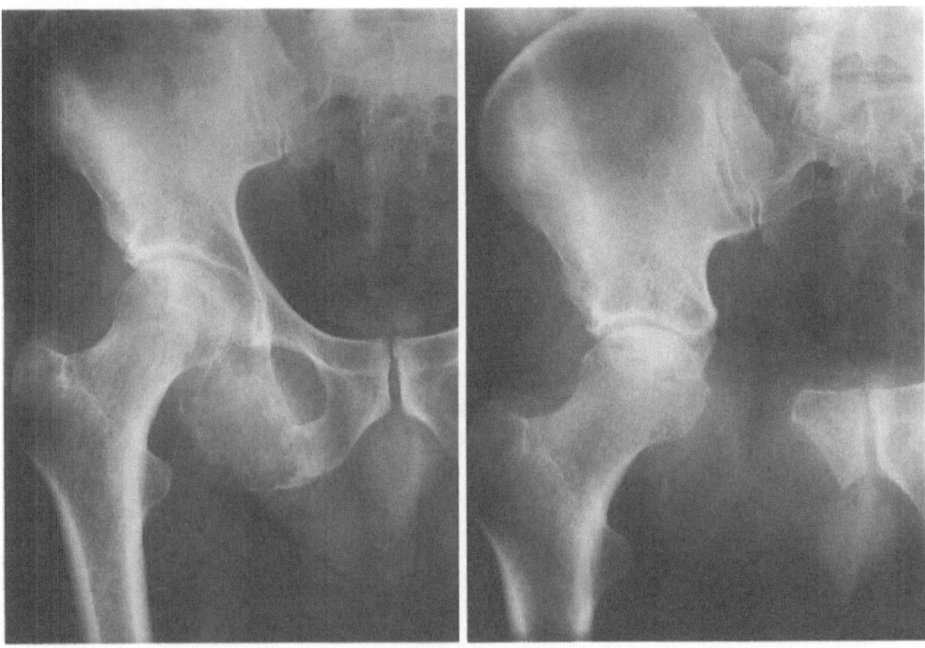

a   b

Fig. 8a, b. Subject H.A., 64 years old, male. **a** Metastasis of a hypernephroma in the right ischium. **b** En bloc resection type IIIA. Soft-tissue reconstruction. Excellent result after 1 year

Table 2. Details of sacral tumors ($n = 11$)

	No. of patients
Diagnosis	
Giant-cell tumor	4
Chordoma	2
Chondrosarcoma	2
Rectum carcinoma	2
Ewing's sarcoma	1
Staging	
IB	6
IIB	1
IIIA	1
IIIB	1
Margin	
Intralesional/marginal	8
Wide	3
Wound complications	6

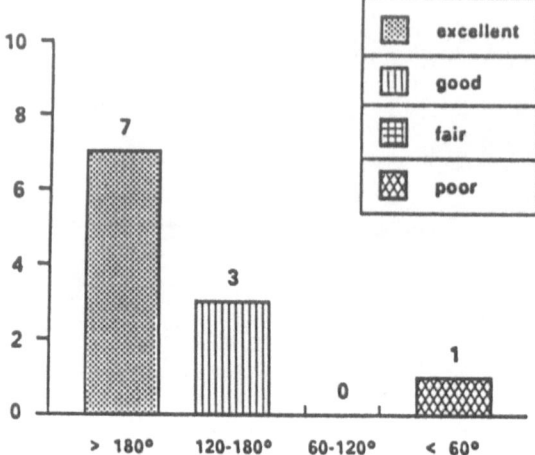

Fig. 9. Results for motion ($n = 11$)

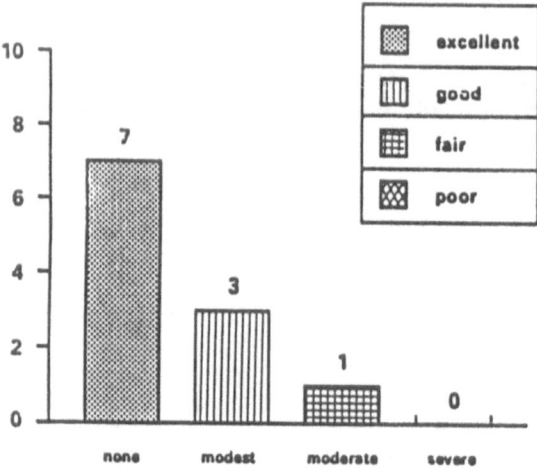

Fig. 10. Results for pain

Discussion

Resection surgery of the pelvis with adequately wide surgical margins is general-ly considered an alternative method to hemipelvectomy today. Nonetheless, it has to be taken into account that in a large percentage of cases the desired goal of a wide en bloc resection is not achieved (in our cases, one-third of the en bloc resections). This carries a considerable prognostic risk for the patient, so that for large tumors and difficult locations hemipelvectomy has still to be regarded as the method of choice.

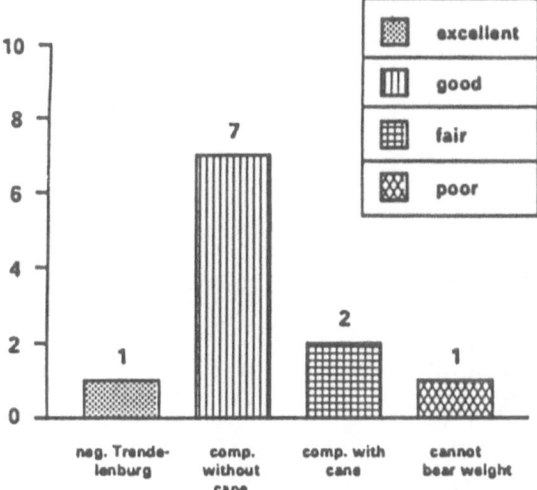

Fig. 11. Results for stability

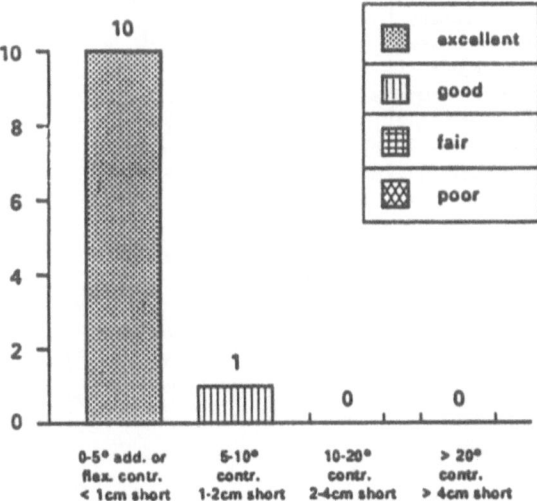

Fig. 12. Results for deformity

Periacetabular resections with removal of the hip joint pose a great functional problem. According to studies by Capanna et al. and Enneking and Mendenez of a major series of periacetabular resections, soft-tissue resection alone with the formation of a flail hip turns out to yield the most unfavorable results. Far better results can be achieved with pseudarthrosis and even better ones with arthrodesis. In both studies, the desired iliofemoral or ischiofemoral arthrodesis could only be achieved in 50% of the cases [1, 4].

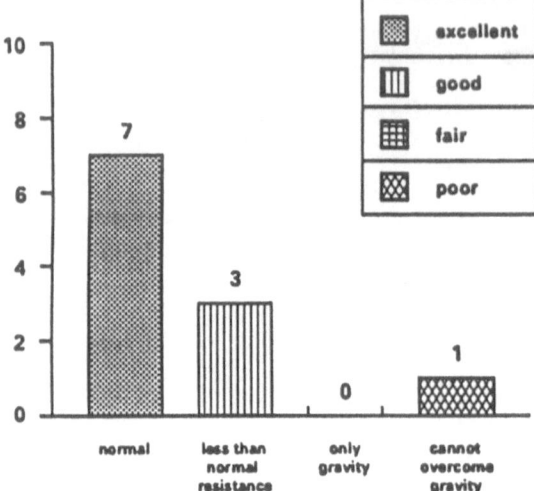

Fig. 13. Results for strength

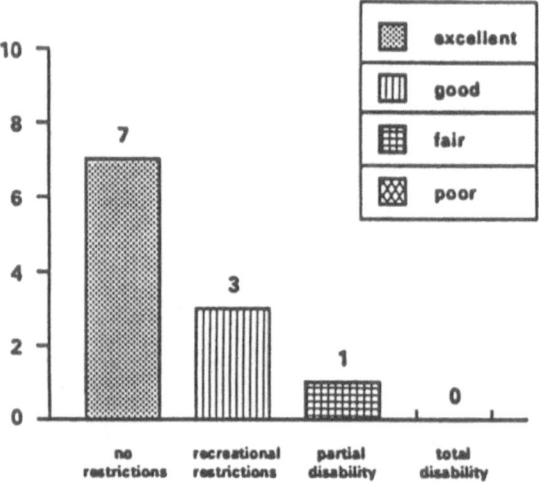

Fig. 14. Results for function

Quite generally, a solid union between the femur and part of the pelvis seems to yield good functional results. Patients who had undergone reconstruction with a saddle prosthesis were generally able to walk and stand well, showed little pain but had distinctly reduced range of motion and muscle power.

Resection of the hip joint still results in the greatest functional problems. In isolated cases, hip rotationplasty achieves a satisfactory functional result after periacetabular resection.

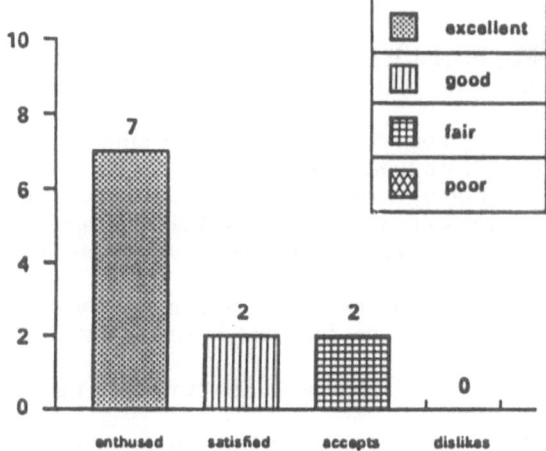

Fig. 15. Results for emotional acceptance

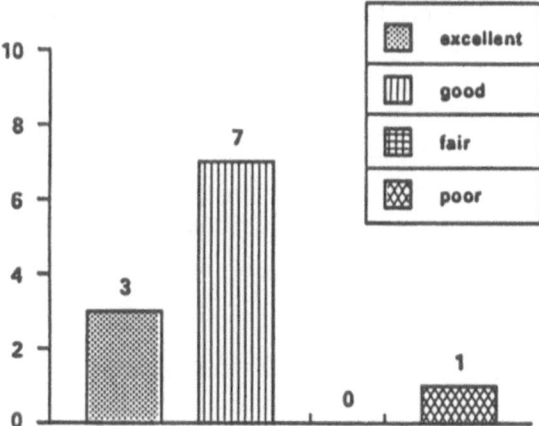

Fig. 16. Results for overall rating

Type-I and type-III resections obtain very satisfactory functional results in general. Stabilization with a bone graft represents a very strong and stable reconstruction method. This grafting procedure can also be carried out later, for example, after a chemotherapy regimen. In many cases, the functional results are better than those obtainable by hemipelvectomy. Even if they are equal or worse, hemipelvectomy puts a considerable psychological strain on the patient, which can be avoided by internal pelvic resections. Despite all this, top priority has to be given to safe and wide resection with adequate surgical margins.

References

1. Capanna R, Guernelli N, Ruggieri P, Biagini R, Toni A, Picci P, Campanacci M (1987) Periacetabular pelvic resections. In: Musculoskeletal Onkology. Churchill Livingstone, New York, pp 141–146
2. Enneking WF, Dunham WK (1978) Resection and reconstruction for primary neoplasms involving the innominate bone. J Bone Joint Surg 60-A: 731
3. Enneking WF (1983) Functional evaluation of reconstruction after tumor resection. In: Kotz R (ed) Proceedings of 2nd international workshop on the design and application of tumor prostheses for bone and joint reconstruction, Vienna 1983. Egermann, Vienna, pp 5–10
4. Enneking WF, Mendendez LR (1987) Functional evaluation of various reconstructions after periacetabular resection of iliac lesions. In: Musculoskeletal oncology. Churchill Livingstone, pp 117–135
5. Kotz R (1983) Possibilities and limitations of limb-preserving therapy for bone tumors today. J Cancer Res Clin Oncol 106: 68–76
6. Nieder E, Engelbrecht E, Steinbrink K, Keller A (1983) Modular system of the total femoral prosthesis—Endo-model. In: Kotz R (ed) Proceedings of 2nd international workshop on the design and application of tumor prostheses for bone and joint reconstruction, Vienna 1983. Egermann, Vienna, pp 231–235.
7. Salzer M, Knahr K, Sekera J, Braun O (1987) Resection treatment of malignant pelvic bone tumors. In: Musculoskeletal oncology. Churchill Livingstone, New York, pp 104–111

Reconstruction of Pelvis and Sacrum After Resection of Bulky Tumors

SHUN-ICHI INOUE[1], NORIHIKO TAKADA[2], and HIROSHI KITAHARA[1]

Reconstructive surgery after extended resection of bulky tumors that arise in the pelvis and sacrum is a challenging task in terms of surgical procedure and functional preservation of the lower extremity. Forty patients with such bulky tumors were treated surgically by us from 1975 to 1986. Of the 40 patients, 11 underwent tumor resection and reconstruction, 29 underwent hemipelvectomy or tumor resection only. The surgical results of the 11 patients who underwent reconstructive operations were studied.

The tumors of the 11 patients consisted of three chondrosarcomas, two osteosarcomas, two giant-cell tumors of the bone, two metastatic bone tumors, and two other diseases. The sites of the tumors were the iliac bone in six, pubic and ischiadic bone in two, and sacrum in three. Six patients who underwent iliac bone surgery received a reconstruction operation by using ceramics in two, acrylic cement and wiring in one, acrylic cement and Luque rod in two, and metal plate and autologous bone graft in one. Two patients who underwent resection of the pubic and ischiadic bone were reconstructed by means of bone grafting in one and Luque rod with acrylic cement in another. Of the three patients who underwent surgery in sacrum, two were reconstructed by using an autologous bone graft Luque rod and one patient was reinforced with an autologous bone graft and a Harrington rod. In terms of surgical complications, two patients had loosening of material and one patient had fracture. At follow-up (range, 12–96 months), 16 patients survived (three locally recurrent tumors) and two patients had died. Site of the tumor and biological character of the tumor were the two key factors in reconstructive surgery of the pelvis and the sacrum after extended resection of bulky tumors.

Two representative cases are shown in figures (Figs. 1, 2).

Case 1. A 40-year-old male patient complained of a painful buttock tumor on the left side. The plain X-ray film findings (Fig. 1a) showed a large sclerotic lesion with a marked periosteal reaction in the left ilium. Following open biopsy, the histological diagnosis was chondroblastic osteosarcoma. After chemotherapy

[1] Department of Orthopedic Surgery, Chiba University, Chiba, Japan
[2] Department of Orthopedic Surgery, Chiba Cancer Center Hospital, Chiba, Japan

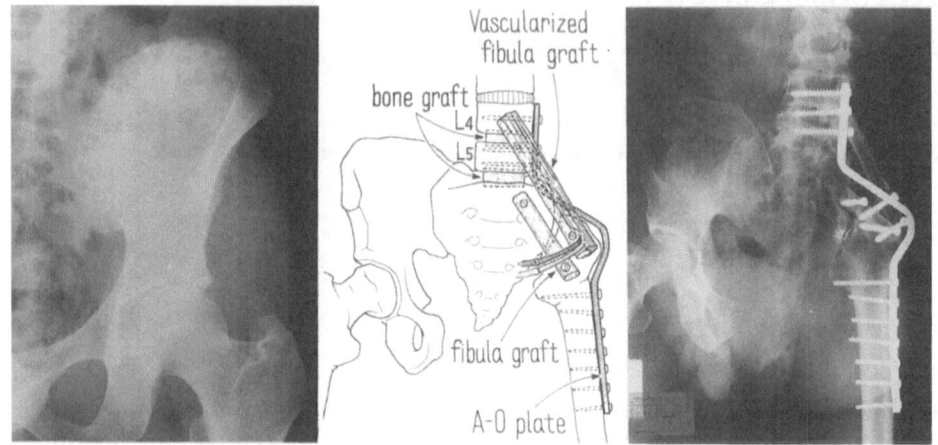

Fig. 1a–c. A 40-year-old male patient. Chondroblastic osteosarcoma of the left ilium. **a** Plain X-ray film. **b** Schematic drawing of the reconstruction surgery. **c** Postoperative X-ray film

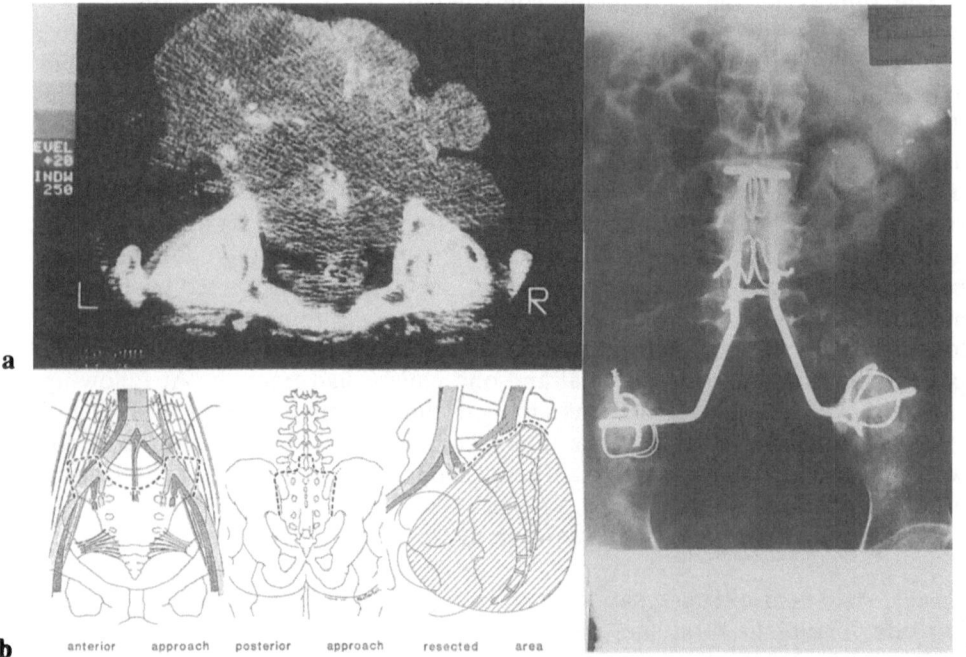

Fig. 2a–c. A 70-year-old male patient. Chordoma of the sacrum. **a** This CT findings shows a bulky tumor destroying the sacrum. **b** Schematic drawing of surgical lines and resected area. The *Shaded area* was removed. **c** Postoperative X-ray film

and irradiation, the left internal pelvis was resected. The pelvis was reconstructed with anterior spinal fusion, A-O plate fixation, and vascularized fibular graftig. One year after surgery, the patient is alive with no local recurrence and no distant metastasis.

Case 2. A 70-year-old male patient unable to sit because of a huge tumor, measuring $35 \times 25 \times 15$ cm, was referred to us. The computed tomographic (CT) findings (Fig. 2a) showed a bulky tumor destroying the sacrum which was compatible with a chordoma. The patient underwent tumor excision. An anterior surgical approach was followed by a posterior surgical approach. Two Luque rods, stainless steel wire, autologous bone grafting, and bone cement were utilized to reconstruct the sacrum. Two months after surgery, the patient was able one again to use a wheel chair. Now, he is fully able to do rehabilitation exercise.

To preserve or obtain function of the lower extremity after operation, the following should be observed: (a) Rigid connection of the spinal column to the pelvic ring is essential for successful reconstruction at the lumbosacral region and iliosacral joint; (b) endurable supporting capability of the acetabulum must be regained; (c) surgery of the pubic joint demands rigid and stable reconstruction of the pelvic ring.

We emphasize the capability of reconstruction after extended resection with sufficient stability by using prosthetic materials, vascularized bone grafting, bone cement, and so on.

Hemipelvis Allograft

Technical Aspects of Three Cases After Tumor Resection

FRANTZ LANGLAIS[1] and CLAUDE VIELPEAU[2]

Summary. Three en bloc resections for malignant tumors of the hip articulation, the periacetabular area, and the iliac wing were reconstructed by irradiated hemipelvis allograft and total hip prosthesis. Oncological and clinical results were favorable with a follow-up of 15–30 months. No luxation was observed: weight bearing was allowed at 3 months, and consolidation seemed to be obtained at 6 months. The walking distance was 500 m to 2 km without pain.

Some technical aspects are described: anterior Campanacci's approach (excising the previous biopsy site through Hueter's approach); osteotomy and reattachment of the iliac crest; fixation of the pubic and ischiatic ramus by large centromedullar screws; stabilization of the prosthesis using a cup with a posterosuperior wall, and three braids of polypropylene: one of them "neck lacing" the prosthesis, and the two others linking the great trochanter and the allograft to control rotations.

Key words: Hemipelvis resection—Hemipelvic allograft—Iliac bone tumors

Introduction

Reconstruction after excision of pelvis tumors extending to the periacetabular area and to the iliac wing poses difficult problems. In three such cases, we performed allograft reconstruction of the hemipelvis, along with a total hip prosthesis, rather than hemipelvectomy or any other conservative procedure. At short follow-up (15–30 months), this operation is proving to be of value because of its low morbidity and its functional results. Some technical aspect of this procedure are discussed.

[1]Service de Chirurgie Orthopédique et Réparatrice, Centre Hospitalier Universitaire, Hôpital Sud, Rennes, France
[2]Service de Chirurgie Orthopédique et Traumatologique, Centre Hospitalier Universitaire Côte de Nacre, Caen France

Clinical Cases

Case 1

The first patient was operated upon in April 1985. The patient was a 30-year-old woman suffering from multiplex exostoses with degeneration in the form of a chondrosarcoma of the pelvis. A computed tomography (CT) scan revealed a voluminous tumor (11×23 cm), extending to the pelvis as well as to the anterior face of the great trochanter.

Campanacci's approach (2) was used, and resection of the tumor was performed along with sacroiliac disarticulation and section of the pubis and ischium under the floor of acetabulum. The hemipelvis was reconstructed with an allograft, screwed onto the sacrum, and fixed by two plates on the remaining pubis and ischium. The hip was reconstructed using a Cochin type resection prosthesis on the shaft of some metaphyseal fragments and fixed by wiring. No ligamentoplasty was used. Postoperatively, the patient was kept in balanced traction for 6 weeks and began to walk with two crutches after 100 days. Consolidation of the allograft was achieved at 6 months. Two years after operation, the walking distance was 2 km. The patient used a walking stick except when at home and had no pain. Passive flexion was over 90°. The hip grading according to Merle d'Aubigné [7] was : pain 5/6, active motion 3/6, stability 4/6. No recurrence or metastases were detected.

Case 2

The second patient was a 41-year-old woman operated on for a pelvic metastasis in October 1985 (Fig. 1). She had been operated on for a carcinoma of the thyroid 2 years previously. Scintigraphy and other tests revealed only one metastasis in the supra- and periacetabular area, with intra- and extrapelvic extensions. She was first treated will radioactive iodine and the pelvic operation was then performed after embolization of the superior gluteal artery. Using the same pproach as in the first case, we performed a similar wide excision, with arthrectomy as far as the intertrochanteric line. Reconstruction was performed using an irradiated hemipelvis screwed onto the sacrum and attached to the pubis and ischium by large centromedullary screws. A total standard hip prosthesis was stabilized using artificial ligaments. The leg was kept in balanced traction for 3 weeks, and weight bearing was allowed at the end of the 3rd month. Eighteen months later, there were no signs of evolutive disease, and the hip grading was pain 5/6, active motion 3/6, stability 4/6. A passive flexion of 100° was achieved, but there was only 45° of active flexion, even though muscular excision was considerable. The patient was able to walk at home without a walking stick and to walk 2 km using one. Standing on the operated leg was possible without tilting the pelvis greatly, perhaps due to a tenodesic effect, as the abductor muscles were not retained (Fig. 2).

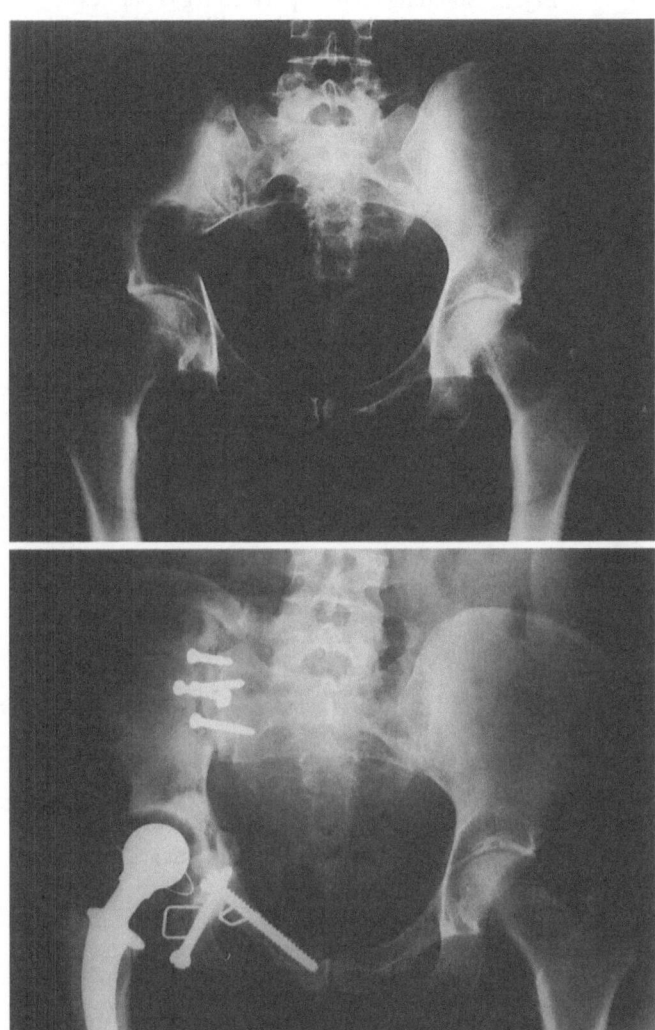

Fig. 1. a Preoperative X ray. Solitary metastasis of a thyroid carcinoma in a women of 41. **b** X-ray at 18 months

Case 3

The third patient was a 60-year-old woman who had been operated on for a total excision of cancer of the kidney 2 years previously. Systematic follow-up revealed a metastatic osteolysis of the supra- and periacetabular area, with no other localization at detailed check-up. Wide excision (performed in July 1986), reconstruction, postoperative care, and rehabilitation were as in the previous case. Evaluation at 8 months revealed no signs of evolutive disease. Functional

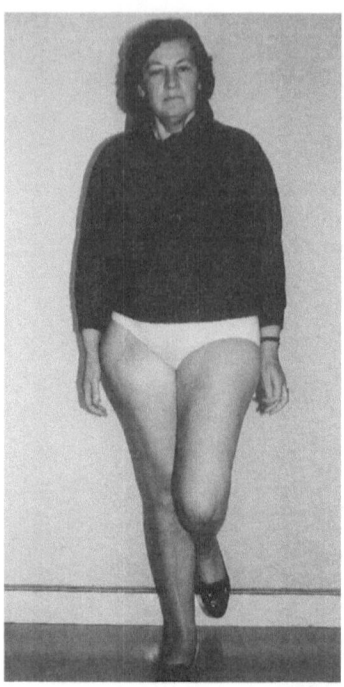

Fig. 2. Standing on the operated leg is painless. Walking distance is over 2 km with a walking stick. Despite extensive muscular excision, there is no major limping and an active flexion of 45° remains possible

grading was: pain 5/6, active motion 3/6 (with 100° of passive flexion), stability 4/6 (the patient walks with a walking stick). the functional result was impaired by the patient's age but mainly by concomitant severe rheumatoid arthritis (a controlateral total knee prosthesis had been performed 3 years earlier).

Technical Aspects

The operation, comprising excision and reconstruction, last about 10 h. The patient is place in a lateral reclining position. Tilting to a three-quarter dorsal position is possible in order to facilitate ligation of the internal iliac artery. The patient is then returned to the lateral reclining position for fixing the allograft and setting of the prosthesis.

The incision begins above the posterosuperior iliac spine, follows the iliac ridges, passes in front of the anterior interspiny notch, and ends at the lateral face of the femur, 10 cm above the tip of great trochanter. This creates a wide cutaneous and muscular flap, including the gluteus maximus, and with a posterior pedicle.

The sciatic nerve is dissected up to the anterior face of the piriformis muscle. The gluteus minimus and medius and the pelvic trochanter muscles (which are removed en bloc with the articulation) are not detached from the tumor in order to excise it without exposing the lesion. The gluteal artery is dissected and ligated. The sacrosciatic ligaments and the posterior sacroiliac ligament are then sectioned.

At the edge of the iliac wing, it is often possible to perform an osteotomy of the iliac ridge, on which insertions of abdominal muscles remain. Sometimes, because of intraosseous extension of the tumor, muscles desinsertion is preferred to osteotomy.

At the anterior and lower part of the incision, the crural nerve is isolated. The iliopsoas, sartorius, and tensor fascia lata are cut at the level of the base of the femoral neck; their iliac insertions are excised en bloc. On the deep face of the psoas major, the branching of the common iliac artery is located and the hypogastric artery is ligated. The iliopsoas is sectioned at the sacroiliac level and the lumbo sacral plexus exposed.

Bone sections are then achieved. The ilioischiatic ramus is sectioned at the upper edge of the tuberosity, and the iliopubic ramus near the acetabulum, leaving the obturator pedicle intact. Manipulation of the lower limb makes the sacroiliac joint gape, making disarticulation easier. The femoral neck is then sectioned at the intertrochanteric lines so that the joint capsule is not opened.

Reconstruction

The reconstruction phase comprises grafting of the hemipelvis, setting and stabilizing of the prosthesis.

The cartilage of the sacrum is abraded in order to facilitated arthrodesis, and the allograft is shape to fit onto the three sacrum, pubis, and ischium sections. The wing of the ilium is shaped to fit the ridge retained. Acetabular fixing slots (for anchoring the cup) are prepared before the graft is fixed.

Fixing of the allograft is achieved: (a) with axial screws for the pubis and ischium; the pubic screw is inserted via the anterior horn of the acetabulum and directed toward the pubis. The ischiatic screw is inserted at the lower point of the tuberosity, entering the posterior wall of the acetabulum. (b) With two screws for the sacrum; they start from the posterior part of the iliac wing: one is directed toward the sacral wing and the other between the first and second anterior sacral foramen.

The iliac ridge is reinserted using a series of strong sutures, passing through the holes of the graft and encircling the ridge. Autografts of cancellous bone are placed around each of the anterior and posterior bone junctions. All these osteosyntheses, notably those of the obturator area and the ridge, produce a very solid fixation.

To set and stabilize the prosthesis, the acetabular cartilage is abraded and the fixing slots prepared. The acetabular cup is set using polymethyl metacrylate (PMMA) bone cement containing antibiotics at an angle of $35°$ of inclination and $10°$ or $20°$ of anteversion. Setting the femoral prosthesis is routine. Artificial ligaments can be used to ensure immediate stabilization of the prosthesis.

The closing is easy: The gluteus maximus is sutured at the iliac ridge level. It is the only muscle covering the graft. The patient is placed in balance traction, using a transtibial pin. After the 5th week, the patient is progressive raised to the vertical position and is allowed to walk in a swimming pool. Placing all of the weight on the foot is allowed after the 3rd month.

Discussion

Allograft: Choice, Conservation, Future

Most pelvic lesions' notably those of the iliac wing at some distance from the acetabulum, can be readily treated by resection of the ala, with or without arthrodesis between the sacrum and the supracotyloid area. But CT scan and nuclear magnetic resonance (NMR) examinations have shown that many malignant tumors extend as far as the acetabulum and even reach the articulation. Such tumors require en bloc resection of all the articulation [arthrectomy], of its capsule, of the pelvi trochanter muscles, as well as the removal of the iliac wing, padded with the medium and small gluteus, and the psoas magnus. But afterward, restoring function poses difficult problems: The allograft seems to be the most promising technique after such large resections.

Other therapeutic solutions include: hemipelvectomy, the poor functional result of which is known [8]; prostheses, which have a high morbidity rate, as they are difficult to fix to the remaining pelvic ring and as musclar reinsertions are impossible [1]; resection of the pelvis without reconstruction, which has only middling results from a functional point of view [2, 9]. As with like femoropubic arthrodesis, the latter is better as a backup procedure in case the allograft fails.

The allograft, therefore, is a valuable tool. It is not very complex, the most delicate part of the operation being the excision. The allograft is a "prosthesis" that is relatively easy to produce. It can be shaped to the required dimensions, fixed, and combined with a standard hip prosthesis. It offers the advantage of being biologically bound to the neighboring bone, as well as favoring muscle reinsertion.

In our bone bank, allografts are aseptically sampled at the same time as the sampling of visceral grafts (kidney, liver, heart). The bone is stored at −40°C and is irradiated with 1.5–2.5 Mrad gamma radiation. This sterilizing process is useful if any contamination occurs during sampling, and it does not seem to influence consolidation with the neighboring bone [5]. Consolidation was obtained in the two younger patients between 3 and 6 months after operation at the pubis and ischium level [where cancellous autografts surrounded the bone/graft junction] and at the iliac ridge level. Consolidation was more diffcult to assess at the sacroiliac level, but after 1 year this junction was stable and painless.

X-ray and technetium scanning examinations tend to show that the allograft rehabilitation is only partial. A biopsy performed more than 1 year after grafting [patient 1] did not demonstrate any colonization by osteocytes. Additionally, an NMR examination performed 1 year after the second operation showed resonance of the allograft, which was characteristic neither of living nor of necrotic bone, but rather of fibrous tissue.

Technique

The technique has the following features. There is vascular control. Two opposing risks are to be faced—peroperative bleeding and necrosis of the flap. The

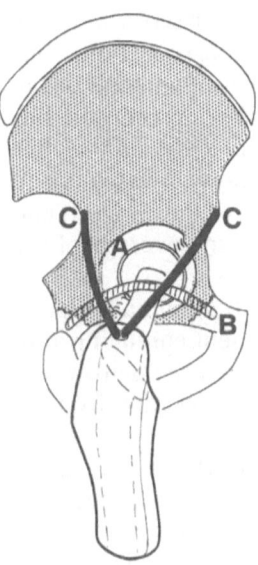

Fig. 3. Stabilization of the prosthesis (case 2 and 3). A Cup with posterior and superior wall. B Polypropylene braid "neck lacing" the neck of the prosthesis, fixed by staples at junctions of the allograft and retained pubic and ischiatic ramus. C Braids controling rotations without limiting abduction or adduction

approach route provides a well-vascularised musculocutaneous flap. Yet in case 3, a skin necrosis over an area of 6 × 1 cm at the anterior edge of the flap occurred and was succesfully treated by simple excision and thin grafting.

To limit bleeding during the excision of a very vascularized thyroid metastasis (case 2), we used preoperative embolization of the superior gluteal artery; there was no complication and there was effective reduction of peroperative blood loss. But in other cases, fearing skin necrosis by embolization of terminal cutaneous arteries, we preferred ligature of the hypogastric artery (which has a substitute celleberal circulation) and of the superior gluteal artery in the sciatic notch (because of its anastomosis with the inferior gluteal artery).

The Campanacci approach is recommended as it enables endo- and exopelvic dissections to be performed under good conditions and permits en bloc excision of the route of the previous biopsy with the tumor. Thus, if such a wide excision is planned, this preliminary biopsy has to be made following the Hueter-type anterior access and using a trephine to collect the supra-acetabular sample.

Stabilization of Graft and Prosthesis

Osteosynthesis of the allograft does not present any particular difficulty (Fig. 3). Both sacroiliac cartilaginous surfaces are abraided, and the length of the pubic and ischiatic ramus and adjusted. The osteosynthesis is accomplished with 7-mm Maconor screws. The screws are 60 or 70 mm long, self-tapping, nozzle-shaped, and are screwed over a 2.5-mm guide wire. They produce a fixation which has several advantages over plate osteosynthesis. It is immovable, does not require deperiostage of the healthy bone, and favors the padding of the osteosyntheses area with cancellous autografts.

Sacroiliac arthrodesis is performed using two 5-mm or 7-mm-diameter screws inserted into the posterior iliac mass at an oblique angle medially and forward.

The upper screw is inserted into the sacral wing and the lower screw emerges between the two anterior sacral foramina, readily located on palpation. This osteosynthesis is not as solid as that of the obturator foramen. Synthesis of the iliac ridge is performed using braided nylon sutures, transfixing the allograft 10 mm under the section slice and passing over the upper edge of the iliac ridge. This fitting enables good setting of the allograft to the well-vascularized osteotomy of the iliac ridge. Fixing of the abdominal muscles to the allograft and reinsertion of the gluteal muscle onto this ridge provides good coverage of the operative site.

Stabilizing the prosthesis is of the utmost importance. A titanium alloy prosthesis was used in these cases and fixed in place by bone cement contaning antibiotics. This cement fixation appears to be more reliable than bone ingrowth as concerns allografts, and the presence of antibiotics provides protection from infection.

The stability of the prosthesis during the first weeks can only be passive as the capsule and all the hip-fixing muscles have been excised. For this reason, a prosthesis with a 32-mm head diameter should be used as it is more stable than smaller heads. The acetabular cup has both posterior and superior walls, limiting the risk of dislocation in these directions [6]. The cup should be placed more horizontally than usual (35°) with very slight anteversion.

In cases 2 and 3, three polypropylene braids were used to obtain double passive stabilization. One encircled the neck of the femur at its upper edge; it was stretched between staples located on the iliopubic and ischiopubic ramus, thus limiting the risk of dislocation of the prosthesis in an upward direction. The two others braids were used to palliate the absence of rotatory control of the hip, with its risk of dislocation by extreme rotation. One braid was placed between holes drilled in the anterior edge of the great trochanter and the anterior part of the pelvis near the puboiliac eminence. It was stretched in intermediate rotation and in adduction, so that abduction and adduction were not limited, but external rotation was. Another braid was stretched in the same way between the ilioischiatic eminence and the posterior edge of the great trochanter to limit internal rotation

Many Unknown Factors Remain

What is the future of these operation from an oncological point of view? The fact that the limb is preserved and the pelvis reconstructed using an allograft did not reduce the extensive nature of the excisions: They would not have been more extensive if hemipelvectomy had been used. Additional treatment was not needed by these patients as at pathological examination these excisions were shown to be "wide" [4] in all cases. Control scanning using iodine 12 months after excision of the thyroid metastasis did not show any fixation, especially at the pelvic level.

What is the future of these allografts? Rehabilitation of the bony graft is hypothetical. Does the large surface of the iliac bone and its cancellous structure promote greater colonization that the dense cortex of diaphysis? This rehabilitation may perhaps increase the risk of fracture due to fatigue of the ilio- and ischiopubic ramus (although these very areas are axially reinforced with screws).

Consolidation seems to be complete in the two younger patients. But it is uncertain at the obturator level in the older patient.

Conclusions

We report three cases of allograft replacement of the hemipelvis after its resection en bloc with the upper extremity of the femur. The perspect of reconstruction did not cause us to limit the importance of tumor excision, which was always "wide." We have not had any case of recurrence or metastasis, but the follow-up extends only over a maximum of 2 years. We were surprised at how trouble-free the postoperative course was in these patients after the 10-h operation. The quality of the functional result was quite good too: After 6 months, the patients were able to walk with a walking stick without experiencing pain. A return to normal family life and even leisure activities was possible after 1 year. The allograft, which is a biologically fixed "prosthesis," appears to be the treatment of choice after thses large pelvic excisions with arthrectomy as the functional results are far better than those obtained with previously used techniques. A few technical precautions need to be taken to obtain these results: absolute sterility of the allograft (we used moderate freezing of minus 40° and gamma radiation); osteosynthesis using a centomedullar screw in the pubic and ischiatic ramus (providing a very solid fixation); conservation of the iliac ridge as a pediculated graft (favoring reinsertion of the abdominal muscles and perhaps allograft colonization); stabilization of the prosthesis, supported by the use of a cup with a posterosuperior wall and artifical ligaments to control rotation amplitude and limit the risks of dislocation.

References

1. Burri C, Gerngros H, Kinzl L, Etter C (1983) Total and partial internal hemipelvectomy. In: Kotz R (ed) Proceedings of 2nd international workshop on the design and application of tumor prostheses for bone and joint reconstruction, Vienna, 1983. Egermann, Vienna, pp 291–293
1 Bis. Rahmanzadeh R, Hahn F, Faenzen M (1983) The endoprosthetic replacement of the pelvis or partial pelvis replacement. In: Kotz R (ed) Proceedings of 2nd international workshop on the design and application of tumor prostheses for bone and joint reconstruction, Vienna, 1983. Egermann, Vienna, pp 294–295
2. Campanacci M, Salzer M, Shives T, Menendez L, Eilbert F, Capanna R, Tomeno B, Dunham W, Mutschler W, Lane J, Nilsonne U, Nieder E (1987) Functional results of reconstruction for periacetabular pelvic resection requiring sacrifice of the hip joint. In: Enneking W (ed) Limb salvage in musculoskeletal oncology. Churchill Livingstone, New York, pp 103–192
3. Campanacci M (1986) Les résections du bassin pour tumeurs. In: Encycl Med Chir (Paris) (ed) Techn Chir Orthop Traumat, 44505, pp 1–7
4. Enneking W, Spanier S, Goodman M (1978) Resection and reconstruction for primary neoplasms involving the innominate bone. J Bone Joint Surg 60A: (6) 731–746
5. Hernigou P, Delepine G, Goutallier D (1986) Massive freeze dried and irradiated bone allografts. Rev Chir Orthop 6: 403–413
6. Langlais F, Aubriot JH, Postel M, Tomeno B, Vielpeau C (1986) Prosthetic recon-

struction of the upper end of the femur after resection for tumors [20 cases]. Rev Chir Orthop 6: 415–425

7. Merle d'Aubigné R (1970) Cotation chiffrée de la fonction de la hanche. Rev Chir Orthop 56: 481–486

8. Michaut E, Rabeux L, Lefevre B, Mazas Y, Pelisse F (1975) Desarticulations de hanche et amputations inter ilio abdominales. Appareillage et résultats fonctionnels. Rev Chir Orthop 61: 547–550

9. Nilsonne U, Kreicbergs A, Olsson E, Stark A (1982) Function after pelvic tumor resection involving the acetabular ring. Internat Orthop [SICOT] 6: 27–33

Chapter 9

Functional Results Following Resection of Tumor in the Proximal Humerus and Tibia

Shoulder Girdle Resections for Bone and Soft Tissue Tumors

Analysis of 38 Patients and Presentation of a Unified Classification System

Martin M. Malawer[1], Isaac Meller[1], and William K. Dunham[2]

Summary. The authors developed a surgical classification system for shoulder girdle resections for patients undergoing limb sparing procedures for bone and soft tissue tumors: Type I, proximal humeral resection; type II, partial scapular resection; type III, total scapulectomy; type IV, total scapulectomy and extra-articular glenohumeral resection; type V, proximal humeral and glenoid resection; and type VI, proximal humeral and total scapular resection. Each type is modified according to the status of the abductor mechanism (A, intact; B, partial or complete removal). This system is based upon the current concepts of oncological surgery and precisely describes the procedures performed, structures removed, and the relation to the glenohumeral joint; it accommodates both compartmental and extracompartmental methods, the status of the abductor mechanism, and indicates the increasing surgical magnitude of the resection. It is not dependent upon the type of reconstruction performed.

Data from 38 patients with an averaged follow-up of 4.6 years are presented (range 2–8.4 years).

Of the 38 tumors, 92% were malignant; 32 were in bone and six in soft tissues. Twenty-four lesions were located in the proximal humerus and 14 in the scapula. Their surgical stages were IA (two), IB (ten), IIA (three), IIB (15), III (five) benign latent (two), and benign aggressive (one). The types of resections were as follows. All operations were easily classified: Type I, 15; II, four; III, four; IV, six; V, eight; and VI, one. The surgical margins achieved were marginal in ten cases, wide in 22, and radical in six. At last follow-up, five patients (12.8%) were dead and two (5%) were alive with disease. There was no evidence of local recurrence in any of the 38 patients.

Type I, II, and III resections were generally used for low-grade sarcoma or benign aggressive tumor, whereas types IV, V, and VI were utilized for high-grade sarcomas. The A and B modifiers correspond to intracompartmental and extracompartmental resections, respectively.

The proposed classification meets all criteria for such systems, is simple, universally applicable, reproducible, and comprehensive. The system is recommended to facilitate uniformity in terminology among surgeons and institutions and to allow prospective comparison of data.

Key words: Shoulder girdle—Sarcoma—Classification system—Tikhoff-Linberg procedure

[1]Children's Hospital National Medical Center, George Washington University School of Medicine and Health Sciences, Washington DC, USA
[2]University of Alabama, Birmingham, AL, USA

Introduction

The shoulder girdle includes the upper end of the humerus, the scapula, and the clavicle as well as the surrounding soft tissues and axillary contents. It is the third most common site of primary bone and soft tissue tumors. Bone tumors of the shoulder girdle occur most frequently in the proximal humerus, followed in decreasing order by the scapula and the clavicle. The deltoid and posterior supraspinal areas of the scapula are the most frequent sites for soft tissue tumors around the shoulder. Only a few large series concerning the epidemiology of tumors of the shoulder girdle have been published. Most them are from major centers, pointing to the rarity of the subject and the need for centralization.

In 1965, Papaioannou and Francis described the following classification for scapulectomies [1]: *Total scapulectomy*, removal of the entire bone, including the glenoid fossa and the acromion and the coracoid processes; *nearly total scapulectomy*, partial removal, leaving the acromion and/or coracoid processes; *radical subtotal scapulectomy*, removal of the entire scapula except for the glenoid fossa and occasionally of the acromion, the coracoid process, or both; *Subtotal or partial scapulectomy*, removal of the tumor-bearing area of bone (usually subspinal) with a margin of surrounding normal bone. In 1968, Samilson et al. revised this earlier classification, adding the classic interscapulo-thoracic resection (Tikhoff-Linberg procedure) and forequarter amputation, thereby establishing a universal classification system that covered virtually all major shoulder girdle operations (resections and amputations) [2] as of that date. These two classification systems were purely descriptive and related almost exclusively to the bone resection only.

These systems do not utilize or reflect the common concepts or terminology that have developed within the field of orthopedic oncology during the past decade. Specifically, they do not clearly reflect the concepts of surgical margin the relation to anatomical compartments (intracompartmental vs. extracompartmental), the status of the glenohumeral joint (intra-articular vs. extra-articular), the magnitude of the individual surgical procedure or precise consideration of the functionally important soft tissue components (the abductor mechanism). In addition, new procedures have been developed that involve mainly tumors of the proximal humerus and not the scapula which have not been classified or only termed "Tikhoff-Linberg" resection.

Since the introduction of adjuvant chemotherapy in the early 1970s, interest in the shoulder girdle and limb sparing procedures has increased markedly. Formerly, most shoulder girdle resections were performed for tumors of the scapula and periscapular soft tissue sarcomas; today, however, the most common indication is the treatment of osteosarcoma of the proximal humerus, which is the third most common site for osteosarcoma. The large majority of osteosarcomas of the proximal humerus are currently treated by limb sparing procedures. Due to the nature of osteosarcoma, its site, and different techniques of reconstruction, a large number of new procedures and modifications of shoulder girdle resections have been developed. Unfortunately, most of these have been reported as a "Tikhoff-Linberg resection" or "modified Tikhoff-Linberg resection"—eponyms that do not accurately describe the procedure performed.

An extensive review of the literature concerning shoulder girdle resections reveals a basic problem: the lack of an accurate and precise classification system for the multitude of modifications and variations of surgical procedures performed to remove tumors of the shoulder girdle. To assess the effectiveness of different treatment protocols and to compare series from different surgeons and centers, the need for a universal classification system based on modern orthopedic oncological concepts is essential. This paper presents a unified classification system based on our experience of over 10 years and a careful analysis of 38 patients.

Historical Review of Shoulder Girdle Resections

Initial reports of shoulder girdle resections were confined to individual bones or portions of the scapula. The first mention of a scapular resection in the literature is a partial scapulectomy performed by Liston for an "ossified aneurysmal tumor" in 1819 [3]. In 1837, Mussey performed a near total scapulectomy with resection of the clavicle for a recurrent chondrosacroma after gleno-humeral disarticulation [4]. Syme performed the first total scapulectomy for a tumor in 1856. In 1909, De Nancrede published a detailed review about "the end results after total excision of the scapula for sarcoma" [5]. He conclusded that anything less than a forequarter amputation for shoulder girdle tumors was inadequate. This brought scapular resections into disrepute for half a century. Pack and Crampton are credited with the revival of the procedure [6]. In 1965, Papaioannou and Francis reported on 26 scapulectomies and described the indications and limitations of the procedure [1]. Between De-Nancrede's paper in 1909 and the most recent one by Adam et al. in 1983, which is called "Scapulectomy revisited . . ." [7], a multitude of case reports and miniseries have been published; these have described modifications of scapular resections and different indications, such as primary benign and malignant bone tumors, soft tissue tumors, and metastases. Any scapular resection is a true limb sparing procedure. The indications are quite limited, since only infra-spinal or distal scapular lesions are amenable to this type of surgery. Nonetheless, the very first limb sparing attempts involved the shoulder girdle.

The early history of the interscapulothoracic (Tikhoff-Linberg) resection, or the triplebone resection was described by two Russian surgeons, Bauman (1914) and Linberg (1928) [8, 9]. Bauman notes a 1908 report by Pranishkov of a case of removal of the scapula and surrounding soft tissues with resection of the head of the humerus and the outer third of the clavicle. The shoulder was subsequently attached to the clavicle by metallic sutures in order to form a new joint. The operation was carried out because of sarcoma of the scapula [8]. Between 1908 and 1913, Tikhoff and Bauman performed three such operations, and Tikhoff was named as the originator [8]. Bauman's original article and subsequent papers were published in Russian, and the procedure became established only after 1928, when Linberg published his classic paper in English in the *Journal of Bone and Joint Surgery* [9]. He accredited Tikhoff as the originator of the operation and Pranishkov was forgotten [8, 9]. Since that time, more than 20 papers, mostly case reports and miniseries (fewer than five cases), describing in total more than 80 cases, have been published. All deal solely with the

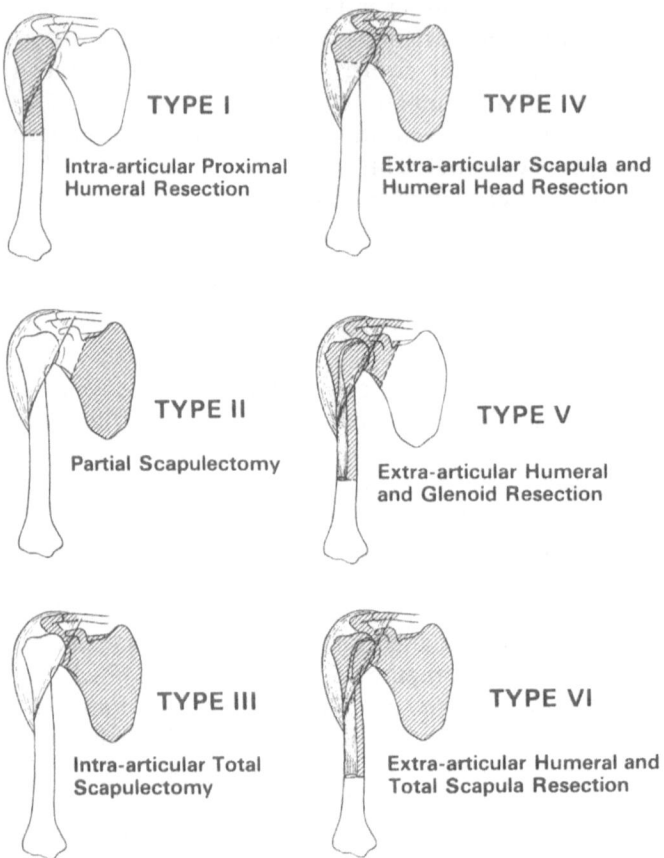

Fig. 1. Surgical classification of shoulder girdle resections

Tikhoff-Linberg resection. Only four large series have been reported, all of them after 1960: Macson (1968), 15 cases [10]; Marcove et al. (1977), 17 cases [11]; Malawer et al. (1985), ten cases [12, 13]; and Guerra et al. (1985), 21 cases [14]. At the same time, countless reports of shoulder girdle amputations have appeared in the medical literature.

When one analyzes reports about the Tikhoff-Linberg resection on a case-by-case basis, it is obvious that a multitude of modifications have been performed. Different amounts of scapula, clavicle, or humerus are resected in any individual case; the same is true for the muscles. A variety of techniques of suspending the humeral stump to the remaining clavicle or scapula or the chest wall have been described, as have different ways of reconstructing the soft tissues.

Surgical Classification

A surgical classification system must be: (a) easy to use; (b) universally applicable; (c) based on staging studies, surgical and functional anatomy; (d) con-

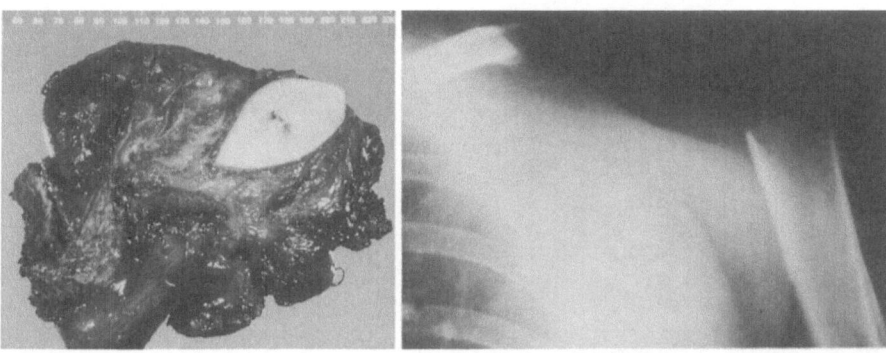

a   b

Fig. 2a, b. Type IVB resection. This is the classic Tikhoff-Linberg resection. **a** Gross specimen. This includes the entire scapula, the proximal humeral head and shoulder joint removed extra-articularlly, and all surrounding muscles. **b** Postoperative radiograph of the defect. The upper extremity is suspended from the clavicle by transfer of the short head of the biceps and Dacron tape

sistent with oncological principles of treatment; (e) correspondent to the magnitude of surgery; and (f) reproducible. To date, a comprehensive surgical classification system for shoulder girdle resections (limb sparing operations) that meets these six criteria has not been described.

We developed a surgical classification system for limb sparing shoulder girdle resections based on the results of 38 patients (Fig. 1).

a) Type I, intra-articular proximal humeral resection
b) Type II, partial scapular resection
c) Type III, intra-articular total scapulectomy
d) Type IV, extra-articular total scapulectomy and humeral head resection (Fig. 2)
e) Type V, extra-articular humeral and glenoid resection (Fig. 3)
f) Type VI, extra-articular humeral and total scapular resection

Each type is further modified according to the status of the soft tissue, especially, the abductor mechanism: A intact; B, partial or complete resection. In the schema in Fig. 1, the "deltoid muscle" represents the abductor mechanism in toto, not only the muscle.

This classification system reflects the type of resection and its relation to the glenohumeral joint and indicates progressive increase in the magnitude of the surgical procedure. Types IA–IIIA usually represent an intracompartmental resection, wheras types I–III (B only) and IV–VI correspond to extracompartmental resection. Types I–III resections are always intra-articular, while types IV–VI are extra-articular. This system is based solely upon the structures removed. The type of resection corresponds to the magnitude of the surgical procedure and thus only infers the type and extent of reconstruction required but does *not* depend upon the type of reconstruction.

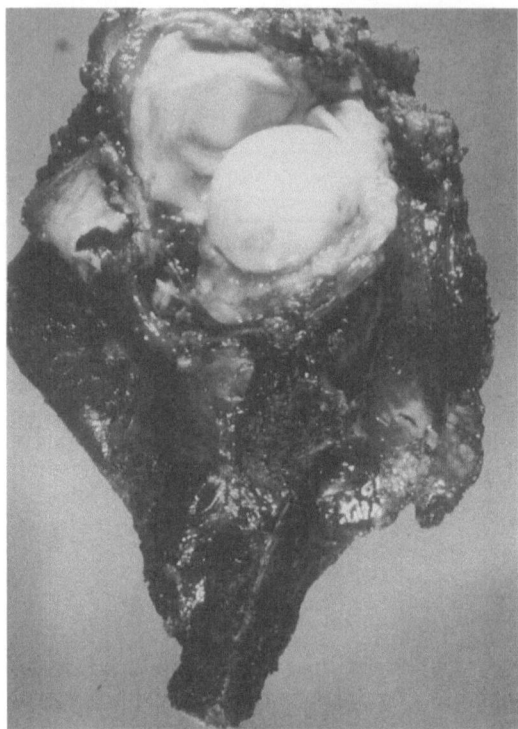

Fig. 3. Type VB resection. Gross specimen following an extra-articular resection of the shoulder and the proximal one-half of the humerus. Note the joint has been opened. The entire abductor mechanism is removed en bloc with the specimen. Reconstruction may be accomplished by a variety of methods: prosthesis, arthrodesis, or allograft replacement. This is the most common procedure performed for stage IIB osteosarcoma of the proximal humerus

Materials and Methods

Thirty-eight major shoulder girdle resections were performed in two orthopedic oncological centers between 1979 and January 1986. There were 22 men and 16 women. The mean age at operation was 33.4 years (range, 3–62 years). The mean age of the male patients was 31.2 years (range, 3–60 years) and that of the females 37 years (range, 15–62 years).

Diagnosis and Stage

Of the 38 lesions, 33 were primary bone tumors and six were soft tissue tumors. There were three primary benign lesions (two osteochondromas and one fibromatosis) and 35 primary malignant tumors including: 12 osteosarcomas; nine chondrosarcomas (eight low-grade lesions and one high-grade lesion); two periosteal ostoesarcomas and two parosteal osteosarcomas; two fibrosarcomas, two malignant fibrous histiocytomas (MFH); two synovial sarcomas (one metastatic to bone); one Ewing's sarcoma; one hemangiopericytoma; one leiomyosarcoma; and one giant cell tumor (GCT). One of the chondrosarcomas was secondary in a patient with multiple hereditary exostosis (MHE). Surgical stages was: IA (two), IB (ten), IIA (three), IIB (15), and III (five). There were three benign tumors—two latent and one aggressive GCT.

Anatomical Site

Twenty-four lesions were located in the proximal humerus (defined as the proximal third of the diaphysis and the head of the humerus, or the proximal diaphysomethaphysis and the head) or the deltoid muscle region. Fourteen lesions were located in the scapula and/or the surrounding soft tissues. Among these scapular lesions, three were located in the distal body and tip of the bone, while 11 were located in or extended to the upper part of the bone (scapular spine, acromial process, coracoid process, glenoid fossa). No lesions of the clavicle were included in the present series.

Adjuvant Treatment

Of the 38 patients, 24 received adjuvant chemotherapy, with or without local radiation therapy, based on the histological type and grade of the tumor and the surgical margins achieved during operation.

Results

The follow-up period was 24 months to 8.4 years, with an average of 4.6 years.

Types of Resection

Types of shoulder girdle resection were: type I, 15 cases (six A, nine B); type II, four cases (all A); type III, five cases (all B); type IV, six cases (all B), type V, eight cases (all B), and VI, one case (B). Twenty-two operations (types III–VI) were done by an extra-articular resection of the glenohumeral joint, while 16 (types I–III) were done via an intra-articular resection.

Margins

Gross and microscopic histopathological examinations of the specimens showed that the surgical margins obtained were marginal in ten cases, wide in 22 cases, and radical in six cases.

Relation of Type of Resection to Diagnosis and Surgical Stage

Type IA resections were utilized for the low-grade sarcomas of the proximal humerus (chondrosarcoma, parosteal osteosarcoma) and for a marginal excision of a previously irradiated Ewing's sarcoma in one patient. Seven of the eight type IB procedures were utilized for high-grade sarcomas (osteosarcoma) of the proximal humerus. All four type IIA procedures were performed for benign tumors; three of these involved low-grade or aggressive benign tumors of the scapula and one was a high-grade sarcoma. All type IV (six cases) resections (by necessity B) were for high-grade sarcomas of the proximal humerus (four) or large stage IB lesions (two). All type V procedures (eight) were for high-grade stage IIB sarcomas (six osteosarcomas, two chondrosarcomas). One type VI resection was performed for a stage IIB osteosarcoma of the proximal humerus.

Relation of Type of Resection to Final Surgical Margin

Types I, II, and III obtained a marginal excision (ME; nine patients) or wide excision (WE; 14 patients), depending upon the extent of soft tissue resection; type IA obtained an ME, whereas all type IB accomplished a WE (Table 1). The margins obtained by type II were marginal (three) and wide (one); those obtained by type III were marginal (two). All six type IV resections were radical. Seven of eight type V resections obtained a WE.

Types of reconstructions. The types of reconstructions were internal prosthetic devices (19 custom-made humeral prostheses and one Kuntscher nail); soft tissue reconstruction was done in 15 cases, and replacement of humerus with an autologous whole fibular graft in four.

Tumor status. Five patients (13.2%) died from metastatic disease within 24 months of surgery. All of these patients had tumors of the proximal humerus; four had osteosarcoma and one had a solitary metastatic synovial sarcoma from an unknown primary site. The metastatic lesion was surgical stage IIA; of the others, four were IIB patients with osteosarcoma: Three underwent type VB resection, and one type VB. The patient with the metastatic lesion underwent a type IA resection. Two additional patients are currently alive with pulmonary disease. Overall, two patients in theis series had late axillary lymph node involvement (one from an osteosarcoma and one from MFH); one died and one is alive with no evidence of disease after lymph node dissection. No local recurrences have occurred.

Complications. There was no flap necrosis, infection, or vascular complications. All extremities were salvaged. There were no secondary amputations. Two patients have required a secondary procedure. One required secondary resection of a promient acromion; the other patient underwent a axillary lymph node dissection 1 month after the initial resection. The patient remains alive with no evidence of disease 43 months later. Transient nerve palsies (mostly the radial nerve and musculocutaneous nerve) and postoperative seromas, the most common complications, usually resolved with conservative treatment.

Revisions. Two prosthesis have required revision: One humeral prosthesis loosened (type V resection) at 3 years and was recemented; a second prosthesis was revised at 6 years due to bending of the stem. Both procedures were done without complication.

Function. No orthotic devices have been required for external support. Patients have not complained of shoulder pain or instability. Hand function was normal in all patients immediately after operation except in those who had transient nerve palsies. A functional range of motion of the elbow was preserved in all patients, although strength was diminished. Cosmetic results are acceptable. Some of the patients use external cosmetic devices to regain shoulder contours. Shoulder motion is normal only following a type IIA resection. Abduction following types III–VI was limited to 0°–30°.

Discussion

The purpose of this paper is to present a new, comprehensive, *unified*, and universal classification system for shoulder girdle resections (Fig. 1). It is based on the results of treatment in 38 patients with a variety of bone and soft tissue tumors, most of which were malignant.

The purpose of this classification system is to standardize terminology for the multitude of surgical procedures for shoulder girdle resections that have been developed within the past two decades. Without such a system, it is difficult to determine the exact nature of the procedure performed and structures removed since many procedures are referred to merely as "Tikhoff-Linberg resections." This is analogous to the confusion in surgical oncology when terms as "mastectomy," "modified mastectomy," and "radical" mastectomy are used. We have analyzed our clinical experience with shoulder girdle resections over the past 10 years and have developed a classification system based on those findings and recently developed principles of orthopedic oncology. We use the term "proposed" classification because we expect as experience is gained in its use, it will of necessity be modified.

Our classification system is based upon the anatomical and functional structures removed. The major modifiers are the presence or absence of the crucial soft tissue structures, the abductor mechanism (A denotes abductors present, B abductors partially or completely resected.) In general, the loss of any component of the abductor mechanism (rotator cuff and/or deltoid muscle) creates a similar functional disability. The abductor mechanism must almost always be resected when there is extraosseous extension by tumor arising from any involved bone. Thus, in reviewing our clinical experience, it became evident that A represented an intracompartmental resection and B an extracompartmental resection, irrespective of histology or primary bone involvement.

Type I, II, and III resections are usually performed with retention of the abductor mechanism (A), and thus are utilized for benign or low-grade lesions of the proximal humerus and scapula, respectively. Conversely, type IV, V and VI resections require removal of the abductor mechanism (B) and are thus most often utilized for the treatment of high-grade sarcomas of the scapula and proximal humerus. Therefore, most type I, II and III resections are performed for intra-compartmental disease, whereas types IV, V, and VI are performed extracompartmentally. Occasionally, type I–III resections can be used for malignant tumors.

Our data show that a marginal excision or wide excision can be accomplished by any of the above procedures, depending upon the extent of the tumor. It is important to note that only type IV can accomplish a true radical resection, since this is the only procedure in which the entire involved bone (scapula) is removed. In addition, this classification system inherently describes the relation of the resection to the status of the glenohumeral joint. Type I–III resections are accomplished intra-articularly, while types IV–VI are performed extra-articularly. In general, the magnitude of the surgical procedure increases as the number assigned to it rises. Similarly, this also parallels the increasing difficulty of the reconstruction that is required following resection. It should be emphasized, however, that this classification system does not depend upon the type of reconstruction performed.

In summary, our proposed classification system considers the status of the structures moved (bone/abductor mechanism) and the type of resection (intra-compartmental vs. extracompartmental) performed, reflects the status of the glenohumeral joint (intra-articular vs. extra-articular), denotes the type of surgical margin achievable, and indicates the increasing surgical magnitude of the resection and, thus also, the reconstructive effort required.

The adequacy of the Tikhoff-Linberg operation and its modifications is underlined by the rarity of local recurrence reported in the literature: 1 in 21 cases at the Rizzoli Institute [14], 1 in 17 cases reported by Marcove et al. [11], and none in our series. However, a shoulder girdle resection is indicated only when staging studies have demonstrated that the neurovascular structures are not involved by the neoplasm. Invasion of the axillary lymph nodes or chest wall is also a contraindication. It is difficult to assess the role of early or late axillary lymph gland involvement since the number of patients with this occurrence is very small (two in our series), but we tend to agree with Marcove et al. [11] that in selected cases it is worthwhile to perform a radical node dissection simultaneously or as a second stage procedure. Chest wall resection is not a part of any known shoulder girdle resection. It is very rare and most authors believe it to be a contraindication to a limb sparing procedure [11, 12]. Such cases are, therefore, not included in our classification system.

The classic Tikhoff-Linberg resection (type IV in the present system) includes the removal of the whole scapula [8, 9]. In carrying out extra-articular resection for tumors of the proximal humerus (usually type V) or deltoid area, we consider it advisable whenever possible, to remove only the lateral part of the scapula (neck and glenoid of scapula with the acromion or coracoid processes) instead of the entire bone. This is the most important modification we propose of the original Tikhoff-Linberg procedure, and it appears as type V in our system. It has been described by Malawer et al. [12, 13] and Guerra et al. [14] recently. Of the triplebone resections in our series, eight were type V. This modification offers much better functional and cosmetic results and makes it possible to anchor an endoprosthesis more firmly by fixing it to the remaining scapula instead of to the stump of the clavicle or rib cage. The scapula osteotomy also permits medialization of the prosthesis and a decrease in bulk in the area to be covered [13].

Our classification system tends to emphasize the importance of an extra-articular rather than intra-articular resection of the glenohumeral joint in order to remove the potentially contaminated joint en bloc. However, either intra-articular or extra-articular resection is easily described. A study of the resected anatomical specimens in the series of Guerra et al. [14] showed that in 20 of 21 cases, the tumor had invaded the subchondral bone and was separated from the joint cavity only by articular cartilage, which was undermined and fissured. In some cases, the invasion also involved the capsule and pericapsular structures. Similar situations are described by Marcove et al. [11] and Malawer et al. [12]. It has been already established that articular cartilage and joints are no longer considered barriers for tumor invasion. In the present series, 15 resections (all types IV, V, VI) were done without opening the glenohumeral joint, although four of ten resections for osteosarcoma of the proximal humerus were intra-articular.

A major determinant of the functional outcome of any shoulder girdle resection is the length of humeral resection. This fact is well expressed in the difference between type IV and types V–VI. A key anatomical consideration is whether the resection is performed distal or proximal to the deltoid tuberosity. We agree with Marcove et al. [11] and Guerra et al. [14] that the resected humeral segment should be reconstructed (in any case where the resection is below the humeral neck or deltoid tuberosity); the goal is to restore length of bone in order to improve the esthetic result, increase the power of elbow movement, and prevent the instability and suspension problem of the limb relative to the trunk. None of our patients has required an external orthosis. Stability is achieved by a combination of skeletal reconstruction and muscle transfer.

The value of any classification system lies in its ability to be simple, universal, reproducible, and consistent with valid surgical concepts. We believe that the new system described in this paper results these criteria. With further prospective evaluation in different centers, however, its validity will be ultimately established.

References

1. Papaioannou AN, Francis KC (1965) Scapulectomy for the treatment of primary malignant tumors of the scapula. Clin Orthop 41: 125–132
2. Samilson RL, Morris JM, Thompson RW (1968) Tumors of the scapula. A review of the literature and an analysis of 31 cases. Clin Orthop 58: 105–115
3. Liston R (1820) Ossified aneurysmal tumor of the subscapular artery. Ediul-Med J 16: 66–70
4. Mussey RD (1837) Removal by dissection of the entire shoulder blade and collar bone. Am J Med Sci 21: 390–394
5. De Nancrede CBG (1909) The original results after total excision of the scapula for sarcoma. Ann Surg 30: 1–22
6. Pack GT, Crampton RS (1961) The Tikhor-Linberg resection of the shoulder girdle. Clin Orthop 19: 148–161
7. Adam YG, Rosen A, Oland J, Halery A (1983) Scapulectomy revisted: soft part sarcomas of the posterior shoulder. Isr J Med Sci 19: 176–179
8. Bauman PK (1914) Resection of the upper extremity in the region of the shoulder joint. Khirurg Arkh Velyaminova S-Peterb 30: 145–149
9. Linberg BE (1928) Interscapulo-thoracic resection for malignant tumors of the shoulder joint region. J Bone Joint Surg 10: 344–349

10. Macson NJ (1968) Modification der resectio interscapulo-thoracalis (Tikhoff-Lunbersche operation). Beitrage zur Orthopadie und Traumatologie 15: 87–88
11. Marcove RC, Lewis MM, Huvos AG (1977) En bloc upper humeral interscaulothoracic resection. The Tikhoff-Linberg procedure. Clin Orthop 124: 219–228
12. Malawer MM, Sugarbaker PH, Lampert MH, Baker AR, Gerger LH (1984) The Tikhoff-Linberg procedure and its modifications. In: Sugarbaker PH (ed) Atlas of sarcoma surgery. JP Lippincott, Philadelphia, pp 205–226
13. Malawer MM, Sugarbaker PH, Lampert MH, Baker AR, Gerber NL (1985) The Tikhoff-Linberg procedure: Report of ten patients and presentation of a modified technique for tumors of the proximal humerus. Surg 97: 518–528
14. Guerra A, Capanna R, Biagini R, Ruggieri P, Campanacci M (1985) Extra-articula resection of the shoulder (Tikhoff-Lunberg). Ital J Orthop Traumatol 11: 151–157

Functional Results Following Resection of Tumors in the Proximal Humerus

Excluding Arthrodesis and Massive Allografts

JEAN P. COURPIED[1], BERNARD TOMENO[1], FRANTZ LANGLAIS[2],
BERNARD AUGEREAU[3], JACQUES H. AUBRIOT[4], SERGE BABIN[5],
DIDIER MOULIES[6], and BERNARD PECOUT[6]

Summary. The authors reviewed 46 cases of resection of the upper humerus for tumor. Of the 46 tumors, 90 % were malignant. The average follow-up was 5 years and the functional evaluation according to Enneking's classification was excellent in one good in seven, fair in 15, and poor in 23. Mechanical complications occurred in 11 cases and reoperation was necessary in eight of these cases.

The length of humeral resection did not seem to affect the functional result. Good and excellent result were only found in cases without arthrectomy, and conservation of the abductor mechanism is a prime factor of shoulder function. To obtain a satisfactory functional result, the best conditions are humeral resection without arthrectomy and conservation of the abductor mechanism.

There were 18 cases with resection restricted to the humerus and abductor preservation: 15 prostheses, and two spacer nails were used and there was one case was without any reconstruction. There were 13 cases with resection restricted to the humerus and abductor resection: eight prostheses and one spacer nail were used and there were four cases were without any resection.

Conservation of the abductor mechanism was unusual when the resection led to arthrectomy. In 15 cases with arthrectomy, three spacer prostheses and five spacer nails were used; for the seven other cases, no reconstruction was performed.

Indications of the kind of reconstruction are discussed according to the type of resection, mechanical complications and functional results of the submitted study.

Key words: Upper humerus—Resection for tumor—Spacer

We reviewed resections of the upper end of the humerus performed in at the Cochin Hospital Orthopaedic Department and at some other departments. After excluding all cases operated on with arthrodesis or massive allografts, we studied 46 cases.

[1] Service de Chirurgie Orthopedique, Hospital Cochin, Paris, France
[2] Hopital Sud, Rennes, France
[3] Hopital St Antoine, Paris, France
[4] Hopital de la Cote de Nacre, Caen, France
[5] Hopital Hautepierre, Strasbourg, France
[6] Hopital Dupuytren, Limoges, France

Materials

There were 20 female and 26 male patients. The ages ranged from 12 to 76 years (mean 35 years). The tumors were chondrosarcoma in 22 cases, osteosarcoma in six, giant cell tumor in five, metastasis in four, and other types in nine. The initial site was mainly the upper humerus (36/46).

Bony resection was performed without arthrectomy in 31 cases (type I in the Malawer classification) and with arthrectomy in the 15 other cases (six type IV, six type V, and three type VI according to Malawer's classification). The margin obtained by the procedure was satisfactory nine times out of ten. After shoulder resection, a prosthesis was used in 25 patients, a spacer in nine patients, and in 12 patients no reconstruction was performed. The average follow-up was 5 years. Twenty-eight patients are continuously disease free, two are, without evidence of disease, two are alive with disease, eight have died of disease, and six are lost to follow-up. Functional evaluation according to Enneking's classification was: excellent, one; good, seven; fair, 15; poor, 23. This classification gives special emphasis to shoulder function, but often in bad results the hand and elbow are useful in some cases if active functional moton of the elbow can be preserved.

Influence of Resection in Functional Result

Length of Humeral Resection

The length of humeral resection ranged from 3 to 17 cm (mean 13 cm) and did not seem to affect significantly the functional result. Long, short, or intermediate lengths of resection were found in each of the three groups (good, fair, poor).

Type of Scapular Resection

Good and excellent functional results were only found in cases without arthrectomy (type I in Malawer's classification). Fair and poor results were found in each kind of bone resection. The best results occurred after resection restricted to the humerus with glenoid cavity conservation, because a good reconstruction was possible in these cases.

Condition of Abductor Mechanism

In the abductor mechanism, the two main parts are the circumflex nerve and deltoid muscle. In our study, there were 22 resections of the abductor mechanism and 24 cases with its conservation. Resection of tumors of the upper humerus very often 2 led to a cut circumflex nerve, even if the tumoral development was not so great (14/22 cases). Deltoid muscle resection was necessary in 15 cases to obtain a satisfactory margin; but in seven of these, the resection was a partial muscle resection without any damage to the circumflex nerve; in these cases, there was conservation of the abductor mechanism. It is quite obvious that conservation of the abductor mechanism is a prime factor in the functional re-

Table 1. Functional result

Resection	Without arthrectomy (31 cases)	With arthrectomy (15 cases)
With abductor conservation (24 cases)		
E + G	8	0
F + P	10	6
With abductor resection (22 cases)		
E + G	0	0
F + P	13	9

E excellent, *G* good, *F* fair, *P* poor, according to Enneking's functional classification

Table 2. Type of reconstruction

Cᵃ Reconstruction	Functional resultᵇ	Mechanical complications
IA		
15 prostheses	E = 1, G = 7, F = 5, P = 2	Asymp = 1
2 nails	P = 2	Reop = 2
1 WR	P = 1	
IB		
8 prostheses	F = 2, P = 6	Reop = 2, No reop = 1
1 nail	P = 1	Reop = 1
4 WR	F = 1, P = 3	
IV 3 prostheses	F = 3	
V 5 nails	F = 2, P = 3	Reop = 3, No reop = 1
VI 7 WR	F = 2, P = 5	

ᵃ Malawer's classification
ᵇ Enneking's classification
Asymp asymptomatic, *Reop* reoperation, *WR* without reconstruction

sult; in 24 cases, there were one excellent, seven good, eight fair, and only eight poor results according to Enneking's classification.

In conclusion, to obtain a satisfactory functional result, the best conditions are humeral resection without arthrectomy and conservation of the abductor mechanism (Table 1). In our study, there were 18 such cases with only five poor functional results. When the resection led to arthrectomy, conservation of the abductor mechanism was unusual—six of fifteen cases.

Reconstruction

The type of reconstruction is very important for the quality of the functional result and depends on the extent of resection [1]. We shall now examine the functional result and the mechanical complications of the various procedures of reconstruction according to the abductor mechanism and bone resection (Table 2).

Scapular and Abductor Mechanism Conservation

In 15 prosthesis, 13 satisfactory were obtained when resection was performed with conservation of the abductor mechanism and without arthrectomy. We used only a humeral prosthesis—Mathy's type, a massive metallic type, or a massive plastic type with a metallic core. In this group, there was one mechanical complication, which was breaking of the cemented stem prosthesis 1 year after the procedure. However, the patient was still asymptomatic 2 years later.

The Length of the humeral resection (5–17 cm) did not affect the functional result. There were two bad functional results. The first was in a 76-year-old man with partial resection of the deltoid muscle and the second in a patient with stiffness of the shoulder. Active rotation of the shoulder was possible in 12 patients, with weight bearing in all cases. All the patients were classified as excellent, good, or fair according to Enneking's system (13 cases); they were able to bring their hands their mouth, back, and perineum, and ten of them were able to bring their hands to the nape of the neck. This shows the importance of motion of the elbow in the functional result. If active flexion of the elbow is preserved or reconstructed, the actual function of the limb will be better, even if the functional score of the shoulder is the same.

Two reconstructions with a cemented nail-like spacer were used. The nail was fixed onto the scapulae with a synthetic ligament. In the two cases, ablation of the nail was necessary: once because of an infection and the second one because of a skin ulceration after breaking of fixation.

In one case without reconstruction, the result was poor; there was no active motion of the elbow [2].

Scapular Conservation with Abductor Mechanism Resection

Eight prostheses were used in type IB of Malawer's classification. There were two cases of dislocation: one was reoperated on (an anterosuperior graft stabilized the humeral prosthesis), and the other is still tolerated. A stem loosening occurred 9 years after the procedure and revision was performed with a good result 4 years later.

One nail-like spacer was reoperated on because of skin ulceration.

Four cases without reconstruction had no mechanical complications. For these patients, the functional score of the shoulder was approximately the same as in cases with a prosthesis, but the actual function of the superior limb was worse. With a prosthesis or spacer, control of the elbow is possible, even if it is low and patients prefer a little stabilized forearm to a nonstabilized one.

Arthrectomy

When resection of the upper humerus tumor required arthrectomy, the abductor mechanism was very often removed. In this group of 15 patients, we used three spacer prostheses and five spacer nails; in the seven other cases, no reconstruction was performed.

The three spacer prostheses were two massive humeral prostheses and one

Table 3. Mechanical complications

Mechanical complications	Reoperation	No reoperation	Assymptomatic
Prosthesis dislocation	1	1	
Loosening of stem prosthesis	1		1
Breaking of nail	1		
Skin ulceration	2		
Pain on nail	2	1	
Infection	1		

prosthesis-like device made with a nail surrounded by cement. They were used for 5–17 cm of humeral resection and fixed to the remaining shoulder girdle. The functional result was fair in the three cases, with no rotational mobility but with active flexion of the elbow in one case.

Five nails were used according to the procedure of Marcove et al. [3] for 12–16 cm of humeral resection. Three patients had to be reoperated on and one had moderate pain. These mechanical complications always had the same cause: The nail brings pressure on the muscles or subcutaneous tissues if it is not firmly fixed. Before the advent of these complications and removal of the nail, the functional result was fair four times out of five, with few movements of the elbow.

In seven patients, no reconstruction was performed for 3–9 cm of humeral resection. There was no mechanical complication but the elbow did not have active mobility.

Conclusions

The length of humeral resection, removal of the glenoid cavity, and conservation of the abductor mechanism depend on the stage of the tumor. Mechanical complications occurred in 11 cases; reoperation was necessary in eight of them (Table 3). When there is only humeral resection without arthrectomy and with conservation of the abductor mechanism, a prosthesis will be the best reconstruction. Often, the active range of motion is very low, but the main action of the abductor mechanism is stabilization of the shoulder. If the abductor mechanism is resected, the functional possibility depends on active rotation of the shoulder and active flexion of the elbow. When the glenoid cavity is conserved, reconstruction with a prosthesis is a good solution, but it must be fixed to prevent dislocation. Arthrodesis can be used if the length of humeral resection is not too great. When arthrectomy is associated with resection of the abductor mechanism, active flexion of the elbow either persists or it does not. In the former case, the use of a spacer prosthesis seems to be a good procedure, allowing a functional and cosmetic result; the pressure of the head prosthesis against subcutaneous tissues will be more tolerable than pressure of a nail if there is breaking of the fixation. In the latter case, a cosmetic result can be looked for with the use of a spacer prosthesis, but resection without reconstruction seems to be better because of the absence of mechanical complications.

References

1. Guerra A, Capanna R, Biagini R, Ruggieri P, Campanacci M (1985) Extra-articular resection of the shoulder (Tikhoff-Linberg). Ital J Orthop Traumatol 11: 151–157
2. Enneking WF (1983) Musculoskeletal tumor surgery. Churchill Livingstone, New York, pp 335–410
3. Marcove RC, Lewis MM, Huvos AG (1977) En bloc upper humeral interscapulothoracic resection. The Tikhoff-Linberg procedure. Clin Orthop 124: 219–228

The Role of Limb Salvage Procedures in Patients with Bone Tumors of the Shoulder Girdle

A.T. AMIRASLANOV[1]

Summary. In the All-Union Cancer Research Center of the USSR AMS, 65 limb salvage procedures were performed for tumors and tumorlike lesions of bones of the shoulder girdle. The choice of a type of surgery was related to morphological structure, site, grade of tumor damage, etc. Forequarter resections were performed in 16 cases, en bloc resections of the humerus with allografting in 25 cases, en bloc resections with autografting in 13 cases, and resections of the superarticular end of the humerus with endoprosthesis application in 11 cases. The results obtained demonstrated that forequarter resection is reasonable for chondrosarcomas of grade 1–2 aplasia, and for parosteal sarcomas of the humerus; in osteogenic sarcoma, however, it is inadvisable as the recurrence rate after surgery is high. Limb salvage procedures in the form of en bloc resection with auto- and allografting are reasonable for benign tumors and giant cell tumors. In the choice of a defect replacement (endoprosthesis, auto- and allograft) after resection of the superarticular end of the humerus, such advantages of endoprosthetic application as the absence of resorption and fracture, as well as shortening the time of limb immobilization should be taken into account.

Key words: Allograft—Autograft—Endoprosthetic application

Introduction

One of the most frequently encountered sites of bone sarcomas of the shoulder girdle is the proximal metaphysis of the humerus. For most patients with primary malignant bone tumors of the humerus, surgery is widespread or takes the leading place in the combination treatment; for benign and tumorlike lesions, it is the only effective means.

Until quite recently, in most cases, patients with bone sarcomas of the humerus underwent exarticulation or forequarter amputation. Modern developments in the diagnosis of bone sarcomas, extensive information on their biological characteristics, and the application of grafts and endoprostheses have enabled limb salvage procedures to be performed in some patients.

With a reasonable approach, limb salvage procedures meet all the principles

---

[1] All-Union Cancer Research Center of the USSR AMS, Moscow, USSR

and standards of surgical treatment of bone tumors, and by results and duration of life may complete with exarticulation and forequarter amputation, having such advantages as retaining the limb and its function.

Material and Methods

In the All-Union Cancer Research Center AMS USSR, 65 patients with tumors and tumorlike bone lesions of the humerus underwent limb sparing operations. All the cases were confirmed morphologically. The choice of the operative was related to morphological structure, character of clinical course, site, grade of tumor damage, and age. Considering the treatment, patients were divided as follows: 16 cases of forequarter resection; 25 cases of en bloc resection of the humerus with allografting; 13 cases; of en bloc resection with autografting; 11 cases of resection of the superarticular end of the humerus with endoprosthetic application.

The most typical tumor site was the proximal part of the humerus (56 cases); less typical sites were the scapula (five cases) and clavicle (three cases).

In the All-Union Cancer Research Center of the USSR AMS, forequarter resections were performed in 16 cases for primary malignant bone tumors of the shoulder girdle, which constituted 24.6% of the overall cases with limb sparing operations. All the operations were performed from the anterior approach by the Tikhov-Linberg method. Of the 16 patients, one patient had an amputation of the limb on the 10th day after an operation to preserve the blood circulation. Eleven patients had tumors in the proximal part of the humerus and five had tumors in the scapula. All patients underwent surgery for primary malignant bone tumors: two cases for parosteal sarcoma, five cases for osteogenic sarcoma, and nine cases for chondrosarcoma. Of two patients with parosteal sarcoma, one patient survived 7 years free of recurrences and metastases. The second patient also survived 7 years but twice developed recurrences in the soft tissues of the operative scar which were excised. This patient used her operated limb constantly and was free of long-term metastases.

In osteogenic sarcoma, one patient had a tumor in the scapula, and four patients had tumors in the humerus. After surgery, all the patients received preventive polychemotherapy. One of five patients underwent an amputation of the limb to preserve the blood circulation and was invaluable for long-term results. Four patients developed recurrences within a year after the operation. for tumor recurrences, two patients underwent amputation of the limb. Two more patients in addition to recurrences developed pulmonary metastases; surgical treatment was not utilized in these cases. The median survival in the four cases averaged 2 years after the operation.

In Chondrosarcoma, five patients had tumors in the humerus, and four patients had tumors in the scapula. of the nine patients, seven underwent surgery alone; two patients received chemotherapy after surgery. Upon histological examination, chondrosarcoma of grade 1 anaplasia was recognized in three cases; there was grade 2 anaplasia in four cases, grade 3 anaplasia in one case, and dedifferentiated chondrosarcoma in one case. Three patients with Chondrosarcoma of grade 1 anaplasia survived for 5 years free of disease. Of four patients with grade 3 anaplasia, one developed an implanted metastasis in the area of the soft tissues of the back 4 years after the operation. The metastasis was excised, and the patient was followed up for 5 years after the operation. A patient with chondrosarcoma of grade 3 anaplasia died from hematogenic metastasizing within 15 months. A patient with dedifferentiated chondrosarcoma received preventive chemotherapy after the operation. As the time of follow-up is too short, it is too early to discuss the long-term results.

For bone tumors and tumorlike lesions of the shoulder girdle, 38 limb-sparing operations with auto-and allografting were performed. In relation to tumor site, the operation were as follows: resection of the superarticular end of the humerus in 31 cases; en bloc resection about the diaphysis in four cases; en bloc resection of the scapula in three cases. Of the 38 patients who underwent limb sparing operations in 13 cases, bone tissue defects were replaced with autografts from the fibula, and in 25 cases with bone allografts conserved by the method of fast-freezing.

The type of fixation was determined individually in relation to the tumor site, form of resection, type of grafting. In most cases (ten patients), a graft was fixed intramedullarly with additional stable osteosynthesis. In four cases, fixation was performed with plate osteosynthesis. In three cases, grafts were fixed intramedullarly with osteosynthesis. In seven patients, an allograft fixation was performed by various modalities during the operation.

For bone replacement, various methods of autoplasty were applied. In five cases, the distal part of the autograft was included in the bonemarrow canal, but with various additional ways of fixation—osteosynthesis, inlay graft. In the rest of the cases, distal part of the autograft was included in the bone marrow of the humerus. In three cases after resection of the clavicle, the defect was replaced with an autograft from the fibula. allografts were fixed intramedullarly with stable osteosynthesis.

Of 25 operated patients with bone allografting, four patients developed recurrences (16%). In two cases with giant cell tumors, forequarter amputation was performed as a repeated operation: in one case with malignant fibrous histiocytoma exarticulation of the limb was performed; in one case with chondrosarcoma, these was excision of a recurrence in the soft tissues. In autoplasty of 13 operated patients, tumor recurrences were noted in two cases (15.4%). The patients needed forequarter amputations for recurrences; there was one patient with chondrosarcoma and one with a giant cell tumor.

Together with the merits of bone plasty, some shortcomings should be pointed out. These are: long immobilization of the limb, resorption and graft fracture, slow adhesion of the graft with the maternal bone. After bone replacement with allografts, various complications were noted in 32% of the cases, and after autoplasty complications were noted in 23% of cases.

All these shortcomings led us to decide to give up bone plasty in favor of endoprostheses in some cases. For bone replacement, we used a Zatsepin endoprosthesis for the humeral articulation.

For bone tumors of the proximal part of the humerus, we performed 11 operations, which were resections of the upper end of the humerus with bone replacement endoprosthetics. Endoprostheses were made individually for each patient.

With regard to the nosological type of the tumor, patients were assigned as follows: parosteal sarcoma in four cases; giant cell tumor in four cases; chondrosarcoma in three cases. Two patients with endoprostheses of the humeral articulation developed a fistula in the operative scar. Following conservative therapy, the fistula was closed in one patient. In another case, despite repeated courses of treatment with various antibiotics and antiseptics, the fistula remained unclosed, and 3 months after surgery the endoprosthesis was removed.

Of 11 operated patients a tumor recurrence was noted in one patient with dedifferentiated chondrosarcoma who underwent resection of the upper end of the humerus with endoprosthetic application.

Of 11 patients who underwent resections of the superarticular end of the humerus with bone replacement endoprosthetics, two died from hematogenic metastasizing within 2 years after the operation: one patient had dedifferentiated chondrosarcoma and the other had parosteal sarcoma. Nine patients upon follow-up were free of metastases at 6 months to 3 years after operation. In endoprosthetic application of the humeral articulation, all the patients underwent rehabilitation measures after removal of the sutures on days 12–14 after surgery.

The functional results of the humeral articulation endoprosthetics were evaluated by a four-point system in nine cases. The results were excellent in one case, good in five cases, fair in two, and poor in one.

Results and Discussion

Summarizing the above, it should be pointed out that forequarter resections are reasonable for affected bones of the shoulder girdle with chondrosarcomas of grade 1–2 anaplasia and parosteal sarcomas. Forequarter resections for osteogenic sarcomas are not feasible, as the recurrence rate postsurgery is high. For benign tumors and giant cell tumors, limb salvage procedures in the form of en bloc resection with auto- and alloplasty or endoprosthetic application are helpful.

In the choice of a defect replacement (endoprosthesis, auto- and allograft) after resection of the superarticular end of the humerus, such advantages of endoprosthetic application as the absence of resorption and fracture as well as shortening the time of limb immobilization should be taken into account.

Proximal Humeral Osteoarticular Allograft Transplantation for Musculoskeletal Tumors of the Shoulder Region

Mark C. Gebhardt, Yolanda F. Roth, and Henry J. Mankin[1]

Summary. Twenty-three osteoarticular allografts were performed for tumors of the proximal humerus. The procedure was successful for benign, aggressive, or ion-grade malignant sarcomas.

Key words: Bone allografts—Proximal humerus sarcomas—Bone tumors—Limb salvage—Chondrosarcoma—Giant cell tumor

Musculoskeletal tumors of the shoulder region present unique reconstructive challenges to the tumor surgeon. Because the functional consequences of amputation are much greater in the upper extremity than the lower, it is usually advantageous to attempt limb salvage wherever possible. In lower grade lesions of the proximal humerus, it is often possible to preserve the deltoid and rotator cuff muscles, making reconstruction of these motors possible. Osteoarticular allografts are seemingly ideal for this location, because they offer sites for attachment of these motors as well as providing an articular surface. Therefore, a retrospective study of 20 patients who underwent 23 osteoarticular allografts of the proximal humerus was undertaken in order to assess the end results of this procedure in a non-weight-bearing limb.

There were ten male and ten female patients with a mean age of 33 years (range 16–63 years). The surgical stage of the patients was stage 0 in one, IA in one, IB in 12, IIA in one, and IIB in three patients. One patients had metastatic disease, and three procedures were done for failed allografts. The majority of the patients had chondrosarcomas (nine) or giant cell tumors (six). Following marginal or wide resection, the defects were reconstructed with osteoarticular proximal humeral, fresh frozen allogrant bones from the MGH Bone Bank. All procedures have been followed by us or the referring physician for at least 2 years or until failure; the follow-up was a mean of 4.7 years (0.5–10.5 years). In addition to monitoring disease outcome and radiographic appearance of the allograft, all patients were functionally graded at latest follow-up by a system

[1]Orthopaedic Oncology Service, Massachusetts General Hospital, The Children's Hospital, Boston, MA, USA

developed by the senior author. The results were excellent in one, good in 15, fair in two, and poor in five of the procedures. There were eight fractures, three infections (requiring removal of the allograft, antibiotics, and a second allograft procedure), one nonunion and two local recurrences. One of four stage II patients developed metastases. Ten patients (43%) had no complications.

There were no problems of shoulder instability in any patient, and all patients demonstrated a reduced but functional shoulder range of motion. Radiographs of the shoulder region showed some narrowing of the joint space with the osteoarticular surface of the proximal humeral allograft demonstrating a moderate irregularity in density, while the patients' glenoid appeared unaltered.

The overall acceptable (good/excellent) rate of the 23 procedures was 79%, and the final result of the 18 patients (accounting for allograft failures that were "salvaged") who did not have local tumor complications was satisfactory in 80%.

We conclude that if adequate tumor resection can be accomplished in low-grade bone neoplasms of the proximal humerus, cadaveric osteoarticular allograft transplants offer a reasonable method of reconstruction of the surgical defect, while preserving a functional upper extremity and some rotator cuff function. This reconstruction is not recommended for high-grade lesions.

Limb Salvage Procedures for Primary Sarcomas of the Humerus

James O. Johnston[1]

Summary. The results of 13 cases of primary sarcoma of the humerus treated by limb salvage procedures with a mean follow-up of 3 years are reported. The tumors included six osteosarcomas, four chondrosarcomas, two malignant fibrous histiocytomas, and one leiomyosarcoma. Following a proximal resection of the humerus, a long-stem Neer prosthesis with varying combinations of bone cement and allograft was utilized for limb salvage reconstruction. The deltoid muscle was preserved in most cases, giving good functional results, with only one local recurrence. We had one postoperative dislocation and one ulnar nerve palsy. There were no stem loosenings no fracture.

Key words: Humerus—Sarcoma—Prosthesis

Introduction

Following the knee and hip area, the proximal humerus is the third most common site for the presentation of primary bone sarcomas. Sarcomas arising from this area, including high-grade lesions such as osteosarcomas, have a lower rate of local recurrence and a better overall survival rate (about 90%) than the same tumor seen in the leg.

One of the earliest limb salvage procedures for tumors of the proximal humerus was that of Tikhor-Linberg, which required aggressive resection of the upper humerus, including the glenoid fossa and distal end of the clavicle. This left the patient with a flail arm and very poor function. With the advent of modern orthopedic technology, this early attempt at limb salvage was replaced by the more popular large bone allografts, prostheses, and shoulder fusions. In this paper, I will stress the use of combined prosthetic devices and large bone allografts.

Prior to our knowledge of the favorable prognosis and low local recurrence rate of humeral sarcomas, limb salvage surgeons sacrificed a great deal of normal tissue about the shoulder joint in order to reduce the local recurrence rate. This frequently involved resection of the entire deltoid muscle, rotator cuff tendon,

---

[1] Department of Orthopedics, University of California, San Francisco, CA, USA

and glenoid fossa, which made reconstructive attempts difficult. Here, I will suggest a more conservative approach by saving the deltoid muscle and glenoid fossa in most cases and still maintain a low local recurrance rate.

Material and Methods

This report includes 13 patients with primary sarcomas in the proximal humerus. The age range was 12–60 years, with a mean of 34 years. Nine patients were males and four were females. The tumor types included six osteogenic sarcomas, four chondrosarcomas, two malignant fibrous histiocytomas, and one leiomyosarcoma. All patients were evaluated at least 2 years after survey and the mean follow-up was 4 years.

Utilizing the new Malawer classification for shoulder resection, nearly all of the cases fall into the IA group, which is the most conservative type of resection and is usually applied to more favorable low-grade lesions such as grade IA chondrosarcoma.

With the patient in a semi-sitting position and the arm draped free, an anterior approach is made to the shoulder joint through the deltopectoral groove. The majority of the deltoid muscle is reflected laterally, leaving a variable cuff of normal muscle tissue depending on the extracompartmental nature of the tumor involved. Care is taken to preserve the axillary and radial nerves posteriorly. In most cases, the rotator cuff is transected proximal to its bony attachment to the humerus. The shoulder is then dislocated. Soft tissue dissection is then carried out distally over the main tumor mass, taken care to leave a thin cuff of normal tissue over the pseudocapsule of the tumor. Once the surgeon reaches the lower pole of the tumor, the humeral shaft is transected about 3–4 cm distal to the lower intramedullary extent of the tumor as determined by preoperative imaging. In none of our cases was the glenoid involved with the tumor and, thus, no glenoids were resected.

In all cases, a long-stem Neer prosthesis was utilized for reconstruction after resection. The average length was 10–11 in. A large head is preferable. In most cases, a large bone humeral allograft is placed over the stem of the prosthesis as a biological spacer for ease of muscle and tendon reattachment postoperatively. If the bone stock of the resected specimen is well preserved, we autoclave the resected humerus in a routine steam autoclave at 137°C for 5 min to kill the tumor and then use the autoclaved autograft as a perfect-fit pseudoallograft. In a very few cases where the bone resection was minimal and in an older patient with a less favorable prognosis, no graft was placed on the Neer stem and we simply filled the defect with bone cement as a spacer.

In all cases, the distal humeral canal was reamed out and the prosthetic stem cemented, but taking care not to allow cement between the allograft and the distal humerus. We attempted to build in as much length as possible in order to hold the large Neer head firmly in place under the acromio-deltoid complex, including the intact coracoacromial ligament. This is critical because no attempt was made to reconstruct the rotator cuff mechanism in most cases. We then attached the anterior and deeper portions of the deltoid shield to the remaining stump of the subscapularis to prevent anterior instability of the humeral head

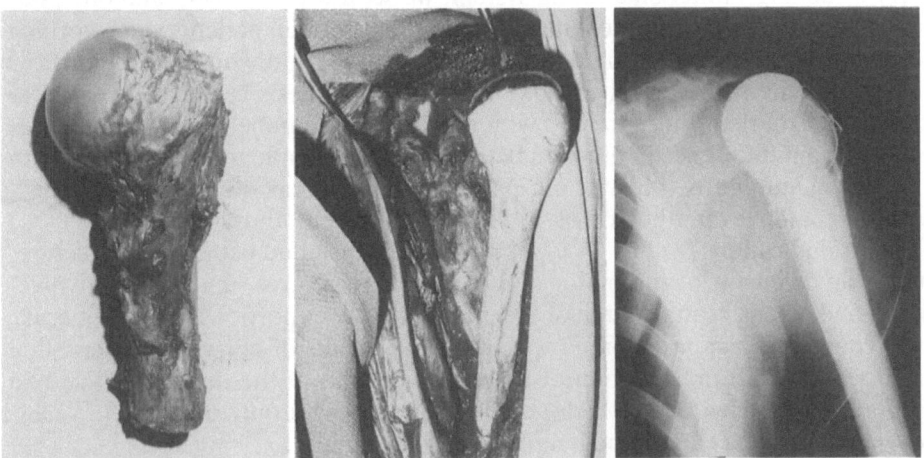

a, b   **c**

Fig. 1. a Typical resection specimen with a thin cuff of normal muscle covering up a IIB osteosarcoma. **b** Appearance of resected specimen after 5 min in autoclave and replaced back in the arm over a long-stem Neer prosthesis with bone cement for fixation. **c** Post-operative appearance

postoperatively. The last suture closure line was the deltopectoral groove and an anterior lateral closure of the remaining muscle cuff at the midhumeral level. No attempt was made to suture specific tendons onto the allograft prosthetic complex (Fig. 1).

The patient was immobilized in a simple canvas shoulder immobilizer for 4 weeks and then started on a range of motion exercise program.

Most of our patients with high-grade tumors received adjuvant chemotherapy postoperatively and a few received irradiation therapy.

Results and Discussion

Of our 13 cases, nine had high-grade IIA or IIB lesions, and of these three with osteogenic sarcoma developed pulmonary metastases and died as a result. We experienced only one local recurrence in our youngest patient, a 12-year-old girl with osteosarcoma who was treated by a IA resection followed by chemotherapy. Six years later, she developed a local recurrence in the upper pole of the surgical scar, which was simply removed with a wide margin and the patient was placed on a second course of chemotherapy. She is still alive and well with no known tumor.

We recently experienced our first anterior dislocation at 6 weeks postoperation in a farmer who returned to work too early and tore out the anterior repair. This required a second operative procedure to repair the anterior instability, following which the patient has continued to work on his farm without difficulty.

Thus far, we have seen no infections. Compared with the leg with its weight-bearing problems, we have seen no prosthetic stem loosenings or fatigue fractures. There was one case of ulnar nerve palsy postoperation.

By Enneking's functional rating system, we scored 12 excellent and one poor result because of pain and weakness. Eight of our thirteen patients were working prior to surgery and all of these have returned to their previous occupations.

The patients with combined bone graft and prosthesis seem to have better muscle control than those treated with only metal and bone cement. There was no significant difference in function between those with allografts compared with autoclaved autografts. Most of our patients showed weak glenohumeral abduction but could elevate the arm to 30° or 40° with scapulothoracic motion.

Contraindications for this IA type limb salvage included pathological fracture, tumor involvement of the major neurovascular structures, major skin involvement, and extensive infiltration of the tumor into lower portions of the humerus.

In conclusion, we are pleased with the early results of our very conservation IA resection with preservation of the major portion of the deltoid muscle and glenoid even in the face of high-grade IIB lesions with only one case of recurrence and with excellent function of the salvaged limb.

Modular Endoprosthesis for Humerus and Tikhoff-Linberg Resection

Rodolfo Capanna, Armando Giunti, Roberto Biagini, Alberto Ferruzzi, Andrea Ferraro, Roberto Casadei, Piero Picci, and Mario Campanacci[1]

Summary. The functional results of 94 modular cemented prosthesis of the proximal humerus are reported. Excellent or good results were obtained in 66% of the patients who had an intra-articular resection but only in 36% of the patients who had a Tikhoff-Linberg resection. Better functional results were observed in atypical (transglenoid) Tikhoff-Linberg resections than in classic types. The overall complication rate was 13% (5% mechanical; 8% infective). No case of aseptic loosening was observed.

Key words: Bone tumors—Proximal humerus prosthesis—Resections—Tikhoff-Linberg procedure

Between 1974 and 1986, 94 modular prostheses were implanted after humeral resection for bone tumor at the Istituto Ortopedico Rizzoli. The prosthesis used from 1974 to 1976 consisted of two parts—the head and proximal body in polyethylene and the distal body and stem in titanium. A free rotational movement was allowed between the two components. The prosthesis had an eccentrically oriented head and a short conical stem; it was custom-made and was inserted only in four patients. From 1976 to 1985, we used a modular multi-component prosthesis, consisting of a large spherical head of polyethylene, a cylindrical spacer, a screw collar, and an intramedullary stem in titanium (Fig. 1). The prosthesis had a free rotational and longitudinal movement at the junction between the head and body components. The size of the assembled prosthesis was adequate for a resection length of 65–170 mm with increments of 15 mm. In 1985, a new type of modular shoulder prosthesis was introduced due to some minor disadvantages of the previous model (Fig. 2). The prosthesis head is now available both in polyethylene and titanium to avoid theoretical wear between the polyethylene head and the acromion. The head of the prosthesis has two holes for anchorage to the scapula (glenoid and/or acromion) in proximal humerus resection or to the clavicle in Tikhoff-Linberg resections. Two additional cylindrical spacers are available for resections longer than 17 cm; the cylindrical spacer is covered with porous ceramic to allow better fixation of muscles to the prosthesis. The prosthesis is now assembled with a conical connection and an axial screw. With this new system, the body of the prosthesis may

---

[1] 1st Orthopaedic Clinic and Bone Tumor Center, University of Bologna, Bologna, Italy

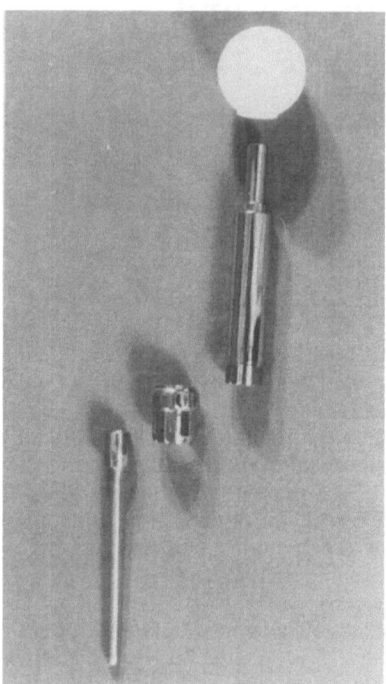

Fig. 1. A modular multicomponent prosthesis consisting of a large spherical head of polyethylene, a cylindrical spacer, a screw collar, and an intramedullary stem in titanium

be changed, if necessary leaving the cemented stem in situ. In the previous model, the elongation caused by pistoning of the body into the prosthetic head was uncontrolled. Although no dislocation resulted, elongation is now restricted without any loss of rotation of the body within the head. The stem is shorter, has an anatomical configuration, and the grooves of the stem are designed to improve cementation to resist rotational and shear stresses.

Materials

Among 94 cases, there were 62% male and 38% female patients, ranging in age from 9 to 75 years. The tumor was located in the proximal humerus (80 cases) or in the scapula (14 cases). There were 75 primary bone tumors: 11 benign tumors (all stage III) and 64 malignant tumors (11 stage IB and 53 stage IIB) [6]. the remaining 19 patients had a metastatic tumor. Histological diagnoses are given in Fig. 3. According to Malawer's classification, there were 60 intra-articular (type I) and 12 extra-articular (type V—modified Tikhoff-Linberg) resections of the proximal humerus, 14 extra-articular resections of the scapula (type IV), and eight extra-articular resections of the proximal humerus and scapula (type VI or classic Tikhoff-Linberg). The abductor muscles were often completely excised, not only in classic Tikhoff-Linberg resections, but also in proximal humerus resections (types I or II). In primary malignant tumors, the deltoid was totally resected, while in metastases and benign tumors it was partially resected. The

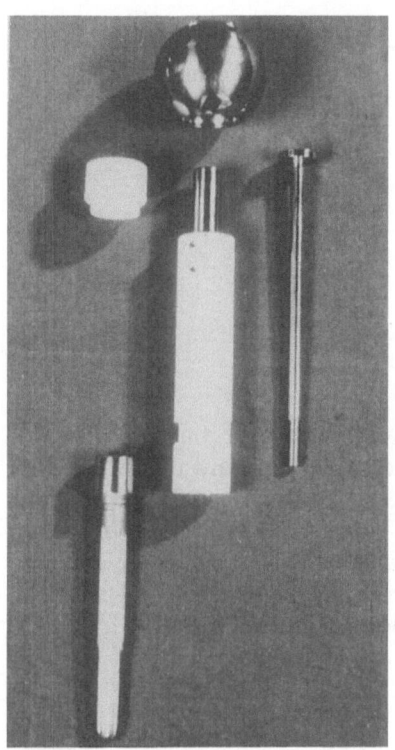

Fig. 2. The new type of modular shoulder prosthesis

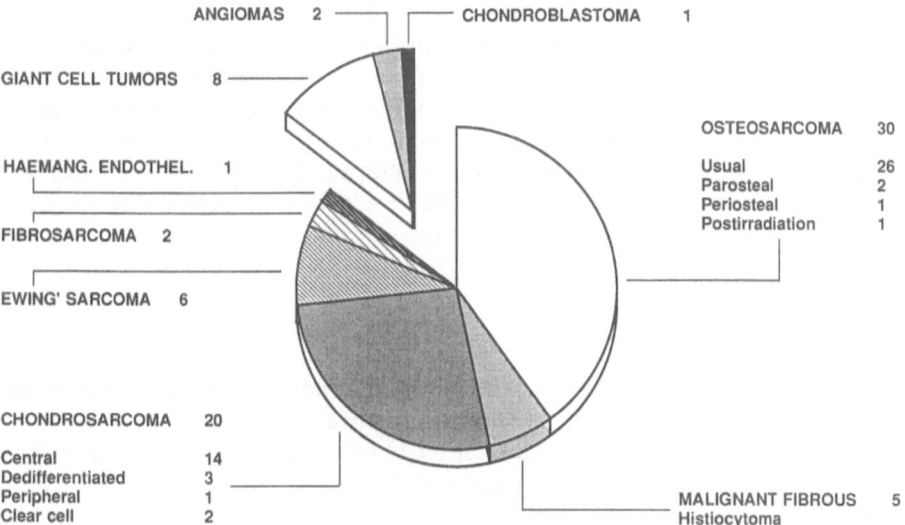

ANGIOMAS   2

CHONDROBLASTOMA   1

GIANT CELL TUMORS   8

OSTEOSARCOMA   30

Usual	26
Parosteal	2
Periosteal	1
Postirradiation	1

HAEMANG. ENDOTHEL.   1

FIBROSARCOMA   2

EWING' SARCOMA   6

CHONDROSARCOMA   20

Central	14
Dedifferentiated	3
Peripheral	1
Clear cell	2

MALIGNANT FIBROUS   5
Histiocytoma

Fig. 3. Histological diagnosis (primary bone tumors)

Table 1. Local recurrences (primary bone tumors)

	Number	Percent
Surgical margins		
Wide	6/56	11
Wide/cont.	1/7	15
Marginal	3/10	33
Intralesional	1/2	50
Preoperative chemotherapy		
Used	2/22	9
Not used	7/24	29

axillary nerve and concomitant vessels were always sectioned, but in eight cases of benign tumors. The rotator cuff and joint capsule were always resected an bloc close to the glenoid. The resection length ranged from 7 to 24 cm (average 14 cm). The surgical margins were wide in 56 cases, wide but contaminated in seven, marginal in ten, and intralesional in two cases. Twenty-two patients had pre- and post-operative chemotherapy (neoadjuvant treatment). The mean follow-up was 4 years (ranging from 1 to 145 months): in 14 cases, the follow-up was over 5 years).

Complications

There were four mechanical complications (5%): three cases of breaking of the cortex with cement extrusion and one case with stem protrusion through the olecranic fossa. Two patients had an impaired elbow extension. These complications occurred in the first group of patients and were avoided later. The stem was shortened intraoperatively when required (33% of the patients) and the new model has a shorter stem. There were eight infections (8%): Four primary infections and four ensuing wound slough or skin necrosis (two patients had previous radiotherapy, and two neoadjuvant chemotherapy). In one case, the infection was controlled with antibiotic therapy, while in seven cases surgical debridement and removal of the prosthesis was necessary.

Oncological Results

At a mean follow-up of 4 years, in primary bone tumors 47 patients are primary NED (63%), five secondary NED (7%), six are alive with disease (7%), while 17 have died (23%). In metastatic tumors, three patients are NED (16%), three are alive with disease (16%), and 13 are dead (68%).

There were 11 local recurrences (12%) with no differences in the recurrence rate between humerus resection (7/60) and Tikhoff-Linberg procedures (4/34). No local recurrence (LR) was found after resection of metastatic tumors, while the LR rate was 15% in the treatment of primary bone tumors. In these, the recurrence rate was 9% (1/11) in stage III tumors, 6% (1/18) in stage IB, and

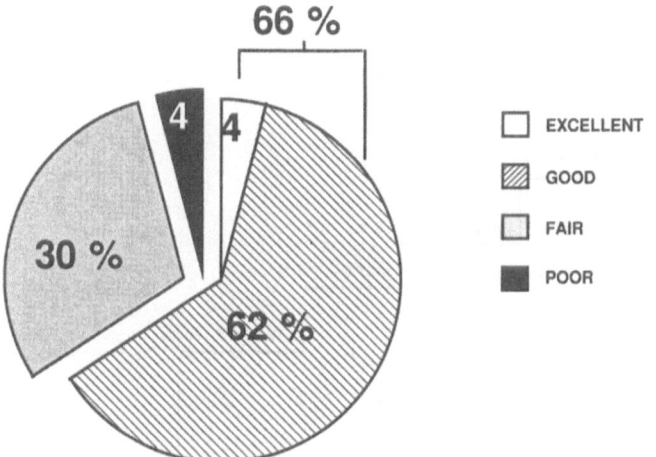

Fig. 4. Functional results in type 1 resections

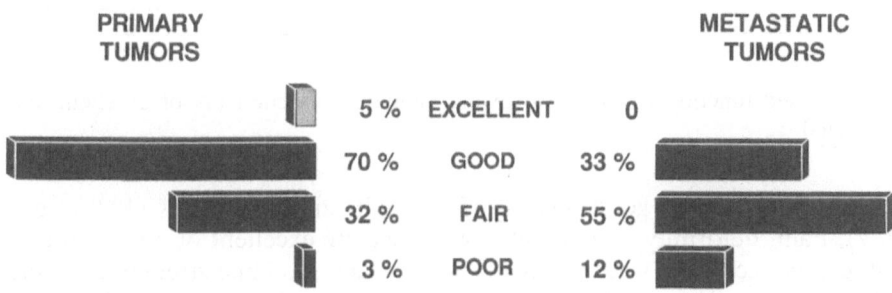

Fig. 5. Results in primary and metastatic tumors

19% (9/46) in stage IIB. Two factors influenced the local recurrence rate: the achieved surgical margins and the use of preoperative chemotherapy in high-grade lesions (Table 1).

Functional Results

Functional results were rated according to Enneking's classification. In type I resections, 66% of patients had excellent (4%) or good (62%) results, while 34% had fair (30%) or poor results (4%; Fig. 4). Better functional results were obtained after resection of primary bone tumors with respect to metastatic tumors (Fig. 5). Regarding the criteria used in evaluating the functional status, "deformity" and "pain" were good or excellent in more than 90% of patients, "emotional acceptance" and "functional activities" in more than 70%., "motion" and "stability" in more than 60%., while "strength in abduction" was good only in 6% of patients (Fig. 6).

Following the Tikhoff-Linberg procedure, the functional results were never

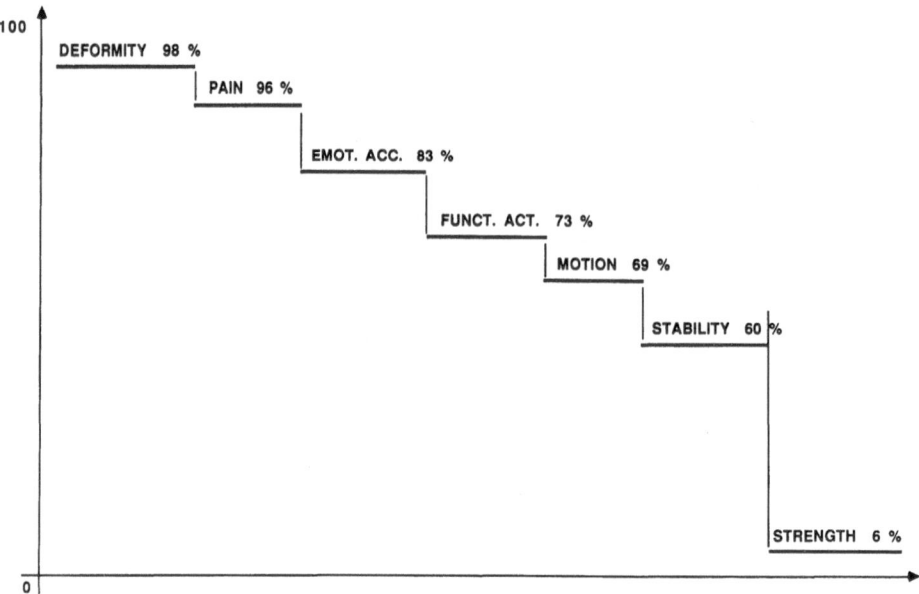

Fig. 6. Detailed functional status in proximal humerus resection (% of excellent and good results)

excellent, rarely (36%) good, usually (54%) fair, and sometimes (10%) poor (Fig. 7). Pain, deformity, and stability were usually excellent or good, motion and functional activities were rarely (40%) satisfactory, while strength as a rule was fair or poor (Fig. 8). Functional results were better in modified than in classic Tikhoff-Linberg resections (Fig. 9). The modified technique allows decrease of the surgical time and blood loss and gives a better esthetic result.

Radiological Appearance

No fractures of bone, cement, or the prosthesis and no radiographical loosening or subsidence of the prosthesis were noted. At the area of contact between the bone and prosthesis, new bone formation was observed in 60% of patients. In prosthetic replacement of the proximal humerus, a normal position of the prosthetic head was present in 60% of patients while a subluxation (usually superior) was seen in 40%.

Discussion

In our experience, local recurrence in shoulder resections for high-grade tumors is more frequent than in lower limb resections. The risk of local recurrence in limited after wide resections (11%), especially following preoperative chemotherapy, and becomes unacceptable after marginal resections. To achieve wide margins in proximal humerus resections, it is usually necessary to excise the

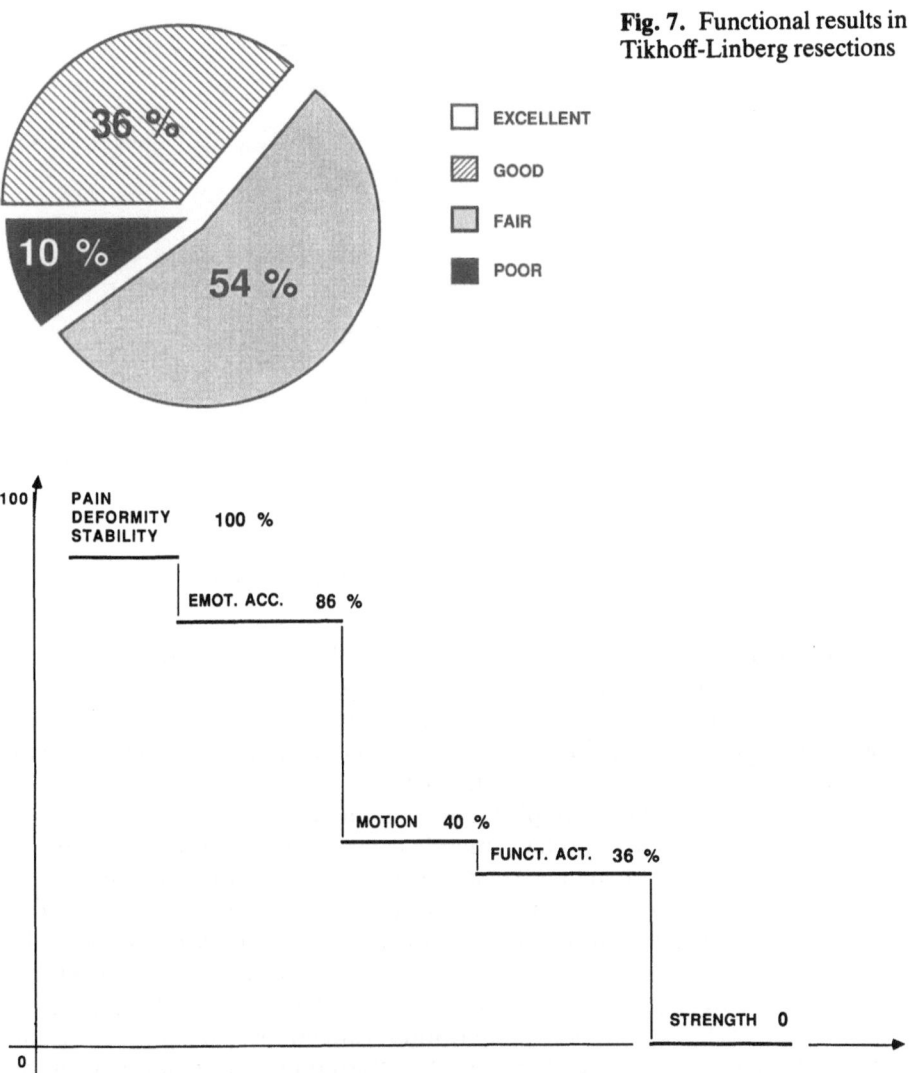

Fig. 7. Functional results in Tikhoff-Linberg resections

Fig. 8. Detailed functional status in Tikhoff-Linberg resection

deltoid subtotally, and it is always essential to sever the blood and nerve supply (which runs close to the bone) and to resect the rotator cuff close to the neck of the scapula. Moreover, a long resection of the bone is usually required. In the Tikhoff-Linberg procedure, the shoulder joint is resected en bloc with all peri-scapular muscles. After this surgical procedure, the abductor mechanism is completely lacking, forward flexion is severely impaired, and the only possible active movement is rotation [1, 2, 4, 11]. After such wide resections, there are several possibilities: no reconstruction, autogenous fibular graft or osteoarticular allograft, shoulder arthrodesis, and prosthesis [1, 4, 7, 10, 12, 13]. In our opinion, the reconstruction technique is preferable, because when no reconstructions are per-

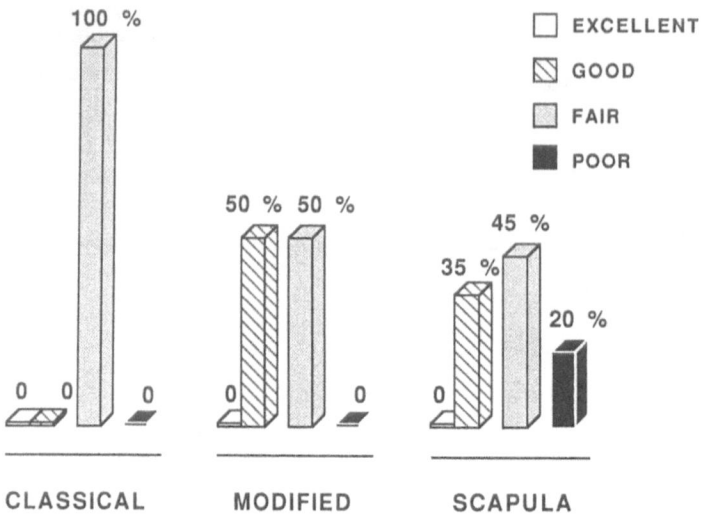

Fig. 9. Functional results in different types of Tikhoff-Linberg resections

formed the shoulder is esthetically poor and unstable, the elbow function (flexion strength) is impaired, and the weight of the upper limb may cause traction of the neurovascular bundle, with consequent parethesias and/or vascular complications of the hand [3, 4]. Prostheses have some advantages compared with the techniques of reconstruction with autogenous fibular graft or osteoarticular grafts [9, 10]. there are fewer complications (less infections, no pseudoarthrosis or fractures), there is no need to have muscle coverage to assist blood supply to the grafts, there is no problem of adverse effects of postoperative chemotherapy or radiation therapy with the incorporation of the grafts. Moreover, reconstruction of the abductor mechanism after complete excision is either impossible (deltoid) or theoretical (axillary nerve), or rarely effective (rotator cuff). In such resections, the prosthesis also has several advantages with respect to shoulder arthrodesis. Again, fewer complications (infections, pseudoarthrosis, or fractures), no need for muscle coverage, no interference of chemotherapy or radiotherapy, and no limitation of the resection length. With an arthrodesis, the shoulder is stable and an active abduction of up to 90° is afforded; the range of rotations is, however, severely limited. We believe that a shoulder arthrodesis is indicated in young active patients having a benign or low-grade tumor, requiring a short resection without important muscle sacrifice. Prosthetic replacement is, therefore, more frequently applicable and reliable (and the only reconstruction in Tikhoff-Linberg resections), allows radiotherapy and chemotherapy after primary healing of the wound, and immobilization is limited to a very short period [4]. The use of a modular prosthesis (to avoid time delay required by a custom-made prosthesis or the need of a large stock) having a cemented intramedullary stem (which showed no significant complications and no loosening in long-term follow-up) is suggested [3–5, 7, 8, 12, 13]. Our model allows the head of the prosthesis to rotate upon the body, with the additional possibility of elongation between the head and body, and has the following advantages: excessive stress of the interface between stem, cement, and bone are avoided, a wider range of rotation is allowed, and the head of the prosthesis may be suspended to the glenoid or clavicle (improving stability) without interfering with the motion (that is between the head and body of the prosthesis). The functional results are satisfactory (good or excellent) in 66% of patients in type I resections and in only 36% of patients having a Tikhoff-Linberg resection. In these cases, the modified technique gave better functional results and other advantages (decreased blood loss and shorter surgical time) versus the classic approach. The use of the modified technique is recommended wherever possible when an extra-articular resection of the proximal humerus is required.

Acknowledgment. This study was supported by grant no. 86.02679.44 Special Project "Oncology" Italian National Research Council.

References

1. Albee FH (1921) Restoration of shoulder function in cases of loss of head and upper portion of humerus. Surg Gyn Obst 32: 1–19
2. Burrows HJ, Wilson JN, Scales JT (1975) Excision of tumours of humerus and femur, with restoration by internal prostheses. J Bone Joint Surg 57-B: 148–159
3. Campanacci M, Capanna R, Cervellati C, Guerra A Calderoni P (1983) Modular rotatory endoprosthesis for segmental resection of the proximal humerus. In: Chao EYS, Ivins JC (eds) Tumor prostheses for bone and joint reconstruction—The design and application. Thieme-Stratton, New York, pp 127–139
4. Capanna R, Van Horn JR, Biagini R, Ruggieri R, Bettelli G, Sola G, Campanacci M (1986) A humeral modular prosthesis for bone tumor surgery. A study of 56 cases. Int Orthop (Sicot) 10: 231–238
5. Capanna R, Van Horn JR, Ruggieri P, Biagini R, Bettelli G, Martell C, De Cristofaro R, Giunti A (1987) Evoluzione interfaccía osso cemento in impianti protesici non sottoposti acarico. Giorn It Ortop Traum 13: 93–101
6. Enneking WF (1985) Staging of musculoskeletal neoplasms. Skeletal Radiol 13: 183–194
7. Kinzl L, Burri C, Mathys R (1983) Isoelastic prostheses for the shoulder joint. In: Chao EYS, Ivins JC (eds) Tumor prostheses for bone and joint reconstruction—The design and application. Thieme-Stratton, New York, pp 383–387
8. Knahr K, Salzer M, Ungethum M, Deutscher K (1983) A modular prosthetic system for the proximal humerus and the proximal femur. In: Kotz R (ed) Proceedings of 2nd international workshop on the design and application of tumor prostheses for bone and joint reconstruction, Vienna, Sept. 5–8, 1983. Egermann, Vienna
9. Mankin HJ (1982) Clinical experience with allograft implantation. In: Modern trends in orthopaedic surgery. Aulo Gaggi Editore, Bologna, pp 65–80
10. Mankin HJ, Doppelt SH, Sullivan TR (1982) Osteoarticular and intercalary allograft transplantation in the management of malignant tumors of bone. Cancer 50: 613–630
11. Rosen G, Murphy ML, Huvos AG. Gutierrez M, Marcove RC (1976) Chemotherapy, en bloc resection, and prosthetic bone replacement in the treatment of osteogenic sarcoma. Cancer, 37 (1): 1–11
12. Salzer M, Knahr K, Locke H, Stark N, Matejovsky Z, Plenk H Jr, Punzet G, Zweymuller K (1979) A bioceramic endoprosthesis for the replacement of the proximal humerus. Arch Orthop Traumat Surg 93: 169–184
13. Sim FH, Pritchard DJ, Chao EYS (1983) Prosthetic replacement of the proximal humerus. In: Chao EYS, Ivins JC (eds) Tumor prostheses for bone and joint reconstruction—The design and application. Thieme-Stratton, New York, pp 279–289

Reconstruction of the Upper Limb by Arthrodesis in Cases of Tumors of the Proximal Humerus

Six Cases of Limb Salvage Procedure of Shoulder Girdle

Hajime Kyogoku, Toshihiko Ogino, Akio Minami, Kimitaka Fukuda, Takeo Matsuno, and Michio Minami[1]

Summary. We describe six cases of a limb salvage procedure for the treatment of malignant and clinically aggressive bone and soft tissue tumors in the shoulder girdle. In two of four cases treated by wide excision, shoulder arthrodesis was performed using a vascularized fibular graft.

If the limb saving procedure of the proximal humerus fails to preserve muscular function, an arthrodesis is superior to a prosthesis. In comparison with a conventional bone graft, an arthrodesis of the shoulder girdle using a vascularized fibular graft has some merits, such as rapid union and the absence of creeping substitution. In cases of arthrodesis, Enneking's evaluation system does not seem to be adequate since the item recording deformity appears inappropriate.

Key words: Limb saving—Vascularized fibular graft—Arthrodesis

Introduction

The concept of nonamputative surgery for the treatment of primary malignant tumors of bone and soft tissue is not a new one. Because of high local recurrence rate, however, attempts to carry out the local resection of malignant tumors was abandoned in the early 1900s [1, 2]. Limb salvage procedure has nevertheless improved because of the development of chemotherapy and the surgical techniques used to treat malignant bone and soft tissue tumors.

The object of this paper is to report the results of six cases of limb salvage and reconstructive surgery in the treatment of malignant tumors and clinically aggressive tumors of the shoulder girdle. Two cases of shoulder arthrodesis using a vascularized fibular graft are also reported. The advantages of arthrodesis and the technical aspects of vascularized fibular graft are discussed.

---

[1] Department of Orthopedic Surgery, Hokkaido University and Hokkaido Orthopedic Memorial Hospital, Sapporo, Japan

Materials and Methods

Between 1948 and 1987, 200 cases of malignant tumors in the shoulder girdle were registered in our clinic. Most of them were treated by traditional fore-quarter amputation, scapulectomy, or shoulder disarticulation followed by chemotherapy. Six of the two hundred patients who had tumors in the shoulder girdle received reconstructive surgery with a limb salvage procedure. There were five males and one female. The length of follow-up ranged from 1 to 11 years, with an average of 85 months.

Our series consisted of one aggressive fibromatosis, one recurred giant cell tumor of the bone, one parosteal osteosarcoma, and a central low-grade osteo-sarcoma.

All patients had a routine history, physical examination, and laboratory deter-mination. Standard anteroposterior and lateral roentgenograms of the involved bone as well as a skeletal survey, bone scanning, and chest tomography were performed. All data were evaluated to determine the size, location, and respect-ability of the tumor, the soft tissue component, and the presence or absence of any metastatic disease and skip areas.

Two scapulectomies and four wide excisions were performed. Two of the four wide excisions were accompanied by shoulder arthrodesis and vascularized fibular graft (Table 1).

Results

By the end of the follow-up periods, none of the patients had any metastasis or local recurrence except for case 4. This patient developed a local recurrence in the humeral shaft; subsequently, the patient underwent a forequarter amputa-tion and remains disease-free 118 months later.

Our post operative results were evaluated according to Enneking's system and are shown in Table 2. In this system, the motion, pain, stability, deformity, strength, functional activity, and emotional acceptance are evaluated [3]. Judged by this grading system, our results are poor with regard to deformity. This is because shoulder arthrodesis was carried out with the patient's arm at an angle of 50° for internal rotation.

However, the two cases which were given shoulder arthrodesis by means of a vascularized fibular graft had a greater range of motion than registered in En-neking's system: 80° in elevation, 80° in abduction, and 30° in extension. At the same time, the patients experienced no pain and had good stability and adequate strength.

Case Report

Case 5

In 1978, a 37-year-old male came to us suffering from a fracture of the surgical neck of the right humerus. X-ray showed radiolucent lesions in the humeral surgical neck, but a biopsy was not performed. In May 1984, a refracture occurred. Radiographs showed an enlarged lytic lesion and scattered calcification areas with ill-defined margins. In June 1984, a biopsy specimen revealed a typical clear cell chondrosarcoma. Wide excision of the proximal humerus including the surrounding healthy muscle and a simultaneous shoulder arthrodesis with a vascularized fibular graft were performed. Since a clear cell chondrosarcoma has a relatively low malignancy, bony union occurred 3 months after the operation. Eight months postoperatively, X-ray showed an apparent fracture at the proximal site of the grafted fibula because of stress concentration. Subsequently, a conventional iliac bone graft was carried out at the site of the lesion. Complete shoulder arthrodesis was achieved 4 months later.

Case 6

A 20-year-old female suffering from pain and swelling of the lateral side of the upper limb presented at our clinic in 1986. X-ray showed an abnormal shadow: a periosteal reaction and a sun-ray appearance in the proximal humerus. A biopsy specimen revealed a central low-grade osteosarcoma. A wide excision and shoulder arthrodesis with a vascularized fibular graft was performed. When a shoulder arthrodesis is performed using a vascularized fibular graft, there is a risk of a stress fracture of the proximal grafted bone. We inserted two pieces of wedge-shaped iliac bone to the proximal site of a grafted fibula and glenoid fossa, since the proximal site of a grafted fibula is subject to stress because of the weight of the upper limb. Complete shoulder arthrodesis was achieved 2 months later.

Discussion

Generally speaking, if the pathological diagnosis of tumors around the shoulder girdle reveals malignancy or a neurovascular bundle, either forequarter amputation or disarticulation is inevitable. If elbow and hand functions are to be preserved, two types of reconstruction may be considered: shoulder prosthesis and arthrodesis. A shoulder prosthesis is suitable in cases with an intact rotator cuff and deltoid muscle. In cases with a malignant tumor around the shoulder girdle, however, it is difficult to preserve sufficient muscle function. For this reason, we prefer an arthrodesis to a prosthesis. Burri has reported 58 cases using a prosthesis for the treatment of tumors around the shoulder [4]. In his report, the postoperative range of motion was 62.4° in elevation and 51.6° in abduction. Our results for arthrodesis are not inferior to those for prosthesis. Enneking's evaluation system does not cover the total upper limb function. Compared with amputation or disarticulation, arthrodesis achieves good stability, good control of the upper limb, and preservation of finger to mouth movement. The preservation of elbow and hand function is a real benefit for patients who undergo arthrodesis. But according to Enneking's evaluation system, the evaluation item marking deformity is definitely poor. This system does not, therefore, seem to be appropriate for use with arthrodesis.

In the current series, a vascularized bone graft was indicated most commonly

Table 1. Limb saving procedures of the shoulder girdle

Case	Age (years)	Sex	Histology	Site	Procedure	Recurrence	Metastasis
1 (R.K)	50	M	Aggressive fibromatosis	Scapular area	Scapulectomy	–	–
2 (Y.S)	34	M	Chondrosarcoma	Scapula	Scapulectomy	–	–
3 (K.K)	33	M	GCT	Proximal humerus	Excision	–	–
4 (S.T)	50	M	Parosteal OS	Humeral shaft	Excision	+	–
5 (T.K)	37	M	Chondrosarcoma (clear cell type)	Proximal humerus	Excision	–	–
6 (M.T)	19	F	OS (central low grade)	Proximal humerus	Excision	–	–

Cases 5 and 6 underwent arthrodesis by vascularized fibular graft
GCT giant cell tumor, OS osteosarcoma

Table 2. Results according to Enneking's evaluation system

Case	Motion	Pain	Stability	Deformity	Strength	Functional activity	Emotional acceptance	Evaluation
1	F	G	F	F	F	G	G	F
2	E	E	E	G	G	E	E	G
3	F	F	G	P	F	P	F	P
4	F	G	G	P	F	P	F	P
5	G	G	G	P	G	G	F	F
6	G	G	G	P	G	G	F	F

In cases of arthrodesis (cases 5 and 6), the item of deformity recorded a definitely poor score
E excellent, G good, F fair, P poor

in patients who were undergoing a limb salvage procedure for malignant or locally aggressive bone and soft tissue tumor [5].

A vascularized fibular graft for arthrodesis is suitable since it preserves the living bone and long bones, achieves rapid union, and prevents creeping substitution.

Conclusion

If in the treatment of a malignant tumor of the shoulder girdle sufficient muscular function cannot be preserved, an arthrodesis is recommended rather than a prosthesis. In cases of shoulder arthrodesis, Enneking's evaluation system is not appropriate for functional evaluation.

References

1. Enneking WF (1981) The effect of the anatomic setting on the results of surgical procedures for soft parts sarcoma of the thigh. Cancer 47; 1005–1022
2. Rosenberg SA (1982) The treatment of soft-tissue sarcoma of the extremities. Ann Surg No. 3: 305–315
3. Enneking WF, Spanier SS, Goodman MA (1980) A system for the surgical staging of musculoskeletal sarcoma. Clin Orth 153: 160–120
4. Burri C (1987) Tumor prosthesis for the shoulder. In: Kölbel R, Helbig B, Blauth W (eds) Shoulder replacement. Springer, Berlin Heidelberg New York Tokyo, pp 181–189
5. Wood MB, Cooney W, Irons GB (1985) Skeletal reconstruction by vascularized bone transfer; indication and results. Kayo Clinic Proc 60: 729–734

Guidelines to Upper Humerus Resections

Frantz Langlais[1], Jean F. Dubousset[2], Jean Dunoyer[3], and André Trifaud[4]

Key words: Upper humerus tumors—Shoulder prostheses—Shoulder arthrodeses—Shoulder spacers—Allograft

The choice of a reconstruction procedure depends on the extension of bone removal [both as concerns the humeral shaft and glenoid fossa] and on the conservation of a functional deltoid muscle [as the rotator cuff may be retained only in some low-grade tumors].

Indications for *four reconstruction procedures* will be discussed:
a) No reconstruction [or simple reattachment of the humerus to the scapula or clavicle by muscular transfer or artificial ligament]
b) Arthrodesis of the shoulder
c) Spacer, the aim of which is reattachment of the humerus to the shoulder girdle but without an actual articulation
d) Prosthesis which may be:
   —Anatomical, with a shape adapted to the glenoid fossa [such as the Neer prosthesis]
   —Total, with an articular scapular component
   —Constrained, sutured to the shoulder girdle to avoid luxations and with built-in intraprothetic mobility [such as Campanacci's prosthesis]

Grafts may be considered from a functional point of view, whether as a spacer (e.g., fibular graft), or as an anatomical prosthesis (e.g., humeral allograft).

Isolated Humeral Resection

In type 1 (Malawer classification), isolated humeral resection, the type of reconstruction depends mainly on conservation of the deltoid muscle.

---

[1] Centre Hospitalier Universitaire Hôpital Sud, Rennes, France
[2] Centre Hospitalier Universitaire St Vincent de Paul, Paris, France
[3] Centre Hospitalier Universitaire Dupuytren, Limoges, France
[4] Centre Hospitalier Universitaire La Conception, Merseille, France

Retention of Deltoid

Here, the mode of reconstruction depends on the level of humerus section.

If bone resection does not involve the lower deltoid insertion, an anatomical prosthesis of the upper third of the humerus will usually give good results.

If most of the deltoid muscle can be retained but its distal tendon has to be severed from the resected bone, reinsertion of the deltoid is necessary to obtain active motion. A global humerus allograft may be used, but there is a risk of fracture and of deterioration of articular cartilage. Thus, we prefer a shoulder prosthesis, the long stem of which may be sleeved by an allograft, since reinsertion of the deltoid tendon seems more reliable on the allograft than on the single prosthesis.

Nonfunctional Deltoid

If the resection includes the upper humerus and if the deltoid muscle is not functional, two types of reconstruction may be considered.

A *prosthesis* is a simple technique, but it has to be constrained in order to limit the risks of subluxation. Association with an allograft has no justification here, as no muscular resinsertion is possible and as it may be easier to cover a thin prosthetic stem than a thick allograft if an significant excision of soft tissues was necessary. However, functional results with these prostheses are only fair, especially as control of active rotation cannot be achieved.

Thus, we advocate arthrodesis, which may be considered for short resections of the upper humerus: It achieves good control over the position of the upper limb and fully justifies conservation of the hand and elbow. Yet, it is a demanding technique; fixation can usually be solved by a long custom-bended plate, screwed into the spine of the scapula. Proximal fusion can be obtained if the glenoid fossa and acromion have been retained; distal consolidation with the lower humerus requires peripheral cancellous autografts. But there is a risk of resorption and of fatigue fracture of the allograft. Thus, we prefer to associate a vascularized fibular autograft.

Both techniques can be successively used in the same patient. First, excision and reconstruction by prosthesis is carried out, as it can be followed without significant risk by chemo- and radiotherapy, if necessary. Later, and if functional results are insufficient [in a patient not requiring anymore adjuvant therapy], removal of the prosthesis and arthrodesis are possible.

Resection of Upper Humerus and Glenoid

Type 5 (Malawer classification) resection includes excision of the upper humerus and glenoid fossa.

Retention of Deltoid

In the rare cases where the deltoid muscle can be retained but the resection of both sides of the articulation is required, a constrained prosthesis, sutured to the remaining scapula, is the best way to utilize the deltoid muscle.

Resection of Deltoid

Generally, the deltoid muscle must be resected, for this "modified Tikkof Lindberg" procedure.

An *arthrodesis* is not recommended as the bony and muscular excision makes fusion of the grafts very uncertain.

Reattachment of the humerus to the scapula by *wiring* the upper part of an intramedullary nail to the scapular girdle was in our experience very disappointing, because usually there was rupture of the suture and subcutaneous protuberance of the nail.

A *spacer* may be the best solution. It has: (a) to be sutured to the girdle and to allow intraprothetic rotation; (b) to have a "humeral head" of large diameter to give a better cosmetic look and to avoid localized zones of hyperpression on the soft tissues and to avoid the risk of skin necrosis; (c) to allow some degree of passive intraprosthetic elongation to reduce traction forces on the scapular suture; care must be taken to limit this stretching to avoid painful traction on the brachial plexus. The Campanacci prosthesis fulfills most of these requirements. An orthesis controlling rotation, as one of the Roehampton type, may improve the functional result.

Is there any indication for *nonreconstruction*? Most cases of nonreconstruction give a poor cosmetic aspect and only a fair functional result, since the flexion of the elbow is impaired. So, we suggest that the indications for nonreconstruction be limited to failures of reconstruction [e.g., removal of a prosthesis] or to excisions with high complication risks [e.g., after a large soft tissue excision, or after severe radiotherapy]. Some good results have then been achieved but not in a predictable manner.

Conservation of the upper limb after shoulder resection gives cosmetic, psychological, and functional benefit compared with amputation. Yet, except in moderate resections of the upper humerus allowing prosthesis or arthrodesis, the main function of the shoulder, which is accurate positioning of the upper limb, has not so far been obtained in the majority of cases.

Functional Results Following Resection Arthrodesis About the Knee

EDMUND Y.S. CHAO and FRANKLIN H. SIM[1]

Summary. Since 1970, 79 patients, ranging in age from 14 to 74 years, have undergone reconstruction of the knee after en bloc resection of a primary tumor at our institute. Among these, 27 had resection arthrodesis. The functional and device evaluation results were analyzed using the rating system adopted by the Musculoskeletal Tumor Society. In this group of patients with knee arthrodesis, 74% had good or excellent results and ten had major or minor complications. Different reconstructive methods were reviewed, but no significant difference in functional results was found. Therefore, segmental bone resection and knee joint arthrodesis can provide good functional results and reconstruction longevity. However, each patient should be judged individually by considering a number of factors before a specific method of knee fusion is selected.

Key words: Knee arthrodesis—Limb salvage—En bloc resection

Introduction

One of the most challenging problems in limb salvage surgery is tumor involvement in the knee joint region [4]. When surgical treatment is contemplated, the first important goal is to achieve local control of the tumor by a wide margin resection. The second goal is to reconstruct the extremity to restore as much useful function as possible. Various techniques for reconstruction include the use of segmental defect replacement (SDR) prosthesis with a mobile knee joint and the utilization of osteochondral allografts. However, in young and physically active patients, knee arthrodesis is preferred, especially when the lesion involves the proximal tibia. Various techniques have been used to achieve segmental arthrodesis of the knee. The most common technique utilizes a hemicylindrical sliding graft with or without vascularized fibular graft augmentation. Metaphyseal segmental grafts from the subtrochanteric area of the opposite femur (cross-leg graft) have also been utilized. Occasionally, an intercalary allograft segment can be used to bridge the defect with autogenous iliac grafts. Finally, modular titanium fibermental SDR prostheses can be used to achieve a resection arthrodesis. The purpose of this paper is to review the functional results of

[1] Orthopedic Biomechanics Laboratory, Department of Orthopedics, Mayo Clinic/Mayo Foundation, Rochester, MN, USA

our knee arthrodesis patients achieved by different surgical techniques. In addition, such results are compared with other types of knee reconstructive procedures without knee arthrodesis. It is hoped that an objective study of our past experience can help to define the proper role of these procedures and their anticipated clinical and functional outcome.

Materials and Methods

Twenty-seven patients with resection arthrodesis of the knee joint were reviewed: 19 were females with a mean age of 24 years (range 12–56 years). Sixteen tumors involved the distal femur with an average resection length of 20.8 cm; 11 involved the proximal tibia with an average resection length of 12.2 cm. Fourteen patients had malignant tumors and 13 patients had benign lesions. Of the 27 patients, 26 had a wide surgical margin of resection, and one had a lesional margin.

A hemicylindrical sliding graft from the ipsilateral tibia or femur was used in 14 patients. Three additional patients had a similar procedure but with vascularized fibular graft augmentation [3]. A subtrochanteric metaphyseal bone segment from the contralateral femur used used in two patients utilizing the cross-leg graft technique. An intercalary allograft segment was used in two patients to achieve a solid resection arthrodesis. Intramedullary rods, a plate, and screws were used to obtain initial fixation of massive grafts to the host bone. In six patients, a titanium fibermetal modular implant was used to achieve an arthrodesis (Fig. 1). The prosthesis has two components joined together by a conical coupling to facilitate implantation. Different lengths and sizes of components can be interchanged to achieve the best replacement and fixation. After each component is cemented into the femoral and tibial intramedullary canals and engaged, set screws are used to achieve additional locking strength. Autogenous iliac grafts are packed around the shoulder regions of the implant to achieve extracortical bone bridging and ingrowth fixation [1].

The functional results were studied using clinical examination parameters rated according to the grading system recommended by the Musculoskeletal Tumor Society with slight modifications [2]. In this system, six parameters pertinent to segmental knee joint arthrodesis are incorporated. Each parameter was rated excellent, good, fair, or poor as related to knee joint motion, pain, joint stability or deformity, strength, emotional acceptance, activities of daily living, and complications. An overall rating was achieved by combining individual ratings on each parameter. Based on this scheme, the functional results of the knee arthrodesis patients were compared with other knee reconstruction procedures after tumor resection based on the same rating scale.

Results

Resection arthrodesis was effective in achieving a pain-free extremity. Patients who underwent this procedure automatically have one parameter rated as poor, i.e., if the procedure is successful there will be no motion. Only 5 of the 27

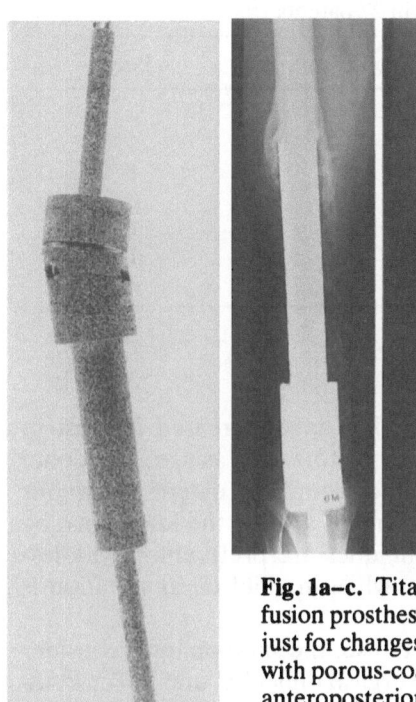

b, c

Fig. 1a–c. Titanium modular fibermetal-coated knee segmental fusion prosthesis. Different sizes and lengths are available to adjust for changes in resection margins. **a** Assembled prosthesis with porous-coated stems. **b** Six-month postoperative knee anteroposterior X-ray view. **c** Six months after knee arthrodesis, lateral view

a

patients used a cane. In the stability/deformity parameter, 21 were rated excellent and six were rated poor. Twenty-four of the patients were rated excellent in the strength parameter, and most of the patients with a resection arthrodesis achieved an excellent functional activity level and seemed to accept the handicap associated with a stiff knee joint.

Complications of varying degrees were present in 13 patients (48%). These included three fractures (two involving the grafts and one in a fibermetal prosthesis), two infections, and one resulted in nonunion of the arthrodesis. In addition, four patients had local recurrence, three of which required amputation. According to the functional evaluation scheme utilized, 20 of the 27 patients had an overall excellent or good rating, three had fair, and four had poor results (Table 1). When comparing these patients' results with those reconstructed with custom knee joint prostheses, similar functional ratings were obtained. However, among different knee resection arthrodesis techniques, there was no significant difference in the functional results associated with each technique.

Discussion

Although amputation has remained the usual treatment for patients with malignant radioresistant tumors, recent enthusiasm for adjuvant chemotherapy and

Table 1. Functional results of resection arthrodesis in 27 patents

Parameter	Excellent	Good	Fair	Poor
Overall	12	8	3	4
Motion	0	0	0	27
Pain	23	1	2	1
Stability/deformity	21	0	0	6
Strength	24	1	1	1
Function/ activity	19	1	6	1
Complications	14	3	6	4

improved techniques of oncological reconstruction have increased interest in limb saving local resections. However, important factors such as age, functional status of the patient, the nature and grade of the lesion, the extent of osseous destruction, and the extent of soft tissue involvement around the knee must be considered. Generally, the reconstructive techniques are preferable in adolescent and older patients with closed epiphyses, while in children amputation is probably a more realistic surgical procedure.

In deciding which reconstructive procedure to use, the surgeon must consider the graft or prosthesis availability, the level of surgical difficulty, and the morbidity and incidence of complications associated with each procedure. Moreover, the effect of adjuvant chemotherapy or radiotherapy on graft remodeling and incorporating must be taken into consideration. Finally, the durability of the reconstructive procedure should also be included in the decision factor.

Our preferred method for restoring skeletal continuity after resection of a lesion around the knee, particularly in young and active patients, is segmental arthrodesis. The high incidence of complications experienced in our patient series is expected to improve with better methods of graft fixation and prosthetic device design. A segmental arthrodesis achieves a stable pain-free weight-bearing extremity. Such a procedure appears to offer the least restriction in strenuous walking and recreation activities. Our recent experience in using the titanium fibermetal SDR prosthesis for knee fusion with extracortical bone bridging appears to provide the most exciting outlook for knee arthrodesis. This technique has the advantage that the ipsilateral tibia or femur is not compromised, and the technique is usually less demanding technically. When a complete modular system of such prostheses is made available during surgery, such a reconstructive technique will no doubt gain more popularity and efficacy. However, important factors governing successful bone graft incorporation and extracortical bone bridging must be identified to ensure its consistent and long-term success.

Although arthrodesis will remain the main stay for reconstruction of bony defects around the knee following tumor resection in certain patients, improvements made in segmental bone and joint prosthesis design with effective soft tissue attachment options and improvements in the biological and biomechanical adaptation of osteochondral allografts may change the future selection preference in limb salvage surgery involving the knee. Each patient undergoing such a procedure should be considered on an individual basis. Every method has its advantages and disadvantages, which must be carefully contemplated by both the surgeons and the patients. The present clinical and functional results in knee arthrodesis following tumor resection should be used as the bench-mark reference to seek future advances in this difficult field of orthopedic oncological surgery.

Acknowledgment. This study was supported by grant number CA 23751, awarded by the National Cancer Institute, DHHS.

References

1. Chao EYS, Sim FH (1985) Modular prosthetic system for segmental bone and joint replacement after tumor resection. Orthopedics 8: 641–651
2. Enneking WF (1987) A system for functional evaluation of the surgical management of musculoskeletal tumors. In: Enneking WF (ed) Limb salvage in musculoskeletal oncology. Churchill Livingstone, New York, pp 5–16
3. Enneking WF, Shirley PD (1977) Resection arthrodesis for malignant and potentially malignant lesions about the knee using an intramedullary rod and local bone grafts. J Bone Joint Surg 59A: 223
4. Sim FH, Beauchamp CP, Chao EYS (1987) Reconstruction of musculoskeletal defects about the knee for tumors. Clin Orthop Rel Res 221: 188–201

The Use of Proximal Tibial Allografts in the Reconstruction of Tumors and Other Defects

MARK C. GEBHARDT and HENRY J. MANKIN[1]

Summary. Fifty-three fresh, frozen cadaveric allografts (50 osteoarticular, three intercalary grafts for arthrodesis) were employed to reconstruct tumors and other defects (e.g., failed prior allografts, trauma) of the proximal tibia. Forty-eight patients had 2 or more years of follow-up. Most patients had low-grade neoplasms (giant cell tumor in 28 cases), although seven patients had high-grade malignancies (osteosarcoma in six). The functional results were judged to be excellent in 44%, good in 26.7%, fair in 2.2%, and to have failed in 26.7%. Tumor complications included two instances of metastases and five local recurrences. Deep infection occurred in 13.2% and fracture in 20.7%. If consideration is given to those patients who failed initially but were salvaged by a second graft, satisfactory results were achieved in 86%. The authors consider this to be a reasonable reconstructive option for tumors and other bony defects involving the proximal tibial articulation.

Key words: Bone tumor—Reconstruction—Proximal tibial allograft

Introduction

Reconstruction of bony defects of the proximal tibia is challenging because it requires reconstitution of the skeleton at a major weight-bearing site and restoration (or substitution) of knee joint function. The causes of bony loss at this site include benign (aggressive), low-grade, and high-grade bone neoplasms, traumatic bone loss, osteonecrosis, pigmented villonodular synovitis, and failed prostheses or allografts performed for arthritis, tumor, or other reasons. Despite the rarity of bone neoplasms, such tumors tend to occur in the knee area and constitute a high percentage of lesions presenting to the orthopedic oncologist, making reconstruction in this area of some import. Oncological considerations include: (a) the extent of bony resection; (b) a decision relative to preservation of the joint (intra- versus extra-articular resection); (c) the need to sacrifice the patellar tendon or fibula; and (d) assessment of the neurovascular bundle. In high-grade neoplasms, particular attention must be paid to this latter point and a decision relative to the safety and functional outcome of a long above-knee

[1] Orthopaedic Service, Harvard Medical School, Massachusetts General Hospital, Boston, MA, USA

amputation compared with that of resection and reconstruction must be made. If a resection is deemed reasonable, the reconstruction options of arthrodesis, custom-made or modular metallic knee prostheses, or osteoarticular allograft are considered. The focus of this presentation will be on the functional and onco-logical results of the use of bone allograft transplantation in reconstructing tumors and other defects of the proximal tibia.

Materials and Methods

From September 1972 until August, 1986, 53 allograft bone transplants were employed to reconstruct bone tumor defects of the proximal tibia by the Ortho-paedic Oncology Service of the Massachusetts General Hospital and The Chil-dren's Hospital, Boston (Table 1). This represents 15.6% of the entire allograft series of 346 patients reconstructed with allografts during that period. Forty-eight patients have 2 or more years of follow-up and will be the focus of this report.

Patients presenting with tumorous lesions of the proximal tibia were carefully evaluated with plane radiographs, bone scans, computed or plane tomograms, and, in selected cases, arteriograms and staged by the system of Enneking et al. [12]. A needle or incisional biopsy was performed to establish the diagnosis. The types of resective procedure were based upon the diagnosis and staging results, and all patients were followed up by the authors or a referring physician post-operatively; the functional results and disease status were recorded. Radio-graphs were assessed for union of the osteosynthesis site at intervals and at the time of last follow-up. Secondary procedures and complications were noted.

For tumorous lesions, the operative procedure was a marginal or wide re-section of the proximal tibia through an extensible longitudinal anterolateral or anteromedial incision. For benign, aggressive lesions with loss of the sub-articular bone plate, or for low-grade (and certain high-grade) lesions, an intra-articular resection was performed. The decision regarding sacrifice of the patellar tendon depended upon the extent of the bony resection and the grade of the neoplasm and its location. For high-grade lesions with potential or dem-onstrated joint involvement, an extra-articular wide resection was performed with sacrifice of the extensor mechanism. For nontumorous lesions, the bony defect was determined by the cause of the destructive process and allograft segments were cut to fit the defect.

Proximal tibial osteoarticular allograft segments were obtained from the MGH Bone Bank. The Bank has been in operation for over 10 years, and the procedures, standards, precautions, and logistics of maintaining it have been presented previously [8, 35] and are in general agreement with the guidelines promulgated by the American Association of Tissue Banks [13, 15]. Selection of donors is in part dependent on the living organ donor program in New England and harvests take place under sterile conditions. The medial, lateral, and pos-terior capsular ligaments and the patellar tendons are retained on the allograft. The donors are screened for syphilis, hepatitis, and AIDS (HTLV-III screening of the donor) and ABO and HLA typing is performed. The bones are cultured for aerobic and anaerobic bacteria at the time of harvest. To preserve the viabil-

Table 1. Demographic data for proximal tibial allografts in 53 patients (26 males, 27 females; mean age 26 years, range 14–64 years)

Diagnosis	No. of patients
Tumor	
Giant cell tumor	28
Osteosarcoma (IIB)	6
Chondroblastoma	2
Chondrosarcoma	1
Parosteal osteosarcoma	1
Fibrosarcoma of bone (IIB)	1
Total	39
Nontumor	
Failed prior allograft	7
Trauma	4
Osteonecrosis	2
Pigmented villonodular synovitis	1
Total	14

ity of the articular cartilage, these surfaces of the skeletal segments were treated with 8% DMSO in ringer's lactate [34, 36, 37] for at least 1 h and the graft stored at −70° to −80° until needed. Selection of the grafts was based on comparison radiographs in two planes of the graft and the patient's tibial joint surface using a metal standard to control for magnification. Prior to reconstruction of the skeleton, aerobic and anaerobic cultures were obtained from the skeletal part, which was then thawed in warm ringer's lactate and antibiotic solution. In cases of osteoarticular reconstruction, the host medial, lateral, and posterior capsular structures and patellar tendon were repaired to the respective locations on the allograft using nonabsorbable sutures. If resection required sacrifice of the knee menisci, the menisci on the allograft were retained. The cruciate ligaments were not reconstructed, but a tight posterior capsular repair was achieved. Osteosynthesis was achieved with a dynamic compression plate or plates and suction drains were used upon closure of the wound. If an extra-articular reconstruction was performed, an allograft was employed to create an arthrodesis using dynamic compression plates. Skin coverage in high-grade lesions was augmented by local gastrocnemius flaps. Postoperatively, the patients received 1 week of intravenous antibiotics (usually a cephalosporin), followed by 2–3 weeks of oral administration. Postoperative immobilization was achieved with a long leg brace or cast for 6–8 weeks or until the osteosynthesis had healed and the joint was considered stable. Following removal of the immobilization, a supervised passive and then active exercise program was begun.

Function was evaluated by a system originally described by the senior author [18, 22] which, although somewhat subjective, is dependent on survival, tumor status, pain, and function. Patients graded as *excellent* are those who have no evidence of disease, are pain-free, and have essentially "normal" function of the part (with the exception of high-performance athletics). Patients are classified as *good* if they also enjoy freedom from disease and pain but have some degree of impairment of function which materially limits their recreational but not oc-

Table 2. MSTS stage for 53 proximal tibial allografts

Stage	Number	Percent
O	11	21
IA	16	30
IB	18	34
IIA	0	0
IIB	7	13
III	1	2

cupational activities. Patients are classified as *fair* if they have sufficient pain or disability as to require aids or supports (crutches, canes, braces, etc.), and/or are unable to return to an appropriate work status. Those patients who require removal of the graft or an amputation as a result of complications or die as a result of failure of local control are considered *failures*.

Results

Demographic Data

There were a total of 53 patients in this series (26 males and 27 females). The average age was 26 years (range 14–64 years) and the average follow-up was 5.5 years (range 2–12.5 years).

The diagnoses (Table 1) included 39 tumorous and 14 nontumorous conditions. In the former category, there were 28 giant cell tumors, six stage IIB osteosarcomas, two chondroblastomas, and one case each of parosteal osteosarcoma, fibrosarcoma of bone, and chondrosarcoma. Proximal tibial allografts were employed to reconstruct failed allografts in seven cases, traumatic defects in four, osteonecrosis in two, and in a single joint destroyed by pigmented villonodular synovitis. The surgical stage of the tumors (Table 2) was benign (or nontumorous) in 11 (21%) cases, stage IA in 16 (30%), stage IB in 18 (34%), and IIB in eight (13%) cases. One patient with a giant cell tumor was initially classified as IA, but the time of revision of the graft for infection, local recurrence and pulmonary metastases were noted. Therefore, for the second allograft procedure the patient was classified as stage III.

Functional Outcome

The functional results were graded by the system described above at the time of last visit (either at the Massachusetts General Hospital or by the referring physician). Patients who required removal of the allograft were rated as failures for their first procedure, and the functional results of the replacement allograft were graded at follow-up as a separate procedure. The results of osteoarticular proximal tibial allografts were graded as excellent in 20 (44.4%) patients, good in 12 (16.7%), fair in one (2.2%), and as failures in 12 (26.7%), giving

Table 3. Results by type of graft in 48 proximal tibial allografts followed up for 2 or more years

Type	Excellent	Good	Fair	Failure	Total
Osteoarticular	20	12	1	12	45
	(44.4)	(26.7)	(2.2)	(26.7)	
Arthrodesis	0	1	1	1	3
	(0)	(33.3)	(33.3)	(33.3)	
Total	20	13	2	13	48
	(41.6)	(27.1)	(4.2)	(27.1)	
Percent satisfactory					68.8
Tumor failures deleted	20	11	1	12	44
	(45.5)	(25.0)	(2.3)	(27.7)	
Percent satisfactory					75.0

Figures in *parentheses* are percentages

Table 4. Complications in 53 proximal tibial allografts

	Number	Percent
Tumor complications (39 patients)		
Total	6[a]	12.8
Recurrence	5[a]	10.2
Metastasis	2	5.1
Death	1	2.5
Allograft complications (53 patients)		
Infection	7	13.2
Fracture	11	20.7
Nonunion	3	5.6
Unstable JT.	5	9.4

Because many of the patients had more than one complication, the numbers shown are not additive. In all, 29 patients (54.7%) had neither tumor nor allograft complications
[a] One patient with giant cell tumor had two recurrences.

an overall acceptable (good or excellent) rate of 68.8% (Table 3). Allograft arthrodeses were performed in three cases and were rated as good, fair, and a failure in one each.

Complications

The complications of the patients can be divided into two categories: (a) tumor complications and (b) allograft complications. Relative to the first category (which is more a function of the tumor type and resection rather than the reconstruction), 6 (12.8%) of the 39 tumor patients developed tumor complications (Table 4): One patient died of metastases during the follow-up period, five (10.2%) developed local recurrence and two (5.1%) developed metastatic disease. Of the eight high-grade lesions, there were no local recurrences and one patient developed metastatic disease. Two of the local recurrences were in the

Table 5. Functional results of 48 proximal tibial allografts with 2 or more years of follow-up showing the effect of complications

Complication	Excellent/good	Fair	Failure	Total
Total series	33 (68.8)	2 (4.1)	13 (27.1)	48
No complications	29 (100.0)	0 (0)	0 (0)	29
Infection	1 (14.3)	1 (14.3)	5 (71.4)	7
Fracture	3 (27.2)	1 (9.1)	7 (63.6)	11
Nonunion	1 (33.3)	3 (33.3)	3 (33.3)	3
Unstable joint	3 (60.0)	1 (20.0)	1 (20.0)	5

Figures in *parentheses* are percentages

same patient with giant cell tumor: A second osteoarticular allograft was employed following resection of a local recurrence 14 months after the initial resection. The subsequently developed multifocal tumor in the native tibia below the second allograft was treated by amputation. Although this behaved more like an intraosseous metastasis, it is counted as a local recurrence.

Allograft complications fell into four categories (Table 4): infection, nonunion, fracture, and unstable joints. There were 25 allograft complications in 20 of the 53 patients; 32 patients (60.1%) escaped complications related to the alloimplant. Seven (13.2%) patients developed infection, 11 (20.7%) sustained a graft fracture, three (5.6%) did not show healing at the osteosynthesis site, and five (9.4%) had an unstable joint.

It should be noted that because many of the patients listed in Table 4 had more than one complication, the numbers are not additive. Of the 53 patients, 29 (54.7%) sustained neither a tumor nor an allograft complication.

The significance of the complications becomes more apparent when the functional results are viewed relative to the complications (Table 5). Of the 48 patients followed for 2 or more years, 29 had no complications and were rated satisfactory (good/excellent) in all cases. In contrast, of the seven patients who developed infection, 71.4% were ultimately failures and only 14.3% were satisfactory. Likewise, the 11 graft fractures resulted in satisfactory results in only three of the patients and failure in seven. Nonunion and unstable joints were less of a problem, with satisfactory results in 33% and 60%, respectively.

Reoperation was required at least once in 30 of the 53 (56.6%) patients and the procedures are listed in Table 6. It is of note that six patients developed loss of articular cartilage, subchondral fracture, or unstable joints necessitating revision to a standard total knee replacement. Five patients required autografting and revision of the osteosynthesis for nonunion or fracture. Amputation was required in three instances (5.6% of the series) for infection in two cases, and local recurrence in one, as noted above. Ten patients required removal of the allograft; in eight patients (seven of whom have been followed for more than 1 year, and one of whom was treated elsewhere), it was possible to revise them with a second osteoarticular allograft. Of the seven, three are excellent, two are good, and two have ultimately ended in amputation (one for infection and one for late recurrence of a giant cell tumor distal to the graft).

If consideration is given to the final outcome (Table 7) of the 43 *patients* ini-

Table 6. Secondary operations

Type of operation	Number of patients
Removal of allograft	10
Second allograft insertion	9
Orif/autograft	5
Total knee arthroplasty	6
Removal of hardware	3
Amputation	3
Resection of recurrence	2
Incision and Drainage	1
Tibial osteotomy	2
Arthroscopy	1

Table 7. End results of 43 patients with proximal tibial allografts (including results of revisions)

Result	Number	Percent
Excellent	20	46.5
Good	17	30.5
Fair	3	7.0
Failure	5	11.6
Satisfactory		86.0

tially entered into the study (as distinct to the 53 *procedures*) and their final outcome after secondary operations and allograft revisions (including the one revision with less than 1 year of follow-up), 20 patients (46.5%) are excellent, 17 (30.5%) are good, two (7.0%) are fair, and five (11.6%) are failures. The overall satisfactory end result, therefore, of patients (including reoperations) is 86.0%.

Discussion

The history of the use of allografts in the reconstruction of bony defects, the immunological considerations, and human and experimental studies have been reviewed elsewhere [14, 22–24, 43] and will not be repeated. Suffice it to say that allogeneic bone and cartilage implants, although clearly less immunogenic than living grafts, are not accepted as readily as autografts and in fact even when frozen excite a significant host immune response. The immune response, which at present cannot be predicted on the basis of studies of blood group and cell surface markers, probably acts not only to diminish variably the manner in which the graft is reconstructed and incorporated by the recipient, but is probably at least in part responsible for the now well-established clinical finding that segments are by most standards excessively prone to infection, fracture, and nonunion [21, 28].

In consideration of the theoretical issues as defined above and the known high complication rate [21, 28], allografting ought to be considered perhaps a less than optimal solution for the patient with massive bone loss. Despite these problems, however, the system has become increasingly popular in dealing with major skeletal defects as created by trauma or resection for musculoskeletal tumors. Furthermore, in recent years, allografting has become an important part of the armamentarium of the total joint surgeon, who finds the technique useful in the treatment of loss of bone stock as a result of failure of metallic devices. In consideration of this seeming paradox, part of the explanation requires that one review the current alternatives available for the treatment of major skeletal loss. Implantation of avascular or, more recently, vascularized autograft is the time-honored solution; clearly, the best tolerated, most predictable and durable substitute for filling a defect in a patient's skeleton is a segment of autogeneic bone [4, 10, 11, 17, 38–42]. The difficulties with this solution are self-evident, however: The amount of autograft is limited in quantity, size, and shape; donor site morbidity can be a significant problem to a patient who is often already severely impaired by the disease and/or the surgery; it is obviously impossible to reconstruct an articular surface. Following the early success of metallic and plastic implants in the treatment of joint disease, numerous custom-made and, more recently, modular artificial devices have been proposed for use in the treatment of massive defects in the skeleton and reports describing the devices and the short-term results of their implantation have begun to appear with increasing frequency [7, 9, 25, 29, 30]. Real concern has, however, been expressed by some of the more thoughtful proponents of this system of skeletal reconstruction, particularly for the treatment of bone tumors in which the average age of the patients in most series is below 30 years. Since the failure rate for the standard hip prosthetic devices has been climbing rapidly and is now believed to be over 20% at 10 years [1, 32, 33] (and as has been suggested by Chandler et al. [5], these values are even greater in younger patients), the threat of failure in young tumor patients who have been treated in many cases with less than optimal custom devices must be considered a significant future problem if the patient survives. These data do not suggest that these systems should not be tried nor that research be discontinued. It is essential, however, that clear reporting of complications and long-term follow-up of any system be completed.

Allograft implantation, although still an imperfect system, represents a biological solution to the problems raised by massive defects in the skeleton. Experience is growing and a number of large series have been reported with results which exceed or are comparable with those of other systems [6, 16, 18, 20, 22–24, 26, 27, 31]. Allograft material despite the immune response is generally well tolerated and nontoxic, and the supply is theoretically unlimited. The shape of the material is usually anatomically correct for the host (especially if sufficient tissues are available in the bank so that a close match can be achieved). Grafts are likely to have appropriate mechanical properties and the structure is relatively easily shaped and implanted. Perhaps the most important issue however is a biological one. Allografts are eventually invaded by host tissues and over time are incorporated, perhaps not completely, but sufficiently to be considered living tissue. This means that if successful, an allogeneic segment represents a permanent implant rather than a temporary spacer, such as the metallic devices.

The use of osteoarticular allografts for reconstruction of skeletal defects of the proximal tibia created from tumor resections or other causes appears to be a reasonable alternative at this site. For situations where the distal femoral articular cartilage can be preserved, it offers the advantage of providing a tibial joint surface of articular cartilage, which although abnormal appears to function satisfactorily for many years. In the case of failure this surface can usually be salvaged with standard metal and plastic total knee arthroplasties. The allograft also offers the ability to reconstruct ligaments, replace menisci, and attach the host patellar tendon to its corresponding site on the allograft. Although the biology of ligamentous and tendon healing to allograft counterparts has not been well studied, the clinical results are quite promising. Extension power and range of motion in this series were acceptable, although we have no means of comparing this series with results following rerouting of the patellar tendon to the fibula or inserting it on a muscular flap.

There were only five instances of unstable joints requiring brace support despite the lack of cruciate reconstruction, although more of these knees would be considered ligamentously normal and none of the patients were encouraged to pursue sports activities. The length of the bony defect does not seem to be an issue as long as the distal tibial articulating surface is preserved and there is enough length to gain fixation of the transplant. In cases of IIB osteosarcomas, we have replaced the proximal two-thirds of the tibia. We, therefore, feel the technique is indicated for benign, aggressive, low-grade, and certain high-grade bone neoplasms as well as for defects of the proximal tibial joint surface arising from trauma, osteonecrosis, pigmented villonodular synovitis, or failed metal and plastic arthroplasties or allografts. The decision in high-grade lesions relative to intra-articular resection in an oncological one, based on assessment of the preoperative staging studies. Likewise, the decisions in benign lesions as to whether to perform a resection rather than more standard reconstruction using autografts will depend upon the extent of the bony and articular surface.

For high-grade lesions with suspected involvement of the knee joint with tumor, it is often necessary to resect the patella and suprapatellar pouch as well as the distal femoral metaphysis and condyles. In these cases, we have elected to perform an arthrodesis using an allograft rather than attempting to restore knee joint function [44]. This appears to offer a stable reconstruction, replacing quadriceps function with a knee arthrodesis. Although seemingly a relatively simple reconstruction, there have been difficulties with wound healing and late infection leading to a satisfactory result in only two of the three cases where arthrodesis was employed for this site. Union, however (despite the use of chemotherapy in these patients), has not been a significant problem and with routine use of local muscle flaps it is hoped that the incidence of wound and infection problems will decrease. The alternative to employing a constrained (standard) rotating hinge prosthesis in combination with a proximal tibial allograft is a theoretical possibility, but we have not as yet performed this for tibial lesions due to concerns of insufficient quadriceps function and distal femoral bone stock. Such a composite reconstruction has proved very satisfactory for use in distal femoral lesions, however [43].

Consideration of resection of the proximal fibula will depend upon the preoperative staging studies and, in particular, on the extent of the soft tissue mass. In general, the proximal fibula has been preserved, but in lesions with large extraosseous lateral masses, especially those of high grade, the fibula should be resected an bloc. Although not routinely performed, consideration should be given to resecting the proximal fibula in extensive resections about the knee in order to aid in skin closure and prevent subsequent skin breakdown over the proximal fibular head. The excised bone could be used as bone graft if not involved by tumor.

The apparently somewhat high incidence of surgical complications clearly deserves further comment. It seems reasonable to consider the allograft bone to be "dead space" (occupied by a nonliving nonvascularized segment of organic "culture medium"), which can serve as a focus for bacterial infection on the basis of transient bacteremia (common in the postoperative period). With even partial revascularization and the introduction of macrophages and other serum factors (including antibiotics), the graft at least in theory becomes less susceptible to infection, and it is hoped that when full incorporation occurs it is as resistant as the adjacent bony tissues. Our data on the incidence of and cofactors for allograft infection support this concept. Although a rather substantial number of the infected patients in the entire allograft series (reviewed by Lord et al. [19]) showed some comorbid conditions (such as skin slough, prior radiation of the bed, postoperative chemotherapy, or, in one case, transmission from the donor), 25% did not and these infections occurred considerably later in the course (8–44 months after the surgery). Furthermore, the flora for these late infections showed a pattern more typical of that resulting from episodes of transient bacteremia. It would seem possible and in fact likely that the grafts in this group of patients were not revascularized at the appropriate rate and hence were more susceptible to late infection than the others who did.

As to the incidence of fractures serving as indicators of immunological failure of the system, the evidence is also tenuous but equally compelling. Three types of fractures were recorded in the recent study by Berrey et al. [2]. Type 1, rapid dissolution, was rare (only two patients in the entire series) and is presumed to represent an immune response in which the graft is rapidly invaded and destroyed by the host tissue [3]. Type 2, shaft fracture, was much more common (about half of the fractures in the series) and was usually associated with more rapid but asymmetrical revascularization of the part as assessed by radiograph and by the rate of healing of the host-donor junction site. Type 3, fractures of the articular surface, occurred somewhat earlier in the course and principally in the distal femur or proximal tibia. The tissue obtained at the time of reconstructive surgery of these fractures showed evidence of demarcation of the osteonecrotic fracture fragment from the major more vascularized segment, suggesting the possibility of a slower and more tenuous course of revascularization. It should be obvious that much of this formulation is speculative, but it seems appropriate to continue to study this issue prospectively by analyzing the host-donor HLA and ABO matches and attempting to correlate these data with the type and rate of complications.

Although the current results of this and other series seem to be "acceptable" and certainly equivalent or perhaps even more suitable than many other methods used in the management of these types of patients and the problems for which they are treated, it is evident to all those in the field that the system could be materially improved by continued investigation. Although numerous studies of graft incorporation have been performed there is an obvious need for a clearer definition of the nature of the cellular processes involved in bone vascularization and host-donor interaction at the junction site and perhaps, more importantly, their optimal rates of occurrence. A second area of research concentration should be in the field of allograft cartilage preservation and joint physiology. Although chondrocytes from fresh allogeneic grafts are more likely to "survive" than those from frozen segments treated with cryopreservatives, the fresh cartilage and bone appears to exert a greater immune response and may in fact invoke a much more profound graft versus host disease.

Study of the long-term results of allograft joint replacements in our patients and in series reported by others show only a slowly progressive joint "deterioration" with relatively few of the patients demonstrating a frank osteoarthritis. To date, the follow-up of the series has been too short to correlate the joint changes (or lack of them) with other factors such as fit, rate of host-donor junction site healing, apparent rate of revascularization on x-ray, but clearly these studies as well as further understanding of the biology of transplanted cartilage and improved cryopreservation techniques will be required if we are to advocate this system as a method of management of joint disease.

In summary, the overall satisfactory (good/excellent) results in this series of 53 proximal tibial allografts were 68.8%, and if tumor failures (which reflect the resection technique more than the reconstruction) are eliminated 75% of the grafts functioned satisfactory. If results are viewed after salvaging the failures in this series, the end results are satisfactory in 86% of the patients. The long-term outcome of the articular surface is as yet unknown, but in this series with an average 5.5 years of follow-up it remains satisfactory. Although problems with infection, fracture, and nonunion exist, it is hoped that these will at least in part be surmountable, allowing this to be a permanent method of reconstruction compared with metallic alternatives. The advantages of restoring a joint surface, knee collateral ligaments, bone stock, and patellar tendon insertion seem to make this a suitable option for reconstruction of tumors and other defects at this site.

Acknowledgments. Supported in part by grants AM 21896 and CA 32968 from the National Institutes of Health.

References

1. Beckenhaugh RD, Ilstrup DM (1978) Total hip arthroplast: a review of three hundred and thirty-three cases with long term followup. J Bone Joint Surg 60A: 306–313
2. Berrey BH, Mankin HJ, Gebhardt MC (in manuscript) Allograft fractures: frequency, treatment and end result.
3. Burchardt H, Jones H, Glowczewskie F et al. (1978) Freeze-dried allogeneic segmental cortical-bone grafts in dogs. J Bone Joint Surg 60A: 1082–1090
4. Campanacci M, Costa P (1979) Total resection of the distal femur or proximal tibia for bone tumours: autogenous bone grafts and arthrodesis in twenty-six cases. J Bone Joint Surg 61B: 455–463
5. Chandler HP, Reineck FT, Wixon RL, McCarthy JC (1981) Total hip replacement in patients younger than 30 years old: a five year follow-up study. J Bone Joint Surg 63A: 1426–1434
6. Dick HM, Malinin TI, Mnaymneh WH (1985) Massive allograft implantation follow-

ing radical resection of high grade tumors requiring adjuvant chemotherapy treatment. Clin Orthop 197: 88–95

7. Dobbs HS, Scales JT, Wilson JN (1981) Endoprosthetic replacement of the proximal femur and acetabulum. J Bone Joint Surg 63B: 219–224

8. Doppelt SH, Tomford WW, Lucas AD, Mankin HJ (1981) Operational and financial aspects of a hospital based bone bank. J Bone Joint Surg 63A: 244–248

9. Eckardt JJ, Eilber, FR, Grant TT, et al. (1985) Management of stage IIB osteogenic sarcoma: experience at the University of California. Canc Treatment Symposia 3: 117–130

10. Enneking WF, Eady JL, Burchardt H (1980) Autogenous cortical bone grafts in the reconstruction of segmental skeletal defects. J Bone Joint Surg 62A: 1039–1058

11. Enneking WF, Shirley PD (1980) Resection-arthrodesis for malignant and potentially malignant lesions about the knee using an intermedullary rod and local bone grafts. J Bone Joint Surg 62A: 1039–1058

12. Enneking WF, Spanier SS, Goodman MA (1980) A system for the surgical staging of musculoskeletal sarcoma. Clin Orthop 153: 106–120

13. Friedlaender GE (1982) Current concepts review: bone banking. J Bone Joint Surg 64A: 307–311

14. Friedlaender GE, Mankin HJ (1984) Transplantation of osteochondral allografts. Annual Rev Med 35: 311–324

15. Friellaender GE, Mankin HJ (1979) Guidelines for the banking of musculoskeletal tissues. Newsletter, Am Assn Tiss Banks 3: 2–7

16. Gross AE, McKee NH, Langer F, Pritzker K (1983) Surgical techniques and clinical experience with articular allografts at the knee. In: Friedlaender GE, Mankin HJ, Sell KW (eds) Osteochondral allografts. Little Brown, Boston, pp 289–300

17. Heiple KG, Chase SW, Herndon CH (1963) A comparative study of the healing process following different types of bone transplantation. J Bone Joint Surg 45A: 1593–1616

18. Hiki Y, Mankin HJ (1980) Radical resection and allograft replacement in the treatment of bone tumors. J Jpn Orthopaed Assoc 54: 475–500

19. Lord CF, Gebhardt MC, Mankin HJ (in press) The incidence, epidemiology and treatment of infection in allograft transplantation. J Bone Joint Surg

20. Makely JT (1985) The use of allografts to reconstruct intercalary defects of long bones. Clin Orthop 197: 58–75

21. Mankin HJ (1983) Complications of allograft surgery. In: Friedlaender GE, Mankin HJ, Sell KW (eds) Osteochondral allografts. Little Brown, Boston, pp 259–274

22. Mankin HJ, Doppelt SH, Sullivan TR, Tomford WW (1982) Osteoarticular and intercalary allograft transplantation in the management of malignant tumors of bone. Cancer 50: 613–630

23. Mankin HJ, Doppelt SH, Tomford WW (1983) Clinical experience with allograft implantation: the first 200 cases. Clin Orthop 174: 69–86

24. Mankin HJ, Fogelson FS, Thrasher AZ, Jaffer E (1976) Massive resection and allograft replacement in the treatment of malignant bone tumors. N Engl J Med 294: 1247–1255

25. Marcove RC, Rosen G (1978) En bloc resections for osteogenic sarcoma. Cancer 45: 3040–3044

26. McDermott AGP, Langer F, Pritzker KPH, Gross AE (1985) Fresh small-fragment osteochondral allografts: long term follow-up study on first 100 cases. Clin Orthop 197: 96–102

27. Mnaymneh W, Malinin TI, Makely JT, Dick HM (1986) Massive osteoarticular allografts in the reconstruction of extremities following resection of tumors not requiring chemotherapy and radiation. Clin Orthop 9: 666–677

28. Rosenberg AG, Mankin HJ (1986) Complications of allograft surgery. In: Epps CH (ed) Complications in Orthopaedic Surgery, 2nd edn, vol 2. Lippincott, Philadelphia, pp 1385–1417

29. Sim FH, Chao EYS (1983) Segmental prosthetic replacement of the hip and knee. In: Chao EYS, Ivins JC (eds) Tumor prostheses for bone and joint reconstruction. Thieme-Stratton, New York, pp 247–266
30. Sim FH, Ivins JC, Taylor WF, Chao EYS (1985) Limb-sparing surgery of osteosarcoma: Mayo Clinic experience. Canc Treatment Symposia 3: 139–154
31. Smith RJ, Mankin HJ (1977) Allograft replacement of the distal radius for giant cell tumor. J Hand Surg 2: 299–309
32. Stauffer RN (1982) Ten year followup study of total hip replacement: with particular reference to roentgenographic loosening of the components. J Bone Joint Surg 64A: 983–990
33. Sutherland CJ, Wilde AH, Borden LS, Marks KE (1982) A ten year follow-up of one hundred consecutive Muller curved-stem total hip replacement arthroplasties. J Bone Joint Surg 64A: 970–982
34. Tomford WW (1983) Cryopreservation of articular cartilage. In: Friedlaender GE, Mankin HJ, Sell KW (eds) Osteochondral allografts. Little Brown, Boston, pp 215–218
35. Tomford WW, Doppelt SH, Friedlaender GE (1983) 1983 bone bank procedure. Clin Orthop 174: 15–21
36. Tomford WW, Duff GP, Mankin HJ (1985) Experimental freeze-preservation of chondrocytes. Clin Orthop 197: 11–14
37. Tomford WW, Mankin HJ (1983) Investigational approaches to articular cartilage preservation. Clin Orthop 174: 22–27
38. Watari S, Ikuta Y, Adachi N et al. (1978) Vascular pedicle fibular transplantation as treatment for bone tumors. Clin Orthop 133: 158–164
39. Weiland AJ, Daniel RK (1979) Microvascular anastamosis for bone grafts in the treatment of massive defects in bone. J Bone Joint Surg 61A: 98–104
40. Wilson PD Jr (1972) Biomechanical behavior of massive bone transplants. Clin Orthop 87: 81–109
41. Wilson PD Jr, Lance EM (1875) Surgical reconstruction of the skeleton following segmental resection for bone tumors. J Bone Joint Surg 47A: 1629–1656
42. Wood MB, Cooney WP, Irons GB (1985) Skeletal reconstruction by vascularized bone transfer: indications and results. Mayo Clinic Proc 60: 729–734
43. Mankin HJ, Gebhardt MC (1987) Allografts in the management of bone tumors: A 1987 update. Surgical Rounds
44. Gebhardt MC, McGuire MH, Mankin HJ (1987) Resection and allograft arthrodesis for malignant bone tumors of the extremity. In: Enneking WF (ed) Limbs salvage in musculoskeletal oncology. Churchill Livingstone, New York

Operative Methods in Functional Reconstruction of Massive Giant Cell Tumors of the Proximal End of the Tibia

NORIYA AKAMATSU[1]

Summary. A 23-year-old female patient was operated on with curettage and bone graft for a giant cell tumor in the proximal end of the left tibia 2 years ago at another hospital. Roentgenograms at our clinic revealed absorption of transplanted bone chips and destruction of the whole proximal end of the tibia invaded by recurrent tumor. She was treated with resection of the proximal end of the tibia including the joint cartilage followed by replacement with a custom-made endoprosthesis designed with reconstruction of the anterior and posterior cruciate ligaments. The patient is able to flex up to 100° with extension lag of 5° and walks without instability of the involved knee 3 years after surgery. The second patient, a 43-year-old female, had a tumor in the proximal end of the left tibia. She was treated by partial resection of the tumor without sacrificing the articular cartilage followed by cryosurgery and transplantation, using a filler of alumina ceramics mixed with bone chips as autograft, which was not sufficient to pack the cavity. This patient has full flexion of the knee without recurrence 8 years after surgery. This is the longest follow-up in the world with this method. Another patient was operated on using the same procedure.

Key words: Tibial endoprosthesis—Iliotibial band—High-density polyethylene

Introduction

The ideal method of treatment of giant cell tumors of the bone is massive resection including the tumor itself. One of the most important problems after resection, however, is functional reconstruction of the involved joint.

Infection and skin necrosis at the site of the proximal end of the tibia are frequently experienced in comparison with the distal part of the femur, although arthroplasty using the hinged type of artificial joint has been performed to reduce the problem [1]. Replacement with an endoprosthesis, however, is not indicated for the knee because of the instability in walking.

We have developed new methods for treatment of giant cell tumors in the proximal end of the tibia.

---

[1] Department of Orthopaedic Surgery, Yamanashi Medical College, Yamanashi, Japan

Material and Method

Case 1

The patient was a 23-year-old female who underwent curettage and bone graft for a giant cell tumor in the proximal end of the left tibia 2 years previously at another hospital. Roentgenograms at our clinic revealed absorption of transplanted bone chips and destruction of the whole proximal end of the tibia invaded by recurrent tumor. She was admitted to our hospital and total resection of the proximal end of the tibia including the joint cartilage was followed by replacement with a custom-made endoprosthesis, consisting of high-density polyethyrene (HDP) and stainless steel. The prosthesis was designed with reconstruction of the anterior and posterior cruciate ligaments using an iliotibial band to reduce instability of the joint. The patient is able to flex up to 100° with an extension lag of 5° and walks without instability of the involved knee 3 years after surgery (Fig. 1).

Case 2

The patient was a 43-year-old female with a giant cell tumor of the bone in the proximal end of the left tibia and was treated by partial resection, involving the tumor without sacrificing the articular cartilage, following by cryosurgery and transplantation. A filler of alumina ceramics mixed with bone chips was used as an autograft, which was not sufficient to pack the cavity after resection. The patient is well and has full flexion of the knee without recurrence 8 years after surgery (Fig. 2). The same operation was carried out on the proximal end of the left tibia in another patient, a 37-year-old male. This patient also has full flexion of the left knee 6 months after surgery without recurrence.

Results and Discussion

The best treatment of giant cell tumors of the proximal end of the tibia is massive resection including the tumor itself, although functional reconstruction of the involved joint after resection is difficult.

The hinged type of artificial joint is not ideal as bone and cartilage in the joint are sacrificed too much. Replacement by an endoprosthesis is not indicated for the knee because of the instability in walking.

The treatment at our clinic for giant cell tumors is as follow. We prefer to perform a partial resection involving the tumor without sacrificing the articular cartilage, followed by cryosurgery [2] and transplantation using a filler of alumina ceramics as biomaterial [3] mixed with bone chips; an autograft is not sufficient to pack the cavity after resection of the tumor [4].

An endoprosthesis with reconstruction of the anterior and posterior cruciate ligaments using an iliotibial band to protect against instability is indicated for such a massive tumor invasion as a recurrent giant cell tumor.

The endoprosthesis consists of the proximal part of the tibia made of HDP with a hold and cavity, in which the anterior and posterior cruciate ligaments are

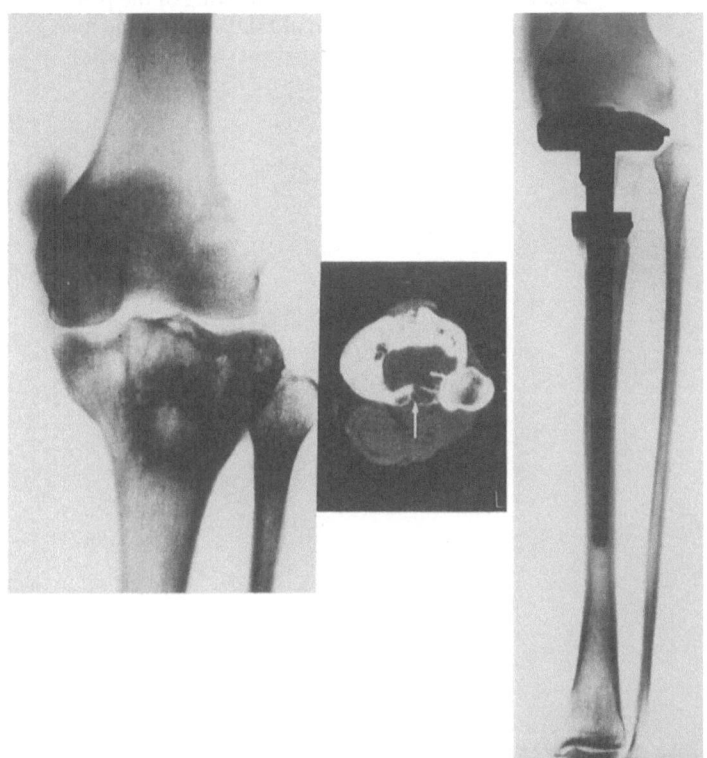

Fig. 1a, b. The result in case 1. **a** At surgery, *arrow* indicates the recurrent tumor; **b** $2\frac{1}{2}$ years after surgery

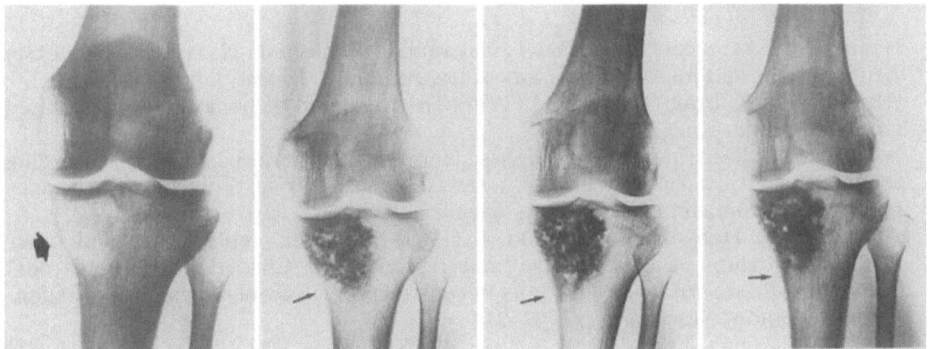

Fig. 2a–d. The result in case 2. **a** At surgery, *thick arrow* location of the tumor; **b** 3 years after surgery; **c** $4\frac{1}{2}$ years after surgery; **d** 5 years after surgery. *Thin arrows* radiolucent area later filled by newly formed bone

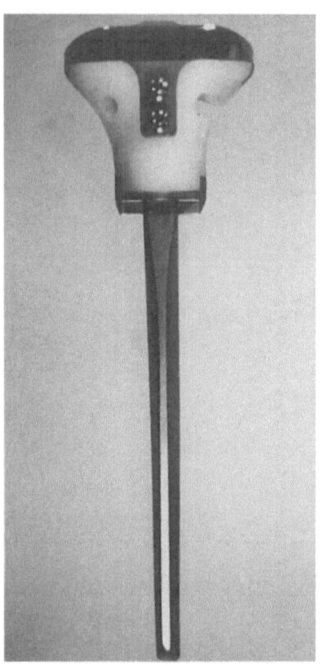

Fig. 3. The endoprosthesis, consisting of the proximal part of the tibia made of HDP with a hold and cavity

inserted using an iliotibial band (Fig. 3). A bone fragment with the patellar tendon is screwed into part of the tuberositas tibiae to reconstruct the extension apparatus.

References

1. Hamada Y, Akamatsu N, Kohzaki T, Nakajima I, Fukushima H, Asanuma K (1981) Artificial bone and joint to the tumors of low extremity. J Joint Surg 1: 57–72
2. Akamatsu N, Kohzaki T, Sawai H (1980) The treatment of bone tumors originated around the knee. Knee 6: 40–45
3. Akamatsu N (1985) Design of multiphase biomechanical materials research regarding ceramics on artificial bone and joint. In: Report of special project research, supported by the Ministry of Education, Science and Culture, Japan. pp 171–174
4. Akamatsu N, Hamada Y, Kohzaki T (1983) Prosthetic replacement and other methods of treatment after massive bone resection. In: Chao EYS, Ivins JC (eds) Tumor prostheses for bone and joint reconstruction—The design and application. Thieme-Stratton, New York, pp 207–214

Total Knee Prosthesis After Upper Tibia Resection for Tumors

Report of 42 French Cases

G. Missenard[1], B. Tomeno[2], F. Langlais[3], J.F. Dubousset[4], B. Augereau[5], E. Schvingt[6], F. Bonnel[7], P. Denayer[8], P. Groulier[9], A. Trifaud[9], and J. Vidal[7]

Summary. Forty-two resections of the upper tibia (average 15.5 cm) were reconstructed by cemented prostheses, either by hinge (23 cases) or rotating hinge (19 cases) Guepar prostheses. Twenty-eight patients were under 19 year of age, and 32 had osteosarcoma. A minimum follow-up of 6 months (average 22 months) was required for the clinical results and of 18 months for the radiological study (up to 9 years).

There were ten cases of metastasis, five of recurrence, and eleven of reoperation for mechanical complications (three with infection, mostly secondary to skin necrosis, five with rupture or adherence of the extensor apparatus, one with slipping of the PE (polyethylene) axle bushings), and two ruptures of femoral component.

The clinical results were satisfactory in 66% of cases (30/42), but in 12 cases an extension lag of 10° or more was observed.

Radiological examination showed no loosening and no modification of the radiological pattern in adults even at long-term follow-up. But in younger patients, proximal bone resorption occurred as a consequence of the rigidity of the stellite stems and thus of stress shielding. No influence, either clinical or radiological, of the prosthetic kinematics (rotating hinge or not) and of sleeving the prosthetic stem with allografts could be demonstrated.

We advocate cement fixation of titanium alloy stems, reinsertion of the extensor apparatus on a medial gastrocnemius flap, no trochleopatellar prostheses in younger patients, and a design of the prosthesis limiting stress shielding. Early mobilization is less important than reliable fixation of the patellar tendon, as a secondary surgical release of the extensor apparatus can improve the range of active flexion if stiffness has occurred.

Key words: Total knee prosthesis—Upper tibia resection—Upper tibia tumors—Gastrocnemius flap

[1] Centre Hospitalier Universitaire St Vincent de Paul, Paris, France
[2] Centre Hospitalier Universitaire Cochin, Paris, France
[3] Centre Hospitalier Universitaire "Hôpital Sud", Rennes, France
[4] Institute Gustave Roussy, Villejuif, France
[5] Centre Hospitalier Universitaire St Antoine, Paris, France
[6] Centre Hospitalier Universitaire Hautepierre, Strasbourg, France
[7] Centre Hospitalier Universitaire La Peyronie, Montpellier, France
[8] Université Catholique de Louvain, Brussels, Belgium
[9] Centre Hospitalier Universitaire La Conception, Marseille, France

Clinical Aspects

General Data

The French series of massive knee protheses for tumors of the upper tibia includes 42 cases (19 females, 23 males) from several French orthopedic centers.

The mean age was 22 years with the following distribution:

<10 years,	1 case
10–19 years,	27 cases
20–29 years,	5 cases
30–39 years,	3 cases
40–49 years,	2 cases
50–59 years,	2 cases
60–69 years,	2 cases

The tumors concerned were:
32 osteosarcomas
4 fibrosarcomas
3 chondrosarcomas
3 other malignant tumors

The postpostoperative follow-up period (average 22 months) was:

0.5–1 years	12 cases
1–2 years	13 cases
2–3 years	9 cases
3–4 years	4 cases
4–5 years	2 cases
>5 years	2 cases

The length of resection mean 15.5 cm (minimum 9 cm, maximum 28 cm) was:

≤10 cm	3 cases
11–15 cm	15 cases
16–20 cm	13 cases
≤20 cm	11 cases

Prothesis

In six patients a modified Lagrange-Letournel prothesis was used; however this rotatory prothesis without a femoropatellar component had to be quickly abandoned because of two ruptures of the femoral component.

For the 36 others patients, a Guepar prothesis was used, though with some minor variations according to the different operators and periods: 13 cases with a rotatory system, four with a system allowing growth, 11 with a trochleopatellar component, and eight with an allograft surrounding the tibial stem. In ten of the cases a metallic axle metallic was used, while in the other 26 the metallic axle was "protected" by a polyethylene cylinder (this latter idea was probably bad: we observed early wear of the polyethylene; one case required reoperation for axle change and some others have shown evolutive axial laxity).

Oncological Results

Five recurrences were observed; four were not reoperated because of metastasis, and one was amputated. Metastatic diffusions were noted in ten cases (five patients have already died).

Orthopedic Complications

No *death* was secondary to surgery but local complications occurred in 18/42 patients (43%).

Five peroneal nerve palsies (four partial, one total) were observed due to the resection; they were related to the extent of the tumor and not to the prosthetic replacement.

There were three cases of *early complications* as a result of infection, isolated or associated with skin nécrosis, leading to: amputation (one case), healing after reoperation (one case), and chronic sepsis (one case), not reoperable because of the poor quality of the soft tissues after massive X-ray therapy.

Late complications requiring reoperation occurred in ten cases: stiff joints in three, ruptures of the extensor system in two, postoperative femur fractures in two, femoral component breakage (Lagrange-Letournel), and axle change in one.

Functional Results

According to Enneking's criteria we noted 13 excellent results in spite of four postoperative complications, 17 good results in spite of seven cases with postoperative complications, seven fair results (two because of complications), and five poor results (four because of complications).

The following is an analysis of 41 cases (the case of early amputation for sepsis mentioned above is excluded.)

The absence of pain was common (36 excellent, 5 good, 0 fair, 0 poor). Strength was less satisfactory (8 excellent, 21 good, 10 fair, 2 poor). Stability was always excellent and deformities were infrequent (four with 1-cm, one with 2-cm, and one with 3-cm shortening). The scores were on the whole satisfactory for acceptance (26 excellent, 10 good, 4 fair, 1 poor) and activity (18 excellent, 16 good, 3 fair, 4 poor).

We experienced some problems analyzing mobility. Using Enneking's functional classification, we observed 20 excellent, 14 good, 4 fair, and 3 poor results, but we are not really satisfied with this grading of mobility, which only considers total range of motion and flexion contracture because in some cases unsatisfactory results are due to a lack of active extension of the knee. This problem of reconstitution of the patellar tendon will be analyzed later depending on the technique used for the extensor system repair.

Discussion on Quality of Functional Results

Age, sex, type of tumor do not influence the length of resection.

The results are stable at follow-up.

The lagrange-Letournel prothesis should not be employed because of the frequent mechanical failures (2/6); we are, however, satisfied with the results using the Guepar prothesis.

With Enneking's criteria the following items were seen to have no influence on the results: the presence or absence of an allograft around the tibial stem, rotatory or nonrotatory system, presence or absence of trochleopatellar component.

Factors having a negative influence on results seemed to be: X-ray therapy before surgery (two cases—one infected and with a stiff joint, one with a poor mobility), presence of postoperative complications, problems of active extension, and axles "protected" by a polyethylene cylinder.

In conclusion, the results are quite good for pain, stability, deformity, activity, and acceptance; they are less satisfactory for strength and mobility (especially in active knee extension). Rehabilitation usually needs 6–12 months (repair of the extensor mechanism, involving postoperative immobilization).

Factors of Tolerance of Knee Prostheses for Upper Tibia Resection

Long-term tolerance of implants may be anticipated from their middle-term radiological pattern: At 5 years, the prognosis of a prosthesis is better if no change has occurred since implantation than if a progressive radiolucency is noticed, even if it is an asymptomatic one. All our 42 prostheses were hinge or rotating hinge total knee prostheses with cemented stems.

With regard to radiological evaluation, we will first describe its usual patterns and then the influence of age, length of resection, sleeving of the stem with allograft, and prosthesis kinematics (hinge rotating or not).

Usual Radiological Patterns

Among the 23 patients with a follow-up of 18 months to 9 years, 16 underwent radiological evaluation at last examination; four others had had a recurrence, and for three there was insufficient X-ray material.

The radiological evolution was very encouraging: Only one femoral component became loose after a traumatic fracture, but the pain remained moderate and did not require revision. The tibial component showed no radiolucency (except two cases with a chronic infection, which presented only a partial proximal osteolysis) and no pain related to impairment of the initial fixation. This good tolerance occurred although 13 of the 16 patients had received intense chemotherapy, and two a radiotherapy of 35 and 72 Gy.

With respect to bone remodeling, there was an obvious difference between two age-groups: Almost no remodeling occurred in adult patients (over 18 years of age, when growth had been completed), but bone resorption, often severe, occurred in most patients less than 18 years. We did not notice among the eight adult patients any significant modification of the remnant tibia: There was no thickening or narrowing of the cortex, nor were there endocortical cysts even at 9 years (Fig. 1). In three cases with a resection of more than 150 mm, we only noted slight bone resorption at the implantation zone (2 or 3 mm).

In the eight younger patients, no loosening could be observed despite the

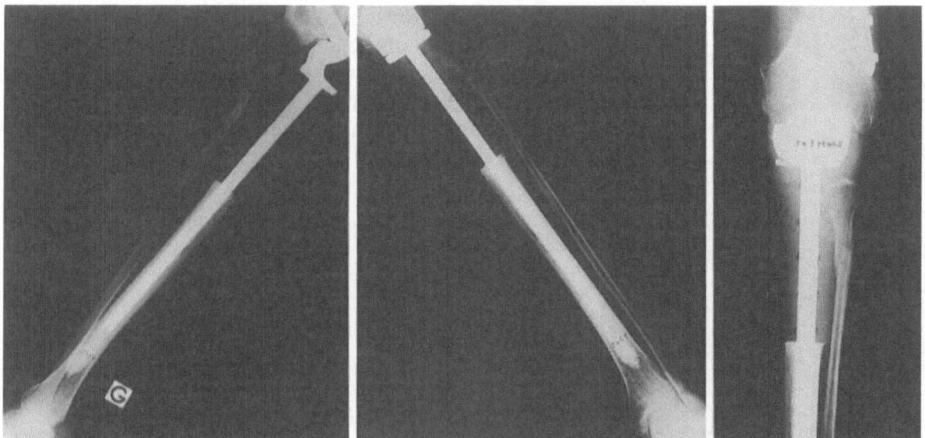

a, b   **c**

Fig. 1a–c. Long-term tolerance of prosthesis. **a** At 1 year; **b** at 6 years; **c** at 9 years. The patient was age 51 when he had a resection of 150 mm for a fibrosarcoma of the upper tibia, reconstructed with a Guepar cemented prosthesis. Despite an active way of life, neither loosening nor bone remodeling can be noticed 9 years later.

patients leading a very active life. However, in five, we detected important bone resorption of 25%–50% of the cortex, with narrowing of the medial cortex of 2 or 3 mm and of the lateral cortex of 1 or 2 mm; it extended from 20–50 mm under the level of resection. This bone resorption could be observed at 6 months; it was asymptomatic and nonevolutive with a similar pattern at 50 months, our longest radiological follow-up (Fig. 2). Resorption was small in three other patients, but although they were under 18 years of age they had already attained adult size at the time of the operation.

A comparison of the development in adult and younger patients suggests that the major factor of bone remodeling is the difference in sensitivity between growing bone and adult bone to the modification of local stresses induced by the prosthesis. However, it may also be noted that the remnant tibia was not subjected to the same mechanical condition in the two groups of patients.

In adult patients, the average level of resection was the middle third of the diaphysis, whereas in younger patients the average level of resection was more distal. Thus, the zone of implantation of the stem in younger patients was in the most poorly vascularized part of the tibia.

In younger patients, the diameter of the tibial stem (average 12 mm) was important compared with the diameter of the tibial shaft. In the five cases with significant resorption, the ratio of stem to shaft was 56%. Such a large stem of very rigid metal, especially as it was made of stellite, induced important stress shielding of the proximal cortex and favored resorption (Fig. 3; Tables 1, 2). With regard to adult patients, the diameter of the shaft was more important, but the average diameter of the stem was only 13 mm, i.e., with a smaller ratio of stem to shaft and thus less stress shielding.

However, the age of the patients remained a more important factor than rigidity of the stem: in the three adults with a resection of over 170 mm and a ratio of 55%, no severe resorption was observed.

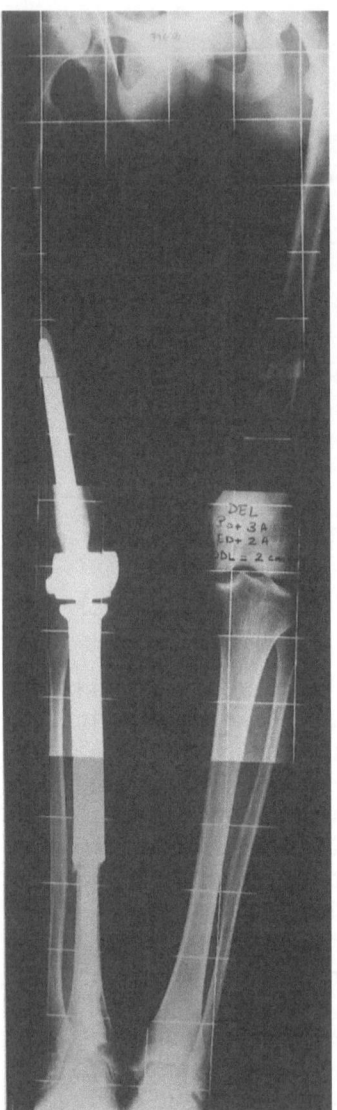

Fig. 2. Bone remodeling in young patient (male). The patient, shown here at age 14 underwent resection of 200 mm of the upper tibia for osteosarcoma and reconstruction with a Guepar rotatory hinge prosthesis 30 months ago. Bone resorption related to stress shielding was noticed at 6 months without further development and clinical influence

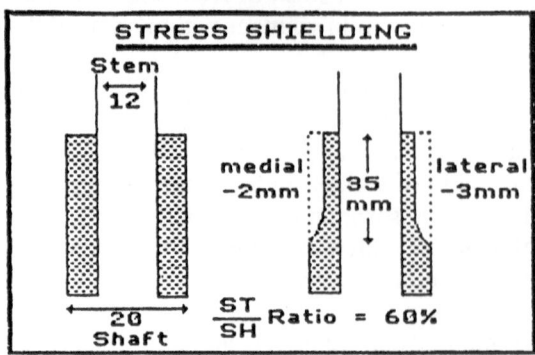

Fig. 3. The stem to shaft ratio and the average radiological pattern after 6 months in younger patients

Table 1. Bone remodeling in 16 cases at middle-term follow-up

Adults[a]		Children[b]	
No modification	Slight resorption	Moderate resorption	Severe resorption
5	3	3	5
	Resection > 170mm, rotatory hinge	Growth achieved	Nonevolutive, asymptomatic for 6 months

[a] Over the age of 18 years
[b] Eighteen years and under

Table 2. Kinematics of the prosthesis

Adults[a]		Children[b]	
No modification	Slight resorption	Resorption	Severe resorption
5	3	5	3
Hinge	Rotatory hinge Resection ≥ 170mm	Hinge Resorption related to age and resection length	Rotatory hinge Resection ≥ 200 mm

[a] Over the age of 18 years
[b] Eighteen years and under

Length of Resection

Is there a maximum length of resection over which there are increased risks of complications, insufficient functional results, or poor fixation of the stem? We studied a group of 11 cases with a resection of 200 mm or more and with an average follow-up of 21 months.

Such a resection was justified by the severe extension of the tumor and explains the four recurrences observed. Yet, despite the importance of resection, no mechanical complication was observed, and the knee functional results were similar to those of other cases of tibial resection: four excellent, four good, two fair, one poor (total results of 42 cases were: 13 excellent, 17 good, 7 fair, 5 poor), with an average range of active motion of 5 to 110 degrees.

Radiological evolution was especially assessed in the four patients who did not show recurrence and with a follow-up of 18–50 months. All were younger patients who had received intense chemotherapy for osteosarcoma. bone resorption of the proximal cortex was important (25%–50%) and occurred before 6 months; however, it showed no development for up to 50 months and was not associated with any pain despite intense activity on the part of the patients.

Thus, if 200-mm resection is necessary for a tumor excision reconstruction with a prosthesis can be used, as it gives generally good functional and radiological results at least in the midterm. Yet to limit bone resorption, improvement of prosthesis design (in order to limit stress shielding) and sleeving of the resection part of the tibial stem with allografts may be useful.

Allograft Sleeved Tibial Stem

In eight cases, the tibial stem of the prosthesis was sleeved with an allograft (average length 125 mm), generally sterilized by gamma radiation (2.5 Mrad) [1, 2]. At short-term follow-up (average 11 months, maximum 24 months), no positive or negative incidence of these allografts was evident.

There was only one complication not related to the allograft, which was one case of sepsis (following resection of a recurrent tumor treated 10 years earlier by 72-Gy irradiations). The functional result of the other cases was favorable but not different from average tibial resection results (three excellent, three good, one fair, one poor).

Radiographic evaluation showed that consolidation was obtained in all cases at 9 months, and at 3 months in most of the cases in which cancellous autografts sleeved the junction between the tibia and allograft. In seven cases, no radiological modification of the allograft was evident (no resorption, densification, radiolucency), but in one case global resorption occurred without clinical consequences.

At short-term follow-up, no disadvantage of reconstruction with allograft and prosthesis was observed, but a longer follow-up is needed to know if rehabilitation occurs and favors long-term fixation of the prosthesis by increasing the bone stock (Fig. 4). Concerning the operative technique, the allograft must be considered as an inert material, not reliable for an exclusive reinsertion of the patellar tendon, which has to be fixed on living tissues, and especially on a muscular flap.

Hinge or Rotatory Articulation?

We studied fixation of the stem and bone remodeling in the 16 patients with a radiological follow-up of over 18 months. Ten prostheses were Guepar II type hinge prostheses (five in adults, five in younger patients) and six prostheses were rotating hinge (either Lagrange-Letournel type, abandoned because of mechanical failures of the hinge bushings, or modified Guepar type). No femoropatellar subluxation or dislocation were observed whatever the type, but the patients with rotating hinges seemed to have better functional comfort than the others.

The rotation possibility of the prosthesis did not modify the radiological patterns of bone resorption, as it is more related to stress shielding and vascularization than to torque stresses.

In the eight adults no resorption was noticed with the five Guepar hinge; but in three cases of long resection with a rotating hinge, the device could not prevent small resorption (2 or 3 mm high) at the level of resection. In the eight younger patients, three rotatory hinges were used in 200-mm resection and did

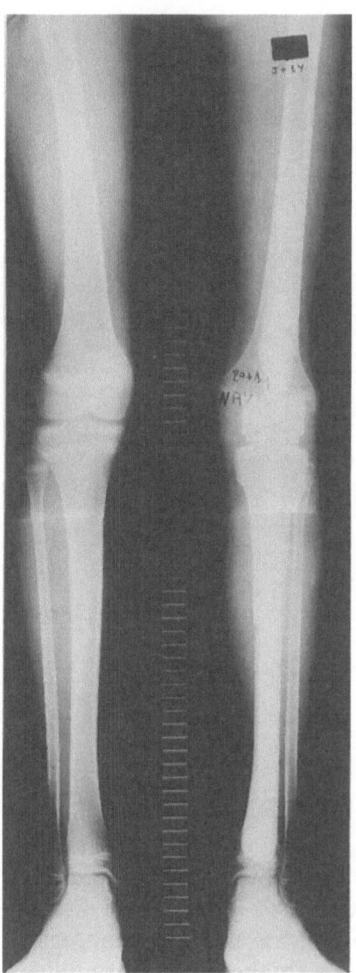

Fig. 4. Allograft of the tibia. The patient was a female at age 13 who underwent resection of 150 mm for osteosarcoma and reconstruction with a rotating hinge prosthesis sleeved by an allograft. At 1 year, the clinical result was good, with fusion of the allograft

not reduce tibial cortex resorption.

Thus, a rotatory prosthesis may be used only if its mechanical resistance is equivalent to a single-hinge prosthesis. Reduction of torque stresses on tibial and femoral fixation has no consequences, as bone remodeling is mainly related to stress shielding due to the rigidity of the stem [3] and to the level of resection needed for tumor excision. Yet a rotatory prosthesis may have the advantage of limiting stresses on the prosthetic components and, thus, the slipping of polyethylene parts.

Discussion

Reconstruction with a cemented total knee prosthesis may be advocated after tibial tumor excisions as it gives good functional results without radiological evidence of deterioration of fixation. No loosening was observed in 16 cases

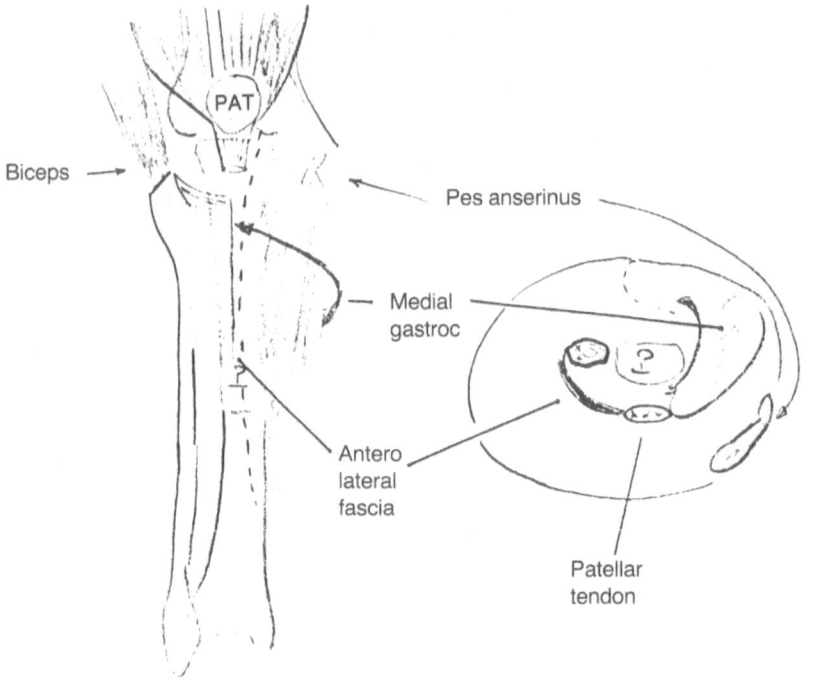

Fig. 5. Preparation stage in procedure A

with a follow-up of 18 months to 9 years, although 13 patients had chemotherapy, even in 11 patients who required a resection of 200 mm or more. There was no obvious consequence with respect to function, complications, and radiological evaluation, either to the kinematics of the prosthesis (hinge or rotatory hinge) [4] or to the allograft sleeving of the stem. However, we continue to use these techniques, the benefits of which may only be assessed after a longer follow-up. Significant resorption is observed in young patient after 6 months. Although no development was noticed and there was no clinical consequence, it would be better to reduce stress shielding: Instead of a rigid stellite stem, we suggest the use of titanium alloy with a lower modulus and the improvement of stress transmissions to the proximal cortex in the design of the prosthesis [5]. For this purpose we plan to use for the upper tibia the titanium conical grafts (TCG) system that we already use for upper femur resection; it has a conical stem, covered at its upper intramedullary part by a titanium mesh, which may favor ingrowth and better transmissions of stresses to the bone at this level.

Proximal Tibia Resection: Reconstruction of Patellar Tendon Complications and Functional Results

Proximal tibia resection creates two serious problems—Primary wound healing and reconstitution of quadriceps insertion.

Fig. 6. After suture in procedure A

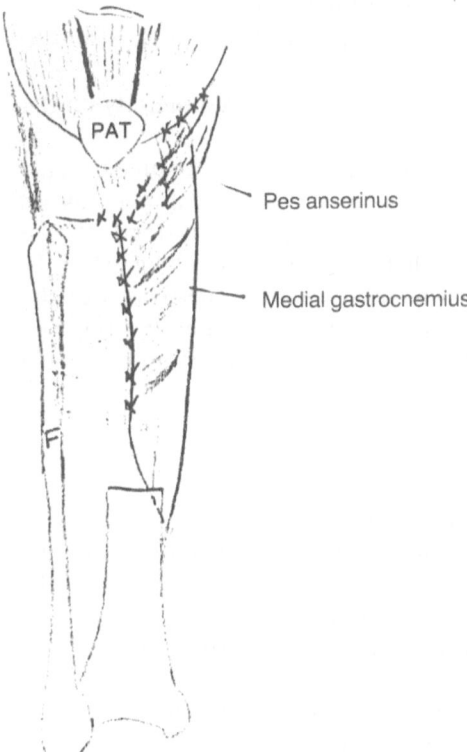

Pes anserinus

Medial gastrocnemius

Forty-two patients (23 males, 19 females) with upper tibia bone sarcoma underwent limb-sparing surgery. The tumors were principally osteosarcoma, fibrosarcoma, and chondrosarcoma. Depending on the surgeon and on the soft tissue resection, four procedures of patellar tendon reinsertion were used: In 28 cases a medial gastrocnemius transposed flap (MGTF) was used. The following two procedures were carried out.

Procedure A

The medial gastrocnemius is released from its femoral and lateral gastrocnemius insertions (Figs. 5, 6). This allows an anterior translation and a suture with the anterolateral fascia, in extension of the knee. Good fixation of the patellar tendon can be done on these fibrous tissues.

The difficulty with this procedure is that the reinsertion has to be done at the right place, avoiding medial or lateral translation and lowering or elevation of the patella.

Procedures B

The medial muscle is divided longitudinally from the lateral one and distally just on its tendinous insertion; the flap is turned down to up, back to front, and medially to laterally over the prosthesis just under the patella.

It is fixed by an interrupted suture to the lateral superficial aponevrosis laterally to the fibula.

The patellar tendon with medial and lateral fascia are sutured directly on the muscle.

Procedure A was used in 17 cases and procedure B in 11 cases. In nine cases, a suture on the prosthesis with the anterolateral fascia and the remaining muscles was done. In three cases, a suture on a prosthetic bioimplant was done: In one case, it was done on an allograft, in the two other cases on a Dacron ligament. In two cases, a pretibial fibula transposition was used for the reinsertions of the tendon. The fibula was transected lower than the tibial resection and screwed onto the remaining tibial shaft. The patellar tendon was sutured on the fibula head.

Postoperative Care

For 4–6 weeks, the knee is immobilized in a cast with 5°–10° of flexion. Full weight bearing with crutches is allowed on the 2nd postoperative day. Gradual rehabilitation begins after the cast is removed with isometric musculation of the quadriceps and passive flexion on a mechanical splint.

The early postoperative complications are evaluated according to different procedures.

The 28 medial gastrocnemius flaps gave one skin necrosis, which healed after surgical excision and suture, and one complete necrosis of the flap with deep infection, which required a secondary amputation after 1 month. For the nine reinsertions on the prosthesis, two deep infections occurred, one of which could be cured by surgical excision. One of the two pretibial fibulas had a skin necrosis, which was treated by a medial gastrocnemius flap. There was no serious complication of the three prosthetic ligaments.

The functional result could be rated 6 months after surgery. There were 13 excellent, 17 good, 7 fair, and 5 poor results.

Discussion

These results, of course, have to be evaluated according to the procedure used for the reconstruction of the quadriceps insertion. The two procedure which are less used (prosthetic ligament and pretibial fibula) do not seem to be very safe. The prosthetic ligament gave three secondary breaks of the patellar tendon with loss of active extension. We know that it is impossible to obtain good healing of living tendon with dead tissue. The pretibial fibula is a difficult procedure and the protrusion of the fibula is dangerous for the skin.

For the two other procedures, the functional results seem to be equal, but MGTF allows the best coverage of the prosthesis. It could avoid postoperative infection.

The different flaps gave the same rate of good and bad results, except perhaps in the case of amputation. This was done in a 9-year-old patient, who had a special growth plate salvage prosthesis, and the tibial component was perhaps too large for his leg. Flap procedure A was used, but it would have been better

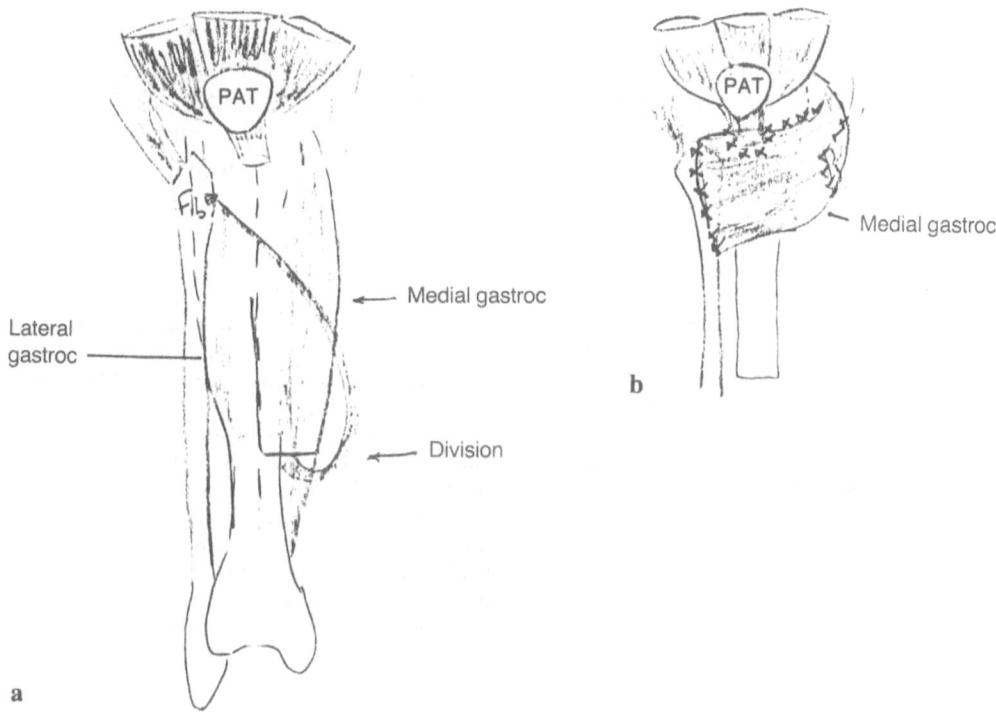

Fig. 7a,b. Procedure B. **a** Preparation stage; **b** after suture

to use B, thereby avoiding the stretching suture.

In fact, the functional results are essentially conditional upon reconstruction of the extensor apparatus and resection of the lateral tissues.

The quadriceps apparatus can give rise to two major problems—stiffness of the knee in extension or loss of active extension.

With regard to the excellent and good results, three were obtained after surgical joint mobilization done for stiffness of the knee. In these cases, the strength of the patellar tendon was good with normal active extension of the knee and flexion of more than 90°. For the six fair results, four were secondary to failures of active extension. In one of these cases, the reason was due to mobilization of the knee being initiated too early, but in the three other cases there was no evident fault. Two of these patients underwent reconstruction of the patellar tendon with a graft. They did not achieve a better result after this procedure. It seems that is more expedient first to have good strength of the patellar tendon, even with some stiffness of the knee. In fact, it is easier to cure this stiffness than to try a new extensor apparatus reconstitution.

The two other patients with fair results had correct active extension but the walk is difficult. In these cases, the tumors involved a large part of the bone (more than 20 cm) and soft tissues. Resection of all the lateral muscles with the sciatic nerve was, therefore, carried out.

Conclusion

Reconstitution of the patellar tendon must be done on a well-vascularised tissue. If there is no remaining soft tissue, a medial gastrocnemius flap can be easily used; it allows prosthesis coverage and optimal healing of the skin. This could perhaps reduce the high rate of complications in this type of surgery.

References

1. Hernigou P, Delepine G, Goutallier D (1986) Massive freeze dried and irradiated bone allografts. Rev Chir Orthop 6: 403–413
2. Poitout D (1985) Homogreffes osseuses massives. Cahiers Enseignement SOFCOT: 23. Expansion Scientifique, Paris, pp 157–177
3. Langlais F, Aubriot JH, Postel M, Tomeno B, Vielpeau C (1986) Prothèse de reconstruction de l'extrémité supérieure du fémur. Résultats à moyen terme de 20 résections pour tumeurs. Orientations actuelles. Rev Chir Orthop 6: 415–425
4. Langlais F, Aubriot JH, Tomeno B, Vielpeau C (submitted) Prothèse Guepar de reconstruction de l'extrémité inférieure du fémur. Résultats à moyen terme de 20 résections pour tumeurs. Orientations actuelles. Rev Chir Orthop
5. Langlais F, Postel M, Aubriot JH, Blanquaert D (1987) The TCG prosthesis system. In: Enneking WF (ed) Limb salvage in musculoskeletal oncology. Churchill Livingstone, New York, pp 88–94

Uncemented Hinge Prostheses with Reinsertion of the Ligamentum Patellae

RAINER KOTZ, NIKOLAUS PONGRACZ, ERICH J. FELLINGER, and PETER RITSCHL[1]

Summary. The possibilities for reconstruction after resections in the region of the knee and coverage of the prostheses by muscles, tendon attachments, and soft tissues are limiting factors to conservative tumor treatment at present. For defect bridging in bone, the Kotz Modular Femur-Tibia Reconstruction (KMFTR) system offers good possibilities. When resecting the proximal tibia, radical removal of the tumor usually also includes the tibial tubercle. The functional result depends very much on successful reattachment of the patellar ligament to the lower leg. In 13 patients with resection of the proximal tibia and endoprosthetic replacement, two different methods of reattachment of the patellar ligament were employed. Medioventral transposition of the double-osteomized fibula was opposed to ventral transposition of the proximal gastrocnemius.

Key words: Tumor endoprosthesis—Patellar ligament reconstruction

Material

From September 1982 to April 1986, a total of 70 patients had lower extremity resections for malignant bone tumors and were treated with a KMFTR system (Table 1) [1]. In 13 cases (proximal tibia in 12, a total knee in one), the tibial tubercle with the insertion of the patellar ligament had to be resected as well. There were eight male and five female patients with an average age of 24.3 years (range 16–62 years). The follow-up for these 13 patients was 31 months (range 18–59 months). The most frequent lesion was osteosarcoma. There was one Ewing's sarcoma and one fibrosarcoma; metastases of a carcinoma were present in three cases, and revision surgery after failed custom-made tumor endoprosthesis was performed in two cases (Fig. 1).

Method

Depending on the location of the tumor, a lateral, medial, ventral, or dorsal reconstruction method was chosen. The preferred method was medial and ven-

---

[1] Department of Orthopedics, University of Vienna, and Viennese Bone Tumor Registry, Vienna, Austria

Table 1. Resections with KMFTR system, September 1982 to April 1986

Resection	Number
Proximal femur	32
Distal femur	22
proximal tibia	12
Total knee	1
Total femur	3
	70

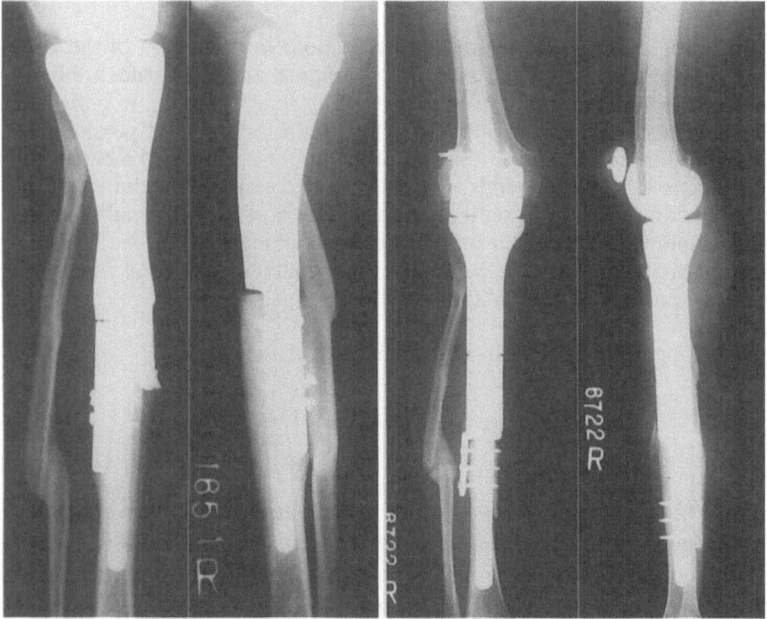

Fig. 1. Failed custom-made tumor endoprosthesis (G.D., aged 16 years, female). Revision surgery with KMFTR system

tral transposition of the fibula after double osteotomy of the fibula and suturing of the fibular collateral ligament to the patellar ligament (Fig. 2) [2]. Here, fixation of the transplant to the bar in the middle of the prosthesis with a few fixation sutures has proved worthwhile. This can keep the fibula in place until the osteotomies have healed. If parts of the pes anserinus remain intact, they can also contribute to the medialization of the "tibial tubercle." Prior to the transposition, the peroneal nerve has to be mobilized from the popliteal fossa to where it gives off a branch to the anterior tibial muscle in order not to be drawn ventrally with the osteotomized fibula. This method is mainly limited by the location of the tumor. If the fibula is also involved, this method is of course precluded after resection.

When the fibula has been resected, proximal gastrocnemius transposition [3,

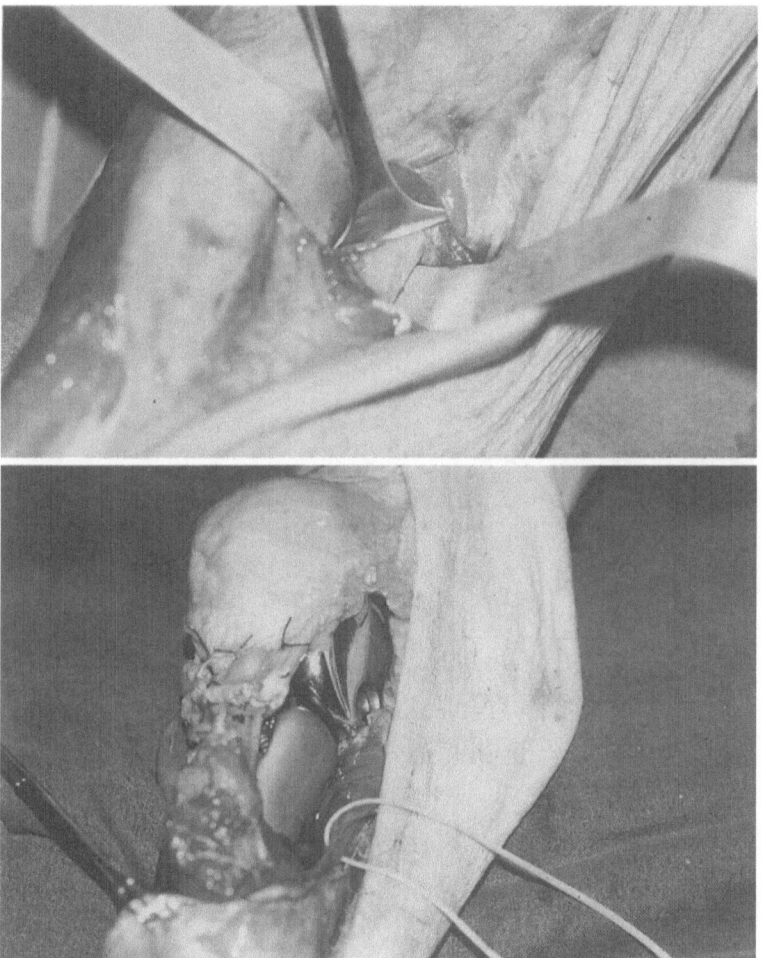

Fig. 2. Patellar ligament reconstruction technique

4,] is available (Fig. 3). The gastrocnemius is detached at its origin from the femur and transferred ventrally and distally. This procedure can be performed unilaterally or bilaterally. The advantage of gastrocnemius transposition lies in the good soft tissue coverage of the prosthesis in the case of large resections; there is, however, the disadvantage of elastic fixation of the patellar ligament to the muscles, which in most cases leads to a cranial dislocation of the patella. Here too, the bar on the prosthesis can serve for temporary fixation in the middle; the tubercle fixation plate and the screws can also occasionally be used for this purpose. The tubercle fixation plate, however, is only a temporary means of fixation and can lead to significant irritations or bursitis under the skin. Of the 13 operated patients with tibial prostheses, there were six fibula transpositions and seven transpositions of the gastrocnemius. Of the patients treated with custom-made prostheses between 1979 and 1982, a further four had fibular transpositions with tibia prostheses.

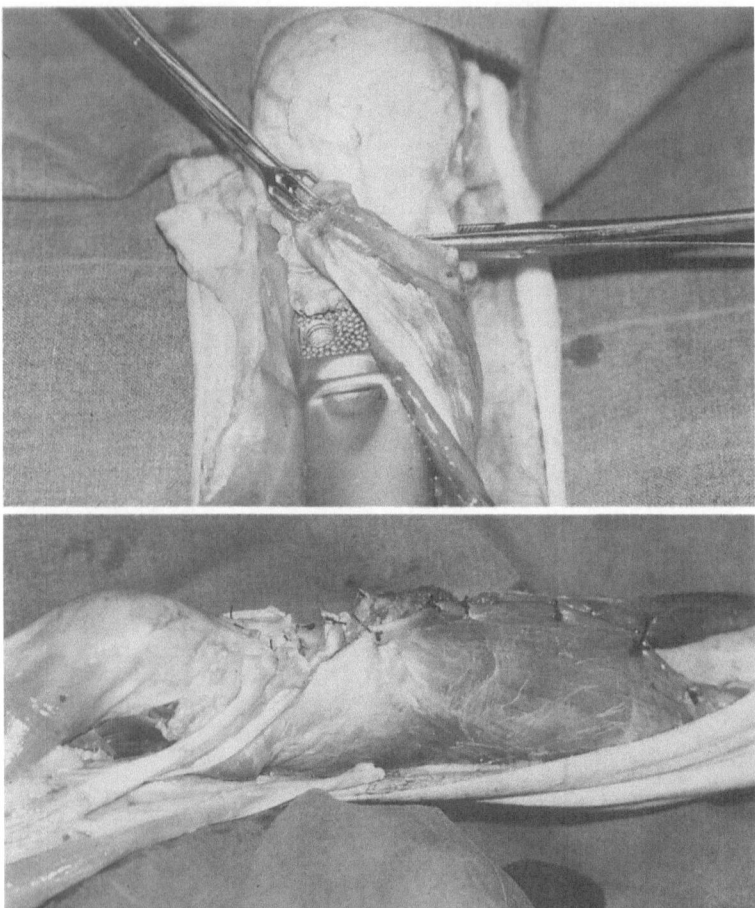

Fig. 3. Ventral and distal transposition of gastrocnemius

Complications

Corresponding to the magnitude of the interventions at the proximal tibia and the extent of the resections, complications such as peroneal palsy—transient and complete (after nerve resections)— as well as avulsions of the patellar ligament, or hematomas in need of revision could be observed (Table 2). In one case with a good clinical result of fibula transposition, amputation had to be performed because of local recurrence of a fibrosarcoma.

Results

Clinical evaluation was carried out according to the modified Enneking system. Nine patients were available for clinical examination and assessment; three pa-

Table 2. Complications

	Fibula transposition ($n = 6$)	Gastrocnemius transposition ($n = 6$)
Peroneal palsies		
Transient	1	1
Complete	2	3
(nerve resection)		
Patellar ligament		
Avulsion (R.R.)	—	2
Hematoma (R.R.)	1	2

R.R. requiring revision

Table 3. Results according to Enneking staying ($n = 9$). Part 1

	Motion	Pain	Stability/ deformity	Strength	Functional activity	Emotional acceptance
Excellent	5	7	6	5	7	8
Good	4	2	2	1	2	1
Fair	—	—	—	2	—	—
Poor	—	—	1	1	—	—

Table 4. Results according to Enneking staging ($n = 9$). Part 2

	Strength		Motion	
	Fibula transposition ($n = 3/4$)[a]	Gas trocnemius transposition ($n = 6$)	Fibula transposition ($n = 3/4$)[a]	Gastrocnemius transposition ($n = 6$)
Excellent	1 (3)[a]	4	2 (3)[a]	3
Good	2 (1)[a]	2	1 (1)[a]	—
Fair	—	—	—	2
Poor	—	—	—	1

[a] Custom-made prostheses with fibula transposition

tients had died from metastases at the time of follow-up. The results with regard to pain on motion, functional ability, and emotional acceptance were excellent in most cases; in others they were good. Only two cases were fair with regard to strength, and stability/deformity and strength were poor in one case each (Table 3). When comparing only motion and adding the four cases with fibula transposition from the custom-made prosthesis of the years, 1979–1982 to the cases with a modular prosthesis, we see a very similar distribution of four excellent and three good results (Table 4).

With regard to strength, the fibula transposition technique is better, having only excellent and good results. In the gastrocnemius transposition group, two fair, one poor, besides three excellent results were found (Table 4).

Discussion

To be able to treat proximal tibial reconstructions with endoprostheses, reconstruction of the extensor mechanism is necessary. The conventional method of gastrocnemius transposition can be compared with fibula transposition and joining of the fibular collateral ligament with the patellar ligament. With regard to radicality, fibula transposition is sometimes precluded since the fibula may have to be resected as well, or very large defects may be bridged better with the large muscle flap than by bone transposition. If, however, fibula transposition with sparing of the peroneal nerve succeeds, the result is not only good fixation of the patella and active extension but also a good cosmetic result since the transferred fibula in front of the prosthesis leads to a configuration similar to the normal tibial tubercle. Overall, one has to say that both methods have to be considered, and that based on the small advantages in function and cosmetic result, fibula transposition should be given preference if it is feasible.

Conclusion

Based on our experience with 70 tumor endoprostheses from 1982 to 1986, the functional results of 13 proximal tibial resections were reported after reconstruction of the tibial tubercle. In half of the cases, gastrocnemius transposition and in the other half fibula transposition were carried out. If fibula transposition is anatomically feasible following resection, this method should be given preference on the basis of the small functional and cosmetic advantages. In the case of large, extensive resections or location of the tumor in the vicinity of the fibula, the gastrocnemius flap procedure can also be performed successfully.

References

1. Kotz R (1983) Modular femur and tibia reconstruction system. In: Kotz R (ed) Proceedings of 2nd international workshop on the design and application of tumor prostheses for bone and joint reconstruction, Vienna, Sept. 5–8, 1983. Egermann, Vienna, pp 64–66
2. Kotz R, Engel A (1983) Cement-free design of a tumor prosthesis for osteosarcoma of the distal femur and proximal tibia with a new fixation technique for the ligamentum patellae In: Chao EYS, Ivins JV (eds) Tumor prostheses for bone and joint reconstruction—The design and application. Thieme-Stratton, New York, pp 399–408
3. Malawer MM (1983) The use of the gastrocnemius transposition flap with limb-sparing surgery for knee sarcomas: Indications and technique. In: Kotz R (ed) Proceedings of 2nd international workshop on the design and application of tumor prostheses for bone and joint reconstruction, Vienna, Sept. 5–8, 1983. Egermann, Vienna, pp 270–274
4. Dubousset J, Missenard G (1983) Insertion by aponevrotic and muscular plasties after proximal tibial replacement in osteogenic sarcoma. In: Kotz R (ed) Proceedings of 2nd international workshop on the design and application of tumor prostheses for bone and joint reconstruction, Vienna, Sept. 5–8, 1983. Egermann, Vienna, pp 275–278

Techniques of Limb-Sparing Resection and Extensor Mechanism Reconstruction for High-Grade Malignant Tumors of the Proximal Tibia

Martin M. Malawer[1] and Kathleen A. McHale[2]

Summary. Limb sparing surgery for high-grade malignant tumors of the proximal tibia is challenging due to anatomical constraints, the surgical approach, the need to reconstruct the patellar tendon/extensor mechanism, and inadequate soft tissue coverage. We report a surgical technique that permits safe resection of a large segment of the tibia and knee joint in continuity with the proximal tibiofibular joint. It includes a new and reliable method of reconstructing the patellar/extensor mechanism and of providing soft tissue coverage. We have successfully treated 11 patients with this technique and report here seven of these patients. The minimum follow-up was two years; the average follow-up was 49.5 months (range 24.6–84.4 months). There were five men and two women: the average age was 28.7 years. The histological diagnoses were osteosarcoma (four cases), malignant fibrous histiocytoma (one), chondrosarcoma (one), and radiation-induced sarcoma (one). There were two high-grade intracompartmental (stage IIA) and five high-grade extracompartmental (stage IIB) tumors. Six intra-articular resections and one extra-articular resection were performed. Four reconstructions entailed customized tibial and knee implants and three involved arthrodesis. Pathological specimens showed meniscal and patellar tendon involvement in two patients and pericapsular tibiofibular joint involvement in six. Local complications were transient peroneal nerve palsy (four patients) and superficial skin sloughs (one patient). All resections obtained negative margins with no local recurrences or metastatic disease. All patients are ambulatory; one requires a cane. Active extension with 0°–15° extension lag was obtained in patients treated by arthroplasty. The medial gastrocnemius flap is essential to provide adequate soft tissue coverage and a reliable method of reconstructing the extensor mechanism. We recommend limb sparing surgery for high-grade tumors of the proximal tibia in carefully selected patients. Routine amputations in these individuals is not justified.

Key words: Tibia—Osteosarcoma—Gastrocnemius flap

Introduction

The distal femur knee is the most common site for high-grade bone sarcomas, and the proximal tibia is the second most common site. In recent years, limb-

[1] Orthopedic Oncology Section, Children's Hospital National Medical Center, George Washington University School of Medicine, and The Washington Hospital Center, Washington DC, USA
[2] Pediatric Orthopedics, Children's Hospital National Medical Center, Washington DC, USA

sparing procedures have become well-established in the treatment of benign and malignant bone tumors. However, limb-sparing surgery for high-grade sarcomas involving the proximal tibia has been reported only rarely. Most cases of proximal tibia resections reported to date have been for giant cell tumors (GCTs) or other aggressive but benign lesions. Most surgeons, pessimistic over the outcome of resection for high-grade sarcomas, continue to recommend amputation [1].

The general lack of enthusiasm for limb sparing surgery for tumors of the proximal tibia has been due to a high rate of complications and secondary amputations following multiple surgical problems. Problems peculiar to the proximal tibia include anatomical constraints, a difficult surgical approach, inadequate soft tissue coverage, and vascular complications. Another problem unique to the proximal tibia is the need to reconstruct the patellar tendon and extensor mechanism if an arthroplasty is utilized.

There have been no specific reports on the use of surgical resection and reconstruction for high-grade sarcomas of the proximal tibia. This study describes the anatomical considerations surrounding surgery at this site and outlines our technique. A new method of extensor mechanism reconstruction is also presented (Fig. 1). We have treated a total of 11 patients with this procedure thus far; this study is limited to seven patients for whom at least 2 years' follow-up data are available.

Patients and Methods

Between 1980 and 1985, seven patients with high-grade sarcomas of the proximal tibia were treated with limb sparing procedures. There were five men and two women, whose ages ranged from 13 to 45 years (average 28.7 years). The histological diagnoses were osteosarcoma (four), male giant fibrous histiocytoma chondrosarcoma (one), and radiation-induced sarcoma (one). All tumors were staged according to the Musculoskeletal Tumor Society Staging System. Five tumors were stage IIB (high grade, extracompartmental), and two were stage IIA (high grade, intracompartmental).

Preoperative Evaluation and Patient Selection

All patients underwent extensive preoperative evaluation to determine whether the tumor was resectable. The primary criterion of resectability was the extent of local tumor; other considerations included the length of bone resection that would be required, the degrees of soft tissue, capsular, and patellar tendon involvement, and the anatomy of the popliteal trifurcation. Patients with a pathological fracture, extensive contamination from a poorly placed biopsy, tumor fungation, local sepsis, or a large posterior extraosseous component were not considered good candidates for limb preservation.

Biplane angiography is essential for local arterial evaluation. The anterior-posterior view is utilized to evaluate the popliteal trifurcation; specifically, the presence or absence of the posterior tibial artery, which may be the sole blood supply to the leg after resection. The lateral view is essential to evaluate the

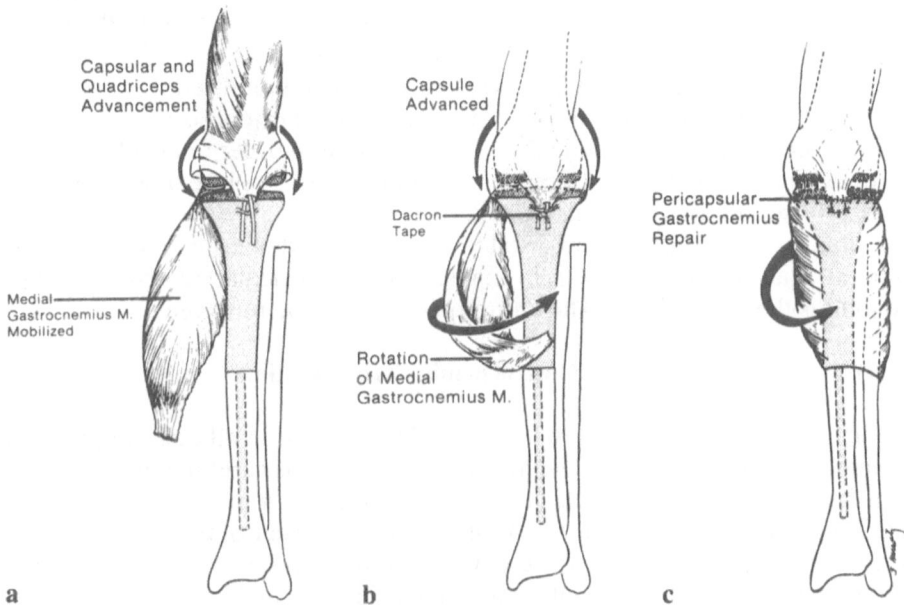

Fig. 1a–c. Schema of extensor mechanism reconstruction. **a** The medial gastrocnemius muscle is mobilized. **b** The patellar tendon is sutured to the prosthesis with Dacron tape and then the medial gastrocnemius muscle is rotated anteriorly to cover the prosthesis and knee joint. **c** the entire knee capsule is sutured to the transferred gastrocnemius muscle. This technique provides for long-term biological reconstruction of the extensor mechanism. The dacron tape (**a**) provides for protection of this suture line in the early postoperative period. The gastrocnemius transfer serves two important functions— coverage of the prothesis and a reliable method of extensor mechanism reconstruction. From [4] with permission

interval between the tibia and the neurovascular bundle. A large posterior tumor component makes resection difficult.

Surgical Technique

The limb sparing procedure has three phases: resection of the tumor, skeletal reconstruction (arthrodesis or prosthetic replacement), and muscle transfer and soft tissue reconstruction.

Resection

The initial step is exploration of the popliteal trifurcation and ligation of the anterior tibial vessels. If this interval is clear, resection proceeds. The patellar tendon is sectioned 2–3 cm proximal to the tibial tubercle, and the entire capsule of the knee is detached circumferentially by electrocautery 2–3 cm from the tibial insertion so as to be removed with the specimen. The cruciate ligaments are sectioned close to the femoral attachments and frozen sections of the proximal stumps are obtained. The capsular excision must be done *prior* to the main tibial resection and osteotomy. The posterior capsule must be dissected carefully under direct vision after the popliteal vessels have been mobilized.

An extra-articular resection of the proximal tibiofibular joint is routinely performed. A sleeve of muscle should be left on the joint in order to avoid inadvertent contamination by tumor. Care should be taken not to place tension on the peroneal nerve; otherwise, a palsy will occur.

The tibia is osteomized 6–7 cm distal to the lesion, as determined by bone and computed axial tomography (CAT) scans. An intra-articular resection of the knee joint is then completed. The entire specimen can be removed en bloc.

Soft Tissue Reconstruction and Gastrocnemius Transposition

A medial gastrocnemius transposition flap (GTF) is used in all cases to provide adequate soft tissue coverage. The medial surgal artery is carefully preserved to the medial gastrocnemius muscle (Fig. 2a). The muscle graft is spread out and rotated anteriorly over the defect and sutured to the border of the anterior muscles, forming a complete soft tissue envelope around the prosthesis (Fig. 2b). Dacron tapes sewn into the patellar tendon are tied to a highly polished loop of the tibial component. The patellar tendon is then sutured to the transferred GTF with nonabsorbable sutures and Dacron tape. The proper tension on the quadriceps mechanism is determined by bending the knee through a 40° range of motion. The medial hamstrings are reattached to the medial gastrocnemius muscle.

The soft tissue posterior to the prosthesis or arthrodesis must be closed to avoid direct contact of the neurovascular bundle with metal or grafts. At the level of the knee joint, the origins of the gastrocnemius heads are approximated; more distally, fibers of the posterior tibialis muscle and/or soleus are approximated.

Rehabilitation. The knee is restricted to 0°–30° range of motion. Rehabilitation emphasizes extensor strength rather than flexion knee flexion is increaed only after full active extension has been obtained.

Results

Type of surgery. Six intra-articular resections and one extra-articular resection were performed. In all cases, negative margins were obtained. All resections were classified as intracompartmental (wide excision). Four patients received a custom-made prosthesis (two stage IIA, two stage IIB), and three primary arthrodeses were performed (stage IIB). All seven patients had primary medial GTF flaps for soft tissue coverage.

Tumor control. There have been no local recurrences, and no patient has developed metastatic disease. One patient developed a metachronous osteosarcoma of the acetabulum 30 months after resection arthrodesis and underwent a hemipelvectomy.

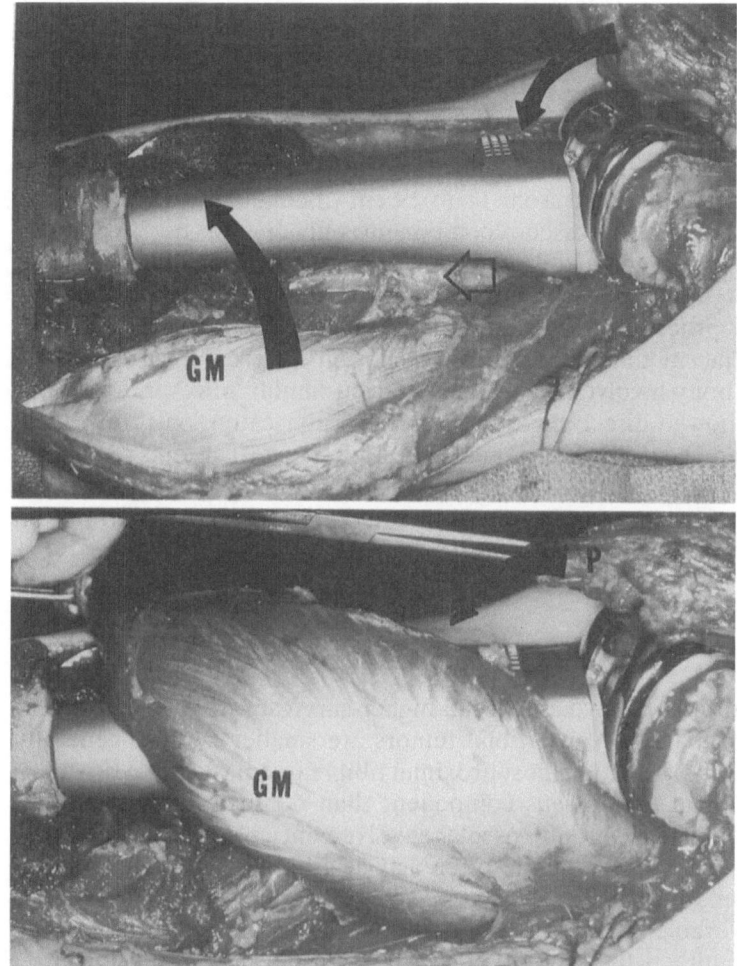

Fig. 2a, b. Proximal tibia replacement for a high-grade sarcoma. **a** Intraoperative photograph following the mobilization of the medial gastrocnemius muscle (*GM*) and the direction of rotation of the gastrocnemius muscle and the extensor mechanism (*solid arrows*). Note the popliteal vessels (*open arrow*). **b** The medial gastrocnemius muscle is rotated anteriorly to cover the prosthesis and to provide soft tissue attachment of the extensor mechanism and patellar tendon (*P*). The muscle is then splayed out to obtain complete coverage (not shown). From [4] with permission

Complications. The common complication was transient peroneal palsy, which occurred in four patients; it resolved in all cases. Skin flap necrosis, which occurred in one patient, healed satisfactorily after superficial debridement and secondary split thickness skin graft. One dislocation, a spherocentric replacement, occurred and required replacement of the tibial tracks.

Function. All patients are ambulatory; five require no orthoses or external support. Range of knee motion in the prosthetic group ranges from 80°–95° of flexion with 0°–15° of extension lag.

Pathological Findings

All gross specimens were reviewed and histological studies were performed. The length of tibial resection ranged from 11 to 19 cm (median 15 cm). Six of the seven tibial tumor had an extraosseous component; only one was not recognized preoperatively. Two patients had gross intra-articular tumor involvement. One patient demonstrated a meniscal tumor implant, presumably resulting from an initial arthroscopic procedure. Evaluation of the tibiofibular joint, pericapsular tissue, and the adjacent tibial atrticual facet showed no gross invasion of the joint by tumor or bony involvement of the adjacent fibula; however, six of the seven specimens showed direct microscopic pericapsular extension through the subchondral and adjacent cortical bone of the tibia facet. The one remaining specimen showed a tumor involving only the medial tibia metaphysis; thus, the tibiofibular joint was not at risk for involvement. Tumor did not penetrate the popliteus muscle posteriorly in any of the specimens.

Discussion

Patients with tibial tumors have an overall higher survival rate than those with femoral tumors, probably because tibial tumors are smaller and are generally detected earlier [2]. Fortunately, most proximal tibial sarcomas tend to be smaller and have less of an extraosseus component than do such lesions in other locations. Posterior extension and vascular involvement are rare; when extension does occur, the popliteus muscle often acts as a barrier to involvement of the popliteal and tibioperoneal arteries.

Given these favorable characteristics, it seems reasonable that limb sparing procedures be attempted for select tibial lesions, despite associated technical difficulties. Since 1978, 11 of 21 patients presenting with such lesions at our institution have undergone limb sparing resection; the remainder underwent an above-the-knee amputation. The majority of amputations were performed prior to 1980. In general, contraindications to resection have been sepsis, local contamination, significant posterior tumor extension, and/or the absence of a posterior tibial artery. We believe that all patients with tibial sarcomas should be considered candiates for limb sparing procedures and should undergo the appropriate staging studies.

The technique of quadriceps reconstruction as described in this study has proven to be a reliable method of soft tissue reconstuction of the extensor/ patellar mechanism [3, 5]. Reconstructing this mechanism has thus far been one of the major barriers to a successful outcome of an arthroplasty. Several techniques of extensor mechanism reconstruction have been reported, including direct suture to the prosthesis or allograft and osteotomy of the fibula with attachment to the lateral collateral ligament. We believe that the technique described in this paper provides immediate stability and allows a biological reconstruction to viable soft tissue. We avoid the preservation of the proximal fibula because of the high risk of tumor involvement of the adjacent soft tissue attachment. We intentionally shorten the extremity by 2 cm to allow the capsule and patellar tendon to reach the gastrocnemius without any tension. Extensor muscle rehabilitation, not flexion, is emphasized postoperatively.

We believe that the routine use of a medial GTF is the single most important factor in decreasing the postoperative morbidity associated with this procedure. Skin flap necrosis and secondary infection, which may be attributed to the normal subcutaneous position of the tibia and lack of adequate muscle and skin for prosthetic or graft coverage, have hitherto posed major barriers to successful resection of the tibia. Skin flap necrosis occurred in one of our seven patients; however, the GTF provided a vascularized bed for salvage by a split thickness skin graft and avoided serious sequelae that would have occurred with an exposed prosthesis. Thus, the transferred medial gastrocnemius serves two important functions: it covers the prosthesis, thereby avoiding secondary infections, and provides a means for reconstruction of the extensor mechanism.

References

1. Eckardt JJ, Eilber FR, Grant TT, Mirra JM, Weisenberger TH, Dorey FJ (1985) Management of stage IIB osteogenic sarcoma: Experience at the University of California, Los Angeles. Cancer Treatment Symposium 3: 117–130
2. Lockshin MD, Higgins TT (1968) Prognosis on osteogenic sarcoma. Clin Orthop 58: 85
3. Malawer MM (1983) The use of the gastrocnemius transposition flap with limb-sparing surgery for knee sarcomas: Indications and technique. In: Kotz R (ed) Proceedings of 2nd international workshop on the design and application of tumor prostheses for bone and joint reconstruction, Vienna, Sept. 5–8, 1983. Egermann, Vienna, pp 270–274
4. Malawer MM, McHale KA (1988) Limb-sparing surgery for high-grade malignant tumors of the proximal tibia: Surgical technique and a method of extensor mechanism reconstruction. Clin Orthop 237: 68–85
5. Malawer MM, Price WM (1984) Gastrocnemius transposition flap in conjunction with limb-sparing surgery for primary sarcoma around the knee. Plast Reconstr Surg 73: 741–749

Moderator's Comment

FRANTZ LANGLAIS[1]

From this second part of the symposium, it appears that with tumors of the upper tibia it is now obviously worth trying limb salvage procedures and that primary amputation or rotationplasty should be limited to cases with a tumoral extension to the tibio peroneal neurovascular bundle. If the bundle is spared but anterior extension of the tumor demands a large excision of the extensor apparatus, knee fusion is a reliable procedure; it can be simplified by the use of an allograft (fixed by centromedullar nailing with a custom femorotibial titanium alloy nail), or by the use of an SDR (segmental defeet reconstruction) prosthesis. If the major part of the extensor apparatus can be retained, the function of the knee should be saved. Articular allograft is of great interest in primary treatment of low-grade tumors, but in high-grade tumors total knee prosthesis seems to be more reliable.

In this global series of 42 total knee prostheses for tibial resection, the radiological survey up to 9 years showed no deterioration of the cemented stem fixations. Reconstruction by prosthesis for tumors of the upper tibia can thus be advocated as there is a low complication rate and a satisfactory average functional result, especially after the use of a gastrocnemius flap [1, 4]; the latter solves the two major difficulties—reinsertion of the patellar tendon and coverage of the prosthesis when a large soft tissue excision is required.

At present, cement fixation remains a safe method for fixation of these prostheses, as there is no evidence of future deterioration [3] and as cement may be a more reliable means of fixation than bone ingrowth in patients requiring intense postoperative chemotherapy or radiotherapy. Moreover, protection against infection by the antibiotics released from bone cement [2] may be very useful in patients with postchemotherapic leucopenia.

Whenever conservation of the femoral epiphysis is possible, it is better to embed the femoral part of the prosthesis in this epiphysis without a prosthetic trochlea and patella: The functional results are the same, and we prefer this conservative procedure, as the long-term tolerance of patellar prostheses is uncertain.

---

[1]Service de Chirurgie Orthopédique et Réparatrice, Centre Hospitalier Universitaire, Hôpital Sud, Rennes, France

Bone remodeling with significant resorption of the proximal cortex is only observed in children and may be a source of concern even though it is nonevolutive and nonsymptomatic. Since it seems to be the consequence of stress shielding by rigid stems, we advocate the use of a low-modulus titanium alloy stem, which could be associated with a design favoring bone ingrowth and better stress transmission at the level of resection.

Only long-term follow-up will enable us to assess the effectiveness of the allograft (does it reduce bone remodeling and preserve bone stock?) and that of the rotating hinge (does it enhance stem fixation and reduce deterioration of the polyethylene parts by limiting torque stresses?). No inconveniences with the allografts and rotating hinges have been observed up to now and clinical trials should be performed.

Even now, tibial reconstruction by total knee prosthesis, especially in adults, is becoming almost as reliable as lower femur reconstruction by prosthesis.

References

1. Dubousset J, Missenard G (1983) Reconstruction of quadriceps insertion by aponeurotic and muscular plasties after proximal tibia replacement in osteogenic sarcoma. In: Kotz R (ed) Proceedings of 2nd international workshop on the design and application of tumor prostheses for bone and joint reconstruction, Vienna, Sept. 5–8, 1983. Egermann, Vienna, pp 275–279
2. Langlais F, Bunetel L, Segui A, Sassi N, Cormier M (1988) Taux osseux d'antibiotiques et ciments prothétiques. Efficacité et durée d'action. Rev Chir Orthop (Paris)
3. Langlais F, Aubriot JH, Tomeno B, Vielpeau C (submitted) Prothèse Guepar de reconstruction de l'extrémité inférieure du fémur. Résultats à moyen terme de 20 résections pour tumeurs. Orientations actuelles. Rev Chir Orthop
4. Malawer MM (1983) The use of gastrocnemius transposition flap with limb surgery for knee sarcomas: Indications and technique. In: Kotz R (ed) Proceedings of 2nd international workshop on the design and application of tumor prostheses for bone and joint reconstruction, Vienna, Sept. 5–8, 1983. Egermann, Vienna, pp 270–274

Chapter 10

Innovative Techniques

Cytostatic Bone Cement

Experimental Studies and First Clinical Experience

Hans-Ulrich Langendorff[1]

Summary. Radical surgery of malignant bone tumors can be limited by anatomical structures and it appears inadequate in bone metastasis. The risks of marginal or intralesional tumor resection are local respreading and spreading of tumor cells. To combat these risks, methotrexate containing bone cement was developed. The data of biomechanical strength the methotrexate release are given. Biological effectiveness was studied in transplanted osteosarcoma and mamma carcinoma in mice. Initial clinical experience using methotrexate bone cement for stabilization of bone metastases and primary liposarcoma of the bone are reported. Indications for methotrexate bone cement are discussed.

Key word: Bone cement—Local chemotherapy—Malignant bone tumors

The surgery of malignant bone tumors: (a) requires careful radical resection of malignant tissue; and (b) aims at the preservation and restoration of function whenever possible. Radical surgery, however, can be limited either by anatomical structures as in the vertebral column or may even be inadequate in bone metastases. While primary malignant bone tumors amount to less than 1% of all cancers, skeletal metastases have to be expected regulary in almost every type of malignant tumor. When there is no prospect of cure, the decreased life expectancy and return to an early functional state must always remain in focus. Radical surgery, which requires extensive reconstructive procedures and long periods of immobilization, is not well tolerated. In these situations, thorough local excision of the malignant tissue, filling of the defect by bone cement, and stabilization with internal fixation devices or endoprosthetic replacement are the methods of choice.

By having to limit the extent of radical surgery, the following problems may result: (a) local respreading of the tumor, followed by progressive bone destruction and secondary instability of the osteosynthesis; and (b) spreading of the malignant tumor intraoperatively.

In a series of 165 impending or pathological fractures due to metastatic disease, we had to reoperate on seven patients after an average time of 13 months

---

[1]Department of Traumatology, Universitätskrankenhaus, Hamburg-Eppendorf, Federal Republic of Germany

becasue of secondary instability casued by local tumor respreading. Harrington et al. [4] reported similar results in hip replacement arthroplasty.

To combat these problems, radiation therapy may be effective. But irradiation is usually carried out when chemotherapy has failed and the first signs of osteolytic destruction are detected; it is not applied, therefore, when a pathological fracture has occurred and operative stabilization is necessary. Another point is that radiation therapy inhibits fracture healing for a very long period of time [5].

This brought up the question of whether the results could be improved by using a cytostatic bone cement. Our aim in developing such a cement was to destroy any remaining tumor tissue, which must always be assumed to exist in a marginal resection, by high local release of a cytostatic drug from the cement. From experimental and clinial investigations in limb perfusion, it is known that the effectiveness of a cytostatic drug does not only depend on the drug or the tumor itself, but also depends on the disposable tissue concentration and the time of delivery. From osteomyelitis therapy, we also know that bone cement can serve as a carrier substance for certain antibiotics.

To our opinion, such a cytostatic bone cement has to fulfill certain conditions:
a) Preservation of biomechanical properties
b) Continuous release of cytostatic substance in tumor-effective concentrations
c) No alterations of cytostatic substance by polymerization of cement
d) No effect on osteogenesis
e) No systemic side effects
f) Possibility of delivery control
Of all presently available cytostatic substances methotrexate (MTX) proved to be the most favorable in fulfilling these conditions MTX is a highly potent substance in the treatment of a great variety of malignant tumors. It gives thermostability and delivery can be controlled by leucovorin rescue therapy.

Our first attempts at simply mixing MTX with bone cement were not successful since the required release of MTX from the cement could not be achieved. By adding certain amino acids, however, MTX release was accomplished. In vitro studies showed that tumor-effective concentrations were obtained. The release of MTX with time resembles the release of gentamycin from bone cement (Fig. 1). The biomechanical properties with regard to bending and compressive strength are slightly decreased compared with plain bone cement but still fulfill the required stability for osteosynthesis or endoprosthetic replacement (Fig. 2).

Biological effectiveness was studied in two different transplantable tumors in mice. Radiation was used to induce mainly osteoblastic osteosarcoma with a large amount of bone formation and a mamma carcinoma. Standard solid plugs containing either normal bone cement or two different concentrations of MTX were inserted into the center of the tumors. Increase of tumor growth was measured and histological examinations were made. Figure 3 shows that tumor growth of the osteosarcoma was not inhibited at the lower dose but was significantly reduced at the higher dose. In mamma carcinoma, this effect was more pronounced so that even at the lower dose tumor growth was reduced (Fig. 4). This difference between osteosarcoma and mamma carcinoma may be due to varying sensitivity of the tumors to MTX or to different penetrating or circulatory conditions. Complete destruction of the tumors was not seen nor could it be expected since the volume and, especially, the surface of the cement plug, which

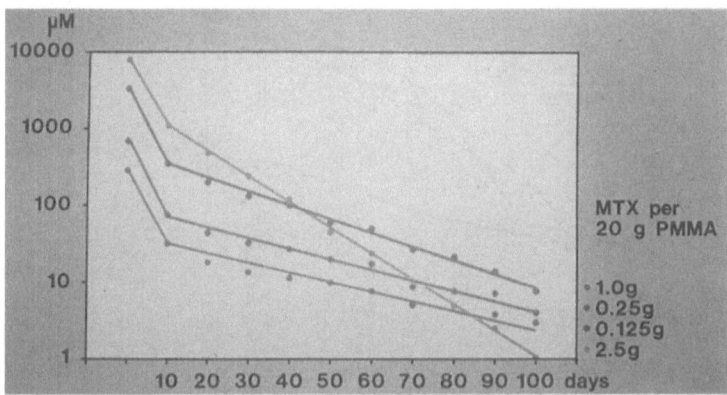

Fig. 1. Release of MTX in vitro from bone cement according various concentrations of MTX and time

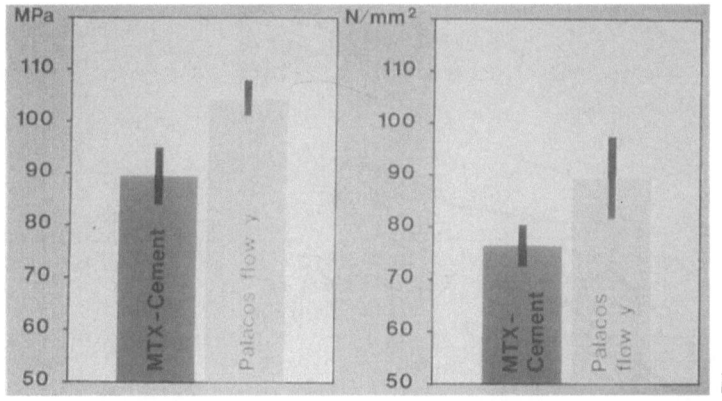

Fig. 2. a Bending and **b** compressive strength of MTX-bone cement compared with plain bone cement

is of great importance for MTX release, were very small compared with the tumor volume.

Further information regarding the penetration and effectiveness was obtained by histological examination. Figure 5 shows that in the osteosarcoma normal bone cement had no influence on the tumor at all. The cement plug was surrounded by vital tumor cells. In contrast to this, the inserted MTX-Palacos plug was surrounded by a wise zone of necrosis (Fig. 6). More distantly, we found highly degenerated tumor cells and only in the periphery was there a vital tumor. This effect was more pronounced in mamma carcinoma than in osteosarcoma and involved nearly three-quarters of the tumor diameter (Fig. 7). The transitional stages from total necrosis to vital tumor implied a declining MTX concentration.

The tissue concentrations of MTX measured in the liver and kidney showed increased levels compared with the muscle tissue next to the tumor and on the

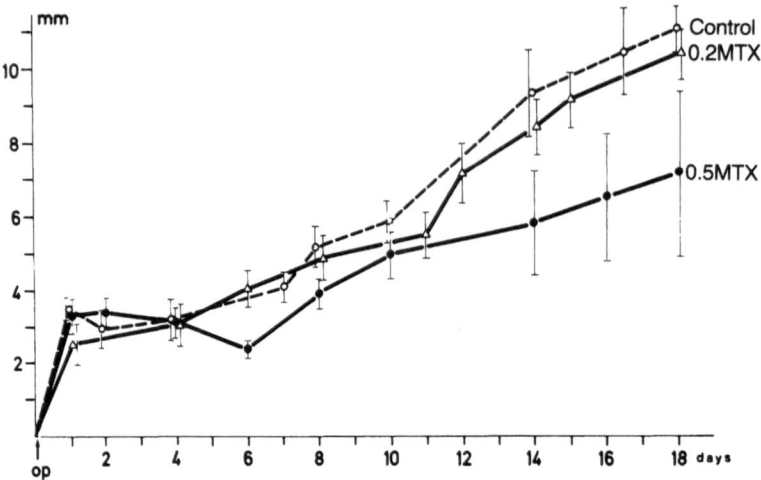

Fig. 3. Increase of tumor growth in osteosarcoma

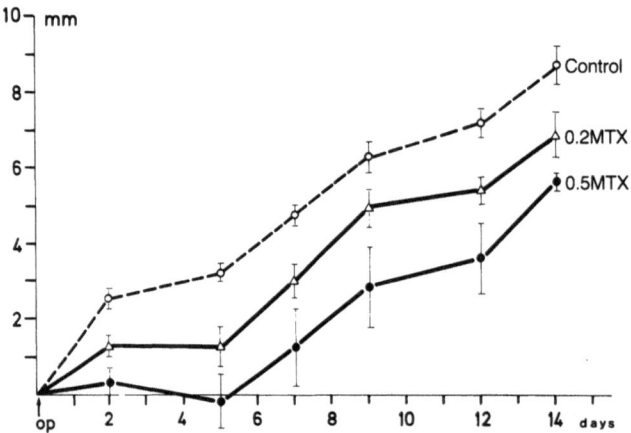

Fig. 4. Increase of tumor growth in mamma carcinoma

contralateral side. Though in the liver, the tissue MTX concentration decreased on days 18 and 21, the MTX concentration in the kidney remained at a constant level. From liver and kidney tissue, it is known that they may retain MTX for several weeks. But altogether, these tissue concentrations are so low that no long-term cytotoxic effects are to be expected.

Systemic tolerance studies were carried out in rabbits with regard to clinical status, body weight serum concentrations, hematology, and histology. Both femura were filled with MTX bone cement containing five different concentrations of MTX. Primary would healing occurred in nearly two-thirds of the animals. At the lower doses, no adverse reactions occurred. At the higher doses, diarrhea was observed regularly during the 2nd and 3rd weeks after implantation and nearly half of the animals died. The other animals recovered after leucovorin rescue therapy.

Body weight, which proved to be a very sensitive parameter regarding sys-

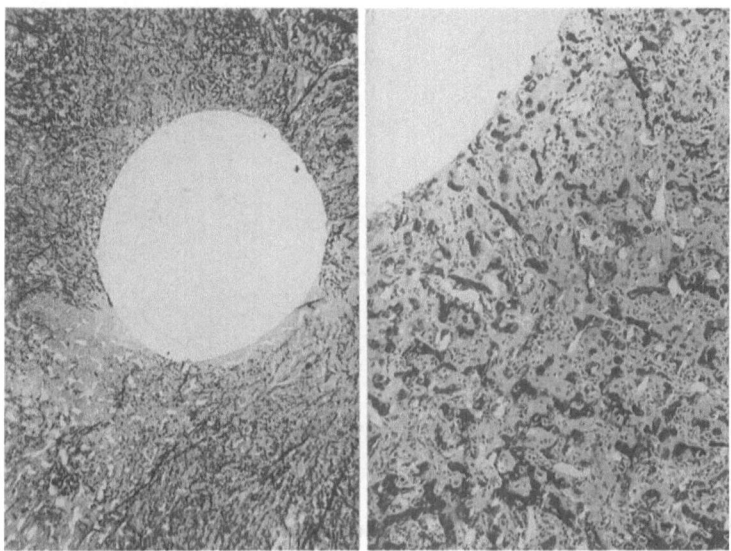

Fig. 5. Histological examination 3 weeks after implantation of plain bone cement in osteosarcoma revealed no effect on the tumor

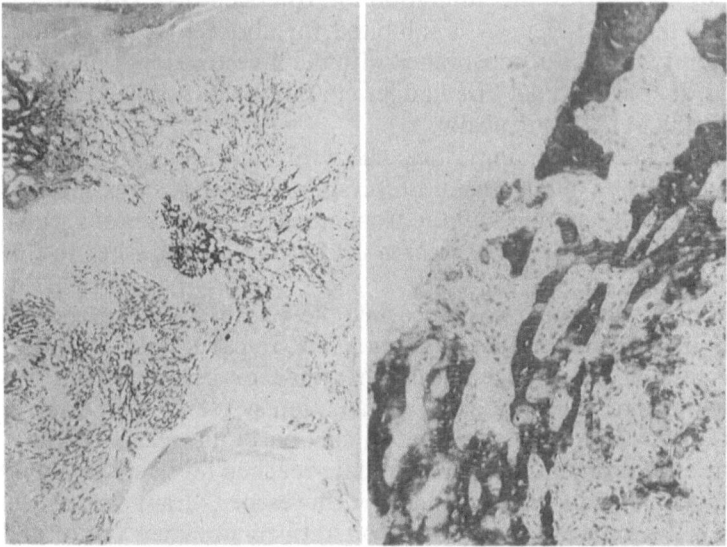

Fig. 6. Histological examination 3 weeks after implantation of MTX-bone cement in osteosarcoma

temic tolerance, decreased especially at the higher concentrations during the first 2 weeks. But by administration of leucovorin twice during the 2nd and 3rd weeks, the animals recovered body weight increased back to normal (Fig. 8). Serum concentrations of MTX decreased with time according to the adminis-

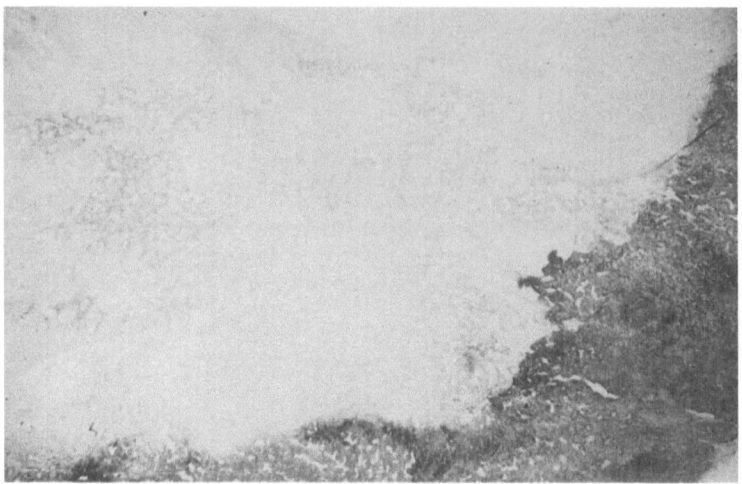

Fig. 7. Histological examination 3 weeks after implantation of MTX-bone cement in mamma carcinoma

tered dose of MTX and were similar to the results obtained in the in vitro studies (Figs. 9, 10).

Another point of interest is the inhibition of osteogenesis. Histological examination showed that osteogenesis is inhibited for about 3 weeks but not suppressed permanently. This is in accordance with the investigations of Nilsson et al. [6, 7], Burchardt et al. [2], and Friedlander et al. [3], who reported similar effects by administering MTX systemically.

Based on these experimental findings, local chemotherapy seemed encouraging to us. In 21 selected cases of malignant osteolysis MTX-Palacos was used for stabilization. All patients except one suffered from metastatic diseases of various origin. One patient had a primary liposarcoma of the bone. I will refer to this below.

An endoprothetic replacement was necessary seven times, a compound osteosynthesis was performed in eight cases, and in six cases only a plug of MTX-Palacos was implanted. The clinical performance postoperatively increased considerably according to Enneking's evaluation system. Postoperatively, the concentration of MTX was measured in suction drainage and plasma. Although MTX concentration in the wound exudate reached levels up to 25000 ng/ml, plasma levels remained low and no leucovorin rescue therapy was necessary. Tissue cultures were made from the intraoperatively obtained tumor and submitted to various concentrations of MTX in vitro. The tumor cell growth decreased with increasing MTX concentration, which was achieved by the local implantation of MTX-Palacos. Especially, in the bronchus carcinoma, where the patient had been treated before the operation by high systemic doses of MTX, these concentrations had practically no effect. This was in accordance with the clinical development of the disease. In this patient, a great osteoloysis of the lower tibia had been stabilized by a compound osteosynthesis. Eight months later, the patient died and autopsy was performed. No signs of local tumor

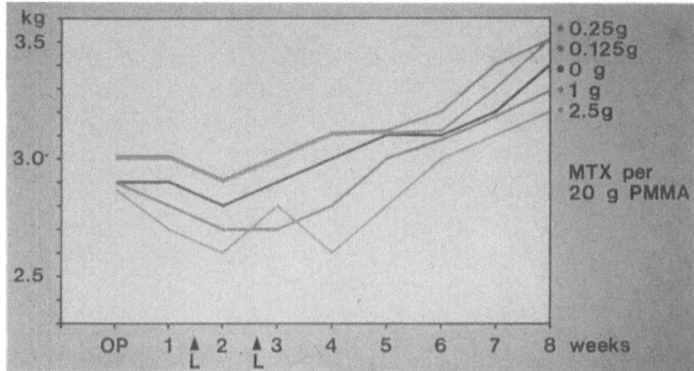

Fig. 8. Body weight in rabbits after implantation of MTX-bone cement into both femora
($n = 8$)

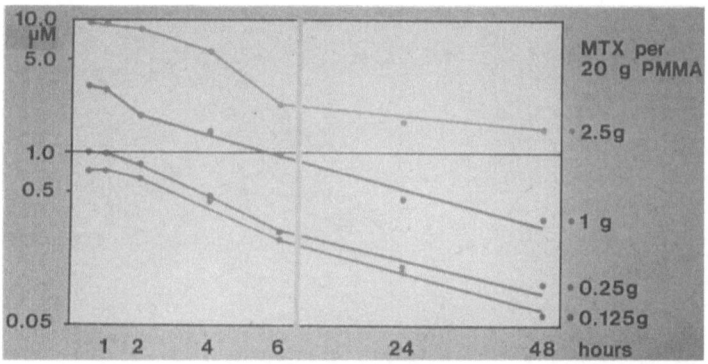

Fig. 9. MTX concentrations in serum of rabbits after implantation of MTX-bone cement
into both femora during the first 48 hours postoperation

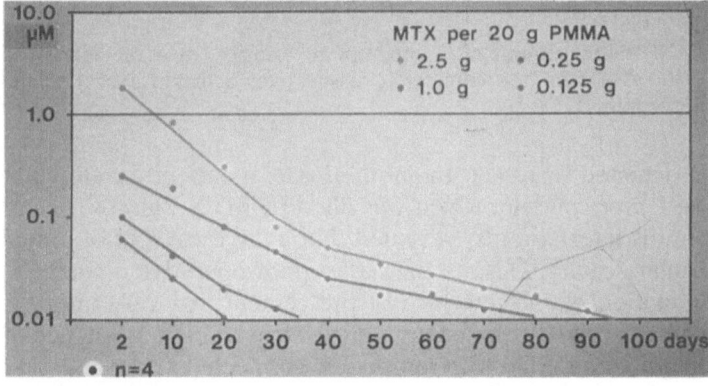

Fig. 10. MTX concentrations in serum of rabbits after implantation of MTX-bone cement into both femora during 100 days postoperation

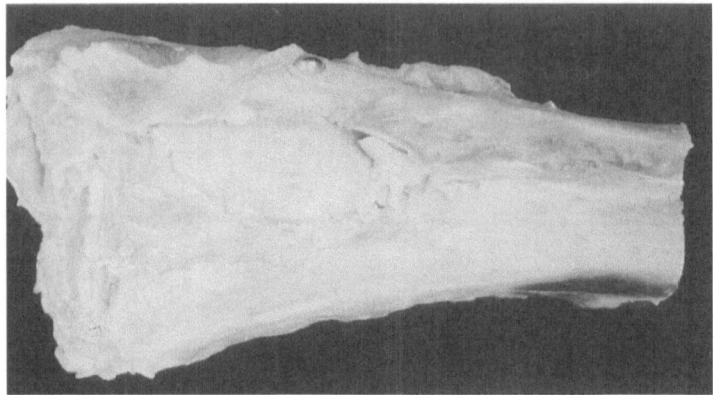

Fig. 11. Eight months after compound osteosynthesis using MTX-bone cement in the lower tibia. Pathological section revealed no local respreading in a metastasis of a bronchus carcinoma

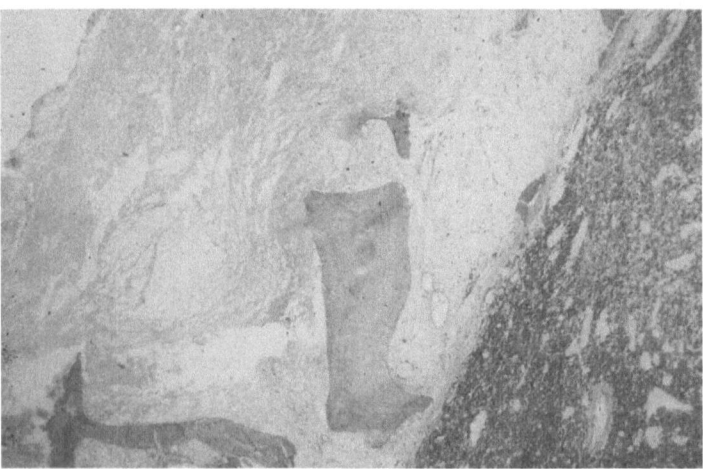

Fig. 12. Interface of MTX-bone cement after incomplete excision of a metastasis of a bronchus carcinoma shows tumor-free connective tissue over a distance of 1.5 cm. Beyond this, vital tumor remains

respreading could be detected (Fig. 11). In another case, a patient developed a great osteolysis in the femur condyle, which was filled by MTX-Palacos. When the patient died 3 months later, autopsy revealed that a large amount of tumor remained in the medullary cavity. Despite the rather poor operative procedure, the histological examination of the interface of the cement was very interesting. It showed that the tumor had been completely destroyed over a distance of 1.5 cm (Fig. 12). The space was filled with tumor-free connective tissue. Beyond this, vital tumor remained. This effect is very similar to our experimental findings.

An interesting course occurred in one of our first patients with a liposarcoma

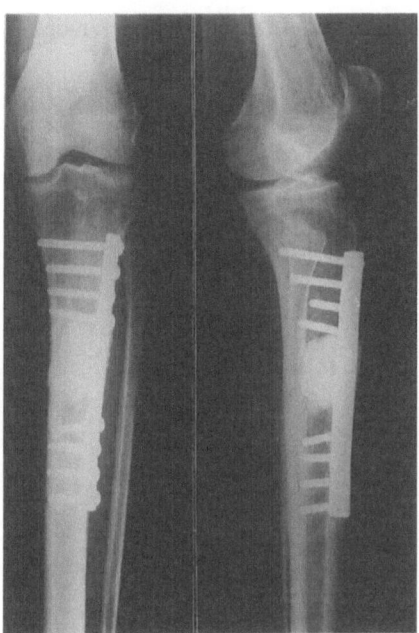

Fig. 13. Liposarcoma of the bone after marginal resection and compound osteosynthesis using MTX-bone cement

of the tibia. Liposarcoma of the bone is an extremely rare tumor and only 35 cases have been described in the world literature. No effective means of chemo- or radiotherapy is known and life expectancy amounts to less than 2 years. Since the patient refused radical resection, we made a local tumor excision and stabilized the tibia by MTX-Palacos and an AO/ASIF plate (Fig. 13). After 2 years, no local respreading or metastasis could be detected. We removed the plug and filled the defect by cancellous bone. Intraoperatively taken biopsies revealed there was no longer any tumor. The ingrowth of the cancellous bone was normal and occurred at the right time (Fig 14).

Complications concerning would healing occurred in one patient, where an osteolysis of the sacroiliac joint was stabilized. The patient developed a decubital ulcer in a previously irradiated field of the back. We doubt whether this was due to MTX.

Close follow-up studies of our patients revealed no radiological signs of local respreading after an average time of 1 year. Twelve patients are still alive; nine died from metastatic disease.

In conclusion, it must again be stressed that malignant tissue should always be removed as far as possible. But MTX-Palacos may give additional safety whenever radical resection is questionable with regard to local respreading. We, therefore, see indications for MTX-Palacos in:

a) Plugging of diagnostic biopsies of malignant bone tumors
b) Marginal resections of primary malignant bone tumors
c) Palliative stabilization of malignant osteolysis

It would also appear to be possible to plug temporarily semimalignant tumors, such as in giant cell tumors, a procedure favored at the last meeting of this society.

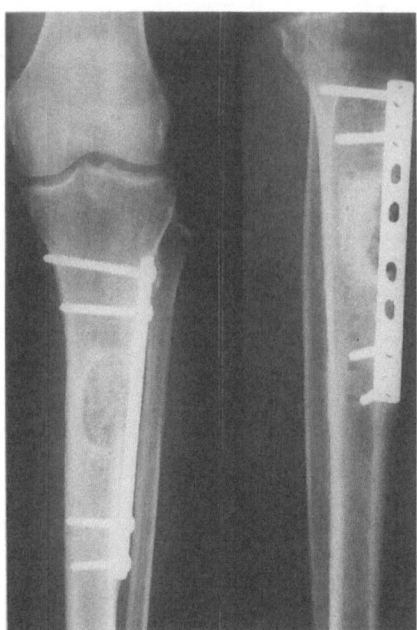

Fig. 14. Ingrowth of cancellous bone 6 months after removal of MTX-bone cement

Other indications for extraosseous tumors, perhaps by using biodegradable carrier substances, are the object of further experimental work. Initial experimental findings in malignant brain tumors studied in the rat showed an increase of the survival rate of over 200% after implantation of an MTX-Palacos plug [8].

References

1. Abrams HL (1950) Skeletal metastases in carcinoma. Radiology 55: 534
2. Burchardt H, Glowczewskic FP, Enneking WF (1983) The effect of adriamycin and methotrexate on the repair of segmental cortical autografts in dogs. J Bone Jt Surg 65-A: 103
3. Friedlaender GE, Tross RB, Doganis AC, Kirkwood JM, Baron R (1984) Effects of chemotherapeutic agents on bone. J Bone Jt Surg 66-A: 602
4. Harrington KD, Sim FH, Enis JE, Johnston JC, Dick HM, Gristima AG (1976) Methylmetacrylate as an adjunct in internal fixation of pathological fractures. J Bone Jt Surg 58 A: 1047
5. Langendorff H, Langendorff G, Sauer HD, Jungbluth KH (1982) Beeinflussung der Frakturheilung durch lokale Bestrahlung. In: Hackenbrach MH, Retior HJ, Jäger M (eds) Osteogenese and Knochenwachstum. Thieme, Stuttgart
6. Nilsson OS, Bauer HCF Broström L-A (1987) Methotrexate effects on heterotopic bone in rats. Acta Orthop Scand 58: 47
7. Nilsson OS, Bauer FCH, Broström L-A (1984) Effects of the antineolastic agent methotrexate on experimental hetertopic new bone formation in rats. Cancer Res 44: 1653
8. Rama B, Mandel T, Jansen J, Dingeldein E, Mennel HD (1987) The intraneoplastic chemotherapy in a rat brain tumor model utilizing methotrexate-polymethyl-methacrylate-pellets. Acta Neurochir (Wien) 87: 70

The Effect of Bone Cement Containing Methotrexate on the Canine Osteosarcoma

A Preliminary Report

L. Hovy[1], B. Tellhelm[2], E. Dingeldein[3], H. Wahlig[3], and A. Enderle[4]

Summary. Spontaneous osteosarcoma is a comparatively common tumor in the long bones of large dogs. The morphological and biological characteristics are similar to those of human osteosarcoma. In six dogs, the primary bone tumor was deliberately excised marginally or intralesionally and the osseous defect was refilled with bone cement containing 125, 250, and 375 mg methotrexate (MTX). Systemic adverse reactions were mild, not dose-dependent, and inconstant but always reversible with low doses of citrovorum factor. The serum concentrations did not exceed 2×10^{-7} mol/l on the 1st day and then decreased continuously. Local tumor recurrence occurred with 1–6 months postoperatively. The histological evaluation showed total cell necrosis surrounding the MTX cement plug, up to 10.8 mm across dependent on the MTX dose, and a varying area of partial necrosis more peripherally. MTX had no effect on the articular cartilage.

MTX bone cement can be considered a potent agent in the local therapy of genuine caine osteosarcoma.

Key words: Canine osteosarcoma—Bone cement—Methotrexate

Introduction

Spontaneous osteosarcoma is a comparatively common tumor entity in the dog, especially in large and giant breeds [1, 6, 7]. Several investigators [1, 6–8] have emphasized the similar morphological and biological characteristics of the disease in dogs to that in humans. In particular, the localization in the long bones, with a tendency occur in the main load-bearing extremities, and the histological morphology are comparable, such that the spontaneous canine osteosarcoma appears to be a suitable experimental model [1].

The poor prognosis of a solely surgically treated osteosarcoma in man and the

---

[1]Department of Orthopedics, University of Frankfurt, Frankfurt, Federal Republic of Germany

[2]Department of Veterinary Surgery, University of Giessen, Giessen, Federal Republic of Germany

[3]Department of Medical Microbiology, Med. Res. E. Merck, Darmstadt, Federal Republic of Germany

[4]Department of Orthopedics, University of Göttingen, Göttingen, Federal Republic of Germany

Table 1. Spontaneous canine osteosarcoma and MTX cement plug

Dog	Sex	Breed	Age (years)	Body weight (kg)	Site	MTX (mg)/ 20 g PMMA	Implanted MTX dose (mg)	Disease-free survival time postop. (months)	Lung metastases
I	F	German shepherd	2 3/4	30	Prox. humerus (r)	250	190	6	No
II	F	St. Bernhard	7 1/2	52.5	Dist. radius (l)	125	190	2	No
III	M	German shepherd/ Labrador mix	2	33.5	Prox. humerus (l)	125	90	1	Yes
IV	F	Pyrenean mountain dog	5	48	Prox. tibia (l)	125	95	1	Yes
V	F	St. Bernhard	5	63.5	Dist. radius (r)	375	940	1.5	No
VI	F	Irish wolfhound	6	48	Dist. radius (r)	375	190	1 (alive)	No

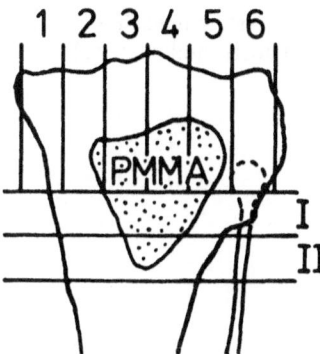

Fig. 1. Scheme of proximal tibia (dog IV) with tumor and cement plug Order of slices in the sagittal and horizontal plane

dog [1] can be improved by adjuvant chemotherapy. High serum concentrations of methotrexate (MTX) proved to be very effective, as noted by Jaffe et al. [4] among. Local administration of MTX seems to be reasonable in order to achieve a high local concentration of MTX ath the target point, i.e., the tumor, and to decrease the systemic toxic side effects of MTX. Bone cement can serve as a drug vehicle with a well-defined release of MTX [2, 5] and at the same time as a bone stabilizer [9].

Materials and Methods

In the time from August 1985 to the present, six dogs within a larger series with spontaneous osteosarcoma of the long bones were operated on in cooperation with the Department of Veterinary Surgery in Giessen. All the dogs were of large breeds with body weights of 30–63 kg and 2–9 years of age (Table. 1) The primary bone tumor was deliberately excised marginally or intralesionally according to the method of Enneking et al. [3] and the central bone defect was refilled with low-viscosity bone cement (Palacos flow Y) containing 125 mg (3x), 250 mg (1x), and 375 mg (2x) MTX/20 g polymethyl methacrylate (PMMA). The serum level of MTX was determined postoperatively by radioimmunoassay.

The dogs were followed up clinically and radiologically.

All dogs were killed at the request of the owners when local recurrence was evident in the X-ray. An autopsy was done to determine bone and lung metastases. The complete bone with the tumor and cement plug was dissected and fixed in formalin (pH 7.0).

The tumor area with the cement plug was cut in two portions and the diaphyseal part was cut in 0.8-cm slices in the horizontal plane. The epimetaphyseal part was cut in 0.8-cm slices in the sagittal plane (Fig. 1). These nondecalcified slices were embedded in methacrylate and serial histological sections of 20 μm were cut and stained according to the methods of Goldner, Giemsa, and Movat.

From the central cement plug area, the neighboring two sections in the horizontal plane and two sections in the sagittal plane were analyzed microscopically in each case.

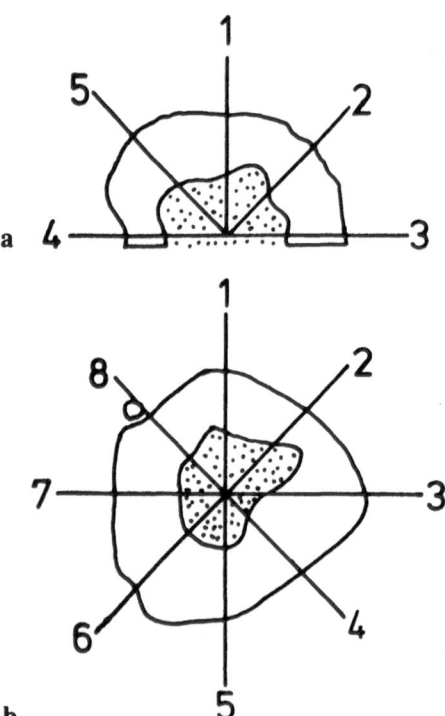

Fig. 2a, b. Measuring system in each section. **a** sagittal plane (*4*); **b** horizontal plane (*1*)

The micromorphological effects around the cement plug were measured along a straight radial line with its center in the middle of the plug (Fig. 2). The range of tissue necrosis was determined at five to eight points (Fig. 2) in each section and measured with a calibrated micrometer eyepiece. Necrosis was defined as an area without any viable cells (tumor, autochthonous bone, or connective tissue). Unfortunately, the specimen of dog III could not be evaluated histologically due to loss after autopsy.

Dog V was killed recently, and histological sections were not available in time for this paper.

Results

Clinical

No complications related to the surgical procedure occurred. Three dogs (I, II, and IV) developed diarrhea with vomiting within 2–6 days postoperatively. These gastrointestinal side effects of MTX were reversible in every case after intravenous administration of 3 × 15 mg citrovorum factor per day for 3 days; in one case (dog II) for 5 days.

The radiological follow-up after onset of lameness revealed local recurrences in five dogs. One dog (VI) is still living free of disease. Tumor recurrence occurred in the first dog (250 mg MTX) after 6 months. Dogs II, III, and IV (125 mg MTX) developed local recurrences and lung metastases with 1–2 months post-

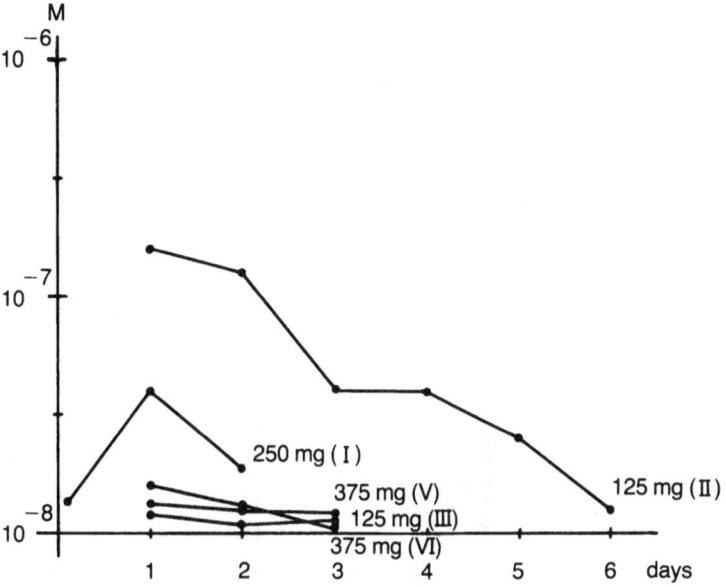

Fig. 3. MTX serum concentration after MTX cement plug

operatively (Table 1).

The tumor in dog V (375 mg MTX) recurred mainly at the site of the large extraosseous part of the primary tumor, which could not be resected radically. At autopsy, no lung metastases were observed.

Serum Monitoring

The highest serum concentrations of MTX, not exceeding 2×10^{-7} mol/l, could be determined on the 1st day postoperatively. The serum levels then decreased continuously (Fig. 3). There was no correlation to the administered MTX dose in this investigation.

Histological

The radiological diagnosis of osteosarcoma was confirmed histologically in the resected tumor mass in every case. Canine as well as human osteosarcoma has pathognomonic tumor areas with sarcoma cells forming a rosette with osteoid in the center or diffuse osteoid deposits and areas with filigree new bone formation and calcification. Besides this there are areas of sarcoma cells without any ground substance. On the other hand, regions with a spindle cell character or even chondroid matrix can be found. Spontaneous tumor necrosis also occurs.

Analysis of the range of tissue necrosis surrounding the MTX cement plug in both planes (horizontal and sagittal) showed a clear cell necrosis dependent on the MTX dose (Fig. 4). The average range of necrosis in the low MTX concentration (125 mg MTX/20 g PMMA) was 1.3 mm and 2.0 mm. The higher MTX concentration (250 mg MTX/20 g PMMA) caused a broad necrosis of 5.3 mm on

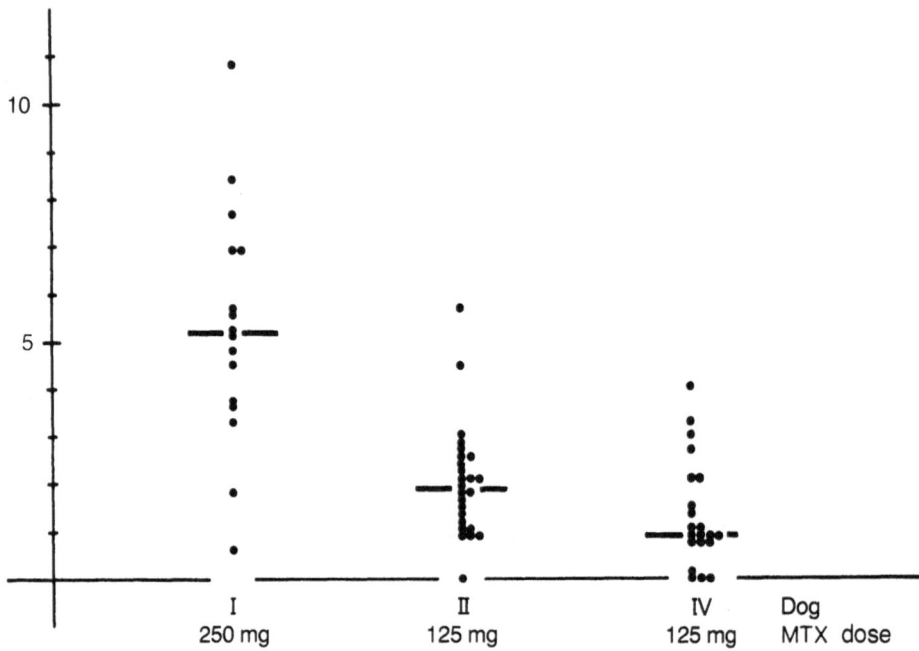

Fig. 4. Median range of tissue necrosis surrounding MTX cement plug

average, ranging up to 10.8 mm (Fig. 4).

The extent of tissue necrosis was the same in areas with tumor cells and in cancellous bone invaded by tumor cells. Bone without tumor invasion did not reach the cement plug.

Adjacent to the zone with definite necrosis, around the cement plug, there was an area with degenerative changes in the nuclei, partial necrosis, and viable tumor cells, varying in amount and depth. This area was separated from the primary necrosis by a relatively distinct margin. Viable tumor or cortical and cancellous bone surrounded the second area without a margin.

In the first dog (I), there was a cone-shaped tumor recurrence in the primary area of necrosis, pointing toward the cement plug, in a small part of one section.

The articular cartilage did not show any signs of cell damage, although the necrosis reached directly to subchondral areas in some parts, leaving only a small distance between the cement plug and joint space.

Invasion of blood vessels by tumor cells in the form of an angiomatosis sarcomatosa was found in one case (dog IV) with lung metastases.

Discussion

Spontaneous canine osteosarcoma can be used as an ideal experimental model [1] on account of similar morphological and biological characteristics to human osteosarcoma [6–8]. Marginal or intralesional excision [3] of the tumor was performed in this study in an attempt to evaluate the effect of locally administered MTX on the genuine osteosarcoma and the adjacent bone as well as the in-

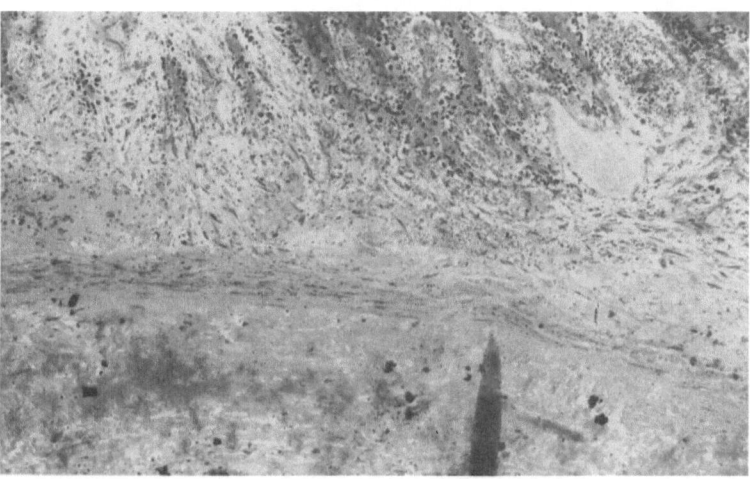

Fig. 5. Total cell necrosis (*lower region*) with margin to the adjacent tumor (*upper region*) and small area with cell degeneration (*middle region*) in dog II. Giemsa, × 63

fluence on the entire organism.

Assessment of the *clinical results* shows that even a nonradical surgical procedure can obtain a disease-free survival time of 6 months without lung metastases. Brodey and Riser [1] found the same time range after radical amputation. Less effective local doses of MTX (125 mg/20 g PMMA) lead to an early local recurrence after 1 or 2 months and have no influence on lung metastases (Table 1). A high MTX concentration (375 mg MTX/20 mg PMMA) seems to prevent the development of lung metastases although the local recurrence is not influenced at the site of the extraosseous part of the primary tumor.

Systemic toxic side effects of MTX are diarrhea and vomiting, which occur occasionally. They are completely reversible with low doses of citrovorum factor and show no relation to the implanted MTX dose.

The *serum analysis* confirms that the serum concentrations of MTX do not exceed 2×10^{-7} mol/l on the 1st day and then decrease continuously (Fig. 3). The in vivo MTX serum concentrations in this study do not correlate with the MTX doses in the cement plug. This is due to various factors, especially different total cement quantity, body weight, and surface area of the cement plug. An in vitro study [2] demonstrated a clear dependence of the MTX release on the MTX concentration in the cement plug. This will be studied in further standardized in vivo investigations in the dog.

The MTX penetration into the surrounding tissue is presumed to be due to a centrifugal diffusion process. Therefore, the *histological evaluation* has to be done in a radial measuring system (Fig. 2).

A clear cell necrosis ranging up to 10.8 mm develops around the MTX cement plug dependent on the MTX concentration (Fig. 4). This area of primary necrosis has a relatively distinct margin to the adjacent more peripheral zone of partial cell necrosis, with degenerative changes in the nuclei but with no signs of definite cell necrosis. This second area of partial necrosis is variable and continues with-

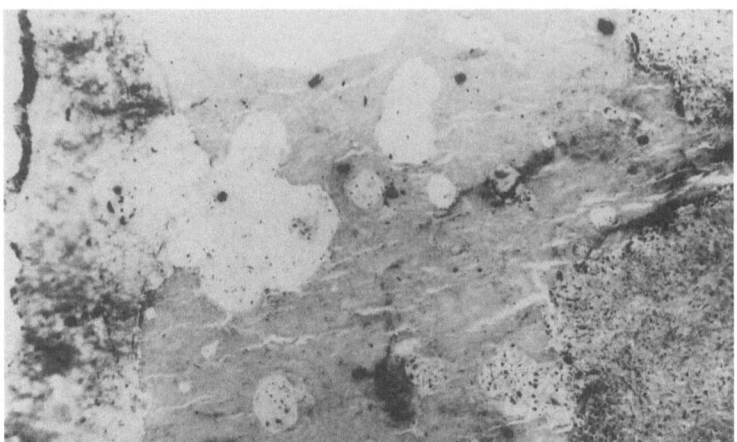

Fig. 6. Total necrosis of tumor and autochthonous bone (*left*) and viable tumor (*right*). Polymethyl methacrylate PMMA (*left*). Dog II, Giemsa, × 25

out a margin into the peripheral tissue (viable tumor or bone). However, it is absent in extensive sections.

Using MTX bone cement pins, Langendorff et al. [5] observed similar effects in a transplanted mouse osteosarcoma. The concentric necrosis and partial necrosis seem to occur on account of the homogeneous tumor tissue compound in this model. The primary area of total cell necrosis can be considered to be the average cytotoxic diffusion distance of MTX in both models, probably due to the initially high release of MTX in the first postoperative days. The second area with partial necrosis seems to be an inconstant effect of the diffusing MTX, depending on the tissue compound and on the decreasing MTX release.

MTX obviously has no cytotoxic effect on the articular cartilage. The effect on the autochthonous bone cannot be evaluated because bone without tumor invasion does not reach the cement plug in this study. Bone with tumor invasion in the marrow adjacent to the cement plug turns necrotic, just like the primary tumor. However, we unpublished data found no bone necrosis after MTX bone cement implantation in the rabbit femur but observed decreased bone remodeling next to the bone cement plug.

In conclusion, MTX bone cement can be considered a potent agent in the local therapy of genuine osteosarcoma in the dog. The most effective MTX concentration in the bone cement and the best-release kinetics will have to be assessed in further investigations.

References

1. Brodey RS, Riser WH (1969) Canine osteosarcoma. Clin Orthop 62: 54–64
2. Dingeldein E, Wahlig H (1986) Methotrexat im Knochenzement—Freisetzung in vitro sowie Serum- und Gewebekonzentrationen im Tierexperiment. Acta Med Aust [Suppl] 35: 25–26
3. Enneking WF, Spanier SS, Goodman MA (1980) A system for the surgical staging of

    musculoskeletal sarcoma. Clin Orthop 153: 106–120
 4. Jaffe N, Farber S, Traggis D, Geiser C, Kim BS, Das L, Frauenberger G, Djerassi I,
    Cassady Jr (1973) Favorable response of metastatic osteogenic sarcoma of pulse high-
    dose methotrexate with citrovorum rescue and radiation therapy. Cancer 31: 1367
 5. Langendorff H-U, Jungbluth KH, Dingeldein E, Wahlig H, Delling G, Senokowitsch
    R (1987) Methotrexate bone cement: new aspects in the treatment of malignant bone
    tumors: I Experimental studies. Langenb Arch Chir 371: 123–126
 6. Misdorp W, Hart AAM (1979) Some prognostic and epidemiologic factors in canine
    osteosarcoma. J Nat Cancer Inst 62: 537–545
 7. Misdorp W (1980) Animal model of human disease: canine osteosarcoma. Am J
    Pathol 98: 285–288
 8. Owen LN (1969) Bone tumors in man and animals. Butterworths, London, pp 29–52
 9. Willert H-G, Enderle E (1979) Temporäre Zementplombe bei Knochentumoren frag-
    licher Dignität. Z Orthop 117: 224–232

Casted Femur-Knee Endoprosthesis with Spongy Metal Surface and Length Adaption In Situ

Ernst Joachim Henssge[1], Erwin Hipp[2], Hans Grundei[3], Thomas Biehl[2], Pavel Dufek[1], and Reiner Gradinger[2]

Summary. Technical innovations in limb salvage surgery are based on four conditions: (a) Development of implant stems adapted to the cavities of the femur and tibia; (b) development of cancellous custom-made alloy based on cobalt-chromium. These implants are incorporated by bone ingrowth; (c) cementless implantation of all stems or acetabular cups. The implants are cast individually with a spongy metal surface for trabecular ingrowth; (d) Lengthening mechanism of the tumor endoprostheses, based on a worm-gearing construction, moved by an inbus screwdriver and controlled by a stop mechanism. The results of seven cases resected between May 1984 and April 1986 (five boys, two girls, aged 10–16 years) were: five osteosarcomas IIB—two excellent, two good, one fair; one osteosarcoma IB—excellent; one chondrosarcoma IIB—initially good, later vertebral metastases, died after 2 years.

The operational guidelines were: prepare the knee and proximal tibia, cut the knee ligaments; implant the tibial and patellar endoprostheses; prepare the femur with soft tissues as necessary in the distal-proximal direction; remove the femur after osteotomy or exarticulation; implant the endoprosthesis and adapt the lengths; examine knee movement and soft tissue tension before closing the fascia and skin.

Key words: Lengthening mechanism for tumor endoprostheses—Spongy metal macroporous surfaces—Cancellous casted alloy

Introduction

The innovations developed in Lübeck and Munich consist of the following: (a) Anatomically adapted stems, fitting well into the cavities of the femur and the tibia; (b) cancellous custom-made alloy based on cobalt-chromium, examined in experiments on sheep. Later, we implanted spongious metal blocks to elevate fresh calcaneum fractures and to make distraction arthrodeses and spondylodeses; (c) adapted stems with macroporous spongy metal surface. The implants show a trabecular ingrowth; (d) a length adaption system based on a worm-gearing construction with a sop mechanism, preventing any motion of the

[1] Klinik für Orthopädie Medizinische Universität, Lübeck, Federal Republic of Germany
[2] Orthopädische Klinik der Technischen Universität, Munich, Federal Republic of Germany
[3] Firma S + G Implants GmbH, Lübeck, Federal Republic of Germany

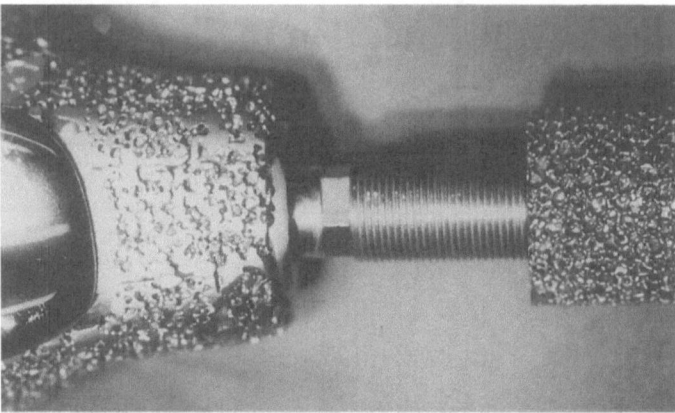

Fig. 1. The lengthening mechanism of a knee-femur endoprosthesis in the fully elongated position

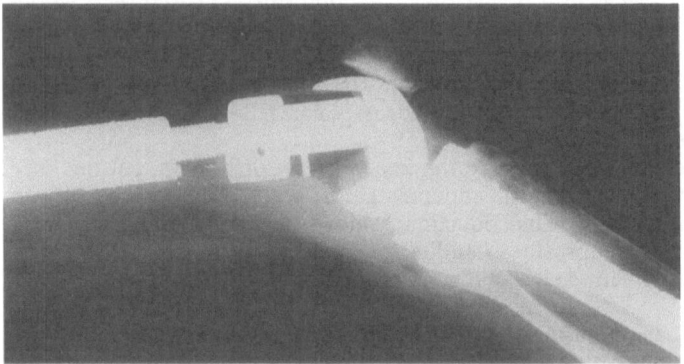

Fig. 2. A 16-year-old boy with osteosarcoma IB at 3 years' follow-up. The lengthening mechanism was moved 2 cm

worm gearing after the implantation. The worm gearing is now protected with a covering.

Material and Methods

Tumor endoprostheses with length adaption are manufactured individually during the time of chemotherapy after biopsy diagnosis. The special macroporous surface of the bridging part of the endoprostheses also allows ingrowth of soft tissues. So, it can be expected that sufficient muscle insertion into the surface of the implant will take place. In the case of total removal of the femur, safe and stable standing using the operated leg will result (Figs. 1, 2).

In the operational technique, the following guidelines are adapted. The operation can start with a pneumatic tourniquet. The lateral approach is adopted. The

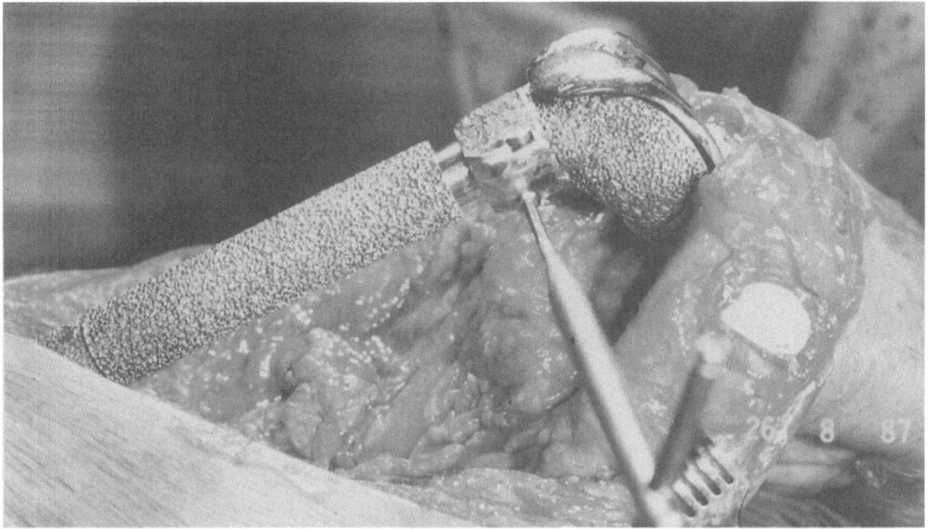

Fig. 3. The lengthening mechanism, now covered, is moved in the last stage of the operation

knee joint is opened and the tibial head prepared. The knee ligaments are cut and the knee is fully bent. The second step is osteotomy of the tibial plateau using the oscillating saw. Templet instruments are helpful here.

After resectioning of spongious bone and rasping the cavity of tibia, the tibial part of the endoprosthesis is implanted without bone cement.

The joint face of the patella is chiseled out, the spongious bone smoothed using high-speed reamer, and the polyethylene inlay implanted using low-viscosity cement.

The block resection of the tumor starts distally. Beginning in the popliteal region, one can follow the main vessels and protect them. The level of the trans-medullar resection is variable to a tolerance of a maximum of 5 cm in compari-son with the planned resection line at the time when the tumor endoprosthesis is ordered. In the case of total exarticulation of the tumor, all the muscle insertions are cut first and, finally, the capsule of the joint.

The next step is implantation of the upper connecting part of the endopros-thesis. In the case of exarticulation, the acetabulum is first, otherwise it is in the femoral cavity.

The knee joint part is coupled with the tibial endoprosthesis in a semicon-strained connection by means of a gliding axis. Proximally, this part of the endo-prosthesis must fit conically with the tumor bridging part. The length adaption mechanism can be moved by an inbus screwdriver (Fig. 3). The definitive length of the leg is checked by connecting with soft tissue tension and knee movement.

In the case of total resection of the femur, a slight elongation of about 2 cm prevents hip joint luxation (Fig. 4).

Length adaption at a later time follows the normal growth and is made by a small incision, again placing the screwdriver. We used this procedure in two cases.

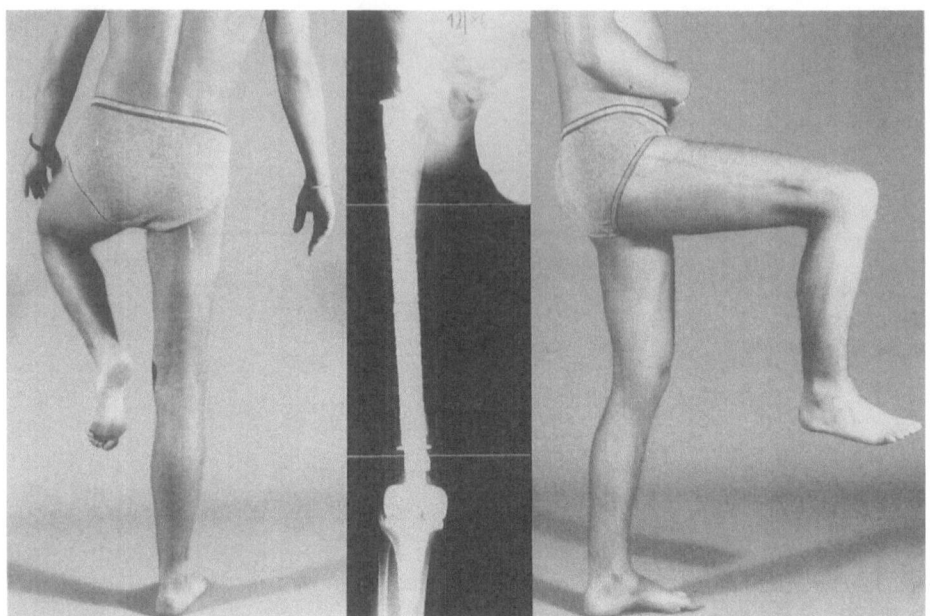

Fig. 4. A 16-year-old boy with diaphyseal osteosarcoma IIB. The femur and knee have been removed. At 3 years' follow-up. Lengthened 2.4 cm

Table 1. Evaluation of prosthetic devices

	Anatomy	Morbidity	Loosening	Failure
Excellent ($n = 3$)	No length discrepancy ($n = 1$)	Active joint motion, weight bearing at 0–2 weeks ($n = 3$)	Bone ingrowth	No
Good ($n = 3$)	<2cm ($n = 4$)	2–4 weeks ($n = 4$)	Bone ingrowth	No
Fair ($n = 1$)	>2cm ($n = 1$)	4–12 weeks	Bone ingrowth	No
Poor	Removal	>12 weeks		

The length adaption during surgery was very helpful for good soft tissue tension, knee movement, and comparing leg length. Toward the end, finally, we did not need more than 3-cm elongation. Thus, we believe that the maximum elongation rate of 5 cm is sufficient.

Results

Between 1984 and 1986, we implanted seven tumor endoprostheses will length adaption. The age of the patients was 10–16 years. There were six osteosarco-

Table 2. Functional anatomy of hip joint

	Motion	Pain	Stability	Strength	Emotional acceptance	Failure
Excellent (n = 2)	Comb. >180° (n = 2)	None (n = 2)	Trendelenburg neg. (n = 2)	Normal (n = 2)	Enthused (n = 2)	No
Good	120°–180°	Modest		Less than normal resistance		No
Fair	60°–120°			Only gravidity		No
Poor	0°–60°					No

Table 3. Functional anatomy of knee

	Motion	Pain	Stability	Strength (s)	Emotional acceptance	Failure
Excellent (n = 2)	90° (n = 2)	None (n = 3)	0°–5° valgus or vagus (n = 5)	Extension 20 (n = 2)	Enthused (n = 1)	No
Good (n = 2)	60°–90° (n = 2)	Modest (n = 3)	5°–10° (n = 1)	10 (n = 4)	Liked (n = 3)	No
Fair (n = 2)	30°–60° (n = 2)		10°–20°	<10	Accepted (n = 2)	Peroneous palsy (n = 1)
Poor	0°–30°		>20°		Disliked	No

mas, five graded IIB and one graded IB. There was one chondrosarcoma graded IIB (Table 1).

The result was good for only $1\frac{1}{2}$ years in the case of chondrosarcoma. However, this patient died 2 years later from vertebral and pulmonal metastases. No loosening was seen, but two patients complained about moderate pain. An important observation was that the best functional result was in the case of the total removal of the femur (Tables 2, 3).

Discussion

Cementless implantation of a tumor endoprosthesis with a spongy metal surface in the region of fixation into the bone and in the region of bridging the block resection can be recommended. After implantation of the endoprosthesis, sensitive and careful length adaption with millimeter steps allows good functional results and can follow the later growth of the patient.

The Development of a Connection Between the Modules of a Modular Femur Endoprosthesis

G.J. Verkerke[1], F.M. van Krieken[2], H.K.L. Nielsen[1], J. Oldhoff[1],
H. Schraffordt Koops[1], R.P.H. Veth[1], A. Postma[1], L.N.H. Göeken[1],
H.H. van den Kroonenberg[2], and H.J. Grootenboer[2]

Summary. To connect the various modules of a modular femur endoprosthesis, e.g., the hip, knee prostheses, growing module, to each other, a universal connection was developed. Prototypes of four designs were built and tested for bending and torsion strength. All of the prototypes survived the test. The most compact connection was selected. The connection can be welded to the modules, which are often hollow. Plasma arc welding is preferred. The strength of the weld was demonstrated by several loading tests.

Key words: Endoprosthesis—Connection—Modules

Introduction

For the treatment of growing children with a malignant bone tumor of the femur, we are developing a modular femur endoprosthesis. One module has the capability of following the growth in the other, healthy leg by means of a non-invasively activated change in length.

Three prototypes were used in the animals and functioned well until they were unfortunately completely bridged by bony overgrowth.

After that, we started to develop a connection between the different modules (growing module, hip prosthesis, and knee prosthesis).

Design

The most important requirements for the connection were: (a) Assembly and disassembly should be possible using established techniques or with methods that can easily be developed. (b) Assembly and disassembly should not require implant elongation greater than 15 mm in order to protest the surrounding tissues and limit the assembly and disassembly force (c) The maximum diameter of the connection should be 30 mm. (d) The maximum length of the connection

---

[1] University Hospital Groningen, Groningen, The Netherlands
[2] Faculty of Mechanical Engineering, University of Twente, Enschede, The Netherlands

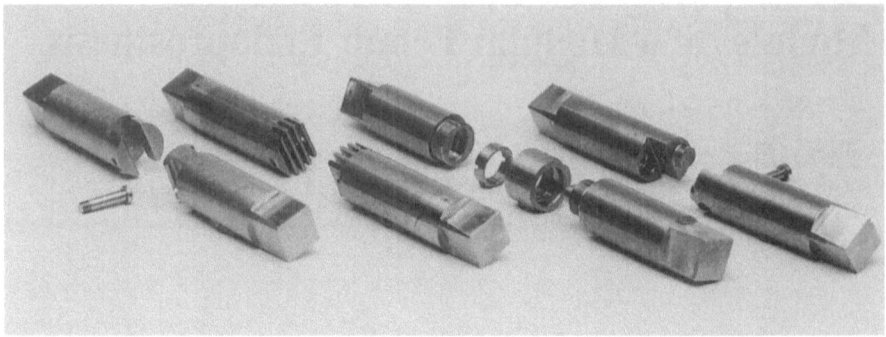

Fig. 1. Four prototypes of a connection

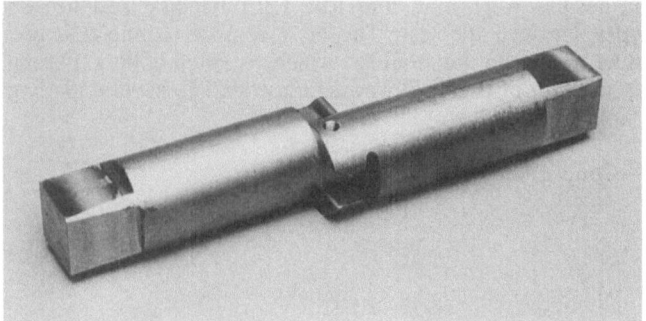

Fig. 2. The selected connection

should be 30 mm. (e) Manufacturing should be sufficiently accurate to insure interchangeability. (f) The connection should not show play that can be sensed by the patient during walking. (g) The connection must be as strong as the growing module. (h) Load carrying, assembly, and disassembly should be possible for at least 65 years.

Because the existing connections, mainly based on conical press-fit, did not meet the requirements, we decided to develop a new connection. A large number of possible solutions were created. The four solutions that met the requirements most closely were selected to be built in prototype (Fig. 1).

Test

The four prototypes, made of Ti-6A1-4V alloy, were tested with: (a) a single torsional loading of 200 Nm in both directions; (b) torsional fatigue loading of 28 Nm (Newton meter) during 10^6 cycles at a frequency of 10 Hz; (c) a single four-point bending load of 320 Nm in four perpendicular directions; (d) bending fatigue loading during 10^6 cycles between 23 and 72 Nm at a frequency of 10 Hz

Result

None of the four prototypes failed. Nondestructive testing did not reveal any cracks. One prototype showed play and slight wear marks. The other three prototypes were judged on their specifications. The prototype shown in Fig. 2 was selected, mainly because it requires no elongation for assembly and disassembly and because it is only 13 mm long.

The connection is manufactured by an electric wire discharge machine, which produces a very accurate connection.

After assembly, possible play is eliminated by using a bolt that pulls the two parts together.

Use

To fasten the connection to the femur endoprosthesis modules, which have often a hollow shaft, the connection parts may be welded to the shaft. Both TIG-welding and plasma arc welding were tried. Plasma arc welding was referred because of the small area of the heat-affected zone. Two plasma arc-welded test pieces were subjected to the loading tests described before. Both test pieces survived the experiments. A nondestructive test did not show any cracks.

Future work

In our endeavor to develop a modular femur endoprosthesis, we are now focusing our attention on other modules, e.g., the hip and knee prostheses and fixation parts connecting the implant to the remaining bone. We will also test this connection and the modified growing module in large dogs. Following this clinical evaluation will be performed.

Amputoresection

An Innovative Technique in Limb Salvage Procedure for Malignant Bone Tumors

Francesco Saverio Santori, Stefano Ghera, Mario Manili, and Giorgio Monticelli[1]

Summary. The indication in the surgical treatment of malignant bone tumors of the limbs with extracompartmental diffusion (IB and IIB stage) is amputation or disarticulation. Infiltration of the soft tissues and neurovascular bundles by the tumor is such that wide resection is often followed by local recurrence. Preoperative adjuvant therapies have permitted the indications for limb sparing procedures to be extended in these types of tumors. Yet, it is sometime impossible to avoid destructive interventions, as in the case of vascular and/or nervous involvement. The technique described consists of resection of the tumor and surrounding structures, such as skin and muscles, with reimplantation of the distal stump onto the proximal one. The intervention follows the classic surgical modalities, with a bone resection in healthy tissue 8–10 cm from the border of the tumor. When the removal has been completed, the distal stump is reimplanted on the proximal part of the limb; this eliminates the limb portion containing the tumor, including the infiltrated vessels, nerves, muscles, subcutaneous structures, and skin. The bone segments are joined by means of an endomedullary nail, the vessels are sutured (terminus-terminally) and, if necessary, a nervous suture is also performed. Following the operation, a leg discrepancy results, which we believe should only be corrected if the lower limb is involved.

Key word: Amputoresection

In the surgical treatment of malignant bone tumors of the limbs, recent studies have confirmed that the prognosis of tumors conservatively treated is comparable with the same forms treated by amputation or disarticulation if the criteria of oncological surgery are observed [1–3]. Today, it is possible to carry out an operation for the removal of the tumor and successive reconstruction with various conservative methods in bone tumors of stage IB and IIB (according to Enneking's staging [4]) that have only slight infiltration in the surrounding soft tissues. Whereas in cases of stage IB or IIB tumor that have amply overrun their own compartments, it is impossible to perform removal correctly. In fact, extensive infiltration in soft tissues, subcutaneous and even cutaneous tissues and/or the invasion of the perivascular and perineural sheaths render effective removal of the neoplasm technically impossible, thus leaving a high risk for local recurrences.

---

[1] Orthopaedic Institute–University "La Sapienza", Rome, Italy

To insure the radicality of the operation for the removal of the neoplasm, it becomes necessary to amputate or disarticulate, or a "segmental" amputation of the limb must be performed, such as a rotationplasty [5]. Our experience has shown, however, that this type of operation is esthetically unacceptable to a large number of patients. We have, therefore, outlined an operation that provides for the amputation of the segment of the limb at the level of the neoplasm, including blood vessels, nerves, muscles, and skin invaded by the tumor process [6]. An additional bone segment is excised proximally and distally to the neoplasm in order to guarantee the radicality of the operation (Fig. 1). An indispensable element in this type of conservative operation is adjunctive preoperative therapy (systemic chemotherapy, endoarterial infusion of antiblastics, hyperthermic antiblastic perfusion in the extracorporeal circulation [7]. The operation always leads to a shortening of the limb, which can be corrected in the lower limb; in the upper limb, however, the functional deficit is such that no correction is generally required.

The aim of this paper is to illustrate the surgical technique in the procedure of resectioning and reimplantation of a limb and to list the possible methods of correcting the differences in leg length in operations on the lower extremity.

Surgical Technique

Initially, two skin incisions are made, running transversely with respect to the main axis of the extremity; one of these incisions is made above and the other below the tumor mass. Starting from the proximal incision, a longitudinal accessory incision is made, running toward the root of the extremity along the projection of the neurovascular bundle; starting from the distal incision, another longitudinal accessory incision is made along the line of projection of the neurovascular bundle toward the distal end of the limb. It is then necessary to prepare the vessels and nerves and to isolate the muscles surrounding the neoplasm; they should be dissected following an oblique plane from the outer surface to the level of bone in a distal-proximal direction above and a proximal-distal direction below in such a way as to dissect the bone as far away as possible from the neoplasm. We generally perform the bone resection 10 cm from the margin of the neoplasm. In this way, once the vessels and nerves have been dissected, the limb segment containing the tumor and all soft tissues surrounding it, including subcutaneous and cutaneous tissues, can be removed as a whole. Once the removal of the mass has been accomplished, the reimplantation of the distal fragment onto the proximal part can begin, accomplishing firstly, the reconstruction of bone continuity, muscle attachments, and dissected blood vessels, and then reconstruction of the muscles and tendons themselves and of cutaneous and subcutaneous tissues. Bone reconstruction can be obtained by osteosynthesis utilizing a blocked intramedullary nail, e.g., Gross and Kempf, prepared in advance based on actual-size X-rays. Normally, bone autografts are done in association with osteosynthesis of the continuity procedure to bridge any residual gap in the bony structure that may result in cases of notable discrepancy between the amount of bone dissected away and that dissected from the soft tissues. If a

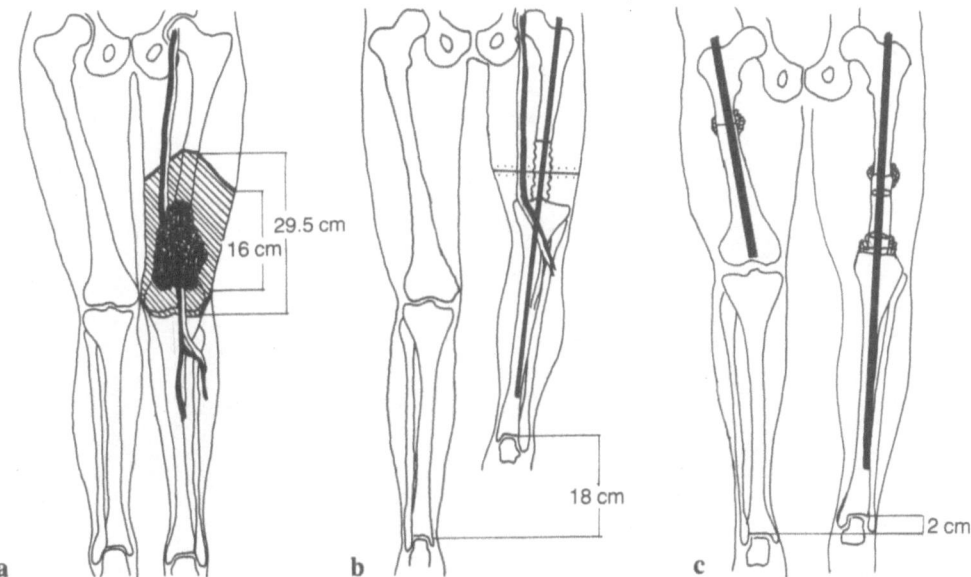

Fig. 1. a Scheme of amputoresection in stage IIB tumors with wide infiltration of the soft tissues and vascular bundles. The shaded area indicates the tissue to be removed. **b** The limb after the first operation; temporary reconstruction with polymethyl methacrylate (PMMA) and vascular suture. **c** Second surgical procedure: shortening of the contralateral limb and application of autografts in replacement of PMMA

second surgical procedure is anticipated to correct the leg discrepancy by shortening the contralateral extremity, it is possible, during the first procedure, to carry out a temporary reconstruction of the bony gap utilizing cement (polymethyl methacrylate) placed around the fixation device. The cement will be removed during the time of second surgery and substituted with bone grafts taken from the diaphysis of the contralateral extremity (Fig. 2).

If, after the first operation, a notable difference in leg length remains, the correction of this difference can be obtained through the application of two alternative methods: (a) by shortening the contralateral extremity, which is generally done for tall patients; (b) by lengthening the affected limb, done by a distractional epiphysiolysis or, if the epiphyses are already sealed, by closed corticotomy and progressive distraction. This correction is indicated in patients of below-average height. Sometimes the reconstruction can be done with uncemented joint modular prostheses [e.g., 8] rather than with bone grafting, as in the case of patients who refuse arthrodesis of the knee.

In situations of reconstruction with bone grafting, the extremity is protected postoperatively in plaster casts for 2–4 months, depending on the case, and then gradually weight bearing is permitted. Removal of the fixation device is carried out when the bone grafts have been completely consolidated (generally after 2 years).

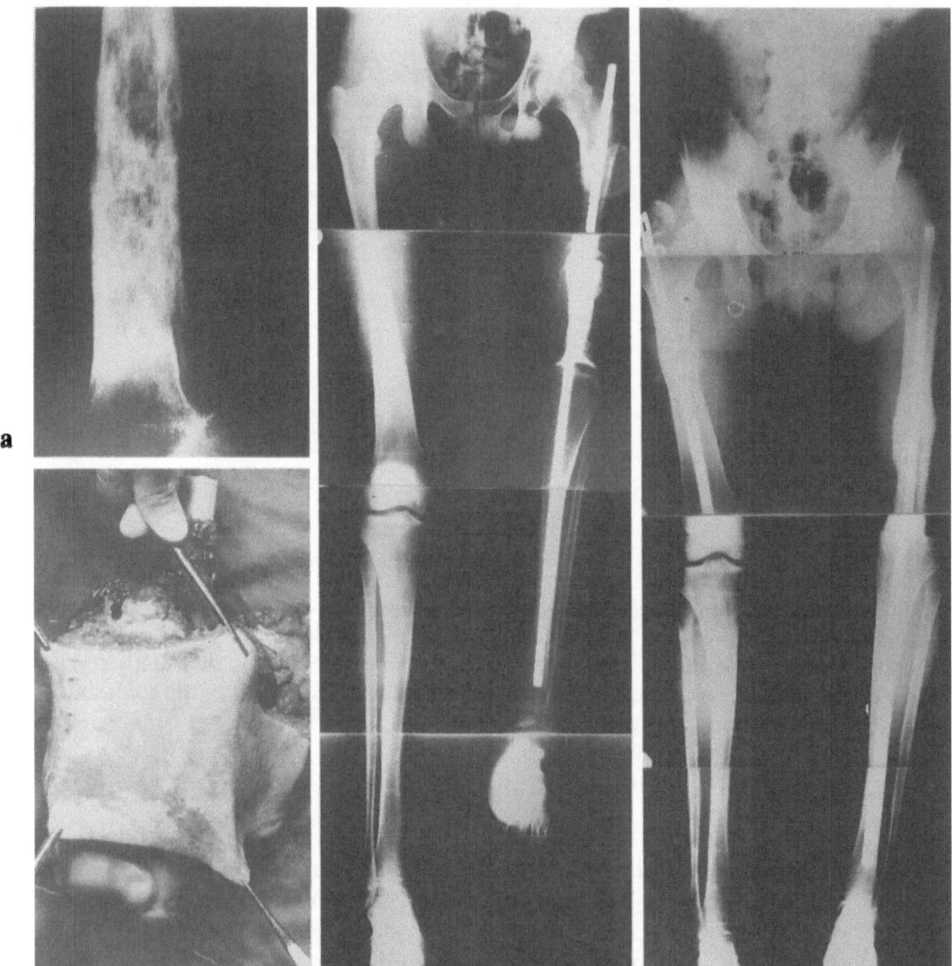

Fig. 2. a Osteosarcoma of the distal femur with wide infiltration of the soft tissues in a tall patient. **b** The removed tumor: note the presence of muscles and skin, wide resection of bone, and, distally, the femoral condyles. **c** X-ray control following amputoresection and synthesis with Kuntscher nail and PMMA. **d** The result following shortening of the contralateral limb and synthesis with a Kuntscher nail. The diaphyseal cortical autografts have been fixed by wiring in substitution of PMMA. Good remodeling of the bone shows graft consolidation at 2 years.

Results

Seven patients, six with diagnoses of classic osteosarcoma and one with malignant fibrous histiocytoma underwent our operation of amputoresection in the period between January 1983 and December 1986. The youngest was 7 years old and the eldest was 45. In one case, the tumor was localized on the distal radius, in four cases it was to be found on the distal end of the femur, in one case on the proximal part of the tibia, and in one case on the distal end (Fig. 3).

The shortest portion of bone excised was 15 cm long and the longest was 29.5 cm. The reconstruction was done with intramedullary osteosynthesis and autoplastic bone grafting in five of these cases; in one case, the reconstructional bone grafting was done in a second operation; the reconstruction in two of the cases was accomplished with a Kotz-type modular prosthesis. In five cases, the collaboration of a vascular surgeon was required, and in two cases that of a microsurgery specialist, reconstruction of neural pathways was not necessary in any of the seven cases. None of the patients operated upon presented vascular disturbances that could compromise the results of the operation. The formation of a thrombosis in the deep venous circulation presented itself in only one case, and that was resolved within 15 days of therapy with anticoagulants. In case no. 2, in which microsurgical suturing was done, the massive edema that occurred in the reattached limb regressed within 21 days of medication. It must be noted, however, that the patient had undergone radiotherapy at the tumor site. In all cases in which autoplastic bone grafting was done, bone growth of these grafts with consolidation of the arthrodesis was obtained in a period varying from 3 to 7 months. Three cases are disease-free at 12, 18, and 36 months. One case of local recurrence was treated with amputation (the patient is still alive with no evidence of disease); in one case, a superficial infection of the soft tissues was controlled with antibiotics. In all cases, systemic postoperative chemotherapy was applied. There were three cases of pulmonary metastasis in the period of 6–14 months following the operation. Three deaths occurred—one at 4 years, one at 2 years, and one at 6 months after the operation.

Discussion

Amputoresection is a new technique that seems to be, in our opinion, a valid alternative to amputation for the treatment of grade IB and IIB tumors (Enneking staging), which have wide invasion of the surrounding soft tissues or infiltrated perivascular tissues. According to our case studies, the risk of local recurrence is very similar to that with amputation if correctly carried out. Amputoresection is made possible by the use of adjunctive preoperative techniques (endoarterial antiblastic infusions or in the presence of hyperthermic perfusion of antiblastics), which permit improved local and general control of the disease.

The local recurrence that occurred in case 2 must be attributed to errors in the surgical resectioning. Otherwise, we did not observe any local recurrences.

The functional result is satisfactory and esthetically it is more than valid. Therefore, in our opinion, this technique is preferable to rotationplasty, which does not have as good an esthetic result and has always been poorly accepted by our patients.

Although amputoresection is to be considered a limb reattachment, with the exception of the nerve, we have never had particular postoperative problems, such as the great circulatory disturbances with massive edema that often undermine the success of reimplantation.

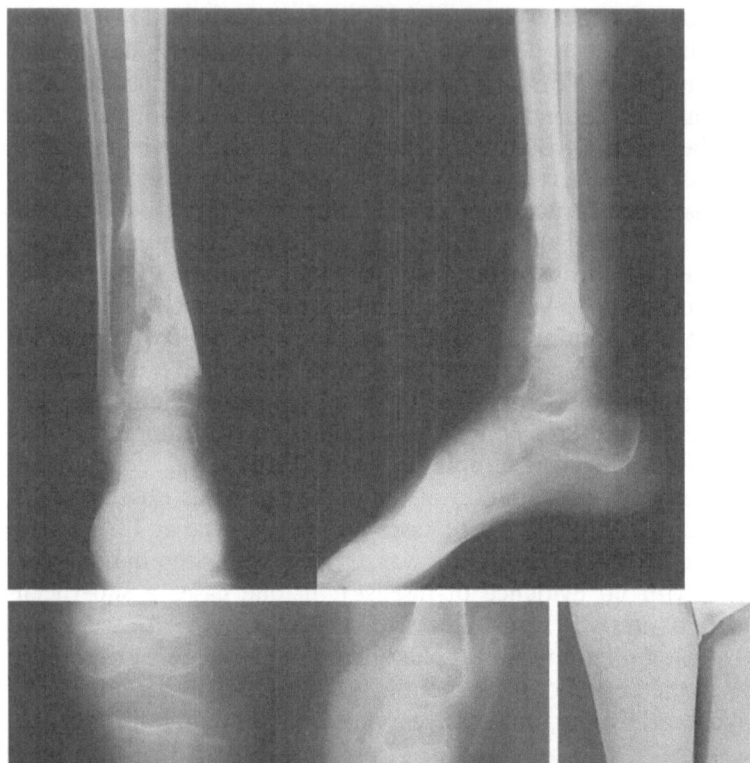

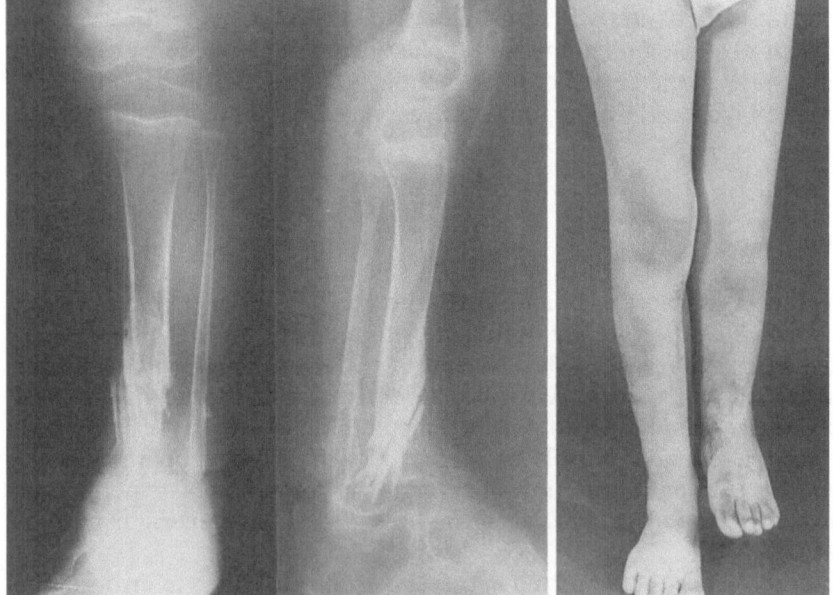

Fig. 3. a Osteosarcoma of the distal third of the tibia in a 7-year-old subject. The tumor has widely infiltrated the surrounding soft tissues. **b** The result after 12 months, following amputoresection and spongy cortical autografts with a tibiotalar arthrodesis. The bone grafts have taken well. **c** The clinical result, with a residual leg-length discrepancy of 10 cm; the wound had no problems of healing. In future, limb lengthening will be performed to correct limb discrepancy

Normally, the appearance of edema in the reattached limb is explained by dissection of lymph vessels causing edema from stasis. In reality, our experience with amputoresection seems to demonstrate that the edema in reattachments is essentially due to local stasis, probably due to dissection of the nerves. The functional result after some time appears to be satisfactory. Even in those patients who did not undergo a second surgical procedure to attain alignment of the extremities, the results have been good. Given the young age of the patients and our reduced sampling, we have not as yet performed limb lengthening, but from the theoretical point of view there should not be any great technical problems. We have had a high incidence of pulmonary metastases (three cases out of seven). This fact seems to be more ascribable to the advanced state of the disease process rather than to the operation. In this regard, we can affirm that the time and application required of the surgeon is not significantly greater to that in normal resectioning and reconstruction by bone grafts. In fact, while more time is required for the vascular and muscular-tendinous reconstruction, initial surgical times are shortened as the tumor does not have to be isolated and freed from the vessels, nerves, etc., but a segment of the limb is simply "amputated." On the whole, we consider the results obtained to be satisfactory and such as to recommend this type of operation in very advanced and selected cases.

Acknowledgment. This work was accomplished with grant no. 860049344 from the C.N.R. project.

References

1. Taylor WF, Ivins JC, Dahlin DC, Edmonson JH, Pritchard DJ (1978) Trends and variability in survival from osteosarcoma. Mayo Clinic Proc 53: 695–700
2. Taylor WF, Ivins JC, Pritchard DJ, Dahlin DC, Gilchrist GS, Edmonson JH (1985) Trends and variability among patients with osteosarcoma; a 7-year up-date. Mayo Clinic Proc 60: 90–104
3. Simon MA, Aschliman MA, Thomas N, Mankin HJ (1986) Limb salvage treatment versus amputation for osteosarcoma of the distal end of the femur. JBJC 68-A: 1331–1337
4. Enneking WF, Spannier SS, Goodman MA (1980) Current concepts review. The surgical staging of neuromuscular sarcoma. JBJS 62-A: 1027–1030
5. Kotz R, Salzer M (1982) Rotation-plasty for childhood osteosarcoma of the distal part of the femur. JBJS 64-A: 959–969
6. Santori FS, Folliero A, Ghera S, Manili M, Pistolesi R, Monticelli G (1986) Reimpianto di arti dopo amputo-resezione di estese neoplasie maligne dell'Osso. Giornal Ital Ortoped Traumatol XII: 13–24
7. Cavaliere R (1983) Regional perfusion hyperthemia. In: Storm FK (ed) Hyperthemia cancer therapy. pp 369–399
8. Kotz R (1983) Modular femur and tibia reconstruction system. In: Kotz R (ed) Proceedings of 2nd international workshop on the design and application of tumor prostheses for bone and joint reconstruction, Vienna, Sept. 5–8, 1983. Egermann, Vienna, pp 64–66

Microsurgical Reconstructions Following Wide Resection of Bone and Soft Tissue Sarcomas in the Extremities

Masamichi Usui[1], Seiichi Ishii[1], Toshikatsu Matsuyama[1], Susumu Asano[1], Shinya Yamawaki[2], Kazuo Isu[1], and Akio Minami[3]

Summary. Nine cases of microsurgical tissue transfer following wide tumor resection are reported. A free vascularized fibula graft was used in six cases, a pedicle fibula graft in two cases, and a free vascularized muscle graft in one. In all cases except one, the grafted tissue survived completely. The average follow-up period was 3.9 years for tumor resection and 2.3 years for reconstructive surgery. Function according to Enneking's grading was found to be excellent in one case, good in five, fair in one, poor in one, and undetermined in one. The oncological status of these cases was disease-free (CDF) in seven cases, no evidence of disease (NED) in one, and alive with disease (AWD) in one.

Key words: Bone tumor—Soft tissue tumor—Microvascular surgery

Limb sparing surgery for malignant tumors in the extremities has been widely attempted. In some cases, however, radical oncological surgery is incompatible with the preservation of limb function. To resolve this problem, the authors attempted to reconstruct the tissue loss caused by radical oncological surgery, using microsurgical tissue transplantation. The authors have already reported on a short-term follow-up study using this same procedure in the upper extremity [1]. The purpose of this paper is to present our increased experience with reconstruction in the lower extremity and to report on the results of functional evaluation in all types of cases.

Materials and Methods

Since 1983, nine microsurgical tissue transplantations following en bloc resection of tumors have been attempted in our department (Table 1). The age of the patients ranged from 12 to 53 years with an average of 24. Three were male and six were female. As for the site or region of the tumor, two cases (cases 2 and 3) were soft tissue tumors and seven were bone tumors. According to the surgical staging system of Enneking et al. [2], five cases were classified as IIB (cases 1–3,

---

[1] Department of Orthopedic Surgery, Sapporo Medical College, Sapporo, Japan

[2] Department of Orthopedic Surgery, National Sapporo Hospital, Sapporo, Japan

[3] Department of Orthopedic Surgery, Hokkaido University Hospital, Sapporo, Japan

Table 1. Summary of cases

Case	Age (yrs)	Sex	Site or region	Diagnosis	Stage	Procedure	Margin	Adjuvant Pre-op.	Adjuvant Post-op.	Removed structures	Reconstruction 1st stage	Reconstruction 2nd stage
1	14	M	Lt. prox. tibia	Osteosarcoma	IIB	En bloc	Wide	CTX	CTX	Tibia (prox. 1/3) muscle (ant. tibial and soleus)	Intercalary prosthesis (ceramic)	Knee arthrodesis (pedicle fibula, split femur, iliac, and bank bone)
2	20	F	Anterior comp. of lt. forearm	Angiosarcoma	IIB	En bloc	Wide	CTX	CTX	Radius (dist. 1/3) muscle (flexor and extensor)	Intercalary bone graft (vascularized fibula) tendon transfer	
3	12	F	Anterior comp.	Malignant hemangiopericytoma	IIB	En bloc	Wide	CTX	CTX	Radius (prox. 1/3) muscle (flexor)	Nerve graft (sural nerve)	Free vascularized muscle graft (gracilis)
4	15	F	Lt. middle ulna	Telangiectatic osteosarcoma?	IIB	Curettage en bloc	Intracapsular wide	None	None	Ulna (middle 1/3) muscle (flexor and extensor)	None	Intercalary bone graft (free vascularized fibula)
5	38	F	Lt. distal radius	Giant cell tumor	IA	En bloc	Wide	None	None	Radius (dist. 1/3) muscle (pron. quad)	Intercalary bone graft (free vascularized fibula)	
6	35	M	Rt. prox. humerus	Chondrosarcoma	IB	En bloc	Wide	None	None	Humerus (prox. 1/3) muscle (deltoid, part of biceps, and triceps)	Shoulder arthrodesis (free vascularized fibula)	
7	53	F	Rt. middle radius	Angiosarcoma	IB	Curettage en bloc	Intracapsular wide	None	CTX	Radius (middle 1/3) muscle (flexor)	Intercalary bone graft (free vascularized fibula) tendon transfer	
8	15	M	Rt. distal femur	Osteosarcoma	IIB	En bloc	Wide	CTX	CTX	Femur (dist. 1/3) muscle (vast. lat. med. and intermed.)	Intercalary prosthesis (ceramic)	Knee arthrodesis (free vascularized double fibula, iliac)
9	12	F	Lt. prox. tibia	Osteosarcoma	IIB	En bloc	Wide	CTX	CTX	Tibia (prox. 1/3) muscle (ant. tibial, gastro, and soleus)	Intercalary prosthesis (ceramic)	Knee arthrodesis (pedicle fibula split femur, iliac, and bank bone)

prox. proximal, *comp.* compartment, *CTX* chemotherapy

8, 9), two were IB (cases 6 and 7), one was IA (case 5), and one more was undetermined (case 4). As for the surgical procedure for tumor resection and its surgical margin, en bloc resection with a wide surgical margin was performed in all cases except cases 4 and 7. In cases 4 and 7, curettage of the tumor with an intracapsular margin was performed at the initial surgery and en bloc resection of the tumor was added at the second surgery. In cases 1–3, 8, and 9, both preoperative and postoperative chemotherapy were applied. In case 7, only postoperative chemotherapy was given. In cases 4–6, neither preoperative nor-post operative chemotherapy was given.

Table 1 shows the structures removed at the time of tumor resection and the details of reconstructive surgery. In cases of osteosarcoma of the lower extremity, an intercalary prosthesis was inserted in the first operation and knee arthrodesis was performed at the second stage (cases 1, 8, and 9). A vascularized fibula was used as the pedicle graft in cases 1 and 9. In case 8, two pieces of free vascularized fibula were used for the knee arthrodesis. In case 3, a free vascularized muscle graft was performed for reconstruction of the flexor muscle of the forearm by using the gracilis muscle. In the remaining five cases, a free vascularized fibula graft was used as an intercalary bone graft.

In cases 2, 4, and 7, multiple tendon transfers were also added for the reconstruction of hand function.

Results and Discussion

The follow-up period from the time of first operation ranged from 3 to 9 years with an average of 3.9 years (Table 2); the period from the second operation ranged from 0 to 3 years with an average of 2.3 years. Microsurgical tissue transfer was successfully performed in all cases except case 2. In case 2, venous thrombosis occurred due to kinking of the vein. The radiofibular junction took 6 months to heal because the grafted fibula failed to revascularize. As for the oncological status of each patient, seven cases have been continuously disease-free (CDF). In case 7, liver metastasis was detected 22 months after tumor resection. In this case, infusion of chemotherapeutic agents into the hepatic artery was effective and the patient remained alive with diseases (AWD) 3 years after surgery. In case 8, pulmonary metastasis was detected 4 months after initial surgery. The metastatic focus was resected and the patient's present status showed no evidence of disease (NED) 3 years after resection of the original tumor. Local recurrence did not occur in any case in this series. These results seem to show that microsurgical tissue transplantation in limb saving surgery is a good procedure procedure from viewpoint of local control of the tumor.

Table 2 shows functional evaluation of all cases. One was rated as excellent (case 4), five were good (cases 1, 2, 6–8), one was fair (case 5), and one was poor (case 3). The final results of case 9 were too early to evaluate. In the patients with osteosarcoma of the lower extremity, function after intercalary prosthesis and knee arthrodesis were evaluated separately. In case 1, the prosthetic limb was rated as poor and the fused knee was good. In case 8, both prosthetic limbs and the fused knee were rated as good. In case 9, the prosthetic limb was rated as poor. There are two different methods of reconstruction of leg function after

Table 2. Results of oncological status and functional evaluation

Case	Diagnosis	Years of follow-up	Status	Reconstruction	Motion	Pain	Stability	Deformity	Strength	Functional activity	Emotional acceptance	Rating
1	Osteosarcoma	1st op.—5	CDF	1st intercalary prosthesis	P	E	P	P	G	F	P	P
		2nd op.—3		2nd knee arthrodesis	P	E	E	E	E	G	G	G
2	Angiosarcoma	3	CDF	Intercalary bone graft and tendon transfer	E	E	E	E	E	G	G	G
3	Malig. hemangiopericytoma	1st op.—9	CDF	Free vascularized muscle graft	F	E	P	P	F	F	G	P
		2nd op.—3										
4	Telangiectatic osteosarcoma	3	CDF	Intercalary bone graft	E	E	E	E	E	E	E	E
5	Giant cell tumor	3	CDF	Intercalary bone graft	G	G	F	F	G	F	G	F
6	Chondrosarcoma	3	CDF	Shoulder arthrodesis	G	E	E	G	E	F	G	G
7	Angiosarcoma	3	AWD	Intercalary bone graft and tendon transfer	E	E	E	E	G	G	G	G
8	Osteosarcoma	1st op.—3	NED	1st intercalary prosthesis	G	E	F	G	E	G	G	G
		2nd op.—0		2nd knee arthrodesis	P	E	E	E	E	G		
9	Osteosarcoma	1st op.—3	CDF	1st intercalary prosthesis	P	E	P	P	F	P	F	F
		2nd op.—0		2nd knee arthrodesis	—	—	—	—	—	—		

CDF continuously disease free, *AWD* alive with disease, *NED* no evidence of disease, *E* excellent, *G good*, *F* fair, *P* poor

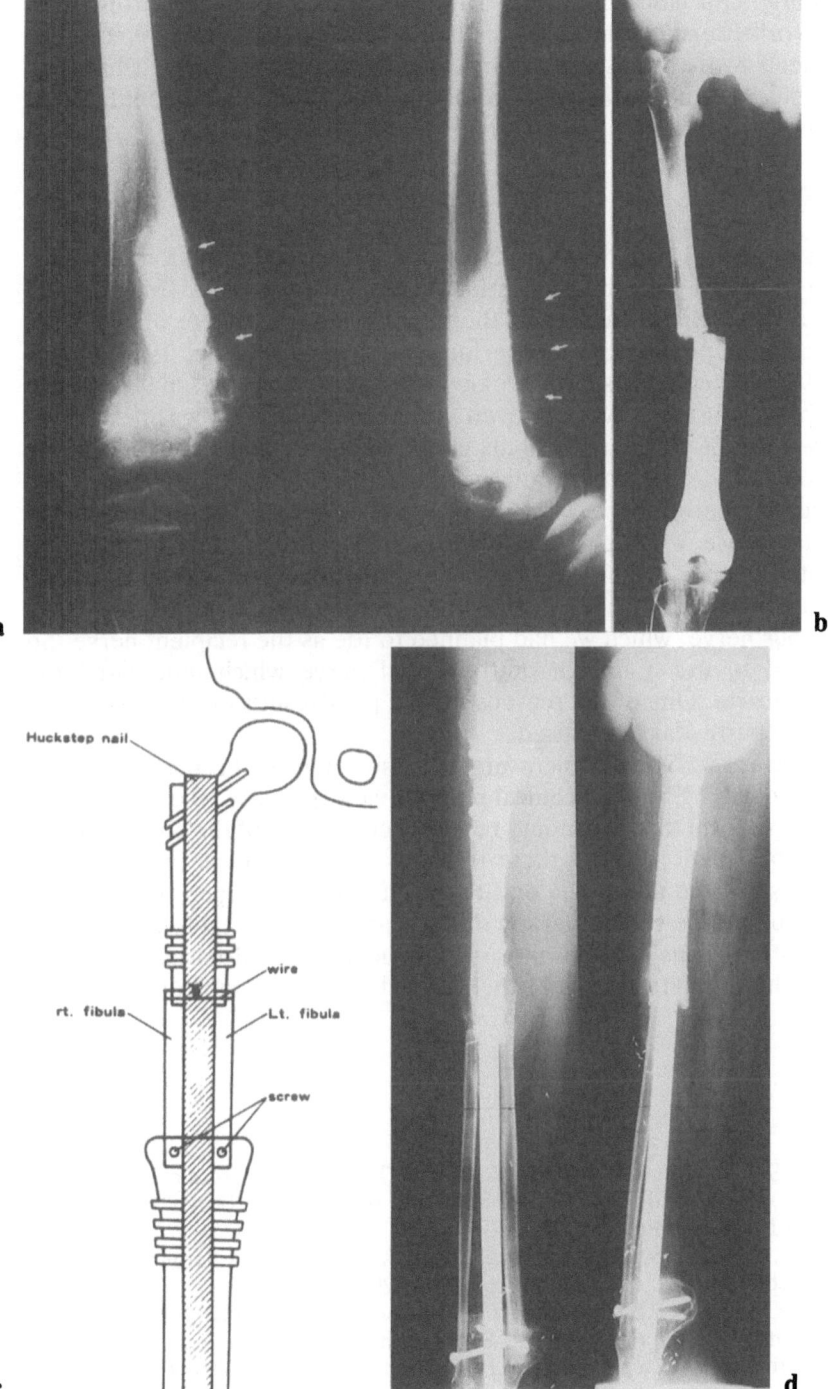

Fig. 1a–d. Case 8. **a** Osteosarcoma of right distal femur. **b** Ceramic spacer was broken. **c** Schema of two pieces of fibula graft. **d** Seven weeks after surgery; bone union is complete

resection of osteosarcoma around the knee joint—prosthetic replacement and knee arthrodesis. Our cases showed that functional results of knee arthrodesis were equal to or better than those of prosthetic replacement. When we consider that the patients with osteosarcoma are usually teenagers, knee arthrodesis seems reasonable. In knee arthrodesis, a vascularized fibula graft is confirmed as a useful method.

Case Reports

Case 8 was a 15-year-old boy with osteosarcoma of the right distal femur. After preoperative chemotherapy by vincristin (VCR), methotrexate (MTX), and adriamycin (ADM), wide resection of the tumor and replacement of the distal femur by a ceramic prosthesis were performed on 25 September 1984. On 15 November 1986, the ceramic spacer broke when the patient fell. On 9 February 1987, the broken prosthesis was removed and knee arthrodesis was performed by using two pieces of vascularized fibula graft. The functional evaluation of the knee was good and the oncologic status was NED (Fig. 1).

Case 5 was fair because the wrist showed 10° of flexion contracture and a defective grasp. Case 3 was poor because stability and deformity of the wrist joint were rated as poor. In this case, secondary reconstruction was performed 5 years after tumor resection. At that time, it was impossible to identify the anterior interosseous nerve, which we had planned to use as the recipient nerve. So we were forced to use a branch of the radial nerve which innervated the brachioradial muscle. One of the reasons for the poor results of this case seems to be due to the particular nerve used.

The question arises: Should microsurgical tissue transfer be performed primarily or secondarily? From a technical point of view, primary reconstruction is much easier to perform than secondary reconstruction. One of the disadvantages of primary reconstruction is that there is a possibility that local recurrence or distant metastasis of the tumor will occur. Another disadvantage is the ill effect of pre- or postoperative chemotherapy on the vascular repair and healing process of the grafted tissue [3]. Primary reconstruction should basically be performed only when we are sure that the surgical margin of the tumor is wide enough.

References

1. Usui M, Ishii S, Yamamura M, Minami A, Sakura T (1985) Microsurgical reconstructive surgery following wide resection of bone and soft tissue sarcomas in the upper extremities. J Reconstr Microsurg 2: 77–84
2. Enneking WF, Spanier SS, Goodman MA (1980) A system for the surgical staging of musculo-skeletal sarcoma. Clin Orthop 153: 106–120
3. Friedlaender GE, Tross RB, Doganis AC, Kirkwood JM, Baron R (1984) Effects of chemotherateutic agents on bone: I. Short-term methotrexate and doxorubicin (adriamysin) treatment in a rat model. J Bone Joint Surg 660A: 602–606

Adipose Venolymphatic Transfer for Management of Postradiation Lymphedema

Robert W.H. Pho[1], Philippe Bayon[1], and Lenny Tan[2]

Summary. The method of adipose venolymphatic transfer is described in a patient who had postradiation lymphedema after excision of a liposarcoma. The technique involved transferring adipose tissue containing lymphatic vessels surrounding the long saphenous vein from the normal healthy leg to the irradiated leg with the creation of an arteriovenous fistula. This technique has the advantages of: (a) transferring lymphatic vessels to provide new drainage without microlymphatic anastomosis; and (b) bypassing the irradiated area when lymphatic vessels are blocked. Two years' follow-up showed there is a reduction in volume of the edematous leg. Postoperative lymphangiogram showed there is evidence of cross-lymphatic drainage from the recipient leg to the opposite normal groin.

Key words: Adipose venolymphatic transfer—Postradiation lymphedema

Introduction

Many methods have been described in the management of lymphedema following radiation. Excision of the deep fascia [1, 2], burying of a dermal flap [3], pedicle skin flap [4–6], myocutaneous flap [7], omental transposition [8], lymphangioplasty [9, 10], and lymphaticovenous anastomosis [11] have been claimed to have partial success.

We describe a new method which we call adipose venolymphatic transfer. This method involves transferring a pedicle, which consists of adipose tissue containing lymphatic vessels surrounding the long saphenous vein, from the *normal healthy leg*, bypassing the irradiated area in which the lymphatic system are obstructed in the lymphedema leg. The long saphenous vein pedicle was tunneled across, above the pubic symphysis subcutaneously to the opposite groin and along the medial aspect of the leg to below the knee of the lymphedema leg. The long saphenous vein was then sutured to the posterior tibial artery at the upper third of the leg to create an arteriovenous fistula; this maintained nutrition of the periadipose lymphatic tissue, allowing lymphatic regeneration and thus providing lymphatic drainage from the irradiated leg with lymphedema to the normal

[1]Department of Orthopaedic Surgery, National University Hospital, Singapore
[2]Department of Diagnostic Radiology, Singapore General Hospital, Singapore

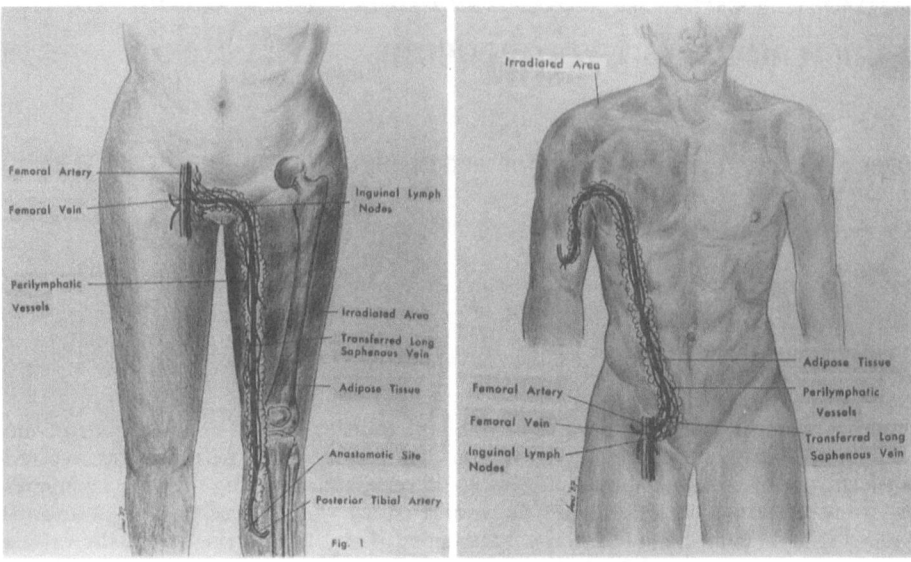

Fig. 1a, b. Adipose venolymphatic transfer. **a** lower limb; **b** upper limb

unobstructed side of the lymphatic system in the opposite groin (Fig. 1).

This concept originated from the senior author's observations in reimplantation surgery and following tumor resection. Lymphedema is not a problem as there is rapid lymphatic reconnection through regeneration, which occurs at the transplanted limb provided the viability of the tissue is not compromised [12]. Lymphatic reconnection and regeneration will occur without any attempt at microlymphatic or lymphatic venous anastomosis [13, 14].

Clinical Case

A 55-year old female had radical resection of a liposarcoma, involving the medial aspect of the left lower half of the thigh, which was first operated on in November 1976. The tumor recurred and further resection was carried out in 1982. The resection was deemed incomplete as the tumor had infiltrated the surrounding muscle and the main neurovascular bundle. She was given a course of radiotherapy (5000 rads) of the left thigh. She developed gross lymphedema of the operated left leg, extending from the mid- thigh down to the foot a year later. There were no palpable lymph nodes in the groin or evidence of recurrence of tumor. The skin and subcutaneous tissue of the irradiated thigh were thickened and indurated. Knee movement ranged from 0° to 90°. The patient had repeated attacks of cellulitis, which required several hospital admissions despite conservative treatment with a pressure garment and elevation. She complained of continuing pain and discomfort from tightness in the calf and thigh. Adipose venolymphatic transfer was carried out on 29 July 1985.

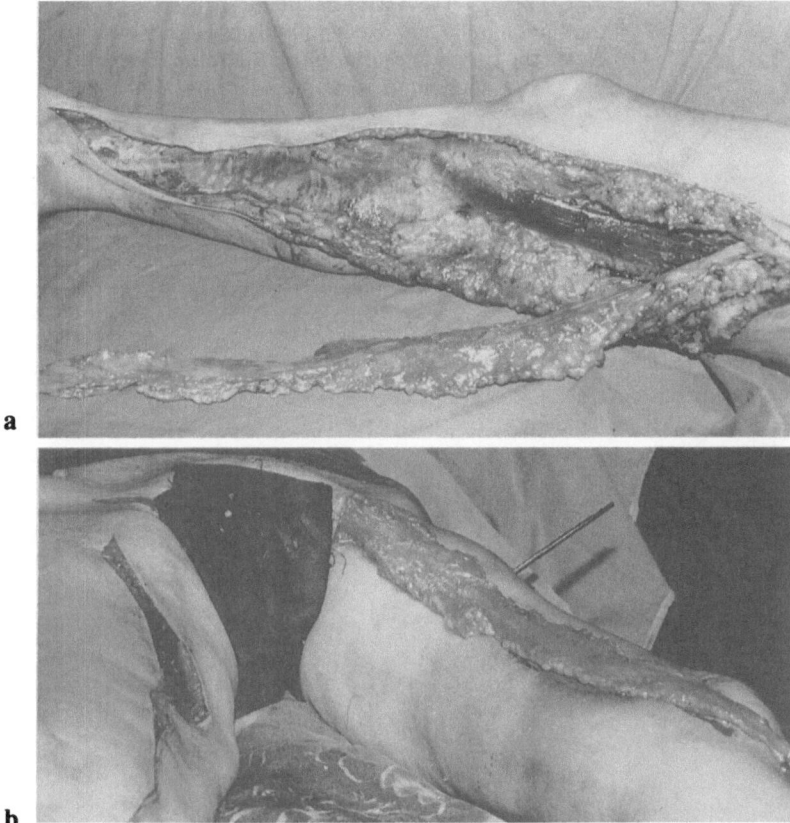

Fig. 2. a Harvesting adipose venolymphatic pedicle based on long saphenous vein from the donor leg. **b** Rerouting pathway of adipose venolymphatic pedicle. Note the swelling in the left thigh before transfer

Operative Technique

The patient was catheterized. Both legs were prepared from the foot up to the groin and the suprapubic region.

In the donor leg, the saphenous vein pathway was outlined with methylene blue from the groin to the ankle. At the level of the medial malleolus, the long saphenous vein was identified. One and a half centimeters of surrounding adipose tissue along the long saphenous vein, containing numerous lymphatic channels, was isolated and harvested together with the vein. The dissection should include the deep fascia and the soft tissue dissection should be placed more anteriorly as it contains more lymphatic channels [11, 15]. The dissection was extended proximally above the knee along the long saphenous pathway, reaching the groin where the long saphenous vein drained into the femoral vein. The superficial and deep inguinal lymph nodes were carefully preserved as they drained the surrounding adipose lymphatic tissues of the long saphenous vein (Fig. 2a).

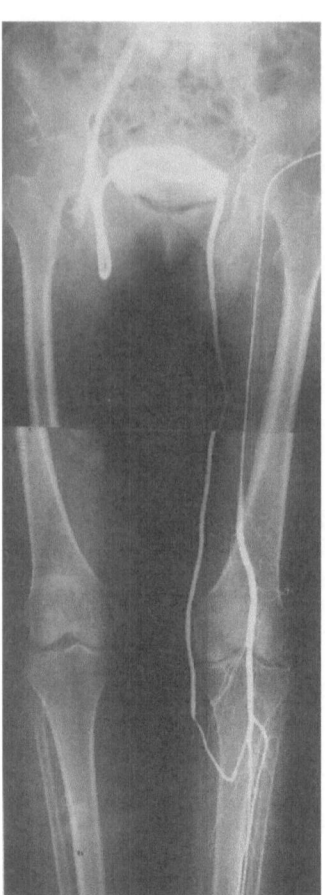

Fig. 3. Arteriogram showing the new pathway of the long saphenous vein with minute branches supplying the surrounding adipose lymphatic tissue. *Arrows* indicate the site of anastomosis between the distal end of the long saphenous vein and posterior tibial artery

A large subcutaneous tunnel was made suprapubically to ensure that the bulky saphenous pedicle together with the surrounding adipose venolymphatic tissue could be tunneled through and lie comfortably without any constriction. The pedicle was then tunneled to the opposite left groin (Fig. 2b) along the antero-romedial aspect of the left leg to the level of $7\frac{1}{2}$ cm below the knee joint, following the long saphenous vein pathway. The adipose venolymphatic pedicle thus effectively bypassed the irradiated scarred area in the thigh, extending from the knee joint to the opposite groin.

An incision was made on the posteromedial aspect of the left leg to identify the posterior tibial artery, which was brought out to the subcutaneous plane. End-to-end anatomosis of the distal end of the saphenous vein to the posterior tibial artery was made to create an arteriovenous (AV) fistula in the pedicle. The saphenous vein thus drained the arterial blood to ensure adequate perfusion for viability of the periadipose lymphatic tissue surrounding the saphenous pedicle, which extended from the left leg below the knee to the opposite right groin of the donor leg (Fig. 3). Primary skin closure was achieved at the donor and recipient legs.

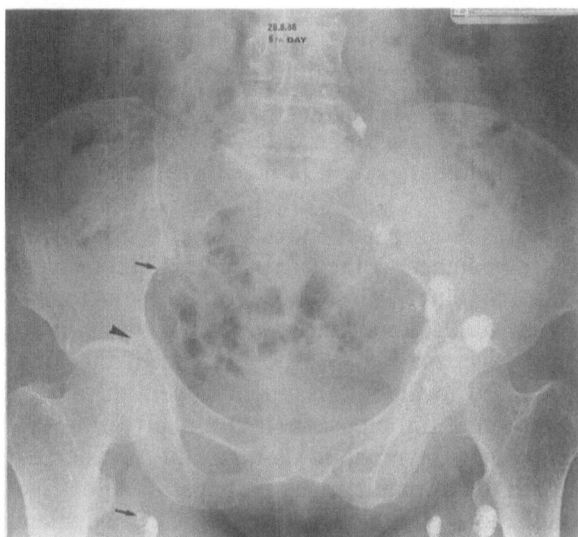

Fig. 4. Lymphangiogram in recipient leg after injection of dye showing evidence of cross-lymphatic drainage to opposite groin (*arrow head*) and the reestablishment of lymphatic channels (*arrows*)

Postoperative Assessment

Postoperatively, both legs were elevated and elastic stockings were applied. The patient was discharged from hospital on the 5th week and advised to continue wearing elastic stockings.

Our follow-up at 26 months indicated that the patient had not suffered from any further episode of cellulitis. She had no leg pain. She had experienced less tightness of the operated left leg. Her cardiac assessment was normal with no evidence of an excessive hypercirculatory dynamic state.

The patient was assessed objectively by measuring the volume and circumference of both legs at two fixed points: (a) 20 cm below the patella with the knee fully extended, where the volume of the leg is a measure of the subfascial and suprafascial compartments; (b) at the level of the lateral malleolus, where the measurement depends on the suprafascial compartment only. Our assessment indicated that there is improvement in measurement of the size and volume reduction of both recipient and donor legs following adipose venolymphatic transfer.

Lymphangiogram was carried out on the recipient leg in August 1986 15 months after transfer. There was evidence of lymphatic reconnection at the suture site below the knee and cross-lymphatic drainage from the recipient (left) groin to the donor (right) groin of the normal area. There was also evidence of increased drainage at the pelvic lymphatic system of the recipient leg (Fig. 4).

Discussion

Adipose venolymphatic transfer is a new concept. Baumeister el al in 1981 reported the use of proximal lymphatic transfer from a normal leg to the opposite leg, in which lymphatic trunks were based on a long saphenous system but the lymphatic was bridged to the dilated lymphatic trunk [16]. Our technique thus differs from this approach.

We believe that the preservation of the long saphenous vein as a splint provides an excellent pedicle in avoiding damage to the surrounding adipose lymphatic tissue during dissection and handling. Anastomosis of the vein to the artery ensures a high flow of arterial blood, supporting nutrition of the periadipose lymphatic tissue to avoid fibrosis formation. We believe that if the long saphenous vein of the pedicle is sutured to the long saphenous vein in the recipient leg a slow circulation will form and thrombosis becomes likely. This will lead to fibrosis of the surrounding adipose lymphatic tissue in the transferred pedicle, thus preventing regeneration of lymphatic tissue and possible blockage of lymphatic drainage along the saphenous lymphatic pedicle. As we are dealing with large vessels, the anastomosis can be done without microscopic magnification. Similarly, there is no tedious work of identifying individual lymphatic channels at the donor pedicle or recipient site for anastomosis. The lymphatic channels will be bridged based on the transfer of healthy tissue and natural regeneration will occur at the transferred site. This is confirmed on postoperative lymphangiogram. Our observation has indicated that adipose venolymphatic transfer does reduce lymphedema in the recipient leg and provides evidence of adequate cross-limb lymphatic drainage.

The loss of the long saphenous vein together with its adipose venolymphatic tissue at the donor site does not constitute great disability to the donor leg as there are sufficient lymphatic channels at the short superficial saphenous system and the deep system. Thus, lymphedema does not persist at the donor leg.

We believe that this technique has the advantage of transferring the normal lymphatic tissue bypassing the irradiated scar area, provides a new lymphatic drainage to the opposite normal area, and increases flow at the recipient lymphatic channels. This technique could also be applied to overcome postmastectomy-irradiated lymphedema in the upper limb by transferring the adipose venolymphatic pedicle and bypassing the irradiated area of the axillary region to the normal healthy tissue in the arm.

Acknowledgments. We are grateful to the Shaw Foundation, Lee Foundation, and Prima Limited for their contributions to the Microsurgery Research Fund, Mr. S.H. Tow for photography, Miss T.M. Mak for the illustration, and Mrs. Janet Han for typing the manuscript.

References

1. Kondoleon E (1912) Die operative Behandlung der elephantiastischen Oedeme nach Quetschung. Munch Med Wchnschr 59: 525
2. Sistrunk WE (1918) Further experiences with Kondoleon operation for elephantiasis. JAMA 71: 800

3. Thompson N (1962) Surgical treatment of chronic lymphoedema of the lower limb—with preliminary report of new operation. Br Med J 2: 1566
4. Gillies H, Fraser FR (1935) Treatment of lymphoedema by plastic operation—a preliminary report. Br Med J 1: 96
5. Mowlem R (1948) Treatment of lymphoedema. Br J Plast Surg 1: 48
6. Smith JW, Conway H (1962) Selection of appropriate surgical procedures in lymphoedema—introduction of hinged pedicle. Plast Reconstr Surg 30: 10
7. Sandor M (1983) A successful operation for lymphoedema using myocutaneous flap as a wick. Br J Plast Surg 36: 64
8. Goldsmith HS, Santos RD (1967) Omental transposition in primary lymphoedema. Surg Gynaecol Obstet 135: 607
9. Handley WS (1908) Lymphangioplasty: a new method for the relief of the brawny arm of breast cancer and for similar conditions of lymphatic oedema: preliminary note. Lancet 1: 783
10. Silver D, Puckett L (1976) Lymphangioplasty—a ten year evaluation. Surgery 80: 748
11. O'Brien BM, Das SK (1979) Microlymphatic surgery in the management of lymphoedema of upper limbs. J Spore Acad Sci 8(4): 474
12. Pho RWH, Lim SML, Satku K (1985) Late metastasis from osteogenic sarcoma. J Bone Joint Surg 67A 1: 147
13. Reichert FL (1926) The regeneration of the lymphatics. Arch Surg 13: 871
14. Danese C, Howard JM, Brower R (1960) Regeneration of lymphatic vessel—a radiographic study. Ann Surg 2156–1–61
15. Gray JH (1940) Studies of regeneration of lymphatic vessels. J Anat 74: 309
16. Baumeister RG, Seifert J, Hahn D (1981) Autotransplantation of lymphatic vessels. Lancet 147

Ceramic Tricalcium Phosphate As a Bone-Graft Substitute for Benign Bone Tumors

Thomas A. Lange[1]

Summary. Tricalcium phosphate (TCP) is a biocompatible ceramic bone graft substitute manufactured by DePuy. Since April 1984, over 80 cases have been entered into an FDA-approved clinical study, in which tricalcium phosphate was used as a bone graft material for fractures, nonunions, miscellaneous bone defects, and tumors. This report details early results of its use in 20 benign bone tumors treated at the University Hospital of Arkansas and the J.L. McClellan Memorial Veterans Hospital, Little Rock, Arkansas. The TCP used was a porous granular (18 patients) or block (two patients) polycrystalline ceramic formed by sintering beta TCP at 2000°C. The particle size varies from 0.4 to 2 mm and has a porosity of 250–400 μm.

Beta TCP is a safe and effective means of grafting and restoring bone in small to large bone defects resulting from benign tumors. The material has a long sterile shelf life, is easily used, avoids graft-donor site morbidity and the potential of allograft disease transmission. Its osteoconductive properties are not fully understood but empirically are effective. Since the material is not osteoinductive, bone will not form in undesirable soft tissue sites. No complications were directly attributable to the material.

Key words: Bone graft substitute—Tricalcium phosphate—Benign bone tumors

Introduction

Tricalcium phosphate (TCP; Orthograft™ Large Granular manufactured in the USA by DePuy) is a biocompatible ceramic bone graft substitute. Since April 1984, over 80 cases have been entered into an FDA-approved clinical study in which TCP was used as a bone graft material for fractures, nonunions, miscellaneous bone defects, and tumors. This report details the early results of its use in 20 benign bone tumors treated at the University Hospital of Arkansas and the John L. McClellan Memorial Veterans Hospital, Little Rock, Arkansas. The TCP used was a porous granular (18 patients) or block (two patients) polycrystalline ceramic formed by sintering beta TCP at 2000°C. The particle size varies from 0.4 to 2 mm and has a porosity of 250–400 μm.

Biomechanically, the material is brittle, which precludes its use in a purely

[1]Department of Orthopaedic Surgery, University Hospital of Arkansas, Little Rock, AR, USA

structural capacity. On the other hand, it can function as a filler for bone defects, particularly in cancellous bone. Biologically, the material is noninflammatory, i.e., its presence in the bone or soft tissue does not induce an antigenic or significant foreign body response. It is considered to be an osteoconductive material rather than osteoinductive. When placed in a bone defect, it serves as a scaffolding upon and around which viable trabecular bone will form [1–6]. Rather than inducing new bone formation, TCP placed in soft tissues such as muscle or subcutaneous fat is resorbed.

Previously published work from our institution has shown TCP to compare favorably with autogenous bone graft in terms of net trabecular bone formed [7]. Surgical defects of 8–12 cm^3 were created in distal femoral or proximal tibial metaphyseal bone in adult pigs and packed with either autogenous cancellous bone or TCP. Quantitative histomorphometric measurements of the bone formed at 5 months and 9 months revealed that net trabecular bone (NTB) formation was comparable in the two groups, the trend favoring TCP, especially at the earlier observation point (26% versus 16% NTB).

Materials and Methods

This report is based on the first 20 patients with benign bone tumors whose defects were grafted with TCP. All tumors met the following conditions; (a) benign histology, (b) sites and lesions were treated by intralesional curettage; (c) the curetted defect was surrounded by normal vascularized bone except for the surgical window; and (d) the absence of infection. The granular form of TCP, known as Orthograft™ Large Granular, was used to fill 18 lesions; the block form (recently discontinued) was used to fill two very large defects. The maximum amount of granular TCP originally allowed by the FDA to fill defects was 5 g (about 6 cm^3). This limit was subsequently raised to 30 g or (about 45 cm^3), making it a more practical alternative to autogenous or allograft bone. The block form of TCP was available in cubes, dowels, and cylinders, with an upper limit of 60 cm^3 permitted to fill a defect. The volume of TCP used varied from 4 to 60 cm^3 in all patients, with a mean of 20 cm^3.

The types of tumors filled with TCP were nonossifying fibromas (five cases), simple bone cysts (four), aneurysmal bone cysts (three), enchondromas (three), chondromyxoid fibromas (two), and one each of giant cell tumor, osteoblastoma, and pigmented villonodular synovitis. Five of the tumors were recurrent, including both chondromyxoid fibromas, one aneurysmal bone cyst, the giant cell tumor, and one simple cyst previously injected several times over 3 years.

The sites of these tumors were in the proximal tibia in five cases, the hip, distal femur, and ankle in four each, and the upper extremity in three. The granular TCP was placed through an intra-articular bone window in three cases—two in the femoral neck and one in the acetabulum. The windows and TCP were covered with thrombin-soaked Gelfoam prior to wound closure. Supplemental bone graft was used in five cases (25%). The type of supplemental bone was fresh-frozen cancellous allograft chips in one (when the amount of TCP allowed was only 6 cm^3), autogenous cancellous bone in one where a tibial osteotomy was done as an associative procedure, and fibular strut grafts in three to support

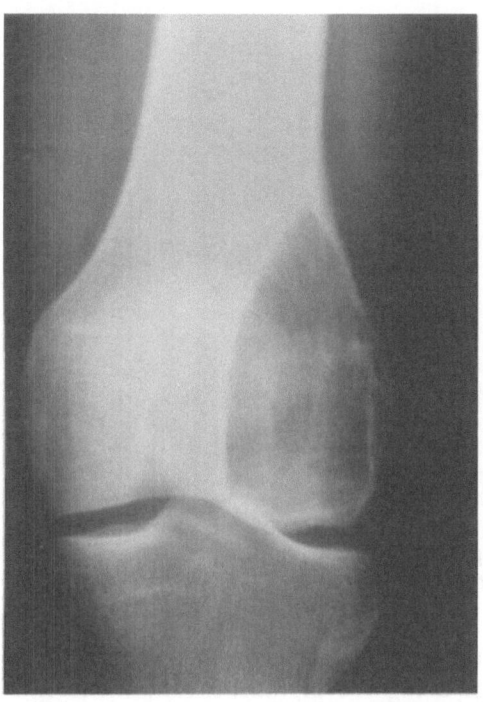

Fig. 1. Preoperative radiograph of an osteoblastoma in the left distal femur of a 26-year-old female

large unprotected areas of subchondral bone considered at risk for fracture.

There were 13 males and seven females, ranging in age from 9 to 53 years (mean age 22). The patients were followed at prescribed intervals of 1, 3, 6, 9, 12, and 24 months, at which time clinical and radiographic examinations were performed. CBC (complete blood count), UA (urinalysis), and SMA-12 (sequential multiple analyzer) laboratory studies were obtained preoperatively and at 3 and 6 months postoperatively. Additional examinations were scheduled as necessary for several patients, and some observation data were provided by the patient's local orthopedist who had examined the patient and forwarded the X-rays for review. Clinical information obtained referred to general activity level of the patient and pain and weight-bearing status of the extremity. The follow-up radiographs were compared with the original postoperative films and most recent prior films to assess qualitatively the amount of resorption of TCP and assess the amount of filling-in of the defect. This exercise was largely subjective. In a few patients, triple-phase bone scans were done to assess vascularity of the primary site (looking for evidence of local recurrence) and bone activity within the zone of repair.

Results and Discussion

The follow-up ranged from 3 to 34 months, with a mean of 10 months. Most patients reported little postoperative pain and were discharged from the hospital in 1–5 days (average 3). No donor-site pain or complications were experienced. In the lower extremity sites, partial weight bearing was begun between days 1

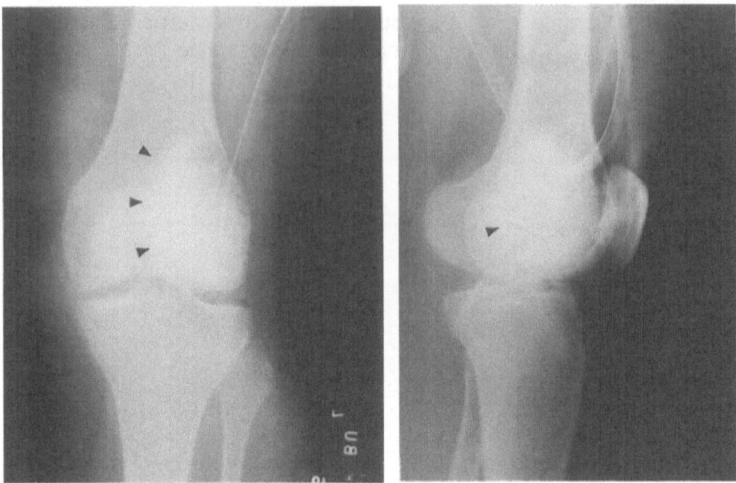

Fig. 2. Postoperative AP and lateral radiographs following curettage of the lesion and placement of TCP. *Arrows* indicate the margin of implant

and 44, the average being at day 12. Full weight bearing was allowed from between day 10 and 4 months, the average being at 2 months. Most patients had more confidence in the reconstruction than the surgeon in that they initiated full weight bearing more quickly than anticipated on an individual basis.

All laboratory studies obtained for our patients remained within normal limits throughout the observation period. Radiographic evaluation for percentage resorption of TCP, as indicated above, was subjective. Disappearance of the granular features of the material varied on the basis of: (a) age of the patient (quicker in younger patients); (b) size of the defect (quicker in smaller defects); and (c) vascularity of the surrounding bone (quicker in well-vascularized sites). The granular radiographic texture usually disappeared after 1–3 months, with an increased homogeneous density usually remaining for several months. Since trabecular bone formation was presumably occurring simultaneously with TCP resorption, it was most difficult to differentiate the two phenomena radiographically. Based on our total experience of 80 cases, we estimate resorption to be at 5%–10% per month, with total resorption requiring between 6 and 24 months.

Limited histological material confirms the osteoconductive nature of TCP. It appear that osteoclasts will resorb TCP directly and that osteoblasts will produce seams of osteoid in immediate opposition to ceramic crystals.

Complications in the series of tumor patients included one soft tissue necrosis related to saline hyperthermia (50°C, 5 min) in the bone cavity, which required a minor wound debridement and reclosure. A more serious problem occurred in a 9-year-old boy with an epiphyseal lesion in the distal tibia. It was curetted and packed with TCP, resulting in a large central growth arrest. No follow-up treatment has been required to date for this child.

Thus far, there have been no pathological fractures of bone defects treated with TCP and no recurrences of tumors, although follow-up is too short to assess either of these with certainty.

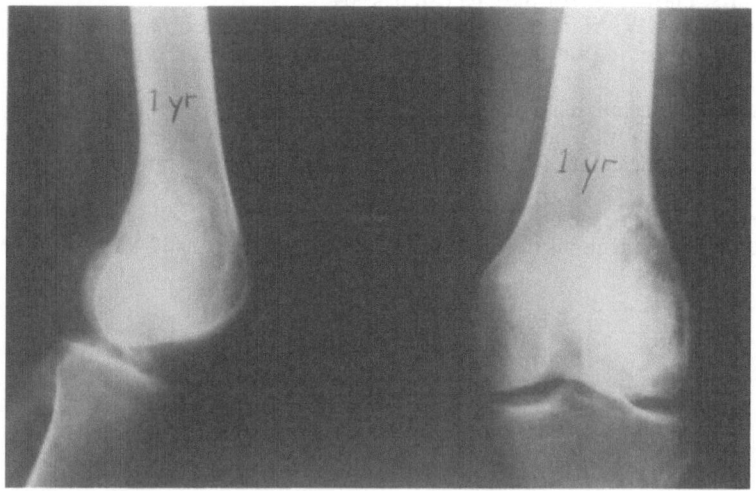

Fig. 3. One-year postoperative radiograph revealed no evidence of recurrence; there is some peripheral resorption of TCP

An illustrative case is that of a 26-year-old housewife with knee pain, who was found to have a large radiolucent defect in the lateral femoral condyle from an osteoblastoma (Fig. 1). Serial follow-up X-rays revealed no evidence of recurrence and some peripheral resorption of TCP 1 year later (Figs. 2, 3). She has normal function of the leg.

In conclusion, beta TCP is a safe and effective means of grafting and restoring bone in small to large bone defects as a result of benign tumors. The material has a long sterile shelf life, is easily used, avoids graft-donor site morbidity and the potential of allograft disease transmission. Its osteoconductive properties are not fully understood but empirically are effective. Since the material is not osteo-inductive, bone will not form in undesirable soft tissue sites. No complications were directly attributable to the material.

Acknowledgments. The author acknowledges study support in part by DePuy, Warsaw, Indiana and the John L. McClellan Memorial Veterans Hospital, Little Rock, Arkansas, USA.

References

1. Renooij W, Hoogendoorn HA, Visser WJ, Lentferink RHF, Schmitz MGJ, Van Ieperen H, Oldenburg SJ, Janssen WM, Akkermans LMA, Wittebol P (1985) Biore-sorption of ceramic strontium-85-labeled calcium phosphate implants in dog femora. CORR 197: 272–285
2. Flatley TJ, Lynch KL, Benson M (1983) Tissue response to implants of calcium phosphate ceramic in the rabbit spine. CORR 179: 246–252
3. Jarcho M (1981) Calcium phosphate ceramics as hard tissue prosthetics CORR 157: 259–278
4. Ferraro JW (1979) Experimental evaluation of ceramic calcium phosphate as a substi-

tute for bone grafts. Plast Reconstr Surg 63 (5): 634–640
5. Moore DC, Chapman MW, Manske D (1987) The evaluation of a biphasic calcium phosphate ceramic for use in grafting long-bone diaphyseal defects. J Orthop Des 5 (3): 356–365
6. Urist MR, Nilsson O, Rasmussen J, Hirota W, Lovell T, Schmalzreid T, Finerman GAM (1987) Bone regeneration under the influence of a bone morphogenetic protein (BMP) beta tricalcium phosphate (TCP) composite in skull trephine defects in dogs. CORR 214: 295–304
7. Lange TA, Zerwekh JE, Peek RD, Mooney V, Harrison BH (1986) Granular tricalcium phosphate in large cancellous defects. Ann Clin Lab Sci 16 (6): 467–472

Autotransfusion with Recovery of Blood Loss in Conservative Surgery for Tumors of Lower Limbs

Battista Borghi[1], Stefano Lari[1], Rodolfo Capanna[2], and Mario Campanacci[2]

Summary. Surgery for tumors of the lower limbs involves large blood loss and great quantities of homologous blood. Transfusions, besides the infectious and immunological risks evaluated in recent studies, adversely affect the survival of patients operated on for bone tumors. We report the technique used for saving blood by combining hemodilution, controlled hypotension, and intra- and postoperative salvage of blood loss. The apparatus used is the Autotrans Dideco BT795/A (or BT795/P) and BT797. The results obtained are evaluated in two groups of patients treated with different methods of perioperative blood loss replacement. In the group treated with the described autotransfusion technique, the average level of preoperative hematocrit was 34%, the homologous blood saved in this group was 82%.

Key words: Bone tumors—Hemodilution—Blood loss salvage

Introduction

Conservative surgery for tumors of the lower limbs may lead to considerable blood loss and thus the need for numerous units of homologous blood. Recent prospective studies on posttransfusional hepatitis in Italy have provided evidence that the risk is about 2% per unit of transfused homologous blood [7]. In about 50% of these cases, the hepatitis becomes chronic. For other infectious diseases transmitted by homologous transfusions, the quantity of transfused blood is not so clearly correlated, but nevertheless it must be considered. Besides the risk of infectious disease, we must keep in mind the immunological reactions and technical errors. More recently, interference with the immunological system has been revealed [2, 3]. In the literature, numerous studies report the relation between the amount of transfusions received and the period of survival in patients with carcinoma of the colon-rectus [4, 5]. In other types of neoplasias, the correlation between perioperative transfusions and survival was less marked but always significant [6]. From 1972 to 1982 at the Istituto Ortopedico Rizzoli, a study with a follow-up of more than 5 years was carried out showing the negative relation between perioperative transfusions and sur-

Department of Anesthesia, Analgesia and Intensive Care[1] and 1st Orthopaedic Clinic and Bone Tumor Center[2], Istituto Ortopedico Rizzoli, Bologna, Italy

vival in 205 patients operated on for osteosarcoma of the long bones [2]. This study took into account various other variables (age, size, grade, interval between diagnosis, surgery, etc.), which in the two groups of patients did not differ significantly. These studies suggest that the use of homologous blood in tumor surgery is a problem to be faced rationally. This could be solved by using techniques of controlled hypotension, autotransfusion, and hemodilution [1]. These techniques though have to be used with particular care, because these patients generally have undergone preoperative chemotherapy and therefore have low values of hemoglobin, hematocrit (Ht), and platelets.

Material and Methods

In 1985, we started studying the possibility of associating autologous transfusions with controlled hypotension. After 3 years' experience, our technique to spare blood is based on the following points.

Preoperative hemodilution. The aim is to dilute the corpuscle part and, especially, the plasma components which in a later phase cannot be recovered from the blood loss. The blood extracted more than 24 h before surgery is separated into plasma and corpuscle components and the plasma is frozen to maintain its properties. When phlebotomy is done immediately before surgery, the Autotrans BT795 DIDECO and BT797 apparatus is used for separation during phlebotomy. If necessary, it is also possible to reinfuse part of the red cells extracted before reinfusing plasma.

Controlled hypotension. To reduce intraoperative bleeding, controlled hypotension is used following protocols of mixed anesthesia (general and epidural) or general anesthesia with inhalant anesthetics in association with labetalol.

Intraoperative hemodilution. When clinical conditions permit, Ht values are maintained at around 20% by infusion of saline solution, hydroxyethyl starch, and hemocomponents. Autologous plasma is usually reinfused at the end of surgery.

Intraoperative recovery

The intraoperative recovery of blood is accomplished with a suitable apparatus, the AUTOTRANS BT795 DIDECO. Recovery is accomplished by two or more means: by suction device and by a plastic collection bag we designed, which can be connected by its adhesive rim to the cloth below the surgical would or sutured to the downward edge of the surgical wound [1]. The blood upon entering the collection bag and the aspiration device is mixed with an anticoagulant solution (ACD), it then passes through the connection tubes, reaching a reservoir with a 40-μm filter. The connection tube going from the collection bag to the reservoir is clamped and opened only at intervals to allow full channel aspiration and to maintain the sponge filter inside the collection bag soaked with anticoagulant solution. A peristaltic pump with adjustable speeds sends the uncoagulated blood into the rotating bowl, where separation and subsequent red cell concentration are effected by high-speed centrifugation, about 5000 rpm. To recover platelets and white cells also, the washing procedure is started when the level of the red cells inside the bowl reaches about 1.5 cm from the rim. Moreover, to facilitate the elimination of hemolysis products and, particularly, of red cell stromas, washing is performed by alternating the passage of the washing isotonic saline solution with a remixing of the bowl contents, until the outlet solution is as clear as the inlet one [1]. This technique can be programmed on a computerized apparatus with the "better quality wash" function. To reduce the trauma to the recovered red cells, besides hemodilution, the following precautions are very important: (a) washing the operative field frequently in order to dilute further the recovered red cells; (b) maintaining the negative aspiration pressure at values around 50 mm/Hg; (c) reducing the distance between the operative field and the reservoir; (d) maintaining the suction tubing as parallel to the ground as possible, always viable, ensuring the unidirectionality (one-way flow) of the fluid by proper positioning of the tubing.

Postoperative recovery. Recovery starts during the suture phase by substituting the aspiration cannule with a simple Y-shaped four-way collector we designed [1], which connects the aspiration and drainage tubes. By connecting this Y-shaped collector to the BT795 apparatus, recovery may continue for a few hours after surgery. If it is necessary to prolong the recovery, we connect the drainage to the aspiration pump, BT797. With this, it is possible to uncoagulate and recover the blood loss. The device can be varied in speed and pressure in the drainage tube.

Results

Firstly, it is necessary to state that the results often depend on the collaboration with the surgeon, who must frequently wash the operative field with saline isotonic solution and try to limit the use of gauzes during surgery. The results obtained are evaluated comparing two groups of patients treated with different methods of replacement of perioperative blood loss.

In Tables 1–3, the data are summarized concerning the first group of patients in whom intra- and postoperative volumic replacement was done with homologous blood without employing the autotransfusion techniques. Here are reported the type and site of the tumor, the kind of resection and reconstruction done, and the quantity of homologous blood used. Tables 1–3 also summarize the data concerning the second group of patients in whom the described autotransfusion technique was used. The differences between the two groups are evident with regard to the average of homologous blood units transfused—6.8 and 1.2 in the perioperative phase. Comparing these two values in the second group, the homologous blood spared was 82%. It must be emphasized that in the second group of 42 autotransfused patients, 35 (83%) did not have homologous transfusions during surgery. Nineteen of these patients (45%) had no intra- and postoperative homologous transfusions. The average value of hematocrit of this group was 34% (range 28%–44%).

Table 1. Location of tumor in 186 patients treated without and with autotransfusion

Resection	Patients without autotransfusion				Patients with autotransfusion			
	Number	Prosthesis (Kotz)	Temporary arthrodesis	Putti. Juvara arthrodesis	Number	Prosthesis (Kotz)	Temporary arthrodesis	Putti. Juvara arthrodesis
Proximal femur	19	19	—	—	6	6	—	—
Distal femur	123	48	49	26	25	16	5	4
Proximal tibia	44	5	20	19	11	5	4	2
Total	186	72	69	45	42	27	9	6

Table 2. Surgical margins and type of reconstruction in patients without and with autotransfusion

	Patients without autotransfusion				Patients with autotransfusion			
	Kotz	Temp. arthr.	P-J arthr.	Total	Kotz	Temp. arthr.	P-J arthr.	Total
Benign								
Wide	7	1	26	34	4	—	2	6
Wide/Contaminated	1	—	5	6	—	—	—	—
Marginal	1	—	3	4	2	—	—	2
Intralesional	—	—	1	1	—	—	—	—
Low grade								
Wide	7	2	5	14	7	—	—	7
Wide/Contaminated	—	—	1	1	—	—	—	—
Marginal	1	—	—	1	—	—	—	—
Intralesional	1	—	—	1	—	—	1	1
High grade								
Wide	44	59	4	107	13	8	2	23
Wide/Contaminated	2	2	—	4	—	—	—	—
Marginal	6	4	—	10	1	1	1	3
Intralesional	2	1	—	3	—	—	—	—
Total	72	69	45	186	27	9	6	42

Temp. arthr. temporary arthrodesis, *P-J arthr.* Putti. Juvara arthrodesis

Table 3. Quantity of homologous blood transfusion in different type of reconstruction

	Patients without autotransfusion						Patients with autotransfusion					
	Number	Homologous transfusion		N° units			Number	Homologous transfusion		N° units		
		Pts.s transfusion	Pts.s intraop. transfusion	Min.	Max.	Average		Pts.s transfusion	Pts.s intraop. transfusion	Min.	Max.	Average
Prosthesis Temp.	72	—	—	1	17	6.3	27	12	25	—	4	1
Arthrodesis	69	1	1	—	22	7.2	9	4	6	—	4	1.4
P/J arthr.	45	1	2	—	21	7.1	6	3	4	—	5	1.6
Total	186	2	3	—	22	6.8	42	19	35	—	5	1.2

Pts.s patients sine, *Pts.s intraop.* patients sine intraoperative

Conclusions

In conclusion, the advantages of autotransfusion with intra- and postoperative blood recovery as described above have reduced by 82% the use of homologous transfusions, thus radically limiting the infectious and immunological risks.

Other important advantages of the method described are the following: (a) reduction of tissue trauma by limiting the use of gauzes during surgery, while frequently washing the operative field with saline isotonic solution diminishes dehydration and conserves tissue vitality; (b) guaranteeing better oxygenation of the tissues due to the better quality of autologous red cells compared with the homologous ones; (c) reducing interference with the immune system; (d) giving the possibility of surgically treating patients who refuse homologous transfusions; (e) reducing the costs, especially when compared with the high social cost due to complications of homologous transfusions.

Acknowledgment. This study was supported in part by a grant from the National Council for Research no. 86.02679.44.

References

1. Borghi B, Fabozzi A, Lari S, Giacomello A, Elmar K, Chesi R (1985) New technique of autotransfusion in hip surgery. In: Salentina-Galatina (ed) Proceedings of international week of updating on anesthesia and Ri., vol 1, pp 761–766
2. Chesi R, Bacci G, Borghi B (submitted) Relations between perioperatory transfusion and distance metastases in osteosarcoma of the extremitities treated with adjuvant chemotherapy. Cancer
3. Fischer E, Lendhard V, Seiffert P, Xluge A, Johannsen R (1980) Blood transfusion induced suppression of cellular immunitary in man. Hum Immunol 3: 187–194
4. Foster RS Jr, Costanza MC, Foster JC, Wanner MC, Foster CB (1985) Adverse relationship between blood transfusions and survival after colectomy for colon cancer. Cancer 55: 1195–201
5. Nathanson SD, Tilley BC, Shultz L, Sneath RF (1985) Perioperative allogeneic blood transfusions-survival in patients with resected carcinomas of the colon and rectum. Arch Surg 120: 734–738
6. Rosemberg SA, Seipp CA, White DE, Wesley R (1985) Perioperative blood transfusions are associated with increased rates of recurrence and decreased survival in patients with high grade soft tissue sarcomas of the extremities. J Clin Oncol 3: 698–709
7. Tremolada F, Chiappetta F, Noventa F, Daifré C, Ongaro G, Realdi G (1983) Prospective study of postransfusion hepatitis in cardiac surgery patients receiving blood or blood products. Vox Sang 44: 25

Author Index

Key Word Index